Periprosthetic Joint Infections

Daniel Kendoff • Rhidian Morgan-Jones
Fares S. Haddad
Editors

Periprosthetic Joint Infections

Changing Paradigms

Springer

Editors
Daniel Kendoff
HELIOS ENDO-Klinik Hamburg
Berlin
Germany

Fares S. Haddad
University College London Hospitals
London
UK

Rhidian Morgan-Jones
University Hospital of Wales
Cardiff
UK

ISBN 978-3-319-30089-4 ISBN 978-3-319-30091-7 (eBook)
DOI 10.1007/978-3-319-30091-7

Library of Congress Control Number: 2016940503

Printed on acid-free paper

This Springer imprint is published by Springer Nature
The registered company is Springer International Publishing AG Switzerland

Dedicated to my family, who allows me the time and energy for these projects. To my beloved wife, Stefanie, and children, Lillie, Viola, and Hugo.

Daniel Kendoff

For Myfanwy, Ioan, and Bronwen, who constantly make me proud.

Rhidian Morgan-Jones

In memory of Sami Fares Haddad and Nina Tamari Haddad, who gave me the tools, the motivation, and the love and support to succeed, and with thanks to Jane, Isabella, Oliver, Florence, Imogen, Alice, and Marina, who make every moment a glorious one.

Fares S. Haddad

Preface

Despite numerous technical improvements in total joint replacement in recent years, an evolution in our understanding of implant biomechanics, and greater clarity on patient, theatre, and surgical optimisation, we have not seen a reduction in periprosthetic joint infection (PJI) or improvements in management commensurate with those seen in other fields. In an era of expanding knowledge, dramatic innovation and great change, our knowledge in the field of periprosthetic infection has yet to translate into a reduced incidence and prevalence or into improved outcomes; this has therefore become an area of great need for the orthopaedic community.

The number of presentations and publications related to PJI has increased dramatically, showing not only the increased interest of orthopaedic surgeons but also a genuine multidisciplinary scientific effort geared to addressing this ever-expanding problem. This increased interest is also noticeable in the growing number of specific infection courses and meetings, the growth of orthopaedic infection societies, and the increased commercial interest of implant suppliers the world over. Current key research strategies and developments focus on prevention, enhanced diagnostics, host stratification and optimisation, biofilm eradiation, implant modifications including coatings, and optimised treatment algorithms.

PJI has been recurrently shown to be a huge economic burden for patients, hospitals, and healthcare systems in many countries. Strategic information on infection incidence and prevalence is needed. Registry data and data from multi-institutional studies are currently limited in their validity and generalisability – a huge push will be needed worldwide in order for us all to speak the same language, agree on definitions, and compare management strategies. Only then will we be able to truly interpret regional, hospital, and surgeon-level data. It is therefore vital that all orthopaedic surgeons engage in this battle that is highly relevant to them, their patients and their institutions, and have a clear understanding of current recommendations supported by published literature.

This comprehensive book should provide an overview scripted by experts in the field of the current status of PJI, summarising current perspectives and potential variations in practice. We have not restricted the remit to surgery but have attempted to cover the entire patient journey and to involve the entire multidisciplinary team that is necessary for successful care. In the past, PJI management had an institutional "historic tradition" or a paradigm based on a surgeon's specific "eminence". A lack of evidence for many important but open questions such as "duration and timing of i.v. antibiotics" or "timing of re-implantation" are topics of ongoing debate. We hope that within these chapters, successful options, based on the best available evidence and practice, can be offered for even the most difficult infection case. This book can be considered one of the keystones for the next stage of evidence gathering that is undoubtedly necessary.

Finally, we should never forget that there are patients suffering at the heart of this problem and that the functional outcomes of successful PJI management, although superficially promising with up to 90 % published "success" in infection control, do not meet the aspirations of patients and surgeons relative to our other interventions. In PJI, "even the winners are losers!" and by reading this book, and joining us on this journey, we will hopefully effect change in this area.

Berlin, Germany — Daniel Kendoff
Cardiff, UK — Rhidian Morgan-Jones
London, UK — Fares S. Haddad

Contents

Contributors

Matthew P. Abdel, MD Department of Orthopedic Surgery, Mayo Clinic, Rochester, MN, USA

V. Antoci Jr., MD, PhD Hip and Knee Reconstruction Surgeon, University Orthopedics, Providence, RI Alpert Medical School of Brown University, Providence, RI, USA

Hany Bedair, MD Department of Orthopaedic Surgery, Massachusetts General Hospital, Harvard Medical School, Boston, MA, USA

Elie Berbari, MD, FIDSA Division of Infectious Diseases, Mayo Clinic, Rochester, MN, USA

Antonia F. Chen, MD, MBA Department of Orthopaedic Surgery, The Rothman Institute of Orthopaedics, Thomas Jefferson University Hospital, Philadelphia, PA, USA

Michael B. Cross, MD Department of Adult Reconstruction Joint Replacement, Hospital for Special Surgery, New York, NY, USA

Carl Deirmengian, BA, MD Department of Orthopaedic Surgery, Rothman Institute/Jefferson, Lankenau, Newton Square, PA, USA

Craig J. Della Valle, MD Department of Orthopaedic Surgery, Rush University Medical Center, Chicago, IL, USA

Lorenzo Drago, PhD Department of Biomedical Sciences for Health, IRCCS Galeazzi Hospital, University of Milan, Milan, Italy

Clive P. Duncan, MB, MSc, FRCSC Department of Orthopaedics, University of British Columbia, Vancouver General and University Hospitals, Vancouver, BC, Canada

Moataz El-Husseiny, MBBCh, MRCS, Dip Sport M, MD (Res) Department of Orthopaedics and Trauma, Great Ormond Street Hospital, London, UK

Donald Garbuz, MD, MHSc, FRCS(C) Department of Orthopaedics, The University of British Columbia, Vancouver, BC, Canada

Eduardo García-Cimbrelo, MD, PhD Department of Orthopaedic Surgery, Hospital La Paz-Idi Paz, Madrid, Spain

Eduardo García-Rey, MD, PhD, EBOT Department of Orthopaedic Surgery, Hospital La Paz-Idi Paz, Madrid, Spain

Kevin L. Garvin, MD Department of Orthopaedic Surgery and Rehabilitation, University of Nebraska Medical Center, Omaha, NE, USA

Thorsten Gehrke, MD Department of Orthopaedic Surgery, Helios ENDO-Klinik, Hamburg, Germany

David A. George, MBChB, BMedSc, MRCS (Eng) Department of Trauma and Orthopaedics, University College Hospital, London, London, UK

Eliza Gil, MA, MBBS, MSc, MRCP Department of Microbiology and Infectious Diseases, University College Hospital, London, UK

Enrique Gómez-Barrena, MD, PhD Department of Orthopaedic Surgery, Hospital La Paz-Idi Paz, Madrid, Spain

Christina J. Gutowski, MD, MPH Department of Orthopaedic Surgery, Thomas Jefferson University Hospital, Philadelphia, PA, USA

Carl Haasper, MD, PhD, MSc Department of Orthopaedic Surgery, Helios ENDO-Klinik, Hamburg, Germany

Fares S. Haddad, BSc, MD(res), MCh, FRCS (Orth) Department of Trauma and Orthopaedics, University College London Hospitals NHS Trust, London, UK

Peter Haiden, MD Department of Traumatology, Landesklinikum Korneuburg, Korneuburg, Austria

Tim Harrison, FRCS (Tr & Orth), MBBS, BSc, Cavendish Hip Fellow Department of Trauma and Orthopaedics, Royal Derby Hospital, Derby Teaching Hospitals NHS Foundation Trust, Derby, UK

Curtis W. Hartman, MD Department of Orthopaedic Surgery and Rehabilitation, University of Nebraska Medical Center, Omaha, NE, USA

Simon S. Jameson, MBBS, MD, FRCS (Tr&Orth) Department of Trauma and Orthopaedics, James Cook University Hospital, Middleborough, UK

Lee Jeys, MBCHB, MSc (Ortho Eng), FRCS Department of Orthopaedic Oncology, Royal Orthopaedic Hospital, Birmingham, UK

Greg Kazarian, BA Rothman Institute/Jefferson, Media, PA, USA

Daniel Kendoff, MD, PhD Orthopaedics and Trauma Department, Helios Klinikum Berlin Buch, Berlin, Germany

Michael M. Kheir, BS Department of Orthopaedic Surgery, The Rothman Institute of Orthopaedics, Thomas Jefferson University Hospital, Philadelphia, PA, USA

Klaus Kirketerp-Møller, MD Department for Dermatology, Bispebjerg University Hospital, Copenhagen Wound Healing Center, Copenhagen, Denmark

Sujith Konan, MBBS, MD, MRCS, FRCS (Tr&Orth) Department of Trauma and Orthopaedics, University College London Hospitals NHS Trust, London, UK

Beau S. Konigsberg, MD Department of Orthopaedic Surgery and Rehabilitation, University of Nebraska Medical Center, Omaha, NE, USA

Konstantinos N. Malizos, MD, PhD Department of Orthopaedic Surgery and Musculoskeletal Trauma, Biopolis,University General Hospital of Larissa, Larissa, Greece

Bassam Masri, MD, FRCS(C) Department of Orthopaedics, The University of British Columbia, Vancouver, BC, Canada

Geert Meermans, MD Department of Orthopaedics, Bravis Hospital, Bergen op Zoom, The Netherlands

Rhidian Morgan-Jones, MBBCh, MMedSci, FRCS(Ed/Tr&Orth) Department of Trauma and Orthopaedics, University Hospital of Wales, Cardiff, Wales, UK

Stephen Morris-Jones, MA, MBBS, MSc, MRCP, FRCPath Department of Clinical Microbiology and Infectious Diseases, University College London Hospital, London, UK

O. Brant Nikolaus, MD Department of Orthopedic Surgery, Mayo Clinic, Rochester, MN, USA

Michael C. Parry, BSC, MBCHB, PGCME, MD, FRCS Department of Oncology and Complex Arthroplasty, Royal Orthopaedic Hospital, Birmingham, UK

Javad Parvizi, MD, FRCS Department of Orthopaedic Surgery, The Rothman Institute at Thomas Jefferson University Hospital, Philadelphia, PA, USA

Vaibhav Punjabi, MBBS, MS, FRACS, FA(Ortho)A Department of Orthopaedics, Princess Grace Hospital, London, UK

Mike Reed, MD, FRCS (T&O) Department of Trauma and Orthopaedics, Northumbria Healthcare, Ashington, Northumberland, UK

Carlo Luca Romanó, MD Department of Reconstructive Surgery of Bone and Joint Infections, Galeazzi Orthopedic Institute IRCCS, Milan, Italy

Delia Romanò, MD Department of Reconstructive Surgery of Bone and Joint Infections, Galeazzi Orthopedic Institute IRCCS, Milan, Italy

N. Amir Sandiford, MSc, FRCS (Trauma/Orth) Department of Orthopaedics, The University of British Columbia, Vancouver, BC, Canada

Sara Scarponi, MD Department of Reconstructive Surgery of Bone and Joint Infections, Galeazzi Orthopedic Institute IRCCS, Milan, Italy

Ian Stockley, MB, ChB, MD, FRCS Orthopaedic Department, Northern General Hospital, Sheffield, UK

Mohamed Sukeik, MD, MRCSEd, PGA Department of Trauma and Orthopaedics, The Royal London Hospital, London, UK

Timothy L. Tan, MD Department of Orthopaedic Surgery, The Rothman Institute of Orthopaedics, Thomas Jefferson University Hospital, Philadelphia, PA, USA

Aaron Tande, MD Division of Infectious Diseases, Mayo Clinic, Rochester, MN, USA

Myra Trivellas, BS Department of Biomechanics, Hospital for Special Surgery, New York, NY, USA

Leo A. Whiteside, MD Department of Surgery, Missouri Bone and Joint Center, Missouri Bone and Joint Research Foundation; Des Peres Hospital, St. Louis, MO, USA

Christopher Peter Wilding, MBBS, BSc (Hons) Department of Orthopaedics, Royal Orthopaedic Hospital, Birmingham, UK

Heinz Winkler, MD *Osteitis Zentrum*, Privatklinik Döbling, Wien, Austria

Akos Zahar, MD Department of Orthopedic Surgery, Helios ENDOKlinik, Hamburg, Germany

Abbreviations

AAOS	American Academy of Orthopedic Surgeons (USA)
ABC	Antibiotic bone compound
AKA	Above-the-knee amputation
ALAC	Antibiotic-loaded acrylic cement
ALBC	Antibiotic-laden bone cement
BMI	Body mass index
CDAD	*Clostridium difficile* diarrhoea
CI	Confidence interval
CRP	C-reactive protein
CRR	Cumulative revision rate
DAIR	Debridement, antibiotics, implant retention
DM	Diabetes mellitus
DMARD	Disease-modifying antirheumatic drug
DSM	Dead space management
EBJIS	European Bone & Joint Infection Society
ESAC-Net	European Surveillance of Antimicrobial Consumption Network
ESR	Erythrocyte sedimentation rate
FAW	Forced air warming
FDA	Food and Drug Administration (USA)
HAI	Hospital-acquired infections
HbA1c	Hemoglobin A1c
HIV	Human immunodeficiency virus
HR	Hazard ratio
IMN	Intramedullary nail
MALDI-TOF	MS matrix-assisted laser desorption ionization time of flight mass spectrometry
MBEC	Minimum Biofilm Eradicating Concentration
MDT	Multidisciplinary team
MIC	Minimal inhibitory concentration
MRSA	Methicillin-resistant *S. aureus*
MRSE	Methicillin resistant *Staphylococcus epidermidis*
MSSA	Methicillin-sensitive *Staphylococcus aureus*
NINSS	Nosocomial Infection National Surveillance Service
NSQIP	National Surgical Quality Improvement Program
OECD	Organisation of Economic Cooperation and Development
OR	Odds ratio

PCR-ESI/MS	Polymerase chain reaction electrospray ionization mass spectrometry
PJI	Periprosthetic joint infection
PMMA	Polymethylmethacrylate
PMNs	Polymorphonuclear cells
PROMS	Patient-reported outcome measures
RA	Rheumatoid arthritis
RCT	Randomized control trial
RR	Relative risk
SII	Surgical invasiveness index
SSI	Surgical site infection
THA	Total hip arthroplasty
TJA	Total joint arthroplasty
TKA	Total knee arthroplasty
TKR	Total knee replacement
TNF	Tumour necrosis factor
WBC	White blood cell

Part I

Incidence and Socioeconomic Impact

1 Incidence and Socioeconomic Impact of Bone and Joint Infections (BJIs): The European Perspective

Konstantinos N. Malizos
and Klaus Kirketerp-Møller

Abstract

Epidemiologic studies demonstrate that population fragmented ageing and increased urbanisation, and motorisation across the globe increase the prevalence of trauma and age-related musculoskeletal conditions, such as fragility fractures and arthritis. The number of primary and revision arthroplasties has increased steadily in the last 20 years and so does the number of fractures treated with implantation of hardware. These numbers are anticipated to further escalate over the next two decades. The prevalence of deep infection following joint replacements and the number of post-traumatic infections is projected to increase at a faster rate as a result of a tendency to operate more on high-risk patients, at greater ages, with diabetes, other comorbidities and immunosuppression. This is further increasing the severity of septic complications and other adverse outcomes, which can often lead to functional impairment, long-lasting disability, or even permanent handicap with an inevitable social and economic burden. Musculoskeletal infections place an additional cost burden on total healthcare expenditures, which are already rising faster than the gross domestic product in most countries, and may also become life-threatening conditions. The scientific community needs to take a more active role to increase awareness and in collaboration with policy makers and funding organisations, collect valid data, construct an action plan and put the scourge of the bone and joint infections higher in the agenda of health care priorities.

K.N. Malizos, MD, PhD (✉)
Department of Orthopaedic Surgery and Musculoskeletal Trauma, Biopolis, University General Hospital of Larissa, Larissa 41110, Greece
e-mail: malizos@med.uth.gr; kmalizos@otenet.gr

K. Kirketerp-Møller, MD
Department for Dermatology, Bispebjerg University Hospital, Copenhagen Wound Healing Center, Copenhagen, Denmark
e-mail: kkm@dadlnet.dk

D. Kendoff et al. (eds.), *Periprosthetic Joint Infections: Changing Paradigms*,
DOI 10.1007/978-3-319-30091-7_1

Keywords
Bone and joint infections • Osteomyelitis • Prosthetic joint infections • Socioeconomic burden of BJIs • Septic arthritis • Necrotising infections • Antibiotic resistance

Introduction

Trauma and disorders of the bone and the joints influence health & quality of life of many millions of people around the globe with enormous costs on the individual, the society and healthcare systems. It is the social and demographic pressures from population ageing, and the effect of massive urbanisation on trauma, alongside with the effects of environmental factors that are driving up an increased demand for new advanced medical applications. This is imposing unprecedented challenges and cost escalation on the health care systems. The technological and scientific advances in health care delivery have been the main drivers for the rising costs. Up to 50 % of the increase in health care spending in market-oriented economies in the last half century is arising from medical technology. Remarkable medical innovations now allow for the treatment of previously untreatable conditions, also increasing medical costs. All these parameters with a significant socio-economic impact are proceeding beyond any control [1, 2].

Over the last 40 years the health care costs in most industrialised countries have been rising at a 1–2 % faster pace than that of the GDP [3]. Trauma, fragility fractures and arthritis, also called "civilisation" diseases, are the most common of the musculoskeletal problems [4]. The current practice of orthopaedic surgery is largely relying on a variety of implants, for the management of trauma, degenerative diseases of the skeleton and deformity correction [5]. Upon implantation the altered local blood supply, together with impairment of the local tissue defence, may facilitate the adhesion of pathogens on their surface. Microorganisms evading local defense mechanisms start colonising the surface of the implant, soon leading to a clinically important infection by biofilm formation. The exo-polysaccharides form a matrix enclosing the bacteria, thus protecting them from phagocytosis, the activity of antibodies, and exposure to antibiotics. The attraction of excited polymorphonuclear cells (PMNs) and macrophages leads to release of proteases and the direct lysis of the adjacent bone. Cytokines released from the excited PMNs induce the formation of osteoclasts, further eroding the bone adjacent to biofilm, leading subsequently to implant loosening [6, 7].

The management of biofilm infections is very demanding, with surgical interventions exerting a severe direct personal burden on patients, including pain and suffering, and an economic impact that stems from the need for more operations, long hospital stays, expensive medical and surgical care and rehabilitation, on top of additional indirect costs for the health care system. With the expanding use of implants for fracture care, arthritis, correction of spinal disorders and deformities, the impact on individuals, together with the social and economic burden, became devastating.

The specific characteristics and the burden from bone and joint infections, though recognised, remain under-appreciated. However, in every process towards solving any type of problem, the first step is to spot and identify it [8, 9]. With the long-lasting recession in the economies of many industrialised countries, the health care budgets are facing reductions, followed by strict regulatory interventions to contain the costs at all stages and levels of care. Recently, there has been a rise in awareness of the cost of musculoskeletal infections among physicians and the public, yet not among policy makers and research-funding agencies. This must be credited to the efforts of the scientific "societies" and "associations" of orthopaedists, infectiologists and microbiologists, although they have not acted in a coordinated line yet.

Current Health Care Policies and BJIs

Between 2000 and 2009, the total health care expenditures in the countries of the Organisation of Economic Cooperation and Development (OECD) have been growing steadily by 4 % annually, compared to only 1.6 % of GDP growth in the same period, leaving a steadily increasing deficit in an ever-accentuating recession [10]. This has forced the payers and governmental agencies to put health care costs under scrutiny, fixated on determining the "true value" of health outcomes achieved for the money spent. Every attempt to reduce the costs needs to focus on value and not on volume. The health care benefits, however, are mostly subjective and the true cost of care within the fragmented system is largely "hidden." Economists and politicians are trying to redefine health care through value-based competition on results. Value measurement will increasingly influence clinical decision-making, payment, and public policy, but it necessitates much more comprehensive and objective assessment of the outcome and cost from all aspects at the patient level. The health benefits accrued to patients for the money spent across the continuum for the full cycle of care must be measured for every patient, also from his/her perspective, with validated disease-specific patient-reported outcome measures (PROMS) and health-related quality of life measures. Following such an approach could reveal not only the true value of care but also the burden of adverse events and unwanted outcomes [11, 12].

Fiscal Challenges and Cost Assessment

Orthopaedic surgery today provides a "health care of true value," but unlike other specialties, orthopaedics lags in using commonly accepted definitions and measures of patient outcomes, agreement on indications for interventions and broadly accepted measures for the quality of this care. Understanding the true value of orthopaedic care delivered, and capturing the costs is a pressing issue but in a fragmented healthcare delivery system collecting and aggregating the patient-reported outcome data is very difficult, and these efforts can be elusive. An additional challenge in calculating "value" is the broad variability in costs configuration together with the lack of reliable cost information. It is difficult for anyone, including consumers, to obtain accurate pricing information for orthopaedic health care services thus limiting our ability to measure and report financial measures [9–12].

The providers do not usually disclose the costs associated with the provision of musculoskeletal services, and fee schedules are often considered proprietary. Contributing factors include provisions imposed by device manufacturers, lack of transparency in hospital billing practices, and large variation in the difference between hospital charges and actual payments made by insurance companies, needless to mention the broad variety in payment policies among the EU country-members' healthcare systems [8]. Collaboration not only with orthopaedists but also with other physicians, and administrators at different levels, is essential in order that widespread outcome assessment and transparent cost accounting be made.

The daily routine in orthopaedics is to care for an abundance of patients in limited number of beds, under pressure for fast treatment. In an ageing population we are expanding the indications for implants and invasive procedures on immunosuppressed patients, within an "environment of pathogens" transported from hospital to hospital, in addition to the emergence and spread of resistant germs due to antibiotic overuse in people, the livestock and in aquacultures. As a result, we are watching a rise in the infections that is reflected on increasing morbidity and mortality rates. In the EU, with more than 2,000,000 hospital-acquired infections (HAI) in a year, 15 % more costly than the community-acquired ones, it is estimated that for 175,000 of the affected patients these complications are lethal [10]. In the UK, 37,000 people die from sepsis every year [13]. The most vulnerable for HAIs are the newborns, patients with indwelling prosthetic devices, and those with bone and joint implants.

According to several reports, about one-third of the HAIs are surgical site infections (SSIs), an unacceptably high rate [13]. Internationally, the frequency of SSI is difficult to monitor because the criteria for diagnosis might not be standardised. A survey sponsored by the World Health Organisation demonstrated a prevalence of nosocomial infections ranging from 3 to 21 %, with wound infections accounting for 5–34 % of the total [14]. The 2002 survey report by the Nosocomial Infection National Surveillance Service (NINSS), which covers the period between October 1997 and September 2001, indicates that the incidence of hospital-acquired infection related to surgical wounds in the United Kingdom is as high as 10 % and costs the country's National Health Service approximately one billion pounds annually [14]. Collated data on the incidence of wound infections probably underestimate the true incidence because most wound infections occur when the patient is discharged, and these infections may be treated in the community without hospital notification [14]. SSIs are associated not only with increased morbidity but also with substantial mortality. Seventy-seven percent of the deaths of surgical patients were related to surgical wound infection [14]. Kirkland et al. calculated a relative risk of death of 2.2 attributable to SSIs, in comparison with matched surgical patients without infection. SSIs also are associated with a significant increase in attributable post-surgical costs, even after adjusting for patient-, surgery-, and facility-level factors. If hospitals at the highest percentage, i.e., 10 % (worst), could reduced their SSI rates to those hospitals at 50 %, the Veteran's Administration hospitals in the US would save approximately $ 6.7 million/year [15–17].

The Burden from the Bone and Joint Infections

More than one-third of the SSIs are bone and joint infections [18]. The increasing numbers of bone and joint infections disable a large number of patients every year worldwide, having a devastating impact on their personal life, on their families and the health care system as they impose a greater demand for additional surgeries, long hospital stays, poor outcomes, chronic disability and even death! Their true incidence remains unknown and due to lack of good epidemiological data, their contribution to the global burden of disease is largely unrecognised.

An epidemiological study of 12,506 culture positive infections from hospitalised patients found that 23 % suffered from osteomyelitis or septic arthritis, 26 % from SSIs, and 7 % from prosthetic joint infections. The 27 % of those were health care – associated infections, 80 % were complicated with higher mortality, longer hospital stay and much higher direct costs [18]. The increased survival after multi-trauma has been linked to an increased rate of post-traumatic osteomyelitis [19, 20]. With an estimated number of more than 7,000,000 fractures annually in the EU countries, mostly affecting the young in their productive life years, osteomyelitis as a post-traumatic complication may often induce irreversible damage with lifelong disability. Most vulnerable are trauma patients with comorbidities, the elderly, and the hosts B and C, imposing an additional burden, thus increased direct expenses, in addition to the productivity loss and the much higher indirect costs. However, accurate data about the socio-economic impact of osteomyelitis are poor due to the difficulties in establishing an acceptable study model as it varies in types, severity, treatment options and rehabilitation needs. A postoperative infection after hip fracture requiring a revision surgery, costs twice as much as the primary operation, three times more than investigation and four times more than hospitalisation in the ward. In addition, to reduce the probability of a life-threatening condition, or even death, stemming from systemic sepsis in a debilitated host, a disarticulation may be necessary, further increasing the burden dramatically [21, 22].

The improved life expectancy among elderly patients with diabetes mellitus is responsible for more neuropathy, vascular insufficiency and the associated local bone and soft tissue complications. Diagnosis and treatment of osteomyelitis improved significantly over the last decades, however, the diabetes mellitus-related infections and the infections of the axial or appendicular skeleton remain as devastating complications, often requiring complex multidisciplinary care with mixed outcomes. Sixty per cent of the diabetes-related osteomyelitis cases result in amputation compared to 6 % in hematogenous infections and 24 % in contiguous infections, mostly affecting the toes, and the tarsal and metatarsal bones. The osteomyelitis incidence rates in the last 40 years remained relatively stable among children, but almost tripled among the elderly, mostly driven by a secular increase in diabetes-related cases. During the same period the overall risk of death in a patient population affected by osteomyelitis was increased at least 2.5-fold. According to a recent randomised controlled trial funded by the French Ministry of Health, in patients aged 18 years or older with microbiologically confirmed pyogenic vertebral osteomyelitis, Louis Bernard et al. demonstrated that duration of 6 weeks of antibiotic treatment is non-inferior to 12 weeks, with respect to the proportion of patients cured at 1 year, which suggests that the standard antibiotic treatment duration for patients with this disease could be reduced to 6 weeks saving costs and burden to the patients [23–25].

Foot ulcers in diabetes is one of the most frequently neglected complications, requiring repeated surgery and usually a long duration for wound healing and not uncommonly an amputation incurring permanent handicap. These problems are commonly encountered in disabled, poorly complying patients, frequently facing financial hardships or unemployment. They often receive poor non-specialised treatment with disappointing outcome but still at high costs. With increasing numbers of patients suffering from diabetes this problem is escalating, while at the same time the diabetic foot clinics are not health care priorities in many public health facilities or they are facing the consequences of the austerity policies and reductions of the health care budgets [25–28].

SSI after spine surgery is a well-known complication that can result in poor outcomes, arthrodesis-site nonunion and neurological injury. It has been directly related to a BMI >35 hypertension, thoracic versus cervical, lumbosacral versus cervical, but the strongest risk factor for SSI of the Spine after adjusting for co-morbidities, age, and other known risk factors is a surgical invasiveness index (SII) more than 21 ($p=0.01$). The SII is a validated instrument that accounts for the number of vertebral levels decompressed, extent of arthrodesis, or instrumentation, as well as the surgical approach employed [29].

In the field of paediatric orthopaedics, in the last decade, pyogenic arthritis follows a trend towards decreased health care utilisation. In a study with a large cohort of patients in a 12-year period (1988–2000), the length of hospital stay decreased significantly from 10 days in 1988 to 5 days in 2000, although the total charges remained unchanged [30].

Necrotizing soft tissue infections (NF) are rare, however, with high mortality rates varying form 7 to 43 %, and even higher when they affect the trunk. They need multidisciplinary management by surgeons, infectiologists, ICU and hyperbaric oxygen unit specialists. These devastating and potentially lethal infections impose high direct in-patient costs and even higher post-discharge costs on the survivors, as they need long rehabilitation periods and coverage of the long-term or permanent disability. Age greater or equal to 44 years was the most powerful predictor of prolonged LOS, elevated TC, and an increased risk of hospital mortality in patients suffering from NF [31]. The financial burden of NF might be significantly reduced by diagnosing the disease in its earliest stages. Clues to the presence of early NF can be gleaned from epidemiological risk factors, associated comorbidities, physical signs and symptoms, and/or specific laboratory markers [32]. Early aggressive medical and surgical management of NF is predicted to reduce the number of bed days and surgical procedures required to control the spread of infection [32], which would translate into reduced cost. An investment on the part of health-care facilities and providers to develop and institute guidelines or clinical care pathways for the evaluation and management of patients presenting with acute skin and soft-tissue complaints might help achieve this goal.

In oncological patients with mega-prosthesis, large series with long follow up report an infection rate of up to 10 %. They are commonly offered to patients with large bone and soft tissue defects, they need long operative time, and they are applied in patients already immunocompromised both from the disease itself and the treatment. Malnutrition, frequent red blood cell and PLT transfusions, neutropenia from the post-operative chemotherapy and bacteraemia from indwelling central venous catheters are major contributors to the high infection rates after implantation of mega-prosthesis. However, lack of accurate data plagues the field. Mega-prosthesis infection is the bane of limb preservation, but it has not attracted major focus of research for infection prevention [33, 34].

Arthritis of various types is one of the world's largest health care problems related to the age, and to trauma, but also to rheumatic and other systemic immune diseases. Their management involves high medical care costs, and at the stage of joint degeneration it leads to disability and early retirement. The long-lasting treatment and the lost working time of patients and their escorting carers exert an immense Socio-economic impact still unrecognised. Major joint degeneration not only markedly reduces health-related quality of life but also generates extensive costs for the community and the patient. Longer waiting time for a THA, female gender, comorbidity, and age younger than 65 years are associated with even higher costs. Available baseline cost data are essential for further health economic analyses and could provide guidance for health care decision makers [35].

The number of patients operated every year with expensive reconstructive procedures, costly implants for deformity correction and joint replacements or re-operations, is steadily increasing. The data from large and old cohorts, such as the Swedish, the Norwegian and the newer UK arthroplasty registers reports, demonstrate a steadily increasing demand for joint replacements in the last three decades with an unprecedented increase in health care expenditures per capita. According to the Swedish Knee Arthroplasty Register (SKAR) report of 2010, in 1990 the 1.6 and 0.9 % of the older women and men in Sweden had at least one knee arthroplasty, and in 20 years (2009) these numbers became five times higher (7.3 % and 5.0 %, respectively). A parallel increase is observed for hip arthroplasties. It will soon be reflected in the need for revisions, risk of peri-prosthetic fractures and Infections [34, 35, 37]. With an estimated number of more than 2,000,000 joint replacements worldwide in 2011, and a prosthetic joint infection (PJIs) rate of 1.65 % at the end of the first year post-op, which increased to 2.35 % at the 3rd year, 2.96 % at the 5th, and 3.35 % at the 7th year of follow up, this problem becomes the most devastating adverse event (after death) for the patient. In the immuno-suppressed patients, as in those receiving an RA with an arthroplasty, prosthetic joint infections are higher than 5 %, and in the revised total joint arthroplasties they reach 7 %. Comparing the cumulative revision rate (CRR) and using only revision for infection as an end point, the SKAR found improvement with time for TKA. However, in TKA (OA and RA) the CRR for infection during 2006–2012 has increased as compared to 1996–2005 (Fig. 1.1).

When this Knee Register estimates the risk of revision due to infection, it counts the first revision due to infection in the affected knee (Fig. 1.2). Over time a reduction in this risk both for OA and RA was noticed, but for the period 2006–2012 the risk of revisions for infections increased compared to the previous 20 years. UKAs have significantly lower risk of infection than TKA, and patients with OA run a lower risk than those with RA [35–37].

In the Swedish Hip Arthroplasty Register 2013 report, peri-prosthetic infection is also the second most common reason for revision THA. The relative proportion of infection increased even more in 2013, i.e., from 13.9 to 14.6 % in primary revisions, and from 23.9 to 25.6 % in multiple-time revisions [37–39]. Infection was also the second most common reason for revision of hemi-arthroplasties, broadly applied in the management of hip fractures. Although the percentage of the prosthetic joint infections was low, compared to

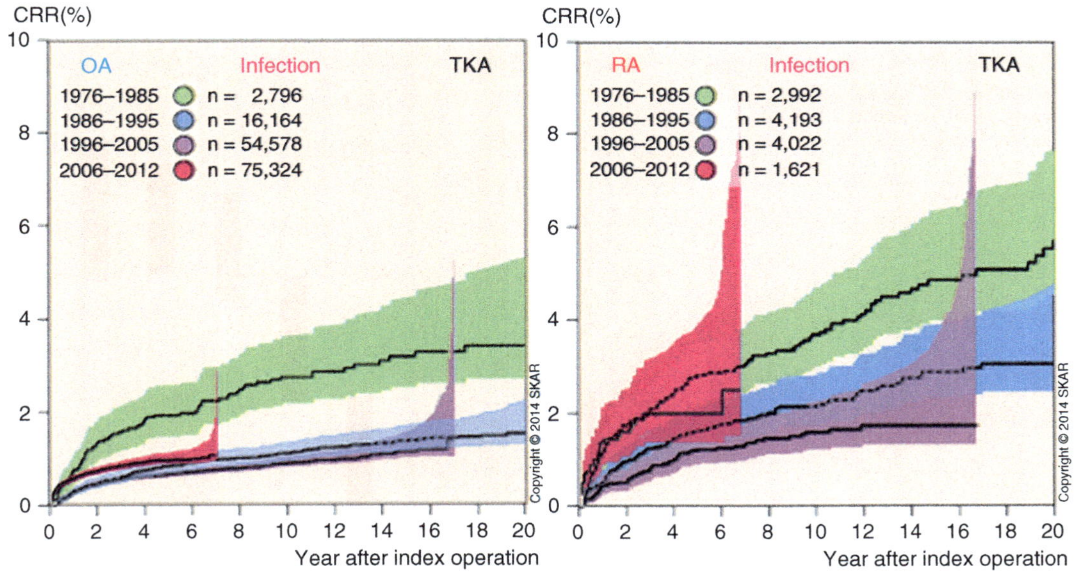

Fig. 1.1 The longer the follow up for the TKA the higher the infection rate in patients with osteoarthritis of the knee. This is even higher for the TKAs in rheumatoid knees (SKAR Report 2014) (Published with permission from the Swedish Knee Arthroplasty Register)

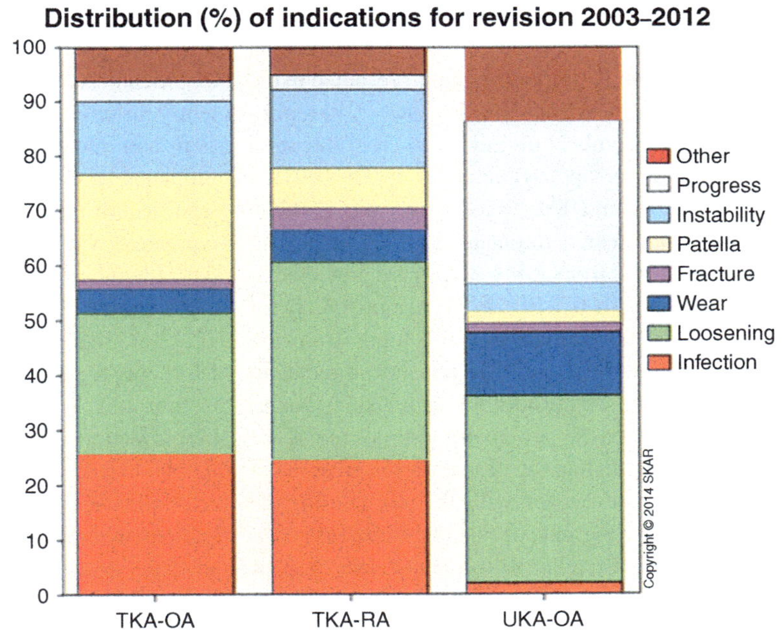

Fig. 1.2 The infection comprised about 25 % of the indications for revision of the TKAs in osteoarthritis, 23 % of the revisions in cases with rheumatoid arthritis and a very low 2.5 % for the UKAs (SKAR Report 2014) (Published with permission from the Swedish Knee Arthroplasty Register)

the large total number of joint replacements, the health care burden and the financial costs dramatically increased due to prolonged hospital stays and suffering of the debilitated patients. This means, among all consequences, a substantial loss of healthy lifetime of the patients, and increased health care expenditures in order that the large number of patients affected are managed. The higher the prevalence of prosthetic knee infections in the Swedish Knee Arthroplasty Register after a

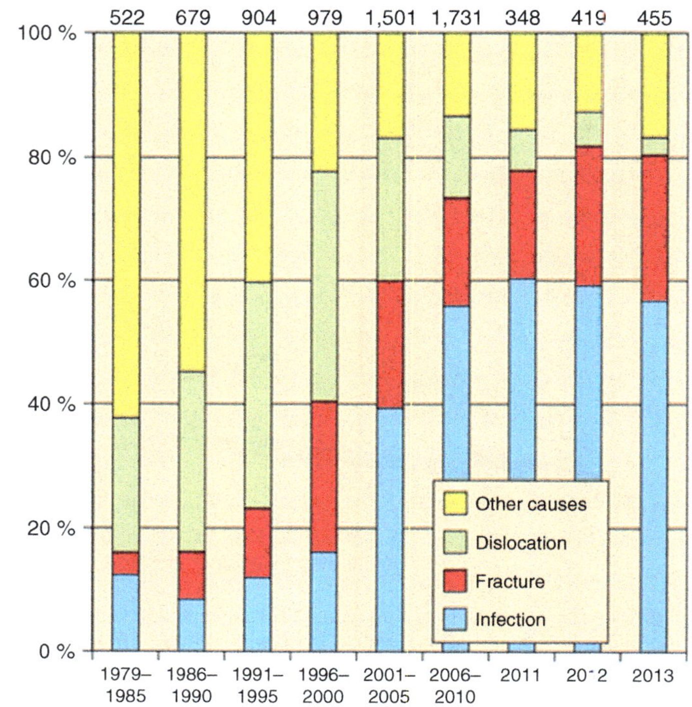

Fig. 1.3 The relative proportion of THA infection increased in 2013 even more, from 13.9 to 14.6 % in primary revisions and from 23.9 to 25.6 % in multiple-time revisions (SHAR Report 2013)

follow-up of 20 years, the longer their survival (Fig. 1.3) [37]. A similar finding is presented in the Norwegian Hip Arthroplasty Register 2010 report, where the number of revisions for infection increased from approximately 6 % in 1997 to nearly 20 % in 2009 [38, 39]. As the absolute number of infected implants is rising, the trend shows that PJIs from 1.4 % (2005) are projected to be increasing to 6.5 % for THA and 6.8 % for TKA in 2030, thus drawing big funds from the ever restricted health care budgets, now directed to fewer patients. The proportion of revisions due to infection increases for multiple-time revisions. After initial revision, the probability is great that a possible further revision will take place during the first year after the index revision. If the first revision is performed due to loosening, infection or dislocation, then the cause for the next revision is, in most cases, the same [39]. Orthopaedic infections from MRSA and other resistant bacteria are responsible for multiple surgical procedures, increased complications, longer hospital stay, 2.5 times higher mortality, 7-fold higher likelihood for the patient to die within 90 days, higher likelihood for him/her to undergo mechanical ventilation, 30-fold higher likelihood to be readmitted, with significantly increased total costs. PJIs are consistently difficult to eradicate, are limiting joint function and have a systemic impact with major influence on fatal outcome, as they demonstrate significantly greater risk of mortality ($p<0.001$), compared with aseptic revision arthroplasty at 90 days (3.7 % vs. 0.8 %), 1 year (10.6 % vs. 2.0 %), 2 years (13.6 % vs. 3.9 %), and 5 years (25.9 % vs. 12.9 %). Independent predictors of mortality in PJIs are the increasing age, higher Charlson Comorbidity Index, history of stroke, polymicrobial infections, and cardiac disease, factors commonly encountered in the population with joint arthroplasties [40]. PJIs from antibiotic resistant bacteraemia may lead to excision arthroplasty and several "years living with disability". Infections from antibiotic susceptible bacteria yield 81 % satisfactory outcomes, while only 48 % of the PJIs from resistant bacteria may be cured [37]. PJIs represent a tremendous economic burden for tertiary-care centres and patients. Measuring the impact of PJIs following primary TKA, with 2-stage revision in the length of hospitalisation, readmissions, and the associated costs, in a 4-year period (2007–

2011) 21 consecutive patients with infected TKAs were matched with 21 non-infected patients who underwent uncomplicated primary TKA. PJIs after TKA compared to the matched group needed significantly longer hospitalisations (5.3 vs. 3.0 days), more readmissions (3.6 vs. 0.1), and more clinic visits (6.5 vs. 1.3). The mean annual cost was also significantly higher in the infected group $116,383 ($44,416 to $269,914) compared to the matched group $28,249 ($20,454 to $47,957) [41]. The SSIs following total hip and total knee replacements are associated with increased number of readmissions. In the first year after these infections have been taken care 1.2 % of the patients are re-hospitalised because of a new SSI for an average of 8.6 days with a cost of $ 26,812. The year after this episode of SSI, 12.5 % of the cases were re-hospitalised due to SSI-related issues, 41 % with SSIs were re-hospitalised for "all cause" reasons, with an average stay of 6.2 days and an additional cost of $31,046. According to the Center for Disease Control & Prevention (CDCP), SSIs associated readmissions are potentially preventable, saving millions $/year to the healthcare system.

The Obstacles

Early diagnosis helps in achieving improved outcomes for patients with infections, however delays are frequent, particularly in the chronic ones, because of their insidious onset with clinical features that may be confused with other conditions and due to lack of specialised and sensitive tests available in the health care settings. More focused research may also improve diagnosis to both speed up treatment and minimise the waste of ineffective drugs. There is an urgent need to educate on and raise awareness of these problems, with organised dissemination of current evidence, and best practices concerning prevention, diagnosis and management of musculoskeletal infections. Unfortunately, only in countries with well-developed health care networks there are specialised centres for the treatment of severe implant-related bone and joint infections, leaving thus a large number of patients in settings where a low volume of cases can be accommodated, with less experienced surgeons, lack of a team approach and understaffed operating theatres and labs. The absence of structured training programs and opportunities in countries with underdeveloped health care systems, results in a paucity of employment of trained orthopaedic surgeons and maintenance of supportive labs for the care of persistent musculoskeletal infections. At all level of education, starting from medical school curricula and following with the various "musculoskeletal" and "bone and joint" infection societies and associations, there is a need for us to strive to train care givers from diverse geographical backgrounds, set up collaborative networks and help develop evidence-based protocols. Modern orthopaedics is expensive, and even personnel trained up to the highest theoretical and practical level have to continuously innovate and improvise when confronted with current economic constraints, austerity and limited resources, the same being the problem in a lot of countries.

The financial problems a lot of tertiary-care referral centres have been facing led to defensive policies, such as restricting access to a patient with an infection. To overcome this obstacle a structure for financial incentives to hospitals with the ultimate goal of better clinical outcomes is needed, and also finding ways to reduce readmissions, re-operations, complications and mortality rates. Influential international organisations like the EU administration, the WHO, the NIH, the "Welcome Trust," the "Bill and Melinda Gates Foundation" do not appear to fully appreciate the burden imposed, the emerging threat posed by the disabling bone and joint infections, and the lack of new effective antimicrobials. The need to raise general awareness of the political decision-making bodies to act against this burden is urgent.

The European Perspective

Europe is not one single country but it consists of 50 independent countries and 6 more that are "partially" recognised. The total population is 742 million people. A European perspective of the socio-economic burden of PJIs has not been established yet. The significant variability of the economic and demographic conditions and cultural convictions throughout Europe differs form north to south, from west to east, and within regions as well as countries. The EU today acts as an international organisation comprising 28 European countries and following common economic, social, and security policies, with a population of 507 million people adhering to a common charter, the Charter of Fundamental Rights of the European Union. Health care in the EU is provided through a wide range of different systems run at the national level. Despite this, the charter states: "A high level of human health protection shall be ensured in the definition and implementation of all Union policies and activities" [42]. All member states have either publicly sponsored and regulated universal health care or publicly provided universal health care. Some countries have universal health care entirely paid by tax and others have hybrid systems, where basic needs are covered through tax-paid systems with additional non-tax covered services. Private funding for health care may represent personal contributions towards meeting the non-taxpayer refunded portion of health care or may reflect totally private (non-subsidised) health care, either paid in cash or met by some form of personal or employer-funded insurance. The regional disparities in health outcomes can be attributable to differences in socio-economic statuses and working conditions, behavioural, cultural factors, and differences in public health policies among member states and regions.

Musculoskeletal diseases are mainly related to ageing, among other aetiologies, and the EU population is currently characterised as rapidly ageing. Increased longevity is one of the main drivers of population ageing, and worries about the sustainability of pensions and health and care systems tend to be exacerbated in recession times. It should be borne in mind that the increased lifespan is clearly an important outcome of the progress in biomedical sciences and technologies, and broadly provided to European citizens by the national health care systems. However, the current crisis raises a lot of issues for individuals and their families regarding the sustainability of social and welfare systems. For these reasons policies are necessary to take this change into account and smooth out the hardest effects of the crisis on the population's health. The economic crisis has very heavy repercussions on life expectancies and health conditions, especially among the elderly. The experts agree that population ageing is, and will remain, the major demographic challenge to the European Union. In the EU-28 countries, the average share of persons aged 65 years and above is projected to increase from the 17.1 % of 2008 to 30 % by 2060, when the number of old people will rise to 151.5 million.

The increasing demand for joint replacements for the benefit of the patients is not only a burden to the healthcare system, but also a lucrative business for private contractors. Due to the different healthcare systems throughout the continent, it is difficult to identify the distribution between private contractors and public service for primary joint replacements. The oldest scientific society in the world studying bone and joint infections, the European Bone & Joint Infection Society (EBJIS), through its board of country representatives, has recently conducted a survey regarding the Orthopaedic health care services each representative presenting results for his/her own country. The figures provided are gross estimates by the country representatives from France, United Kingdom, Germany, Greece, Czech Republic, Switzerland (non-EU), Spain, Denmark, Sweden, Belgium, The Netherlands and Azerbaijan (non-European), with a total of 401 million inhabitants.

Private Versus Public Contractors in Primary Arthroplasties

Primary prosthetic joint implantations are in their vast majority performed in public hospitals in the Nordic countries, whereas in countries like Germany about 20 %, and France or Belgium more than 50 %, are provided by private contractors. Revision surgery for an arthroplasty, after loosening or fracture, is much more demanding in terms of hospital and human resources, skills, hardware and recovery, and this is especially so when the revision is due to an infection. The survey findings demonstrate the clear tendency that revision surgery and overall revisions due to an infection are preformed preferably in the public hospital. A simple explanation could be that private contractors either do not have the facilities or avoid taking the risk for an unpredictable outcome of septic joints surgery in terms of length of stay, expensive antibiotics, and the subsequent increased burden. There are very few reports on the actual direct costs of septic joints revision arthroplasties, revealing significant differences in service charging and coding, and reimbursement policies among countries and regions within countries. There are vast variations among reimbursements by public health care providers and those insurance companies make for the increased costs of treatment.

Financial Incitement

Financial incitement is a very powerful tool used by health care authorities to induce changes. In some countries a flat-rate system has been implemented. By "flat-rate system" it is meant that in case of readmission within a defined timeframe the provider of the index operation cannot charge for any extra costs. In some counties this is expanded allowing even admission to another hospital to be invoiced to the index department (UK). The timeframe of the quarantine period differs from 18 (Confederation Helvetique) to 44 (Italy) days. The survey revealed that United Kingdom, Czech Republic, the Netherlands, Italy and France have a flat-rate policy. This policy is apparently aiming at providing the patient with the incentive of a free-of-charge re-examination with the ultimate goal of preventing complications. The flat-rate system focuses on reduction of early and short-term adverse events like SSIs and dislocations, but might have very little effect on the long-term complications like late infections, loosening of the prosthesis and hardware failure. There are no studies proving the true savings derived by this type of health care management, and moreover, the flat-rate policy has also some drawbacks. Use of implants that could reduce long-term complications, such as the coated ones, is not encouraged, and also withholding of readmissions until the patient is out of the quarantine period may appear.

In the management of infected joint arthroplasties today, the dominating treatment option follows the two-stage exchange procedure. The time between the first stage with implant removal, surgical debridement, and local antibiotic delivery, and the subsequent second stage of re-implantation varies from 2 to 6 weeks, or sometimes more. In some countries the optimal time to implement stage two is within the quarantine period, hence hindering the surgeon from obtaining reimbursement for the second procedure. But the approach of "the flat-rate system" carries the risk of encouraging re-implantation at a sub-optimal time, with a questionable benefit for the patient. It appears that this type of financial incitement could be a way to induce changes, but it needs much stronger advocacy on the part of the clinicians and the scientific societies to optimise the structure of incentives and evaluate its true benefits.

The Global Financial Crisis in 2007–2008

Economists have characterised the Global Financial Crisis of 2007–2008 as the worst global recession since the Great Depression of 1929. Surprisingly, most of the responses to the EBJIS Survey do describe that the financial crisis had little or no impact on the health care system. In Greece and Spain, on the contrary, under a major influence of such a crisis the implementation of "salvage" programs with dramatic budget reductions and stringent austerity measures, is suffering from shortage of health care personnel, hospital resources and service accessibility, having a direct negative effect on the public healthcare quality indices. The same survey has also revealed that within the communities, there is an ongoing effort to reduce cost and increase effectiveness, and in this respect, the health care systems are not by-passed.

The Long-Fought Battle with the Antibiotic-Resistant Bacteria

Antibiotics paved the way for unprecedented medical and societal developments in the previous century, and are today indispensable in most health scare systems throughout the world. Achievements in modern medicine, including use of implants in musculoskeletal surgery, which today are taken for granted, would not be possible without access to effective prophylaxis and treatment against bacterial infections. The antibiotic resistance is a rapidly progressing and complex issue with consequences affecting everybody in the world. However, coordinated action is largely limited, both at national and international levels. The ongoing effort to control infections in clinical practice has yielded inadequate results, and no single solution has been successful. Although various strategies are being implemented worldwide, between 2000 and 2010 the consumption of antibiotics increased by 36 %. Most antibiotics are intended for use in commercially driven livestock to help promote growth and prevent disease, in agriculture, aquaculture and horticulture. Unnecessary prescription by physicians, uncertain of a diagnosis or treating largely self-limiting bacterial or viral infections, is also a major contributing factor to the development of antimicrobial resistance. The European Surveillance of Antimicrobial Consumption Network (ESAC-Net) for 2010 reports a use ranking from 11.1 (Estonia) to 39.4 (Greece) daily doses/1000 inhabitants/day [43]. In low-income countries, antibiotics are given as a substitute for provision of clean water and safe waste disposal. In Nigeria, 88 % of the staphylococci are methicillin-resistant. The 95 % of adults in India and Pakistan carry bacteria resistant to β-lactams.

Anderson et al. reported that health care and community acquired-MRSA infections have surpassed HIV as the most deadly pathogen in the US and Europe, accounting for more than 100,000 deaths per year [42]. The high burden of resistant infections results from the increasing costs of treatment, longer duration of illness and higher rates of mortality, as well as the inability to follow procedures that rely on effective antibiotics to prevent infection [43, 44].

A recent report entitled "*Tackling a Crisis for the Health and Wealth of Nations, from the Review of Antimicrobial Resistance*" led by the economist Jim O'Neill and informed by two other reports prepared by KPMG and RAND Europe, as well as the 1st annual progress and implementation report on antimicrobial resistance for the UK Government, following their 2013 5-year strategy plan, estimates that 300 million people will die as a result of drug resistance within the next 35 years. If this happens, it would have a catastrophic knock-on effect on the world's economy, reducing global GDP by 2–3.5 %, more than it should otherwise have been in 2050. In addition to antibiotic resistance, the review projects also revealed resistance to antimalarial, HIV, and tuberculosis drugs. However, the consultants admit the data are unreliable, and state that "These were considered as proxies in the absence of better data or forecasting tools; much more details and robust work will no doubt be done by academic researchers and clinicians in the future." The authors also admit that their "teams experienced significant problems with data collection because of the lack of consistent sources monitoring the number of bacterial infections globally" [44–46]. According to a recent report from the United Kingdom, the human cost of the antibiotic-resistance crisis is estimated to 300 million cumulative premature deaths by 2050, with a loss of up to $100 trillion (£64 trillion) to the global economy. This dire situation has been highlighted for years by the Infectious Diseases Society of America [45–47].

Achievements in modern medicine including the use of implants in musculoskeletal surgery, which today are taken for granted, would not be possible without access to effective prophylaxis and treatment for bacterial infections. With the rising awareness about the antibiotic resistance threat among policy-makers and the public, there comes an increasing demand for action.

As with other such assets, for keeping it available the first step is conservation, making better antibiotic stewardship by reducing demand through vaccination, infection control, diagnostics, public education, incentives for clinicians to prescribe fewer antibiotics, restrictions on access to newer, last-resort antibiotics, and implementation of strict rules to ban their use for the growth of livestock. This needs top-down political action from the part of governments, regulatory agencies and medical associations, implementing a structure of incentives for conservation if they really mean to match their rhetoric [46].

Innovative concepts improving the efficacy of current drugs and replenishing effectiveness by developing new drugs should be the second step, where scientists have the biggest role to find ways to maximize the impact of the existing stocks, such as scanning all compound libraries for new drugs, or for combinations to reverse resistance to existing medicines and so to extend their useful life, a concept that has proven successful in the treatment of HIV. Discovery of new antibiotics is a necessary but not sufficient solution because of the high cost of research towards this direction and lengthy timelines.

This brings up the third step, i.e., increasing the number of antibiotics that reach the market. From the 30 new antibiotics approved by the FDA between 1983 till 1992, there were only seven between 2003 and 2012. Restructuring of the incentives given to the firms that are called to do that work might be an effective approach to overcome this problem. World Health Organisation is in the process of a draft preparation on antibiotic resistance, proposing new business models for the development of new drugs, driven by the public need rather than market forces [47]. *Antibiotic resistance should be on the global political agenda, not just the agendas of infectious disease meetings.*

The Impact of Bone and Joint Infections on Global Health

The BJIs constitute a set of problems, which although it is spread globally as a challenge, is seen through different lenses at the different parts of the world. Resource-rich countries are challenged to design effective prevention of infections, and provide affordable access and quality of care for their patients with infected implants and other musculoskeletal infections, while the resource-poor countries are challenged to understand and develop sustainable services from scratch. One of the most pressing concerns in resource-poor settings is trauma and infection complications, requiring the attention and service of sub-specialist surgeons. Goals concerning global health equity, as well as ready access to basic medical care are priorities, but it is not possible without the development of safe and effective surgical care. Providing orthopaedic care through volunteerism to local, national, and international patients who are unable to pay or cannot easily access care is not only an ethical responsibility but also a professional one. Surgery in low-income and middle-income countries, however, faces implementation challenges. Compared with vaccination or antiretroviral treatment, surgery needs more infrastructure, such as clean operating rooms, anaesthesia, electrical power for monitoring equipment, and ancillary laboratory services. It also requires more specialized human resources and infrastructure than many traditional public health interventions. Cost-effectiveness should not be perceived as a barrier to expansion of surgery in resource-poor settings. When these challenges are met, surgery can produce health benefits with similar cost-effectiveness ratios [48–51]. Education is key for the medical students who are going to be the next generation of researchers, and public health professionals, the general public, and the decision makers. A first step is to train the legislators and policy makers and give them access to good evidence, and also give them the ability to interpret it. However, competing influences are frequently raising hindrances to evidence-informed policy making [52].

Europe today is facing an unprecedented pressure from huge numbers of immigrants flooding the southern countries, seeking after better living conditions, bringing thus the problem of the health care equity into its ground. This is further increasing the burden on the health care system and the restricted budgets. Several key principles should guide efforts to reduce disparities. First, we should look for hidden disparities, reporting clinical performance data that are stratified according to patients' race, ethnic group, and socioeconomic status. Reducing and even more, eliminating racial and ethnic disparities in health outcomes is more difficult than simply standardising the health care provided to patients. It is our professional responsibility as clinicians, to collaborate with the administrators and policymakers to improve the way we deliver care to diverse patients, including patients of any racial or ethnic background. Scientists' job is not over once a paper is published. We can reach at a point in our career when we should decide, in a world of limited resources and time, to focus on making a difference, thus we can definitely do better [53–55].

The Future

For such devastating impact from the long fought battle against the germs, there is a definite need to forge a new "social contract" between health care, the medical innovation system with its basic scientists and clinical researchers, and the "society" as a key to the development of sustainable health-care systems that take maximum advantage of the power of modern medicine and reduce its socioeconomic burden. The future is likely to be shaped by the 4P medicine that is **p**redictive, **p**re-emptive, **p**ersonalised, and **p**articipatory. Such an approach has the potential to transform health care from disease-orientated provision to a true health maintenance service [54]. For a more effective and efficient management of the bone and joint infections, we are proposing six priority issues requiring immediate attention: (1) As most diagnostic tests suffer from inadequate specificity and/or sensitivity combined with subtle clinical presentation of most bone and joint infections, often resulting in missed or delayed diagnosis and thus compromising clinical care; the development of rapid, simple, cheap and robust diagnostic tests is a priority. (2) Education and training of the medical community on the value of rapid intervention with surgical treatment of the BJIs and effectively targeted antibiotics, should be addressed in a systematic way from the academia and the specialty societies. (3) Focus on translational work to develop biofilm-resistant implants through collaboration of specialty groups from surgeons and basic scientists from the fields of biology, chemistry, physics, and funding agencies. (4) A better understanding of the "host at risk" for infection. This will lead to targeted preventive measures and more optimal clinical practices. (5) Implementation of policies to reduce unemployment and poverty as fundamental causes of poor health with higher incidence of infections and increased morbidity and mortality; and (6) Accurate data accumulation in registers at national and international level with emphasis on the socio-economic impact of musculoskeletal infections to obtain indisputable and convincing evidence and raise much higher the scientific interest, attract committed grants and increase global investments to reduce the burden.

Progress will be made against the scourge of bone and joint infections if all parties, politicians, funding agencies and the scientific community establish a collaborative action plan through surveillance and research, public and patient education, implementation of strategies for prevention and control, advocacy and partnerships with public health institutions, both private and public funding and academia, to increase awareness and raise priority for bone and joint infections on the global health agenda. Our patients' safety and our professional integrity depend on it!

Acknowledgements The authors wish to thank the following for providing data for the EBJIS Survey:

Dr. med Volker Alt, Germany, Dr. Martin Clauss, Switzerland, Prof/Dr. Chingiz Alizada, Azerbaijan

Prof/Dr. Lorenzo Drago, Italy, Dr. Dirk Jan Moojen, The Netherlands, Dr. Guillem Bori, France

Prof. MUDr. David Jahoda CSc, Czech Republic, professor Jos Stuyck, Belgium, Anna Stefansdottir, Sweden, Mr. Martin McNally, United Kingdom, Mr. Rhidian Morgan-Jones, United Kingdom.

References

1. Smith S, Newhouse JP, Freeland MS. Income, insurance, and technology: why does health spending outpace economic growth? Health Aff (Millwood). 2009;28(5):1276–84. doi:10.1377/hlthaff.28.5.1276.
2. Beyer F, Costa-Font J, Felder S. Ageing, health, and health care. Oxf Rev Econ Policy. 2010;26:674–90. In: The Lancet, August 2013, editorial.
3. Jenkner E, Leive A. Technical notes and manuals: health care spending issues in advanced economies. Washington, DC: International Monetary Fund; 2010.
4. Stengel R. The high cost of care. Time. 2013;181:3.
5. Eldenburg L, Krishnan R. Management accounting and control in health care: an economics perspective. In: Handbooks of management accounting research, vol. 2. Philadelphia: Elsevier; 2006. p. 859–83.
6. Kurtz SM, Lau E, Watson H, Schmier JK, Parvizi J. Economic burden of periprosthetic joint infection in the United States. J Arthroplasty. 2012;27:61–5.
7. OECD Health Statistics 2014 [Internet]. Available from: http://oecd.org/els/health-systems/health-data.htm.
8. Bozic KJ, Kurtz SM, Lau E, Ong K, Vail TP, Berry DJ. The epidemiology of revision total hip arthroplasty in the United States. J Bone Joint Surg Am. 2009;91:128–33.
9. Rosenthal JA, Lu X, Cram P. Availability of consumer prices from US hospitals for a common surgical procedure. JAMA Intern Med. 2013;173:427–32.
10. Bozic KJ, Kurtz SM, Lau E, Ong K, Chiu V, Vail TP, Rubash HE, et al. The epidemiology of revision total knee arthroplasty in the United States. Clin Orthop Relat Res. 2010;468:45–51.
11. Ruiz Jr D, Koenig L, Dall TM, Gallo P, Narzikul A, Parvizi J, et al. The direct and indirect costs to society of treatment for end-stage knee osteoarthritis. J Bone Joint Surg Am. 2013;95(16):1473–80. doi:10.2106/JBJS.L.01488.
12. Mather 3rd RC, Koenig L, Kocher MS, Dall TM, Gallo P, Scott DJ, Bach Jr BR, Spindler KP, MOON Knee Group. Societal and economic impact of anterior cruciate ligament tears. J Bone Joint Surg Am. 2013;95(19):1751–9. doi:10.2106/JBJS.L.01705.
13. Alexander JW, Van Sweringen H, Vanoss K, Hooker EA, Edwards MJ. Surveillance of bacterial colonization in operating rooms. Surg Infect (Larchmt). 2013;14(4):345–51. doi:10.1089/sur.2012.134.
14. Pearson A. Reports on surgical site infections and hospital acquired bacteraemias from the English Nosocomial Infection National Surveillance Scheme. Euro Surveill. 2002;6(16):pii=2121. Available online: http://www.eurosurveillance.org/ViewArticle.aspx?ArticleId=2121.
15. Kirkland KB, Briggs JP, Trivette SL, Wilkinson WE, Sexton DJ. The impact of surgical-site infections in the 1990s: attributable mortality, excess length of hospitalization, and extra costs. Infect Control Hosp Epidemiol. 1999;20(11):725–30.
16. Mangram AJ, Horan TC, Pearson ML, Silver LC, Jarvis WR. Guideline for prevention of surgical site infection, 1999. Hospital Infection Control Practices Advisory Committee. Infect Control Hosp Epidemiol. 1999;20(4):250–78; quiz 279–80.
17. Schweizer ML, Cullen JJ, Perencevich EN, Vaughan Sarrazin MS. Costs associated with surgical site infections in veterans affairs hospitals. JAMA Surg. 2014. doi:10.1001/jamasurg.2013.4663.
18. Lipsky BA, Weigelt JA, Gupta V, Killian A, Peng MM. Skin, soft tissue, bone, and joint infections in hospitalized patients: epidemiology and microbiological, clinical, and economic outcomes. Infect Control Hosp Epidemiol. 2007;28(11):1290–8.
19. Cierny G 3rd. Infected tibial nonunions (1981–1995). The evolution of change. Clin Orthop Relat Res. March 1999;(360):97–105.
20. Mayon-White RT, Ducel G, Kereselidze T, Tikomirov E. An international survey of the prevalence of hospital-acquired infection. J Hosp Infect. 1988;11 Suppl A:43–8.
21. Mader JT, Crops MW, Calhoun JH. Adult posttraumatic osteomyelitis of the tibia. Clin Orthop Relat Res. 1999;360:14–21.
22. Edwards C, Counsell A, Boulton C, Moran CG. Early infection after hip fracture surgery: risk factors, costs and outcome. J Bone Joint Surg Br. 2008;90(6):770–7. doi:10.1302/0301-620X.90B6.20194.
23. Bernard L, Dinh A, Ghout I, Simo D, Zeller V, Issartel B, et al. Antibiotic treatment for 6 weeks versus 12 weeks in patients with pyogenic vertebral osteomyelitis: an open-label, non-inferiority, randomised, controlled trial. Lancet. 2015;385(9971):875–82. 7.
24. Lipsky BA, Berendt AR, Cornia PB, Pile JC, Peters EJG, Armstrong DG, et al. Infectious diseases society of america clinical practice guideline for the diagnosis & treatment of diabetic foot infections. Clin Infect Dis. 2012;54(12):1679–84.
25. Age-adjusted hospital discharge rates for non-traumatic lower extremity amputation (LEA) per 1,000 diabetic population, by level of amputation, United States, 1993–2009. Centers for Disease Control and Prevention (CDC), 2010 [Internet] (updated: October 2, 2014). Available from: http://www.cdc.gov/diabetes/statistics/lealevel/fig8.htm.
26. Jeffcoate WJ, Lipsky BA, Berendt AR, Cavanagh PR, Bus SA, Peters EJ, et al. Unresolved issues in the management of ulcers of the foot in diabetes. Diabet Med. 2008;25(12):1380–9. doi:10.1111/j.1464-5491.2008.02573.
27. Apelqvist J, Eneroth M. Costs of deep foot infections inpatients with diabetes mellitus. Pharmacoeconomics. 2000;18(3):225–38.
28. Cizik AM, Lee MJ, Martin BI, Bransford RJ, Bellabarba C, Chapman JR, et al. Using the spine surgical invasiveness index to identify risk of surgical site infection: a multivariate analysis. J Bone Joint Surg Am. 2012;94(4):335–42. doi:10.2106/JBJS.J.01084.

29. Freedman J, Guller U, Benjamin DK, Higgins LD, Pan D, Cook C, et al. National trends in health care utilization and racial and socioeconomic disparities in pediatric pyogenic arthritis. J Pediatr Orthop. 2006; 26(6):709–15.
30. Mulla ZD, Gibbs SG, Aronoff DM. Correlates of length of stay, cost of care, and mortality among patients hospitalized for necrotizing fasciitis. Epidemiol Infect. 2007;135(5):868–76. Epub 2006 Nov 3.
31. Young MH, Engleberg NC, Mulla ZD, Aronoff DM. Therapies for necrotising fasciitis. Expert Opin Biol Ther. 2006;6:155–65.
32. Sudarsky LA, Laschinger JC, Coppa GF, Spencer FC. Improved results from a standardized approach in treating patients with necrotizing fasciitis. Ann Surg. 1987;206:661–5.
33. Racano A, Pazionis T, Farrokhyar F, Deheshi B, Ghert M. High infection rate outcomes in long-bone tumor surgery with endoprosthetic reconstruction in adults: a systematic review. Clin Orthop Relat Res. 2013;471(6):2017–27. doi:10.1007/s11999-013-2842-9.
34. Rolfson O, Ström O, Kärrholm J, Malchau H, Garellick G. Costs related to hip disease in patients eligible for total hip arthroplasty. J Arthroplasty. 2012;27(7):1261–5.
35. No authors listed. The Swedish knee arthroplasty register: annual report 2014. http://www.myknee.se/en/. Date last accessed Mar 2015.
36. Healey JHCORR, Insights TM. High infection rate outcomes in long-bone tumor surgery with endoprosthetic reconstruction in adults: a systematic review. Clin Orthop Relat Res. 2013;471(6):2028–9. doi:10.1007/s11999-013-2893-y.
37. Bozic KJ, Lau E, Kurtz S, Ong K, Rubash H, Vail TP, et al. Patient-related risk factors for periprosthetic joint infection and postoperative mortality following total hip arthroplasty in Medicare patients. J Bone Joint Surg Am. 2012;94(9):794–800. doi:10.2106/JBJS.K.00072.
38. Kilgus DJ, Howe DJ, Strang A. Results of periprosthetic hip and knee infections caused by resistant bacteria. Clin Orthop Relat Res. 2002;404:116–24.
39. Kurtz SM, Ong KL, Schmier J, Mowat F, Saleh K, Dybvik E, et al. Future clinical and economic total hip and knee arthroplasty. J Bone Joint Surg Am. 2007;89 Suppl 3:144–51.
40. Robertsson O, Ranstam J, Sundberg M, W-Dahl A, Lidgren L. The Swedish knee arthroplasty register a review. Bone Joint Res. 2014;3(7):217–22.
41. Zmistowski B, Karam JA, Durinka JB, Casper DS, Parvizi J. Periprosthetic joint infection increases the risk of one-year mortality. J Bone Joint Surg Am. 2013;95(24):2177–84. doi:10.2106/JBJS.L.00789.
42. eur-lex.europa.eu. [webpage on the internet]. Article 35: health care. official journal of the European union. [updated 26.10.2012; cited April 2015]. Available from: http://eur-lex.europa.eu/legal-content/EN/TXT/?uri=CELEX:12012P/TXT.
43. Anderson DJ, Kaye KS, Chen LF, Schmader KE, Choi Y, Sloane R, et al. Clinical and financial outcomes de to methicillin resistant Staphylococcus aureus surgical site infection: a multi-center matched outcomes study. PLoS One. 2009;4(12), e8305. doi:10.1371/journal.pone.0008305.
44. O'Neill J. Review on antimicrobial resistance. Antimicrobial resistance: tackling a crisis for the health and wealth of nations [Internet]. December 11, 2014. Available from: http://amr-review.org/.
45. ECDC. Summary of the latest data on antibiotic consumption in the EU. Nov 2012 [Internet]. Available from: http://ecdc.europa.eu/en/eaad/Documents/ESAC-Net-summary-antibiotic-consumption.pdf. Accessed 31 Oct 2013.
46. Smith R, Coast J. The true cost of antimicrobial resistance. BMJ. 2013;346:f1493. doi:10.1136/bmj.f1493.
47. UK government report: UK 5 year antimicrobial resistance (AMR) strategy 2013–2018, Annual progress report and implementation plan, 2014 [Internet].
48. Kapadia BH, McElroy MJ, Issa K, Johnson AJ, Bozic KJ, Mont MA. The economic impact of periprosthetic infections following total knee arthroplasty at a specialised tertiary-care center. J Arthroplasty. 2014; 29(5):929–32. doi:10.1016/j.arth.2013.09.017.
49. Lee N. The lancet technology: august, 2014. Surgical training through the looking glass. Lancet. 2014;384(9943):573.
50. Marseille E, Morshed S. Essential surgery is cost effective in resource-poor countries. Lancet Global Health. 2014;2(6):e302–3.
51. Chao TE, Sharma K, Mandigo M, Hagander L, Resch SC, Weiser TG, Meara JG. Cost-effectiveness of surgery and its policy implications for global health: a systematic review and analysis. Lancet Glob Health. 2014;2(6):e334–45. doi:10.1016/S2214-109X(14)70213-X.
52. Marshall HC. How to achieve health equity. N Engl J Med. 2014;371:2331–2. doi:10.1056/NEJMe1412264.
53. Chin MH. Improving care and outcomes of the uninsured with chronic disease… Now. Ann Intern Med. 2008;149(3):206–8.
54. Orton L, Lloyd-Williams F, Taylor-Robinson D, O'Flaherty M, Capewell S. The use of research evidence in public health decision making processes: systematic review. PLoS One. 2011;6(7):e21704. doi:10.1371/journal.pone.0021704. S2214-109X(14)70213-X.
55. Tooke J. Seizing the potential of scientific advance. Lancet. 2015;385(Suppl):S1–2.

2 The Incidence and Socioeconomic Impact of Periprosthetic Joint Infection: United States Perspective

Christina J. Gutowski, Antonia F. Chen, and Javad Parvizi

Abstract

Periprosthetic joint infection (PJI) following total joint arthroplasty leads to prolonged hospitalization, considerable morbidity, loss of productivity in the workplace, and a significant financial burden. The incidence of PJI domestically is rising yearly at an alarming rate, and deep infection is among the most frequent indications for performing revision hip or knee arthroplasty in this country. Revision for infection has been shown to cost more than double that of a revision procedure performed for aseptic loosening or mechanical failure. Infection with resistant organisms has also becomes more prevalent, which is associated with worse treatment outcomes and a higher cost of care. The government is the primary payer for the majority of cases of PJI, through Medicare spending, and several proposals for various reimbursement strategies are on the horizon that will impact provider compensation for physicians and hospitals. This chapter explores the clinical and financial implications of the rising incidence of PJI in this country, and considers the future impacts these trends may have on the American healthcare system.

Keywords

Periprosthetic joint infection • Cost • Reimbursement • Cost-effectiveness

C.J. Gutowski, MD, MPH (✉)
Department of Orthopaedic Surgery, Thomas Jefferson University Hospital, Philadelphia, PA, USA

A.F. Chen, MD, MBA
Department of Orthopaedic Surgery, The Rothman Institute of Orthopaedics, Thomas Jefferson University Hospital, Philadelphia, PA, USA

J. Parvizi, MD, FRCS
Department of Orthopaedic Surgery, The Rothman Institute at Thomas Jefferson University Hospital, 925 Chestnut St., Philadelphia, PA 19107, USA
e-mail: parvj@aol.com

D. Kendoff et al. (eds.), *Periprosthetic Joint Infections: Changing Paradigms*,
DOI 10.1007/978-3-319-30091-7_2

Introduction

Periprosthetic joint infection (PJI) is a truly devastating complication of total joint arthroplasty (TJA) [1]. It adversely impacts the patient, by causing functional disability, increased morbidity and also mortality [2]. The management of PJI currently is far from optimal, often resulting in the need for prolonged hospitalization, administration of long term intravenous antibiotics, and the need for multiple surgical interventions [3]. The protracted course of treatment results in a massive financial burden on the treating institution and the health system on a national level. The incidence of PJI has been increasing steadily over the last decade, both in terms of the absolute number of cases, as well as the proportion of primary total hip and knee arthroplasties that succumb to infection [3, 4]. The resistance profile of infecting organisms has also changed over the recent years with an increase in the number of surgical site infections and PJIs being caused by antibiotic resistant organisms [5, 6]. While recurrence of PJI after treatment is not common, eradication rates as low as 16–37 % have been shown with infection of certain organisms treated with less-aggressive strategies [7, 8]. The extensive treatment required to appropriately treat a patient with PJI is significantly more expensive than that for aseptic loosening after primary TJA [3], and treating institutions are experiencing a decline in reimbursement along with the development of penalties for infection-associated readmission [9, 10]. Together, these trends have created a worrisome situation for physicians, economists, and policymakers looking ahead at the future of PJI in the United States. The purpose of this chapter is to critically examine the incidence, treatment paradigms, and the impact of the microbial profiles involved in PJI, and to investigate the current and future socioeconomic impact these trends may have on the American healthcare system.

Incidence of Infection

Domestic Incidence of Musculoskeletal Infection

The incidence of generalized musculoskeletal infection, including PJI, osteomyelitis, soft tissue infection, and septic arthritis, is increasing largely due to the aging population and an increase in the number of patients with preexistent comorbidities such as diabetes and obesity, that may predispose them to infection [11, 12]. For PJI, the absolute numbers of cases per year is rising, which is attributed to the increase in the number of primary TJA that is being performed. Other factors that may also explain the rise in the prevalence of PJI may relate to the increase in awareness regarding PJI and development of better diagnostic strategies. Data extracted from the Nationwide Inpatient Sample (NIS) demonstrated that the absolute number of PJIs increased from 2001 to 2011, as infected total hip arthroplasties (THAs) grew from 4545 to 8858, and total knee arthroplasties (TKAs) increased from 7113 to 17,773 [13]. The odds of developing PJI after TJA also rose over this time period. PJI is the most common indication for performing revision TKA and third most common reason for revision THA in the United States [14, 15].

Infecting Organism Profile

In recent years, there has been an increase in the number of both postoperative surgical site and deep PJI caused by methicillin-resistant organisms [5, 16]. This change in microbial resistance profile is concerning from a clinical standpoint, because infection with an antibiotic resistant organism is associated with an increased rate of treatment failure, longer hospitalizations, and worse overall outcomes [8, 16]. The optimal treatment for these patients has been stated to be two-stage exchange arthroplasty that includes resection arthroplasty, placement of a static or dynamic antibiotic-impregnated spacer, and administration of prolonged course of intravenous antibiotics prior to reimplantation,. The surgical management of patients with PJI, and particularly those infected with antibiotic resistant organisms, leads to a profound decreases in quality of life, socioeconomic contribution, and earnings potential [17]. The shift in virulence of these organisms may explain an interesting paradigm shift that has been witnessed within American hospitals: the average length of hospitalization for treatment of PJI has declined steeply over the last 20 years,

However, the average charges per case have been consistently rising [4]. This may reflect the more aggressive and expensive nature of treatment that has recently been undertaken by clinicians when treating PJI, the extended and costly nature of pursuing a two-stage exchange arthroplasty with intravenous antibiotics, and other aggressive methods of treatment. The financial impact of these clinical trends will be discussed in more detail in the next section.

Economic Impact of Infection

Costs of Revision Arthroplasty for PJI

For many reasons, PJI places a major financial burden on the patient, the payer, the treating institution, and the healthcare system as a whole. The direct medical costs of a revision THA performed for PJI range from $68,000 to over $107,000, according to one report [16], depending on the infectious organism and the type of treatment undertaken. These costs are 2.8 times higher than the cost associated with revision arthroplasty for aseptic loosening or mechanical failure, and 4.8 times higher than costs for primary THA [18]. The comparisons are similar among TKA patients [19] In their 2005 report, *Bozic and Ries* were able to identify several key drivers of this difference between cost in patients undergoing revision THA for infection, as compared to those undergoing revision for aseptic loosening, as delineated in Table 2.1 [18].

Table 2.1 Clinical characteristics of revision total hip arthroplasty (THA) for infection, compared to revision THA for aseptic loosening and to primary THA

Longer operative time
More operative blood loss
Higher post-operative complication rate
More total hospitalizations
More days in hospital
More total surgeries
Higher total hospital costs
More outpatient visits
Higher outpatient charges during 12-month period following procedure

Table adapted from Gutowski and Bozic [25]

Association Between Microbial Resistance and Cost

The cost of treatment is dependent on several factors. Parvizi et al. showed that the mean cost of treatment for infections caused by methicillin-resistant organisms is $107,264, as compared to $68,052 for treatment of sensitive strains [16]. Interestingly, even when controlling for surgical treatment performed (irrigation and debridement, versus one-stage exchange arthroplasty, versus two-stage exchange arthroplasty), PJI caused by antibiotic resistant organisms was associated with higher costs (Table 2.2). Among patients undergoing irrigation and debridement (I&D), for example, those with a methicillin-resistant infection were associated with 1.7 times higher cost. This is partly explained by a nearly two-fold longer length of hospital stay in these patients with resistant organisms.

Financial Considerations of Clinical Decision-Making

Treatment strategy does play a role in determining the overall cost for management of PJIs. The cost of treatment must be weighed against the chances of successful outcome. For example, resection arthroplasty followed by staged reimplantation after several weeks of intravenous antibiotics is the most aggressive and costly treatment protocol. It is also associated with considerable morbidity, loss of function, and cost of time lost from work and leisure. However, it appears to provide more favorable long-term outcome versus I&D [20]. I&D with retention of components, followed by several weeks of antibiotics, is much less expensive to perform and quality of life and the socioeconomic productivity is not as profoundly affected, but is associated with a much higher rate of infection recurrence [21]. If these patients require future surgeries for a failed debridement attempt, the overall cost can escalate above that associated with the two-stage exchange arthroplasty strategy. Fisman et al. utilized cost-effectiveness analysis modeling techniques to examine these two management strategies, and found that the

Table 2.2 Cost per treatment procedure for periprosthetic joint infection (PJI) with sensitive or resistant strains

Procedure	Mean cost, methicillin-resistance	Mean cost, methicillin- sensitive	p-value	Resistant: sensitive quotient
I&D	$32,720	$18,734.20	0.001	1.7465
Resection arthroplasty	$30,387.40	$23,459.50	0.0199	1.2953
1-stage exchange	$36,606.60	$25,886	0.033	1.4141
Reimplantation	$35,022.40	$26,775.70	0.0105	1.3080

parameter with the greatest impact on overall cost is the relapse rate of infection [22]. In a patient with a high risk of recurrence, such as those with PJI caused by a highly-virulent organism, the recommended strategy both from a clinical and cost-effectiveness standpoint would be two stage exchange arthroplasty. However, in a frail, elderly patient who has a higher risk of morbidity and mortality, a less aggressive treatment strategy, namely I&D with retention of the components, may be undertaken to achieve higher cost-effectiveness.

Reimbursement Considerations

In 2009, the average cost to a hospital for treating a single case of hip PJI was $30,300 and knee PJI was $24,200 [23]. Higher cost of care was found to be associated with patients of minority race and patients who lived in the West or Northeast parts of the United States. The financial burden associated with treatment of PJI is disproportionately assumed by the high-volume referral centers [24]. A disincentive exists among low-volume surgeons and hospitals to provide care to these patients, due to the clinically-challenging nature of these cases and probably lack of appropriate multidisciplinary teams. This phenomenon is compounded by an economic disincentive derived from increased pressures to minimize risk and improve cost-effective healthcare delivery. Insufficient reimbursement for these cases results in an average net loss of approximately $15,000 per revision TKA. If the patient's care is reimbursed through Medicare, one form of government insurance in the United States, the institution's average net loss per case approaches $30,000 [25].

Reimbursement for revision TJA, specifically PJI, has been a source of policy debate in recent years. Medicare coding and reimbursement practices were only changed in 2005 to reflect the complexity of revision and infected cases, after sufficient data were released that demonstrated increased hospital and surgeon resource utilization for these cases [26]. Medicare reimbursement policy is particularly relevant to this patient population because the majority of patients undergoing arthroplasty are funded by Medicare [27], as TJA already accounts for more Medicare spending than any other inpatient procedure. Five billion USD of the 2006 Medicare budget was spent on these TJA codes, and by 2030, TJA is projected to cost Centers for Medicare and Medicaid Services more than $50 billion annually [28]. Focusing on PJI specifically, data from the National Inpatient Sample revealed a relatively constant proportion of PJI patients covered by Medicare and Medicaid: from 2008 to 2011, 60.7 % to 63.26 % and 5.33 % to 6.73 %, respectively [29]. Interestingly, Medicare bears a disproportionate amount of the financial burden associated with these patients. Medicare covers nearly 60 % of those patients who fall victim to PJI, while private insurers or self-pay accommodates the remaining subgroup (Table 2.3). Meanwhile, Medicare covers only 37 % of patients with successful primary arthroplasties, while private insurers represent a much larger proportion of these less-expensive, uncomplicated patients. The "national bill," or the aggregate annual charges to Medicare for treatment of PJI across the nation, has risen steadily and was reported to be over $2 billion in 2011. This is over twice the amount of overall charges to private insurers for this condition.

Table 2.3 Percentage of hospital discharges for PJI, reimbursed by various payers

	2008	2009	2010	2011
Medicare	61	63	60	62
Medicaid	5	6	6	7
Private	28	26	26	27
Uninsured	1	1	1	1
Other	5	4	4	3

HCUP NIS Database. http://hcupnet.ahrq.gov/HCUPnet.jsp?Id=791E0204CFD43716&Form=DispTab&JS=Y&Action=%3E%3ENext%3E%3E&__InDispTab=Yes&_Results=Newquery

Looking Towards the Future

In consideration of the trends outlined above, concern has intensified regarding the sustainability of the current paradigm surrounding treatment of PJI. In 2009, the total hospital cost incurred across the United States for treating patients with PJI was $566 million. By 2020, it is projected to reach $1.62 billion, for nearly 60,000 cases (Figs. 2.1 and 2.2) [23, 30].

The current reimbursement model for PJI is undergoing a transition, as payers attempt to anticipate and adjust to the future financial burden. The Patient Protection and Affordable Care Act contains several provisions for improving delivery and reimbursement of healthcare services in the United States. Specifically, the movement away from fee-for-service reimbursement models towards a lump-sum payment for a bundled episode of coordinated care has been initiated. TJA lends itself well to testing this payment model [31], which represents a shift of financial risk from payer to provider. However, it is concerning that the financial aspects of PJI have not been explicitly reconciled in any of the four proposed bundled payment models currently being trialed [32]. Postoperative infection, as an unexpected and to some extent uncontrollable event, can be costly and would not be covered under the proposed models, which offer lean reimbursements based off costs for uncomplicated primary TJA. Development of one infection in the hospital could quickly eliminate any cost savings and gain-sharing that providers are working towards capturing. Patients with several comorbidities, deemed at high-risk for developing PJI, may undergo surgical delay until optimization could be achieved [33], or theoretically deprived of elective arthroplasty, as a result of the economic disincentives created by bundled payment schemes.

Policies have been implemented to financially motivate providers to prevent postoperative infections. In 2008, Centers for Medicare and Medicaid Services introduced the "Do Not Pay" rule, which outlined the withholding of additional reimbursement for certain "preventable" conditions; postoperative PJI was included on this list. By the time the Final Rule was passed, strong advocacy from the orthopaedic community managed to convince the Centers for Medicare and Medicaid Services (CMS) to remove PJI from the list [34]. While review of hip and knee PJI continues for future addition to the "Do Not Pay" list, this has not been adopted to date.

The Hospital Readmissions Reduction Program launched in fiscal year 2013, where hospitals with excess readmissions for acute myocardial infarction, heart failure, and pneumonia within 30 days of discharge were penalized with a cut of 1 % of Medicare inpatient payments. This penalty increased to 2 % in fiscal year 2014. The Centers for Medicare and Medicaid Services estimates that in its second year, the Hospital Readmissions Reduction Program would impose penalties on 2225 hospitals for an excess of $227 million [35]. In October 2014, the Department of Health and Human Services announced that the maximum penalty increased to 3 %, and that the program would expand to include readmissions for chronic obstructive pulmonary disease and complications after TJA. In consideration of already-high costs and resultant financial losses associated with treating complicated PJI, these penalties can have far reaching consequences. A concern that is becoming increasingly relevant involves the development of medical refugees: patients who have either developed PJI, or those who are candidates for TJA but have several risk factors for postoperative PJI, and are unsuccessful in finding a provider willing to treat them. More and more hospitals and surgeons may resort

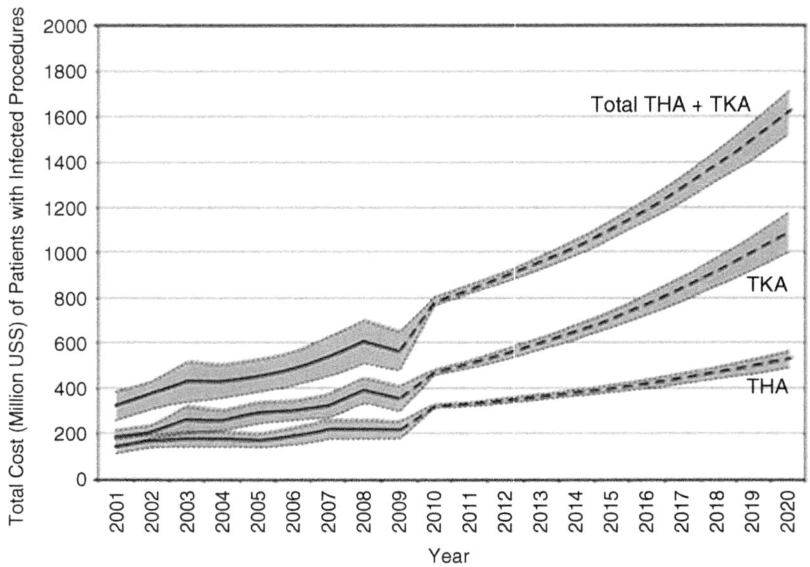

Fig. 2.1 Historical and projected total inpatient cost of infected arthroplasty procedures in the United States, 2001–2020 (Adapted from Kurtz et al. [23], Copyright 2012, with permission from Elsevier)

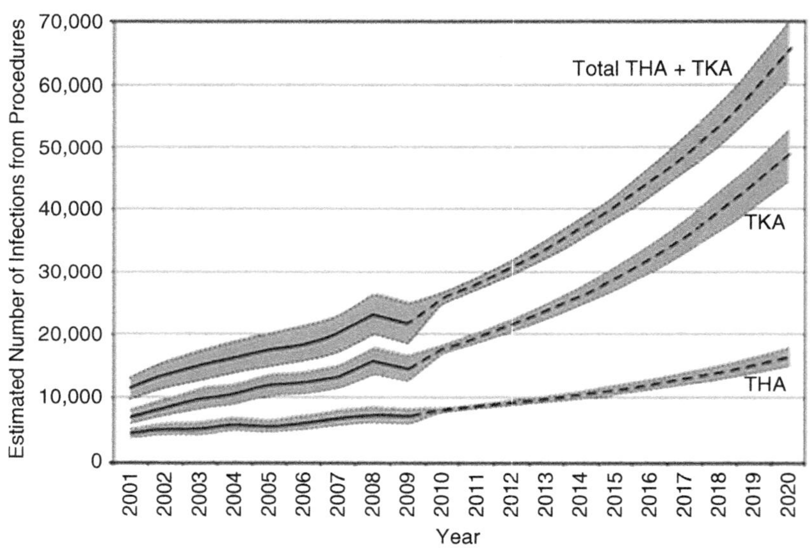

Fig. 2.2 Historical and projected number of infected arthroplasties in the United States, 2001–2020 (Adapted from Kurtz et al. [23], Copyright 2012, with permission from Elsevier)

to "cherry-picking" in order to minimize risk and thereby mitigate financial loss [36].

Conclusion

Currently, TJA accounts for more Medicare spending than any other inpatient medical procedure [28, 37]. Government payers, namely Medicare, also fund over 60 % of all cases of PJI treated in the country annually. As the incidence of primary arthroplasty and the rate of postoperative infection continue to increase, the clinical and financial burden placed on the healthcare system will become ever more pervasive [23]. Implementation of the Affordable Care Act will bring adoption of new models of care delivery, payment, and penalties that may give rise to economic disincentives for both hospitals and surgeons against treating patients with PJI or with risk factors for developing infection, potentially leading to exclusion of patients from the healthcare system. Looking ahead, a multipronged approach to minimizing the economic burden of PJI must include cost-effective care starting on an individual patient basis, while creating a global incentive structure that rewards value, effective prevention, and evidence-based treatment. With the present state of affairs, and in an effort to provide a cost effective care, considerations should be given to building specialized centers of care for management of PJI, akin to oncology centers, that bring together a multidisciplinary team of experts.

References

1. Kurtz SM, Lau E, Watson H, Schimier JK, Parvizi J. Economic burden of periprosthtic joint infection in the United States. J Arthoplasty. 2012;27(8 Suppl 1):61–5.
2. Berend KR, Lomardi AV, Morris MJ, Bergeson AG, Adams JB, Sneller MA. Two-stage treatment of hip periprosthetic joint infection is associated with a high rate of infection control but high mortality. Clin Orthop Relat Res. 2013;471(2):510–8.
3. Bozic KJ, Ries MD. The impact of infection after total hip arthroplasty on hospital and surgeon resource utilization. J Bone Joint Surg. 2005;87(8):1746–51.
4. Kurtz SM, Lau E, Schmier J, Ong KL, Zhao K, Parvizi J. Infection burden for hip and knee arthroplasty in the United States. J Arthroplasty. 2008;23:984–91.
5. Anderson DJ, Sexton DJ, Kanafani ZA, Auten G, Kaye KS. Severe surgical site infection in community hospitals: epidemiology, key procedures, and the changing prevalence of methicillin-resistant Staphylococcus aureus. Infect Control Hosp Epidemiol. 2007;28:1047.
6. Parvizi J, Ghanem E, Azzam K, Davis E, Jaberi F, Hozack W. Periprosthetic infection: are current treatment strategies adequate? Acta Orthop Belg. 2008;74:793.
7. Bradbury T, Fehring TK, Taunton M, Hanssen A, Azzam K, Parvizi J, et al. The fate of acute methicillin-resistant Staphylococcus aureus periprosthetic knee infections treated by open debridement and retention of components. J Arthroplasty. 2009;24(6 Suppl):103–7.
8. Parvizi J, Azzam K, Ghanem E, Austin MS, Rothman RH. Periprosthetic infection due to resistant staphylococci: serious problems on the horizon. Clin Orthop Relat Res. 2009;467(7):1732–9.
9. National Quality Measures Clearinghouse. Total hip arthroplasty (THA) and/or total knee arthroplasty (TKA): hospital 30-day, all-cause, unplanned risk standardized readmission rate (RSRR) following elective primary THA and/or TKA. Centers for Medicare & Medicaid Services/The Joint Commission. Endorsed 1/31/13, available online at http://www.qualitymeasures.ahrq.gov/content.aspx?id=46501#Section615, found 3/5/15.
10. Centers for Medicare & Medicaid Services. Readmissions reduction program. Available online at http://www.cms.gov/Medicare/Medicare-Fee-for-Service-Payment/AcuteInpatientPPS/Readmissions-Reduction-Program.html, found 3/5/15.
11. Patel A, Calfee RP, Plante M, Fischer SA, Arcand N, Born C. Methicillin-resistant Staphylococcus aureus in orthopaedic surgery. J Bone Joint Surg (Br). 2008;90:1401–6.
12. Trampuz A, Widmer AF. Infections associated with orthopaedic implants. Curr Opin Infect Dis. 2006;19:349–56.
13. Jaekel DJ, Ong KL, Lau EC, Watson HN, Kurtz SM. The epidemiology of total hip and knee arthroplasty infection. In: Springer BD, Parvizi J, editors. Periprosthetic Joint Infection of the Hip and Knee, vol. 1. New York: Springer; 2013. p. 1–14.
14. Bozic KJ, Kurtz SM, Lau E, Ong K, Chiu V, Vail TP, Rubash HE, Berry DJ. The epidemiology of revision total knee arthroplasty in the United States. Clin Orthop Relat Res. 2010;468:45–51.
15. Bozic KJ, Kurtz SM, Lau E, Ong K, Vail TP, Berry DJ. The epidemiology of revision total hip arthroplasty in the United States. J Bone Joint Surg. 2009;91:128–33.
16. Parvizi J, Pawasarat IM, Azzam KA, Joshi A, Hansen EN, Bozic KJ. Periprosthetic joint infection: the economic impact of Methicillin-resistant infections. J Arthroplasty. 2010;25(6-S):103–7.
17. Parvizi J, Adeli B, Zmistowski B, Restrepo C, Greenwald AS. Management of periprosthetic joint infection: the current knowledge. AAOS exhibit selection. J Bone Joint Surg. 2012;94:e104(1–9).
18. Bozic KJ, Ries MD. The impact of infection after total hip arthroplasty on hospital and surgeon resource utilization. J Bone Joint Surg. 2005;87-A(3):570–6.
19. Herbert CK, Williams RE, Levy RS, Barrack RL. Cost of treating an infected total knee replacement. Clin Orthop Relat Res. 1996;331:140–5.
20. Hansen E, Tetreault M, Zmistowski B, Della Valle CJ, Parvizi J, Haddad FS, Hozack WJ. Outcome of one-stage cementless exchange for acute postoperative periprosthetic hip infection. Clin Orthop Relat Res. 2013;471(10):3214–22.
21. Cockarell JR, Hanssen AD, Osmon DR, Morrey BF. Treatment of infection with debridement and retention of the components following hip arthroplasty. J Bone Joint Surg. 1998;80:1306–13.
22. Fisman DN, Reilly DT, Karchmer AW, Goldie SJ. Clinical effectiveness and cost effectiveness of two management strategies for infected total hip arthroplasty in the elderly. Clin Infect Dis. 2001;32:419–30.
23. Kurtz SM, Lau E, Watson H, Schmier JK, Parvizi J. Economic burden of periprosthetic joint infection in the United States. J Arthroplasty. 2012;27(8-S):61–5.

24. Sculco TP. The economic impact of infected total joint arthroplasty. Instr Course Lect. 1993;42:349–51.
25. Gutowski CJ, Bozic KJ. Chapter 8. Economic aspects of total hip arthroplasty. In: Parvizi J, editor. The hip. Towson: Data Trace Publishing; 2013.
26. Bozic KJ, Katz P, Certernas M, Ono L, Ries MD, Showstack J. Hospital resource utilization for primary and revision total hip arthroplasty. J Bone Joint Surg. 2005;87-A(3):570–6.
27. Inc, MA. Medicare physician payment up slightly. Orthopedic Network News. 2010;21(1).
28. Wilson NA, Schneller ES, Montgomery K, Bozic KJ. Hip and knee implants: current trends and policy considerations. Health Aff. 2008;27:1587–98.
29. HCUP NIS database. http://hcupnet.ahrq.gov/HCUPnet.jsp?Id=791E0204CFD43716&Form=DispTab&JS=Y&Action= %3E%3ENext%3E%3E&__InDispTab=Yes&_Results=Newquery.
30. Kurtz SM, Ong KL, Lau E, Bozic KJ. Impact of the economic downturn on total joint replacement demand in the United States: updated projections to 2021. J Bone Joint Surg. 2014;96:624–30.
31. Froimson MI, Rana A, White Jr RE, Marshall A, Schutzer SF, Healy WL, et al. Bundled payments for care improvement initiative: the next evolution of payment formulations. AAHKS bundled payment task force. J Arthroplasty. 2013;28(1-S):157–65.
32. Hackett DJ, Rothenberg AC, Chen AF, Gutowski C, Jaekel D, Tomek IM, et al. The economic significance of orthopaedic infections. J Am Acad Orthop Surg. 2015;23(Suppl):S1–7.
33. Ng VY, Lustenberger D, Hoang K, Urchek R, Beal M, Calhoun JH, et al. Preoperative risk stratification and risk reduction for total joint reconstruction: AAOS exhibit selection. J Bone Joint Surg. 2013;95:e191–5.
34. Bozic KJ, Rubash HE, Sculco TP, Berry DJ. An analysis of Medicare payment policy for total joint arthroplasty. J Arthroplasty. 2008;23:133–8.
35. Health policy brief: medicare hospital readmissions reduction program. Health Affairs. 12 Nov 2013.
36. Parvizi J. Just say 'no' to operating on patients at high risk for periprosthetic joint infection. Orthopedics Today. January 2012
37. Bumpass DB, Nunley RM. Assessing the value of a total joint replacement. Curr Rev Musculoskelet Med. 2012;5:274–82.

Part II

Prevention of Periprosthetic Joint Infection

Prevention of Periprosthetic Joint Infections: Minimizing the Risks

3

David A. George, Eliza Gil, and Stephen Morris-Jones

Abstract

Although typical published rates for periprosthetic joint infection are only about 1–2 % of all total joint arthroplasties, these infections have come to represent an increasingly significant burden on society. Financial estimates may be made for the economic loss associated with periprosthetic infection, but the personal cost of morbidity, whether psychological or physical, is often incalculable. This chapter examines the risk factors for development of periprosthetic infections, and discusses which of these factors are modifiable. By developing strategies that target those risks which are controllable, orthopaedic teams can seek to reduce periprosthetic joint infection rates to minimum levels. Risk factors may be considered as being either associated with individual patient characteristics or with the operative procedure itself and the environment in which it is performed. Risk reduction interventions will often require input from multidisciplinary teams, and the timing for interventions can be categorized as occurring in the pre-operative, immediate peri-operative or post-operative phases.

Keywords

Total joint arthroplasty • Periprosthetic joint infection • Prosthetic joint infection • Risk reduction strategies • Screening • Antibiotic prophylaxis • Operative environment

D.A. George, MBChB, BMedSc, MRCS (Eng) (✉)
Department of Trauma and Orthopaedics, University College Hospital, London, 250 Euston Road, London NW1 2PG, UK
e-mail: DAVIDGEORGE@DOCTORS.ORG.UK

E. Gil, MA, MBBS, MSc, MRCP
Department of Microbiology and Infectious Diseases, University College Hospital, London, UK

S. Morris-Jones, MA, MBBS, MSc, MRCP, FRCPath
Department of Clinical Microbiology and Infectious Diseases, University College London Hospital, London, UK

D. Kendoff et al. (eds.), *Periprosthetic Joint Infections: Changing Paradigms*,
DOI 10.1007/978-3-319-30091-7_3

Introduction

Periprosthetic joint infection (PJI) is a clinical condition where there are never any winners. A cloud without a silver lining, PJI brings no benefit to patient, surgical team or society. The costs of PJI are profound, and some are incalculable. To a patient, PJI may involve prolonged and persistent pain, loss of function, emotional distress or, rarely, more serious complications. Not surprisingly, the patient-surgeon bond of trust is often threatened. Surgical teams may feel an onus of responsibility to perform revision arthroplasty themselves, although the evidence is that referral to specialised centres improves outcome. Perhaps the most straightforward cost to calculate is the financial one, borne by society. Even ignoring potential economic productivity losses, a recent Australian study demonstrated that cases of PJI managed with debridement and implant retention, still cost over 3 times as much as age-, sex- and arthroplasty site-matched controls [1]. Although total joint arthroplasty (TJA) infection rates are low at between 1 and 2 % per prosthesis-lifetime, an expanding older population will lead to increasing prevalence of PJI. Over the period 2001–2009, the annual cost to hospitals in the United States of America for infected knee and hip arthroplasties rose from $320 million to $566 million; the estimated projection for 2020 exceeds a staggering $1600 million [2]. Against this sobering backdrop, it is not surprising that there is a growing appreciation of the need to focus on "getting it right first time" [3]. As in so much else of medicine, prevention is better than cure.

The first step in the challenge to reduce PJI rates is to identify those risks that are modifiable; strategies can then be developed to focus on minimizing these risks.

Risk factors for development of PJI following TJA are usually divided into two categories: those associated with the patient, and those associated with the surgical intervention itself [4, 5]. However, it is also very useful to consider when the opportunities for risk minimization may occur, as this will help dictate the timing of interventions. In this way, different risk reduction strategies may be targeted to the three different time blocks: the pre-operative period, the operative and immediately peri-operative window, or the post-operative convalescent stage.

Patient-Associated Risk Factors for Periprosthetic Joint Infections: Screening and Management

Patient-associated risks are summarized in Table 3.1. These should be identified in the pre-operative period and those that can be modified should be reviewed. This is likely to require multidisciplinary input and may necessitate careful peri-operative management and surgical scheduling. Modification of patient-associated risks are discussed.

Active Infection

Patients should be assessed for evidence of ongoing infection, in particular for symptoms of dental or urinary tract infection, as these are common infections that carry a risk of haematogenous seeding [4, 6, 7]. Patients with evidence of current infection should be actively investigated, including with a midstream urinary culture, and those with positive results should be treated with a suitable antibiotic prior to their arthroplasty. Microbiological guidance regarding the choice of agent should be sought if needed.

Medical Co-morbidities

Diabetes Mellitus

Maintaining good glycaemic control in the peri-operative period is essential in the prevention of PJI; however, there is currently little evidence regarding the utility of routine screening of elective TJA patients for hyperglycaemia and/or diabetes, and this is not currently recommended.

Chronic Liver or Kidney Disease

TJA has been shown to be safe even in patients with cirrhosis [8] and routine pre-operative

Table 3.1 Patient-associated risk factors

	Risk Factor[s]	Is risk modifiable?	Intervention
Gender	Male	No	
Presence of active infection	Infection of the joint or surrounding soft tissues	Yes	Tissue sampling to ensure identification of causative pathogen. Treat infection prior to surgery
	Infection at a distant site	Yes	Screen for infective symptoms. Treat infection prior to surgery
Medical Co-morbidities	Inflammatory arthropathy	Yes	Minimize active inflammation and optimize bone density
	Immunodeficiency	Possibly	Optimize viral load and CD4 count of HIV+ patients
	Diabetes – glucose >180 mg/dl or >10 mmol/l	Yes	Diabetes control should be optimized
	Chronic kidney disease	No	
	Liver Disease	No	
	Malignancy	Possibly	Optimize treatment with immunosuppressants and leukocyte (particularly neutrophil) count
Medical or Surgical History	Previous surgical intervention	No	
	Recent hospitalization	No	
	Prolonged admission to a rehabilitation facility	No	
	Immunosuppressive medication	Yes	Minimize immunosuppression, stop in the pre-operative period and optimize agents used
Nutritional status	Morbid obesity (BMI >40 kg/m^2)	Yes	Weight loss and dietetic advice
	Malnutrition	Yes	Nutritional supplements and dietetic advice
Social history	Smoking	Yes	Smoking cessation
	Excessive alcohol consumption	Yes	Abstinence or reduction of alcohol intake
	Intravenous drug use	Yes	
Commensal flora	Nasal colonisation with Methicillin-resistant *Staphylococcus aureus*	Yes	MRSA suppression

screening for liver disease is not advised [4]. Pre-operative identification of kidney disease is imperative as it allows for safe drug dosing, including of antibiotics.

Inflammatory Arthropathy

The patient's underlying condition and bone density should be optimized or stabilized, if possible, and immunosuppression reviewed, as discussed below. Patients with rheumatoid arthritis (RA) are at particular risk of PJI and suffer worse outcomes than non-RA patients with PJI; vigilance must be maintained in these patients for evidence of PJI, which must be treated promptly and aggressively.

Immunodeficiency

It is advisable to liaise with the infectious disease or HIV specialist responsible for the ongoing care of any HIV-positive patient when planning for TJA, with a particular view to optimizing the patient's CD4 count and viral load pre-operatively.

Table 3.2 Recommendations for when to stop immunosuppression pre-operatively

Drug	Prior to surgery
Hydroxychloroquine	Do not stop
Non-steroidal anti-inflammatories Methotrexate	Within 1 week
Sulfasalazine Azathioprine	>1 week
Etanercept	>10 days
Infliximab	3 weeks
Tocilizumab Abatacept Adalimumab	4 weeks
Leflunomide	6 weeks
Rituximab	8 weeks

Medical/Surgical History

Immunosuppressive Treatment

Disease-modifying agents should be stopped prior to elective TJA; the timing of drug cessatioin varies from drug to drug according to its half-life in the body, and recent recommendations are listed in Table 3.2 [4].

Nutritional Status

Morbid Obesity

These patients should be given advice to reduce their weight prior to surgery and should be referred for dietetic advice. Many of these patients will also have diabetes: their glycaemic control and diabetic management should also be optimized pre-operatively. In order to ensure that obese patients receive sufficient antibiotic prophylaxis and avoid underdosing [9], it is imperative that this should be considered as part of the pre-operative planning, involving the hospital pharmacists if necessary..

Malnutrition

Patients suspected to be malnourished pre-operatively should have their nutritional status assessed [10], including measurement of height and weight, calculation of body mass index and measurement of serum albumin levels. Patients identified as being malnourished should be referred for dietetic assessment and considered for nutritional supplements.

Behavioural Risks and Substance Misuse

Smoking

Smoking cessation prior to surgery has been shown to substantially reduce the risk of post-operative complications and mortality [11, 12]. Furthermore, the longer the duration of smoking cessation the lower the post-operative complication rates [12, 13], but even a reduction in total tobacco intake may be beneficial [14]. Again, the pre-opearative assessment should be used as an opportunity to pick up on patient smoking habits and to educate patients of the associated PJI risks, offering strategies to stop, or reduce, smoking in order to minimize these avoidable risks.

Excessive Alcohol Consumption

The optimal pre-operative period of abstinence from alcohol is not known, and may be longer than 4 weeks [15]. The pre-operative assessment provides a useful opportunity to assess alcohol intake and to provide health promotion advice regarding reduction or cessation. It is prudent to delay elective TJA in alcohol dependent patients until they have been assessed by alcohol support services and have managed to reduce their intake.

Intravenous Drug Use

The current international consensus suggests that these patients should not be offered elective TJA [4] due to their grossly elevated risk of PJI, with rates approaching 30 % [16].

MRSA Carriage and Suppression

Rapid screening and suppression of patients with nasal carriage of methicillin-resistant *S. aureus* (MRSA) should be implemented to minimize the risk of PJI with this organism. Although the use of suppression therapy will also reduce colonization with methicillin-susceptible *S.aureus* (MSSA), at present the practice of screening pre-operatively for MSSA carriage remains controversial [17].

Prophylactic Antibiotics

The aim of using prophylactic pre-operative antibiotics is to minimize viable microbial contamination of the surgical site. Within each orthopaedic centre, the antibiotic selected should cover the organisms most commonly found as causes of post-operative infections for that location. Sufficient time should be allowed after administration to ensure that adequate drug concentrations in the tissues will have been reached by the time of surgical incision. Ongoing microbiological surveillance of wound organisms and their antimicrobial susceptibilities is imperative to ensure appropriate prophylaxis and minimize the risk of PJI.

Choice of Antibiotic

Pre-operative antibiotic prophylaxis should be prescribed according to local guidelines, which will take into account the local epidemiology and antibiotic resistance patterns. Typically a first (cefazolin) or second generation cephalosporin (cefuroxime) or isoxazolyl penicillin is used [4]. These agents are chosen because they are rapidly bactericidal to the commonest Gram-positive and Gram-negative bacterial agents causing PJI and have excellent penetration of soft tissue, bone and haematoma. They also have favourable pharmacodynamics – achieving therapeutic concentrations from incision to closure.

Surgical prophylaxis with these antibiotics is preferable to the use of newer, broader spectrum agents in order to minimize the risk of emergence of resistance.

In patients with anaphylaxis to penicillin, a glycopeptide (vancomycin or teicoplanin) should be used. Patients with non-anaphylactic reactions to penicillin can usually be safely treated with cefuroxime (second-generation cephalosporin) but not cefazolin (first-generation), which has a side chain structurally similar to penicillin.

Neither cefazolin, cefuroxime nor isoxazolyl penicillin provide any coverage against MRSA. Patients who are identified as MRSA positive during preoperative screening should receive prophylactic vancomycin or teicoplanin. These agents may also be used as first line operative prophylaxis in the context of MRSA outbreaks and in areas with a high MRSA prevalence; however, they provide inferior activity against MSSA so outside of these settings they should only be used first-line in the context of penicillin allergy. There is currently no universal guidance on modifications to preoperative prophylaxis in patients colonized with other drug resistant pathogens [4].

In patients with previous septic arthritis or a history of PJI, microbiological guidance should be sought and a pre-operative antibiotic should be selected that has activity against the previous infecting organism. The choice of antibiotic does not need to be changed for patients with other pre-existing prostheses, including those with prosthetic heart valves.

Dosing

The dose of pre-operative antibiotics should be adjusted according to the patient's actual body weight to ensure suitable concentrations are reached. In adults, cefazolin doses are 1 g for patients who weigh <60 kg and 2 g for patients who weigh >60 kg; vancomycin is dosed at 10–15 mg/kg up to a maximum of 1 g; the cefuroxime dose in adults is 1.5 g and teicoplanin 400 mg, independent of the patient's weight.

Timing of Administration

Several studies have identified an increased risk of infection in patients who received antibiotics greater than 60 min prior to surgical incision [18–20] and there is some evidence of an additional benefit of administering antibiotics within 30 min of incision compared with an hour [21, 22].

Accordingly, current US guidance advises administration of antibiotic prophylaxis within an hour before incision whilst European guidelines suggest administration within 30 min [21, 23]. Vancomycin and fluoroquinolones require prolonged infusion and should be administered within 2 h of the surgical incision [4]. If a proximal tourniquet is used, antibiotic prophylaxis must be completely infused prior to application of the tourniquet [24, 25].

An additional dose of antibiotic should be administered following loss of ≥2 l blood, administration of ≥2 l intravenous fluid or after two half-lives of the antibiotic have elapsed (if surgery is ongoing): this equates to cefazolin 2–5 hourly, cefuroxime 3–4 hourly, isoxazolyl penicillin 3 hourly and vancomycin 6–12 hourly [4].

Table 3.3 Operative factors influencing the risk of PJI

Prophylactic antibiotic	Inappropriate drug or under-dosed
Surgery	Prolonged operative time
	Prolonged bleeding
	Blood transfusion
	Choice of prosthetic material (possible risk modifier)
	Use of antimicrobial coatings/antibiotic impregnated cement (possible risk modifier)
	Suture material
Wound care	Use of a wound drain
	Wound dehiscence
	Choice of wound dressing
	Superficial surgical site infection

Duration

There is no evidence of benefit from prolonging the administration of antibiotics post-operatively beyond 24 h in clean, elective cases [26–30]. There are also numerous disadvantages to prolonging the duration of antimicrobial therapy that include the increased risk of side effects, the direct drug costs, the risk of development of *Clostridium difficile* diarrhoea, and the often unnoticed selection of resistant organisms.

The Operative Environment

The risk of PJI is also influenced by the surgery itself, the environment in which the operation is conducted, and post-operative wound care. The main modifiable peri-operative risks are summarized in Table 3.3.

Air Cleanliness

Particulate matter in the air of the operative room (OR) is a potential source of surgical wound contamination [31] and the incidence of PJI correlates with the number of airborne bacteria present in the environment around the surgical site [32].

OR personnel shed particulate matter, including bacteria, into the environment; increased numbers of OR personnel leads to increased bacterial air contamination [33, 34] and the movement of staff and objects in the OR, as well as the opening and closing of doors, causes air currents that increase the movement of particulate matter in the air and the deposition of bacteria onto the surgical site [35, 36]. Door opening to the OR should be minimized, and all required equipment, including sizes of implant, should be available within the OR prior to the commencement of surgery [4]. In spite of the documented effects of air currents, the evidence for laminar flow remains mixed, and in some studies its use appears to be associated with an increased risk of surgical site infection [37, 38]. There is currently insufficient evidence to support the routine use of space suits during TJA [39, 40].

The longer the duration of surgery the greater the probability of bacterial contamination of the wound and the higher the risk of infection after TJA [41–44]. It is therefore essential that efforts are made to minimize length of surgery, without compromising the surgical procedure itself. There is also a direct correlation between how long instrument trays are open and the likelihood of bacterial contamination [45]. Instrument trays should be opened as close as possible to the start of surgery.

There is no evidence that performing clean cases after infected cases leads to an increased risk of PJI, however, most centres order the list with possible infected cases timetabled last to minimize the chance of cross-contamination between cases. The OR should be cleaned thoroughly after suspected or confirmed cases of infection [4].

Operator Preparation

All OR personnel who come into contact with the patient should wash their hands for two to five minutes with an antiseptic wash prior to the first case [46, 47]. There is no evidence that any particular handwashing antiseptic agent is superior. There is also little consensus regarding the duration of handwashing between cases and a shorter duration of washing or hand cleaning with alcohol handrub may be sufficient [48, 49], although if there has been possible contamination the initial handwashing process should be repeated [4].

Gloves must be used, changed between cases, and hand hygiene must be performed prior to putting gloves on and following their removal. There may be additional benefit in changing gloves at least every 90 min and following cementation as methacrylate cement damages the integrity of surgical gloves [4]. Consideration should also be given to possible soiling of gloves from handling OR lights, since handles have been shown to be a source of bacterial contamination [50].

All OR personnel should wear surgical masks, minimizing the risk of contaminating the surgical site with oropharyngeal flora [4, 46].

Skin Site Preparation

Whole body skin cleansing with chlorhexidine gluconate should start at least the night before elective TJA, following which patients should sleep in clean nightwear and bedding and should avoid the application of topical skin products [4, 46]. Chlorhexidine wash should not be used excessively as this can cause skin irritation; in patients who are allergic to chlorhexidine, antiseptic soap can be substituted.

There remains ongoing debate about the relative benefit of chlorhexidine gluconate in alcohol versus aqueous povidone-iodine scrub in preparing the skin site, and there is no conclusive evidence regarding additional efficacy in preventing infection [51].

Active skin ulceration in the vicinity of the surgical site has been demonstrated to be a significant risk factor infection for PJI [52]. Skin lesions are frequently heavily colonized with bacteria, and thus elective TJA is discouraged in patients with active skin lesions, including ulcers, eczema or psoriasis, in the vicinity of the surgical site until these lesions have been optimized [7].

Hair at or around the incision site should be removed by clipping (rather than shaving) on the day of surgery and not before, as this has been demonstrated to minimize the risk of infection [53, 54].

The Prosthesis

Whether the choice of prosthetic material used in TJA has a role in the prevention of PJI remains uncertain [43, 55, 56]. A recent study of revision total hip arthroplasty procedures demonstrated a protective role for tantalum compared with titanium, when used for the acetabular component [57], suggesting that the choice of prosthetic material may be a modifiable risk factor. However, currently the optimal choice for PJI risk minimization remains to be elucidated. Similalry, prostheses themselves can also be coated with materials that have antimicrobial properties, supplementing the infection-preventing effects of systemic prophylactic antibiotics. Antimicrobial coatings are typically used with uncemented implants, whereas cemented implants may be used in conjunction with antibiotic-impregnated cement.

Uncemented Implants

Uncemented implants require adaptations to enable sufficient osseointegration [58] and have a potential role in infection prevention via antibacterial coatings and through the release of metal ions, which also have antimicrobial properties.

Hydroxyapatite is commonly used to coat the interosseous segments of implants, supporting direct bone integration and mineralization of the implant surface [59] as well as reducing foreign body reactions and bacterial adhesion [60, 61], the evidence suggests, however, that it does not appear to confer any benefit in the prevention of PJI [62, 63].

Metal ions such as iron, zinc, titanium, carbon and silver have broad-spectrum antibacterial properties, reducing microbial adhesion and proliferation, whilst enhancing osteoblastic integration [64–67]. The use of coatings that take advantage of these properties might aid in the prevention of PJI. Indeed mid-term trial results where oncology patients underwent two-stage exchange arthroplasty with silver treated implants demonstrated lower rates of PJI compared with matched controls [68]. No study has yet investigated the use of sliver-coated prostheses in low risk primary procedures, but there may be a role for using such implants in higher risk primary and revision procedures.

Only one implant is commercially available that utilizes these properties, by incorporating silver ions into the surface of the prosthesis [69], protecting the implant from infectious organisms [67]. There are several postulated mechanisms by which this may work, including the active disruption of bacterial amino acids or DNA with subsequent enzyme and critical cellular dysfunction, through alterations to the cellular membrane and receptor function inhibiting bacterial replication, or by organism destruction via hydroxyl-radical formation [70].

An alternative mechanism for PJI prevention through modifications to the prosthesis is by the addition of antibiotics or antibiofilm coatings. Although still in their early developmental stages, these strategies give a glimpse into the future of infection prevention.

Antibiotics may be added to, and released from, the implant surface in a number of ways [71–73] creating a high concentration of antibiotics at the bone-implant or cement-implant interface, theoretically preventing bacterial adhesion, colonization and biofilm formation [74–77]. Such high local concentrations of antibiotics cannot be achieved via systematic routes without complications and toxicity [78, 79]. Clinical trials have still not been undertaken to assess the efficacy of this method of prevention of PJI.

There are several methods of local antibiotic therapy that are currently in use. These techniques aim to release high levels of antibiotics over a prolonged period of time, preventing bacteria from establishing a biofilm, before the antibiotic concentration falls to a sub-inhibitory level [80]. These methods are rarely utilized in primary elective arthroplasty, and are mostly reserved for revision procedures where there is established PJI. Notwithstanding this, biodegradable options may have a role in primary procedures as they do not require further surgery in order to be removed, in contrast to non-biodegradable alternatives.

Cancellous allograft bone impregnated with microbe-specific antibiotics has long been used in this way [81]. The bone graft becomes integrated into the surroundings whilst the antibiotics are eluted in a controlled manner. A variety of antibiotics can be used; vancomycin has been shown to be significantly better than tobramycin, and rifampicin can be released for up to 21 days [82, 83].

Bovine collagen sponge can also be impregnated in gentamicin and used to form a fleece to surround the implant, enabling a controlled release of gentamicin; a peak in concentration is seen within the first 48 h and the sponge is fully resorbed by 2 weeks [84, 85]. This technique has been used successfully in the treatment of septic arthritis, open fracture fixation and PJI, however some studies have noted increased rates of infection following its use and again, its role in the prevention of PJI has not been ascertained unequivocally [86–89].

Fewer side-effects have been noted from the use of a disposable antibacterial coating (DAC), which is currently undergoing level 1 trials in Europe [90]. DAC is a biodegradable hydrogel with antibacterial and antibiofilm properties, which releases high concentration of antibiotics at the point of application [91]. It can be applied to the femoral components in uncemented hip prosthesis, or even upon the wound during closure. *In vitro* studies demonstrate that the antibiotics are released for up to 96 h [92].

Cemented Prostheses

Cemented implants require polymethylmethacrylate (PMMA) cement, which has a role in PJI prevention. The cement itself does not possess any inherent antibiotic properties, as its action is solely to secure the implant in position; however, the addition of antibiotics to the cement has demonstrated a reduction in PJI rates during primary elective arthroplasty [93, 94]. The antibiotic of choice depends upon local guidelines, but should provide broad spectrum antibacterial cover. The most commonly used antibiotics are gentamicin and tobramycin (targeting both gram-negative and some gram-positive bacteria) and vancomycin (with activity exclusively against gram-positive bacteria) [79, 95]. During revision procedures for an infective source, the choice of antibiotic will depend upon preoperative microbiological susceptibility patterns.

Despite the theoretical advantage of using antibiotic impregnated cement in preventing PJI in primary arthroplasty, the clinical evidence is mixed. The Norwegian registry demonstrated a lower relative risk for a PJI with antibiotic-impregnated cement, compared with uncemented implants; the Swedish hip arthroplasty registry, however, failed to demonstrate any difference in rates of revision due to infection in uncemented versus cemented total hip arthroplasty [96, 97].

The matter is complicated further by the perception that addition of antibiotics may compromise the mechanical properties of the cement; this has been demonstrated in some *in vitro* studies, but refuted in others [95, 98, 99]. There has also been speculation that the overuse of antibiotics in cement may lead to the selection, and proliferation, of antibiotic-resistant bacteria and therefore that it may not be justifiable to use antibiotic-impregnated cement in low risk patients undergoing primary procedures. In light of this speculation, some practitioners advocate that only higher risk patients should receive antibiotic-impregnated cement; this would include immunosuppressed patients and those with diabetes, rheumatoid arthritis and malnutrition [99, 100].

With such conflicting information and divided opinions, it currently remains the orthopaedic surgeon's decision whether to use antibiotic-impregnated cement or not. This decision should take into consideration their local factors – policies, PJI rates, bacterial epidemiology and susceptibilities, patient co-morbidity and immunosuppression, and personal clinical experience.

There are alternative, or even additional strategies to achieve local delivery of antibiotic other than via the bone-prosthetic interface or antibiotic-impregnated cement,: placement of antibiotic-impregnated synthetic calcium pellets onto the wound prior to closure, irrigation of the soft tissue with diluted antibiotics, or use of an antibiotic intra-wound powder have all been described [101–103]. Calcium pellets have been shown to remain within the wound for 3 months, enabling the prolonged release [>30 days] of therapeutic concentrations of antibiotics, typically vancomycin [101, 104].

Wound Management

Closure

Following the insertion of the implant, purposeful wound closure must be undertaken to help reduce the risk of deep PJI by creating a physical barrier to infection. Inappropriate wound closure can result in an abundance of dead-space or direct communication of the implant with the external environment, resulting in higher PJI rates. The presence of a haematoma, dead-space and unnecessary foreign bodies within the wound all may act as a nidus for infection, and every effort must be undertaken to limit these insults. Closure of the wound should be undertaken in a systematic manner from deep to most superficial layer, closing all fascial planes.

Suture Material

A variety of suture materials is available for closure, and choices include single or multi-filament, absorbable or non-absorbable, and plain or antibiotic-impregnated. Several studies advise against the use of non-absorbable sutures as they can act as a foreign body and therefore increase the risk of infection [105, 106].

The use of antiseptic-impregnated sutures may have a role in preventing PJI. Coated vicryl plus (polyglactin 910) sutures utilise triclosan, a broad-spectrum antiseptic effective against *Staphylococcus aureus* (including MRSA) and *Staphylococcus epidermidis*, to reduce bacterial adherence and viability [107–110]. Use of these sutures has been shown to reduce surgical site infections following general surgical procedures, cerebrospinal-fluid shunt-implantation and cardiothoracic surgery [111–115]. Although no randomised control trial has yet formally determined the role for impregnated sutures in orthopaedic surgery, benefit would seem likely since surgical site infections are a known risk factor for development of PJI.

Wound Drains

Operative drains are used to reduce post-operative haematoma formation, but may also provide a portal of entry for bacteria into the wound; the advantage of draining such collections, therefore, needs to be balanced against the potential increased risk of PJI [116]. Reassuringly, a meta-analysis pooling the results of 18 studies demonstrated no significant difference between wounds treated with a drain and those without, with respect to superficial or deep infections, wound haematoma, or reoperations for wound complications [117]. However, given the associated risks it is recommended that drains be removed within 24 h after total joint arthroplasty [118, 119].

Dressings

Following closure, operative wounds should be protected with sterile dressings. Various such dressings are available, acting to preserve the sterile field for prolonged periods. The ideal dressing should be able to absorb excess exudate from the wound, whilst maintaining a moist environment and preventing postcperative contamination. The post-operative wound environment is ideal for healing via growth factor proliferation and subsequent growth and migration of fibroblasts, endothelial cells and keratinocytes, yet it is also a favourable environment for microbial colonization.

Inappropriate dressing and wound care can lead to high infection rates [120]. A systematic review of the literature identified no single postoperative dressing regimen as being superior to others for hip and knee arthroplasty wounds; however, one study demonstrated Aquacel and Tegaderm dressing to be almost 6 times more likely to result in a wound with no complications compared with Cutiplast, irrespective of patient co-morbidity [120, 121].

Dressings vary widely in their features; they may allow the movement of air, be completely waterproof, or provide negative pressure as seen with PICO dressings (Smith and Nephew Healthcare, Hull, United Kingdom). Such single-use negative pressure wound therapy devices are placed upon the closed incision and encourage angiogenesis, growth of granulation tissue, removal of exudate and reduction of bacterial bioburden. Early findings have demonstrated promising improvements in surgical site infection rates following primary and revision joint arthroplasty [122–125].

Irrespective of the type of dressing adopted, dressings should be left undisturbed for as long as possible to maintain the sterile micro-environment. However, the critically important caveat to this is that inspection is mandatory if significant wound discharge is present.

References

1. Peel TN, Dowsey MM, Buising KL, Liew D, Choong PFM. Cost analysis of debridement and retention for management of prosthetic joint infection. Clin Microbiol Infect. 2013;19(2):181–6.
2. Kurtz SM, Lau E, Watson H, Schmier JK, Parvizi J. Economic burden of periprosthetic joint infection

in the United States. J Arthroplasty. 2012;27(8 Suppl):61–5.
3. Briggs TW. Improving the quality of orthopaedic care within the National Health Service in England: getting it right first time. Br Orthopaed Assoc News. 2011;50:8.
4. Parvizi J, Gehrke T. Proceedings of the international consensus meeting on periprosthetic joint infection [Internet]. 2013. Available from: http://www.msis-na.org/wp-content/themes/msistemp/pdf/ism-periprosthetic-joint-information.pdf.
5. Zhu Y, Zhang F, Chen W, Liu S, Zhang Q, Zhang Y. Risk factors for periprosthetic joint infection after total joint arthroplasty: a systematic review and meta-analysis. J Hosp Infect. 2015;89(2):82–9.
6. Cruess RL, Bickel WS, von Kessler KL. Infections in total hips secondary to a primary source elsewhere. Clin Orthop. 1975;(106):99–101.
7. Schmalzried TP, Amstutz HC, Au MK, Dorey FJ. Etiology of deep sepsis in total hip arthroplasty. The significance of hematogenous and recurrent infections. Clin Orthop. 1992;(280):200–7.
8. Cohen SM, Te HS, Levitsky J. Operative risk of total hip and knee arthroplasty in cirrhotic patients. J Arthroplasty. 2005;20(4):460–6.
9. Freeman JT, Anderson DJ, Hartwig MG, Sexton DJ. Surgical site infections following bariatric surgery in community hospitals: a weighty concern? Obes Surg. 2011;21(7):836–40.
10. Jensen JE, Jensen TG, Smith TK, Johnston DA, Dudrick SJ. Nutrition in orthopaedic surgery. J Bone Joint Surg Am. 1982;64(9):1263–72.
11. Singh JA, Houston TK, Ponce BA, Maddox G, Bishop MJ, Richman J, et al. Smoking as a risk factor for short-term outcomes following primary total hip and total knee replacement in veterans. Arthritis Care Res. 2011;63(10):1365–74.
12. Mills E, Eyawo O, Lockhart I, Kelly S, Wu P, Ebbert JO. Smoking cessation reduces postoperative complications: a systematic review and meta-analysis. Am J Med. 2011;124(2):144–54.e8.
13. Sørensen LT. Wound healing and infection in surgery. The clinical impact of smoking and smoking cessation: a systematic review and meta-analysis. Arch Surg Chic Ill 1960. 2012;147(4):373–83.
14. Sadr Azodi O, Bellocco R, Eriksson K, Adami J. The impact of tobacco use and body mass index on the length of stay in hospital and the risk of post-operative complications among patients undergoing total hip replacement. J Bone Joint Surg Br. 2006;88(10):1316–20.
15. Tonnesen H, Rosenberg J, Nielsen HJ, Rasmussen V, Hauge C, Pedersen IK, et al. Effect of preoperative abstinence on poor postoperative outcome in alcohol misusers: randomised controlled trial. BMJ. 1999;318(7194):1311–6.
16. Lehman CR, Ries MD, Paiement GD, Davidson AB. Infection after total joint arthroplasty in patients with human immunodeficiency virus or intravenous drug use. J Arthroplasty. 2001;16(3):330–5.
17. Chen AF, Hely AE, Xu PZ, Rao N, Klatt BA. Preoperative decolonization effective at reducing staphylococcal colonization in total joint arthroplasty patients. J Arthroplasty. 2013;28(8 Suppl):18–20.
18. Classen DC, Evans RS, Pestotnik SL, Horn SD, Menlove RL, Burke JP. The timing of prophylactic administration of antibiotics and the risk of surgical-wound infection. N Engl J Med. 1992;326(5):281–6.
19. Galandiuk S, Polk HC, Jagelman DG, Fazio VW. Re-emphasis of priorities in surgical antibiotic prophylaxis. Surg Gynecol Obstet. 1989;169(3):219–22.
20. Hawn MT, Richman JS, Vick CC, Deierhoi RJ, Graham LA, Henderson WG, et al. Timing of surgical antibiotic prophylaxis and the risk of surgical site infection. JAMA Surg. 2013;148(7):649–57.
21. Van Kasteren MEE, Manniën J, Ott A, Kullberg B-J, de Boer AS, Gyssens IC. Antibiotic prophylaxis and the risk of surgical site infections following total hip arthroplasty: timely administration is the most important factor. Clin Infect Dis Off Publ Infect Dis Soc Am. 2007;44(7):921–7.
22. Steinberg JP, Braun BI, Hellinger WC, Kusek L, Bozikis MR, Bush AJ, et al. Timing of antimicrobial prophylaxis and the risk of surgical site infections: results from the Trial to Reduce Antimicrobial Prophylaxis Errors. Ann Surg. 2009;250(1):10–6.
23. Bratzler DW, Houck PM, Workgroup SIPGW. Antimicrobial prophylaxis for surgery: an advisory statement from the National Surgical Infection Prevention Project. Am J Surg. 2005;189(4):395–404.
24. Prokuski L. Prophylactic antibiotics in orthopaedic surgery. J Am Acad Orthop Surg. 2008;16(5):283–93.
25. Johnson DP. Antibiotic prophylaxis with cefuroxime in arthroplasty of the knee. J Bone Joint Surg Br. 1987;69(5):787–9.
26. Mauerhan DR, Nelson CL, Smith DL, Fitzgerald RH, Slama TG, Petty RW, et al. Prophylaxis against infection in total joint arthroplasty. One day of cefuroxime compared with three days of cefazolin. J Bone Joint Surg Am. 1994;76(1):39–45.
27. Wymenga AB, Hekster YA, Theeuwes A, Muytjens HL, van Horn JR, Slooff TJ. Antibiotic use after cefuroxime prophylaxis in hip and knee joint replacement. Clin Pharmacol Ther. 1991;50(2):215–20.
28. Niederhäuser U, Vogt M, Vogt P, Genoni M, Künzli A, Turina MI. Cardiac surgery in a high-risk group of patients: is prolonged postoperative antibiotic prophylaxis effective? J Thorac Cardiovasc Surg. 1997;114(2):162–8.
29. Turano A. New clinical data on the prophylaxis of infections in abdominal, gynecologic, and urologic surgery. Multicenter Study Group. Am J Surg. 1992;164(4A Suppl):16S–20S.

30. Tang WM, Chiu KY, Ng TP, Yau WP, Ching PTY, Seto WH. Efficacy of a single dose of cefazolin as a prophylactic antibiotic in primary arthroplasty. J Arthroplasty. 2003;18(6):714–8.
31. Edmiston CE, Seabrook GR, Cambria RA, Brown KR, Lewis BD, Sommers JR, et al. Molecular epidemiology of microbial contamination in the operating room environment: Is there a risk for infection? Surgery. 2005;138(4):573–9; discussion 579–82.
32. Lidwell OM, Lowbury EJL, Whyte W, Blowers R, Stanley SJ, Lowe D. Airborne contamination of wounds in joint replacement operations: the relationship to sepsis rates. J Hosp Infect. 1983;4(2):111–31.
33. Ritter MA, Eitzen H, French ML, Hart JB. The operating room environment as affected by people and the surgical face mask. Clin Orthop. 1975;(111): 147–50.
34. Andersson BM, Lidgren L, Schalén C, Steen A. Contamination of irrigation solutions in an operating theatre. Infect Control. 1984;5(7):339–42.
35. Whyte W, Hodgson R, Tinkler J. The importance of airborne bacterial contamination of wounds. J Hosp Infect. 1982;3(2):123–35.
36. Friberg B, Friberg S, Burman LG. Correlation between surface and air counts of particles carrying aerobic bacteria in operating rooms with turbulent ventilation: an experimental study. J Hosp Infect. 1999;42(1):61–8.
37. Breier A-C, Brandt C, Sohr D, Geffers C, Gastmeier P. Laminar airflow ceiling size: no impact on infection rates following hip and knee prosthesis. Infect Control Hosp Epidemiol Off J Soc Hosp Epidemiol Am. 2011;32(11):1097–102.
38. Gastmeier P, Breier A-C, Brandt C. Influence of laminar airflow on prosthetic joint infections: a systematic review. J Hosp Infect. 2012;81(2):73–8.
39. Hooper GJ, Rothwell AG, Frampton C, Wyatt MC. Does the use of laminar flow and space suits reduce early deep infection after total hip and knee replacement?: the ten-year results of the New Zealand Joint Registry. J Bone Joint Surg Br. 2011;93(1):85–90.
40. Miner AL, Losina E, Katz JN, Fossel AH, Platt R. Deep infection after total knee replacement: impact of laminar airflow systems and body exhaust suits in the modern operating room. Infect Control Hosp Epidemiol Off J Soc Hosp Epidemiol Am. 2007;28(2):222–6.
41. Carroll K, Dowsey M, Choong P, Peel T. Risk factors for superficial wound complications in hip and knee arthroplasty. Clin Microbiol Infect Off Publ Eur Soc Clin Microbiol Infect Dis. 2014;20(2):130–5.
42. Namba RS, Inacio MCS, Paxton EW. Risk factors associated with deep surgical site infections after primary total knee arthroplasty: an analysis of 56,216 knees. J Bone Joint Surg Am. 2013;95(9):775–82.
43. Pulido L, Ghanem E, Joshi A, Purtill JJ, Parvizi J. Periprosthetic joint infection: the incidence, timing, and predisposing factors. Clin Orthop. 2008;466(7):1710–5.
44. Skråmm I, Saltytė Benth J, Bukholm G. Decreasing time trend in SSI incidence for orthopaedic procedures: surveillance matters! J Hosp Infect. 2012;82(4):243–7.
45. Dalstrom DJ, Venkatarayappa I, Manternach AL, Palcic MS, Heyse BA, Prayson MJ. Time-dependent contamination of opened sterile operating-room trays. J Bone Joint Surg Am. 2008;90(5):1022–5.
46. Mangram AJ, Horan TC, Pearson ML, Silver LC, Jarvis WR. Guideline for Prevention of Surgical Site Infection, 1999. Centers for Disease Control and Prevention (CDC) Hospital Infection Control Practices Advisory Committee. Am J Infect Control. 1999;27(2):97–132; quiz 133–4; discussion 96.
47. WHO | About SAVE LIVES: Clean Your Hands [Internet]. WHO. (cited 2015 Jan 13). Available from: http://who.int/gpsc/5may/background/5moments/en/.
48. Parienti JJ, Thibon P, Heller R, Le Roux Y, von Theobald P, Bensadoun H, et al. Hand-rubbing with an aqueous alcoholic solution vs traditional surgical hand-scrubbing and 30-day surgical site infection rates: a randomized equivalence study. JAMA. 2002;288(6):722–7.
49. Weight CJ, Lee MC, Palmer JS. Avagard hand antisepsis vs. traditional scrub in 3600 pediatric urologic procedures. Urology. 2010;76(1):15–7.
50. Davis N, Curry A, Gambhir AK, Panigrahi H, Walker CR, Wilkins EG, et al. Intraoperative bacterial contamination in operations for joint replacement. J Bone Joint Surg Br. 1999;81(5): 886–9.
51. Dumville JC, McFarlane E, Edwards P, Lipp A, Holmes A. Preoperative skin antiseptics for preventing surgical wound infections after clean surgery. Cochrane Database Syst Rev. 2013;(3):CD003949.
52. Penington A. Ulceration and antihypertensive use are risk factors for infection after skin lesion excision. ANZ J Surg. 2010;80(9):642–5.
53. Tanner J, Norrie P, Melen K. Preoperative hair removal to reduce surgical site infection. Cochrane Database Syst Rev. 2011;(11):CD004122.
54. Alexander JW, Fischer JE, Boyajian M, Palmquist J, Morris MJ. The influence of hair-removal methods on wound infections. Arch Surg Chic Ill 1960. 1983;118(3):347–52.
55. Bozic KJ, Lau E, Kurtz S, Ong K, Rubash H, Vail TP, et al. Patient-related risk factors for periprosthetic joint infection and postoperative mortality following total hip arthroplasty in Medicare patients. J Bone Joint Surg Am. 2012;94(9):794–800.
56. Berbari EF, Hanssen AD, Duffy MC, Steckelberg JM, Ilstrup DM, Harmsen WS, et al. Risk factors for prosthetic joint infection: case-control study. Clin

Infect Dis Off Publ Infect Dis Soc Am. 1998;27(5):1247–54.

57. Tokarski AT, Novack TA, Parvizi J. Is tantalum protective against infection in revision total hip arthroplasty? Bone Jt J. 2015;97-B(1):45–9.
58. Mavrogenis AF, Dimitriou R, Parvizi J, Babis GC. Biology of implant osseointegration. J Musculoskelet Neuronal Interact. 2009;9(2): 61–71.
59. Cook SD, Thomas KA, Kay JF, Jarcho M. Hydroxyapatite-coated porous titanium for use as an orthopedic biologic attachment system. Clin Orthop. 1988;(230):303–12.
60. Arciola CR, Montanaro L, Costerton JW. New trends in diagnosis and control strategies for implant infections. Int J Artif Organs. 2011;34(9):727–36.
61. Goodman SB, Yao Z, Keeney M, Yang F. The future of biologic coatings for orthopaedic implants. Biomaterials. 2013;34(13):3174–83.
62. Parker MJ, Gurusamy KS, Azegami S. Arthroplasties (with and without bone cement) for proximal femoral fractures in adults. Cochrane Database Syst Rev. 2010;(6):CD001706.
63. Beaupré LA, al-Yamani M, Huckell JR, Johnston DWC. Hydroxyapatite-coated tibial implants compared with cemented tibial fixation in primary total knee arthroplasty. A randomized trial of outcomes at five years. J Bone Joint Surg Am. 2007;89(10):2204–11.
64. Taylor E, Webster TJ. Reducing infections through nanotechnology and nanoparticles. Int J Nanomedicine. 2011;6:1463–73.
65. Colon G, Ward BC, Webster TJ. Increased osteoblast and decreased Staphylococcus epidermidis functions on nanophase ZnO and TiO2. J Biomed Mater Res A. 2006;78(3):595–604.
66. Puckett SD, Taylor E, Raimondo T, Webster TJ. The relationship between the nanostructure of titanium surfaces and bacterial attachment. Biomaterials. 2010;31(4):706–13.
67. Ellis JR. The Meany roles of silver in infection prevention. Am J Infect Control. 2007;35(5):E26.
68. Wafa H, Grimer RJ, Reddy K, Jeys L, Abudu A, Carter SR, et al. Retrospective evaluation of the incidence of early periprosthetic infection with silver-treated endoprostheses in high-risk patients case-control study. Bone Jt J. 2015;97-B(2):252–7.
69. Agluna, Accentus Medical Ltd, Oxford, UK [Internet]. Available from: www.accentus-medical.com.
70. Gordon O, Slenters TV, Brunetto PS, Villaruz AE, Sturdevant DE, Otto M, et al. Silver Coordination Polymers for Prevention of Implant Infection: Thiol Interaction, Impact on Respiratory Chain Enzymes, and Hydroxyl Radical Induction. Antimicrob Agents Chemother. 2010;54(10):4208–18.
71. Sinclair KD, Pham TX, Farnsworth RW, Williams DL, Loc-Carrillo C, Horne LA, et al. Development of a broad spectrum polymer-released antimicrobial coating for the prevention of resistant strain bacterial infections. J Biomed Mater Res A. 2012;100(10): 2732–8.
72. Lee CT, Lee CW, Hu CW, Lai KA, Yeh ML. PLGA encapsulating antibiotic loaded titanium prosthesis in osteomyelitis prevention in rats. 2012 annual meeting of the Orthopaedic Research Society, San Francisco; 2012.
73. Stewart S, Barr S, Engiles J, Hickok NJ, Shapiro IM, Richardson DW, et al. Vancomycin-modified implant surface inhibits biofilm formation and supports bone-healing in an infected osteotomy model in sheep: a proof-of-concept study. J Bone Joint Surg Am. 2012;94(15):1406–15.
74. Lawson MC, Bowman CN, Anseth KS. Vancomycin derivative photopolymerized to titanium kills S. epidermidis. Clin Orthop. 2007;461:96–105.
75. Edin ML, Miclau T, Lester GE, Lindsey RW, Dahners LE. Effect of cefazolin and vancomycin on osteoblasts in vitro. Clin Orthop. 1996;(333):245–51.
76. Parvizi J, Wickstrom E, Zeiger AR, Adams CS, Shapiro IM, Purtill JJ, et al. Frank Stinchfield Award. Titanium surface with biologic activity against infection. Clin Orthop. 2004;(429):33–8.
77. Hickok NJ, Shapiro IM. Immobilized antibiotics to prevent orthopaedic implant infections. Adv Drug Deliv Rev. 2012;64(12):1165–76.
78. Garvin KL, Evans BG, Salvati EA, Brause BD. Palacos gentamicin for the treatment of deep periprosthetic hip infections. Clin Orthop. 1994;(298):97–105.
79. Stevens CM, Tetsworth KD, Calhoun JH, Mader JT. An articulated antibiotic spacer used for infected total knee arthroplasty: a comparative in vitro elution study of Simplex and Palacos bone cements. J Orthop Res Off Publ Orthop Res Soc. 2005;23(1):27–33.
80. Anagnostakos K, Schröder K. Antibiotic-Impregnated Bone Grafts in Orthopaedic and Trauma Surgery: A Systematic Review of the Literature. Int J Biomater. 2012;2012:e538061.
81. Winkler H, Stoiber A, Kaudela K, Winter F, Menschik F. One stage uncemented revision of infected total hip replacement using cancellous allograft bone impregnated with antibiotics. J Bone Joint Surg Br. 2008;90(12):1580–4.
82. Winkler H, Janata O, Berger C, Wein W, Georgopoulos A. In vitro release of vancomycin and tobramycin from impregnated human and bovine bone grafts. J Antimicrob Chemother. 2000;46(3):423–8.
83. Witsø E, Persen L, Løseth K, Bergh K. Adsorption and release of antibiotics from morselized cancellous bone. In vitro studies of 8 antibiotics. Acta Orthop Scand. 1999;70(3):298–304.
84. Hayes G, Moens N, Gibson T. A review of local antibiotic implants and applications to veterinary orthopaedic surgery. Vet Comp Orthop Traumatol VCOT. 2013;26(4):251–9.

85. El-Husseiny M, Patel S, MacFarlane RJ, Haddad FS. Biodegradable antibiotic delivery systems. J Bone Joint Surg Br. 2011;93(2):151–7.
86. Jerosch J, Hoffstetter I, Schröder M, Castro WH. Septic arthritis: Arthroscopic management with local antibiotic treatment. Acta Orthop Belg. 1995;61(2):126–34.
87. Chaudhary S, Sen R-K, Saini U-C, Soni A, Gahlot N, Singh D. Use of gentamicin-loaded collagen sponge in internal fixation of open fractures. Chin J Traumatol Zhonghua Chuang Shang Za Zhi Chin Med Assoc. 2011;14(4):209–14.
88. Swieringa AJ, Goosen JHM, Jansman FGA, Tulp NJA. In vivo pharmacokinetics of a gentamicin-loaded collagen sponge in acute periprosthetic infection: serum values in 19 patients. Acta Orthop. 2008;79(5):637–42.
89. Hayes GM, Gibson TWG, Moens NMM, Monteiro B, Johnson RJ. Intra-articular pharmacokinetics of a gentamicin impregnated collagen sponge in the canine stifle: an experimental study. Vet Surg VS. 2014;43(2):166–73.
90. Romano C. Biofilm-related infections in orthopedic and trauma surgery: international collaborative projects ahead, Milan; 2013.
91. Implant Disposable Antibacterial Coating (I.D.A.C.): a Novel Approach to Implant-Related Infections in Orthopaedics and Trauma Surgery [Internet]. Available from: http://www.i-dac.eu/news/4.
92. Drago L, Boot W, Dimas K, Malizos K, Hänsch GM, Stuyck J, et al. Does implant coating with antibacterial-loaded hydrogel reduce bacterial colonization and biofilm formation in vitro? Clin Orthop. 2014;472(11):3311–23.
93. Chiu F-Y, Chen C-M, Lin C-FJ, Lo W-H. Cefuroxime-impregnated cement in primary total knee arthroplasty: a prospective, randomized study of three hundred and forty knees. J Bone Joint Surg Am. 2002;84-A(5):759–62.
94. Espehaug B, Engesaeter LB, Vollset SE, Havelin LI, Langeland N. Antibiotic prophylaxis in total hip arthroplasty. Review of 10,905 primary cemented total hip replacements reported to the Norwegian arthroplasty register, 1987 to 1995. J Bone Joint Surg Br. 1997;79(4):590–5.
95. Jiranek WA, Hanssen AD, Greenwald AS. Antibiotic-loaded bone cement for infection prophylaxis in total joint replacement. J Bone Joint Surg Am. 2006;88(11):2487–500.
96. Hailer NP, Garellick G, Kärrholm J. Uncemented and cemented primary total hip arthroplasty in the Swedish Hip Arthroplasty Register. Acta Orthop. 2010;81(1):34–41.
97. Dale H, Skråmm I, Løwer HL, Eriksen HM, Espehaug B, Furnes O, et al. Infection after primary hip arthroplasty: a comparison of 3 Norwegian health registers. Acta Orthop. 2011;82(6):646–54.
98. Dunne NJ, Hill J, McAfee P, Kirkpatrick R, Patrick S, Tunney M. Incorporation of large amounts of gentamicin sulphate into acrylic bone cement: effect on handling and mechanical properties, antibiotic release, and biofilm formation. Proc Inst Mech Eng H. 2008;222(3):355–65.
99. Hanssen AD. Prophylactic use of antibiotic bone cement: an emerging standard--in opposition. J Arthroplasty. 2004;19(4 Suppl 1):73–7.
100. Bourne RB. Prophylactic use of antibiotic bone cement: an emerging standard – in the affirmative. J Arthroplasty. 2004;19(4 Suppl 1):69–72.
101. McPherson E, Dipane M, Sherif S. Dissolvable antibiotic beads in treatment of periprosthetic joint infection and revision arthroplasty – the use of synthetic pure calcium sulfate (stimulan®) impregnated with vancomycin & tobramycin. reconstr rev [Internet]. 2013 Mar 19 (cited 2015 Mar 5);3[1]. Available from: http://reconstructivereview.org/ojs/index.php/rr/article/view/27.
102. Sørensen TS, Andersen MR, Glenthøj J, Petersen O. Pharmacokinetics of topical gentamicin in total hip arthroplasty. Acta Orthop Scand. 1984;55(2):156–9.
103. Sweet FA, Roh M, Sliva C. Intrawound application of vancomycin for prophylaxis in instrumented thoracolumbar fusions: efficacy, drug levels, and patient outcomes. Spine. 2011;36(24):2084–8.
104. Kallala R, Nizam I, Haddad F. Outcomes following use of antibiotic-eluting, absorbable, calcium sulphate beads in revision hip and knee surgery for periprosthetic infection. Bone Joint J Orthop Proc Suppl. 2013;95-B[Suppl 34]:364.
105. Edlich RF, Panek PH, Rodeheaver GT, Turnbull VG, Kurtz LD, Edgerton MT. Physical and chemical configuration of sutures in the development of surgical infection. Ann Surg. 1973;177(6):679–88.
106. Blomstedt B, Osterberg B, Bergstrand A. Suture material and bacterial transport. An experimental study. Acta Chir Scand. 1977;143(2):71–3.
107. Edmiston CE, Seabrook GR, Goheen MP, Krepel CJ, Johnson CP, Lewis BD, et al. Bacterial adherence to surgical sutures: can antibacterial-coated sutures reduce the risk of microbial contamination? J Am Coll Surg. 2006;203(4):481–9.
108. Rothenburger S, Spangler D, Bhende S. Burkley D. In vitro antimicrobial evaluation of Coated VICRYL* Plus Antibacterial Suture (coated polyglactin 910 with triclosan) using zone of inhibition assays. Surg Infect. 2002;3 Suppl 1:S79–87.
109. Gómez-Alonso A, García-Criado FJ, Parreño-Manchado FC, García-Sánchez JE, García-Sánchez E, Parreño-Manchado A, et al. Study of the efficacy of Coated VICRYL Plus Antibacterial suture(coated Polyglactin 910 suture with Triclosan) in two animal models of general surgery. J Infect. 2007;54(1):82–8.
110. Storch M, Perry LC, Davidson JM, Ward JJ. A 28-day study of the effect of Coated VICRYL* Plus Antibacterial Suture (coated polyglactin 910 suture with triclosan) on wound healing in guinea pig linear incisional skin wounds. Surg Infect. 2002;3 Suppl 1:S89–98.

111. Ford HR, Jones P, Gaines B, Reblock K, Simpkins DL. Intraoperative handling and wound healing: controlled clinical trial comparing coated VICRYL plus antibacterial suture (coated polyglactin 910 suture with triclosan) with coated VICRYL suture (coated polyglactin 910 suture). Surg Infect. 2005;6(3):313–21.
112. Mingmalairak C, Ungbhakorn P, Paocharoen V. Efficacy of antimicrobial coating suture coated polyglactin 910 with tricosan (Vicryl plus) compared with polyglactin 910 (Vicryl) in reduced surgical site infection of appendicitis, double blind randomized control trial, preliminary safety report. J Med Assoc Thail Chotmaihet Thangphaet. 2009;92(6):770–5.
113. Fleck T, Moidl R, Blacky A, Fleck M, Wolner E, Grabenwoger M, et al. Triclosan-coated sutures for the reduction of sternal wound infections: economic considerations. Ann Thorac Surg. 2007;84(1):232–6.
114. Rozzelle CJ, Leonardo J, Li V. Antimicrobial suture wound closure for cerebrospinal fluid shunt surgery: a prospective, double-blinded, randomized controlled trial. J Neurosurg Pediatr. 2008;2(2):111–7.
115. Justinger C, Moussavian MR, Schlueter C, Kopp B, Kollmar O, Schilling MK. Antibacterial (corrected) coating of abdominal closure sutures and wound infection. Surgery. 2009;145(3):330–4.
116. Degnim AC, Scow JS, Hoskin TL, Miller JP, Loprinzi M, Boughey JC, et al. Randomized controlled trial to reduce bacterial colonization of surgical drains after breast and axillary operations. Ann Surg. 2013;258(2):240–7.
117. Parker MJ, Roberts CP, Hay D. Closed suction drainage for hip and knee arthroplasty. A meta-analysis. J Bone Joint Surg Am. 2004;86-A(6):1146–52.
118. Drinkwater CJ, Neil MJ. Optimal timing of wound drain removal following total joint arthroplasty. J Arthroplasty. 1995;10(2):185–9.
119. Willemen D, Paul J, White SH, Crook DW. Closed suction drainage following knee arthroplasty. Effectiveness and risks. Clin Orthop. 1991;(264):232–4.
120. Ravenscroft M, Harker J, Buch K. A prospective, randomised, controlled trial comparing wound dressings used in Hip and knee surgery: aquacel and tegaderm versus cutiplast. Ann R Coll Surg Engl. 2006;88(1):18–22.
121. Collins A. Does the postoperative dressing regime affect wound healing after hip or knee arthroplasty? J Wound Care. 2011;20(1):11–6.
122. Malmsjö M, Gustafsson L, Lindstedt S, Gesslein B, Ingemansson R. The effects of variable, intermittent, and continuous negative pressure wound therapy, using foam or gauze, on wound contraction, granulation tissue formation, and ingrowth into the wound filler. Eplasty (Internet). 2012 Jan 24 (cited 2015 Mar 5);12. Available from: http://www.ncbi.nlm.nih.gov/pmc/articles/PMC3266212/.
123. Weed T, Ratliff C, Drake DB. Quantifying bacterial bioburden during negative pressure wound therapy: does the wound VAC enhance bacterial clearance? Ann Plast Surg. 2004;52(3):276–9; discussion 279–80.
124. Karlakki S, Brem M, Giannini S, Khanduja V, Stannard J, Martin R. Negative pressure wound therapy for managementof the surgical incision in orthopaedic surgery: a review of evidence and mechanisms for an emerging indication. Bone Joint Res. 2013;2(12):276–84.
125. New clinical data shows PICO canister-free NPWT system has positive benefits for high-risk orthopaedic patients. Available from: http://www.smith-nephew.com/news-and-media/media-releases/news/pico-npwt-high-risk-orthopaedic-patient-benefits/.

Prevention of Periprosthetic Joint Infection: What Is the Current Evidence?

4

Simon S. Jameson and Mike R. Reed

Abstract

Periprosthetic joint infection is a disastrous complication following routine joint replacement surgery. The cause is often multi-factorial. In order to minimise risk, a team-based approach should be followed to optimise modifiable patient risk factors and adhere to best surgical practice, informed by robust evidence. This chapter discusses the current best evidence.

Keywords

Surgical site infection • Periprosthetic joint infection

Introduction

Periprosthetic joint infection (PJI) is a major, but infrequent complication of arthoplasty surgery and is associated with substantial morbidity and economic cost [1–3]. A number of patient, surgical and environmental specific risk factors may contribute to the development of a PJI [4, 5] (Table 4.1). The common pathogenic organisms responsible for orthopaedic SSIs are shown in Fig. 4.1 [6]. In this chapter we discuss the current evidence for best surgical practice to reduce the risk of PJI.

S.S. Jameson, PhD, FRCS (T&O)
Department of Trauma and Orthopaedics, James Cook University Hospital, Middlesbrough, UK

M.R. Reed, MD, FRCS (T&O) (✉)
Department of Trauma and Orthopaedics, Northumbria Healthcare, Woodhorn Lane, Ashington, Northumberland
NE63 9JJ, UK
e-mail: mike.reed@nhs.net

Modifiable Patient Risk Factors

Patient-related factors, such as diabetes mellitus (DM) and rheumatoid disease (RA), are modifiable and certain aspects of management can be optimised to reduce infection.

Diabetes Mellitus

Wound infection has been shown to be more common in patients with diabetes after arthroplasty, and in non-diabetic patients who developed transient post-operative hyperglycaemia [7]. Hyperglycaemia is associated with increased

D. Kendoff et al. (eds.), *Periprosthetic Joint Infections: Changing Paradigms*,
DOI 10.1007/978-3-319-30091-7_4

Table 4.1 Risk factors for surgical site infection

Patient factors	Operative factors
Systemic:	ASA score >2
Obesity	Long duration
Diabetes	Poor surgical technique
Immunosuppression	Contaminated or dirty wound
Smoking	Lack of systemic antibiotic prophylaxis
Rheumatoid arthritis	Lack of local antibiotics/antiseptic
Psoriasis	Hypothermia
Poor nutritional status	Poor diabetic control
Advanced age	MSSA/MRSA colonisation
Local:	
Previous arthroplasty	
Arthroplasty following fracture	
Type of joint	
Peri-operative wound complications	

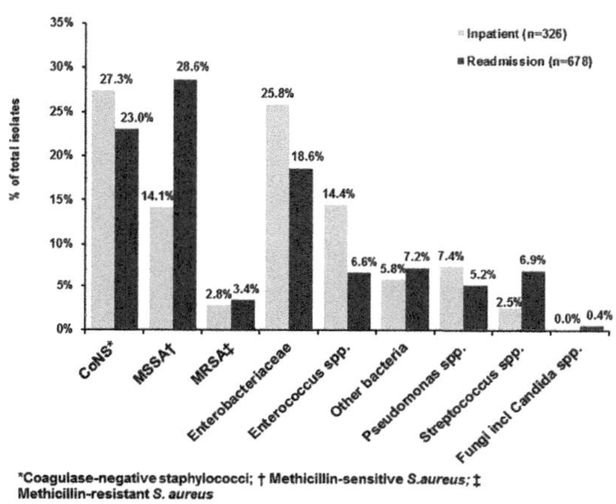

Fig. 4.1 Micro-organisms reported as causing SSIs (all orthopaedic patients, England). *SSI* surgical site infection, *MSSA* methicillin-sensitive *Staphylococcus aureus*, *MRSA* methicillin-resistant *Staphylococcus aureus* (Adapted with permission from the Health Protection Agency)

monocyte susceptibility to apoptosis [8] and impaired neutrophil function (impaired chemotactic, phagocytic and bactericidal capability) [9]. Blood glucose levels above 11.1 mmol/l are associated with SSIs in cardiac surgery [10], and in general surgical patients immediate post-operative hyperglycaemia is associated with SSI [11]. The potential to improve *in vivo* neutrophil phagocytic function by aggressive glucose control (using infusion delivery) has also been demonstrated in cardio-pulmonary bypass patients [12]. However, the effect on SSI is likely to be modest – a recent large study of 40,000 patients undergoing knee replacement found no additional risk for patients with either controlled or uncontrolled diabetes, compared to non diabetics [13].

Rheumatoid Arthritis

RA is an independent risk factor for infection in arthroplasty, but also for revision and subsequent re-infection. This is especially significant as RA patients often present earlier for arthroplasty.

Local and systemic corticosteroids have been shown to delay wound-healing, increase the risk of wound infection [14] and cause adrenal insufficiency. A recent Cochrane review has questioned the historical practice of providing long-term users with additional perioperative steroids (which may amplify immunosuppression at time of surgery) [15].

Although disease-modifying antirheumatic drugs (DMARDs) increase the risk of prosthetic joint infection [5], the British Society for Rheumatology (BSR) guidelines suggest that in most cases these should not be stopped prior to joint replacement [16]. Methotrexate is a commonly used first-line drug [17] and, despite its inclusion within the DMARD group, is not considered by some authors to increase wound infection risk and should not be discontinued prior to orthopaedic surgery [18]. Other randomised trials show a clear reduction in risk when methotrexate is stopped prior to joint replacement [19]. However, nitrous oxide should be excluded from the anaesthetic regimen as the interaction can induce immunosuppression [20].

Tumour necrosis factor (TNF)-alpha is an inflammatory cytokine (highly concentrated in the synovial tissue of RA patients) implicated in joint destruction [21]. Any increase in risk of infection in patients who received anti-TNF therapy prior to surgery is debatable [22, 23]. The BSR state that the potential benefit of preventing post-operative infections (by stopping treatment) should be balanced against the risk of a peri-operative disease flare. If anti-TNF therapy is to be withheld, it should be discontinued 5–20 days before surgery (3–5 times the drug half-life), restarting when there is good wound healing and no evidence of infection [24].

The recent consensus statement on PJI recommends all disease-modifying drugs should be stopped prior to surgery – specifically methotrexate should be stopped a week before surgery, and recommenced 2 weeks after surgery [25]. The authors discuss each case with the rheumatology team.

Patient Weight and Obesity

The effect of obesity (body mass index, BMI $\geq$30 kg/m^2) on SSI is well documented [26]. Self-reported wound complications and reoperations after hip replacement are 1.5–3 times higher in obese patients [27] and there is a 3–7 times higher risk of PJI [28, 29]. Increased length and complexity of surgery and poorer vascularisation of the subcutaneous layer may contribute to this elevated risk. Obese patients also require a significantly higher fraction of inspired oxygen (FiO_2) to reach an adequate arterial oxygen level [30]. In super obese patients ($\geq$50 kg/m^2) bariatric surgery may be indicated. In patients that underwent both bariatric surgery and lower limb arthroplasty, the wound infection rate was 3.5 times lower in patients who had bariatric surgery first [31]. Communication with the anaesthetist to evaluate the risk and to discuss increased doses of peri-operative antibiotics is recommended [32].

Low BMI (<18 kg/m^2) may also increase the risk of PJI, most likely as a result of poor nutrition [29]. As with obese patients, referral to a dietician may be necessary prior to surgery.

Smoking

Smoking is associated with impaired wound healing and infection [33]. Patients randomised to a cessation programme 6–8 weeks prior to arthroplasty had significantly fewer wound complications (5 % vs. 31 %), shorter length of stay, fewer re-operations and cardiovascular benefits [34]. A large non-randomised study found a 3.2 times greater risk of developing wound complications in patients who smoked [35].

Screening for and Decolonisation of *Staphylococcus aureus*

The costs associated with treatment of infections due to methicillin-resistant organisms are 1.5 times higher compared to sensitive organisms [36]. A methicillin-resistant *Staphylococcus aureus* (MRSA) screening programme for all planned NHS surgery was implemented in April 2009, with a positive result prompting decolonisation prior to admission.

Nasal carriers of methicillin-sensitive *Staphylococcus aureus* (MSSA) also have an increased risk of SSI. In a large, randomised, multi-centre trial, the risk of developing a *S. aureus* infection in MSSA-carrier patients who were decolonised on admission to hospital (mupirocin nasal ointment and chlorhexidine soap) fell by nearly 60 % compared with placebo – a significant reduction from 7.7 to 3.4 % [37]. Nasal carriage of MSSA is common (~20 %) [37] and UK hospitals are beginning to decolonise patient carriers prior to joint replacement – this has been demonstrated to be cost effective [38].

Other Considerations

Urogenital and periodontal foci of infection are important sources for haematogenous spread of sepsis and must be eradicated prior to joint replacement [39]. Pre-operative serum albumin levels of less than 3.5 g/dl also increase the risk of post-operative infection [40].

Pre-operative Phase Surgical Risk Factors

Patient Preparation Prior to Theatre

Admission to hospital prior to surgery should ideally be the same day to reduce the risk of colonization of the patient's skin with possibly resistant hospital-acquired bacterial strains. Patients should shower with soap on the morning of surgery [41]. Washing with an antiseptic reduces skin bacteria (microflora), but there is little evidence of a reduction in risk of SSI [42, 43]. There is no evidence that removing hair reduces the risk of SSI [44]. Dry shaving with a razor may irritate the skin and increase the bacterial count so if hair removal is necessary, electric clippers or depilatory creams on the day of surgery are favoured [41, 45].

Patients should be pre-warmed prior to surgery, to avoid hypothermia during the operation and particularly in recovery [46, 47]. A UK randomised trial published in the Lancet demonstrated pre-warming reduces the risk of infection by approximately 65 % in clean surgery [48].

Antibiotic Prophylaxis

The role of parenteral prophylactic antibiotics has been studied and accepted across most surgical specialties [49, 50], and may be the single most significant factor in the prevention of deep wound infection following lower limb arthroplasty [51].

Although many different groups of antibiotics can be used for prophylaxis, there is insufficient evidence of a significant difference in the efficacy of cephalosporins, teicoplanin or penicillin-derivatives, or a benefit of one generation of cephalosporins over another [52]. Cephalosporin use has been associated with *Clostridium difficile* colitis, especially in the elderly, but rates are low after joint replacement (1.7 per 1000 replacements) [53].

Aminoglycosides, such as gentamicin, can be administered locally (in the cement) or parenterally. In a review of 15,000 primary total hip replacements from the Norwegian Arthroplasty Register the lowest risk of revision was found in patients who received both systemic and local (in cement) antibiotics [54]. Although there were no significant differences in superficial wound infection, a meta-analysis examining the benefit of antibiotic-laden bone cement (ALBC) in over 6000 arthroplasties identified a lower deep infection rate [55]. ALBC is used in primary arthroplasties throughout Europe but only approved for use in revision arthroplasty after PJI in North America. Despite concerns, there remains no good evidence of changing microbial profiles and greater resistance following routine prophylactic use of ALBC [56]. Preventing deep infection with antibiotic prophylaxis and ALBC has shown improvements in health outcomes among hospitalized patients, with reduced mortality risk and lower costs [57].

The National Institute for Health and Care Excellence (NICE) recommends a single intravenous dose of antibiotic prophylaxis on starting anaesthesia, with a repeat dose if the operation is longer than the half-life of the antibiotic, or if blood loss is a significant [58]. The American Academy of Orthopaedic Surgeons (AAOS) state that the administration of antibiotic should precede the skin incision by 1 h and duration of prophylaxis should not exceed the 24 h. Rates of infection have been found to be lowest for patients who received an antibiotic within 2 h of the incision [49], and there was no difference between 1- and 3-day courses of prophylactic antibiotics in terms of deep-infection rate [59]. In over 32,000 major procedures (including THR and TKR), risk of SSI was not significantly associated with prophylactic antibiotic timing [60]. Administration of antibiotics as early as possible in the anaesthetic room, and well before (at least 5 min) tourniquet inflation (in order to limit any further rise in tissue antibiotic concentration) seems logical [61].

Unfortunately, there are risks of prophylaxis and there is a delicate balance between reducing risk of SSI and the adverse effects of antibiotics, such as anaphylaxis, interactions with other drugs and antibiotic-associated diarrhoea, including Clostridium difficile (CDAD) and thrush. However, whilst recommended antibiotic prophylaxis has shifted from cephalsporins to dual therapy in order to reduce the incidence of CDAD, data suggests acute kidney injury is higher and SSI has remained unchanged [62–65].

The choice of antibiotic should take into account resistance patterns and cover microorganisms most likely to cause SSI. Patients undergoing high-risk surgery who are MRSA positive should receive a suitable antibiotic active against local strains of MRSA. The combination of vancomycin and cefazolin appear to reduce the incidence of MRSA infections, but the number needed to treat to prevent a single MRSA infection is very high [66]. Another study of over 6000 joint replacements concluded that Gentamicin 4.5 mg/kg alone should not be used as prophylaxis for primary joint arthroplasty as it did not reduce CDAD significantly but increased the risk of other postoperative complications [67].

The most suitable prophylaxis should be the most-narrow spectrum to cover the most common organisms and should be cost-effective. A team-based approach to antibiotic prophylaxis policy is desirable, with knowledge of evidence and information about resistance and drug costs informing recommendations about specific drug regimens.

Peri-operative Phase Surgical Risk Factors

Theatre Etiquette

The World Health Organisation recommends that all surgical staff should keep doors to the operating room closed, except as needed for the passage of equipment, personnel and the patient. Staff should store essential equipment in the operating room to decrease theatre traffic [68]. Frequency of theatre door-opening is a positive predictor of raised bacterial counts [69]. The International Consensus on Periprosthetic Joint Infection Meeting in 2013 reiterated the importance of this: of the 207 questions asked, only the question 'should operating room traffic should be kept to a minimum?' received a unanimous vote with 100 % agreement among the assembled 400 international PJI experts [25].

Although chlorhexidine gluconate has not been demonstrated to reduce SSI rates, it is associated with a more prolonged and effective reduction in colony forming units following surgical hand scrub than povidone-iodine. Alcohol rub used in preparation for surgery may be as effective as hand scrubbing in preventing SSIs [70]. There is no evidence to suggest that any particular alcohol rub is better than another [71, 72].

Surgical Site Preparation in Theatre

Skin moisturisers appear to inhibit the ability of aqueous preparations to decolonise the skin, and may increase skin bacteria counts. Avoidance of oil based moisturisers and de-greasing with alcohol pre-wash is recommended [73].

A large randomised trial of 849 patients undergoing clean-contaminated surgery in which preoperative skin preparation was performed with either 2 % chlorhexidine-alcohol or aqueous povidone-iodine and paint found that the rate of SSI was significantly lower in the chlorhexidine-alcohol group [74]. However, when 41 variables were examined in over 4000 cardiac patients, risk of SSI was not influenced by skin preparation (alcohol betadine or chlorhexadine) [75]. There are currently a number of ongoing clinical trials examining the influence of skin preparations [76]. Further data are likely to emerge in the next few years but the current evidence for skin preparation in joint replacement is limited. NICE support the use of either povidone-iodine or chlorhexidine, but state that alcohol-based solutions may be more effective than aqueous solutions [44].

Theatre Design

Airborne contaminants are said to be the largest single contributor to infection [77]. One billion skin cells are shed daily per person [78] with up to 10 % carrying bacteria [79]. For orthopaedic surgery, laminar-flow ventilation systems have been advocated although they are not in universal use. These employ high-efficiency particulate air filters where particles greater than 0.3 μm are removed (5 μm for conventional theatres). Ultra-clean air can reduce bacterial and particle concentrations [80]. Evidence from the past supports ultra-clean air in conjunction with prophylactic antibiotics to reduce infections after joint arthroplasty [81]. There is no dispute that the air within an effective laminar flow theatre is extremely clean. However, more recent evidence has questioned the benefit. Brandt et al. found laminar flow to have no protective effect against SSI in 99,230 patients [82]. When 88,311 arthroplasty patients from the New Zealand joint registry where analysed, revision rates for deep infection were significantly higher in laminar flow theatres, despite adjustment for other known variables [83]. A systematic review of 123,788 joint replacements found laminar flow did not reduce the occurrence of SSI [84]. However, before abandoning laminar flow the interaction with forced air warming should be examined. A recent study demonstrated that air from outside the canopy may be drawn into the surgical wound area when forced air warming (FAW) devices are used, and deep infection rates were reduced when FAW was abandoned in favour of contemporary conductive fabric warming in joint replacement [85]. The infection control hazards associated with forced air warming have recently been collated and many units, including the authors', use alternative warming systems [86].

Operating Personnel Clothing

NICE recommends double gloving in arthroplasty surgery [87]. Glove perforation increases the risk of transmission of blood-borne diseases and breaks the asepsis barrier, potentially allowing contamination of the wound and thus increasing the risk of infection [88, 89]. Studies have shown that use of a blunt needle compared to sharp needle during surgery reduces glove perforation rates significantly [90, 91]. Most perforations are unnoticed (61.5 %) and are caused by shearing rather than penetration by sharps [88]. A Cochrane systematic review supported the use of double gloving, despite no evidence of a reduction in SSI [92]. Surgical teams should use scrub staff assisted closed gloving to reduce the risk of gown contamination [93]. Glove changing at regular intervals is an effective way to decrease the length of exposure to bacterial contamination [89]. Latex-free gloves have significantly higher perforation rates when compared with latex gloves [94].

Modern space suits contribute to a higher revision rate for infection compared with a normal theatre gown and mask, when analysed independently of laminar flow [83].

Surgical Drapes

If an incise drape is to be used, NICE recommend that an incise drape impregnated with iodophore should be placed unless the patient has an iodine allergy. Although a Cochrane review concluded that these drapes did not make any difference to infection rates [95], only one trial involved orthopaedic surgery, which showed no difference in post-operative wound infection rates following hip fracture surgery with or without non-impregnated Opsite (Smith & Nephew Wound Management, Hull, United Kingdom) [96].

Surgical Equipment

Commonly used equipment can become desterilised in the theatre environment during a procedure, and may be a source of surgical field contamination. Davis et al. found contamination rates of 11.4 % for sucker tips, 9.4 % for skin (outside) blades, 3.2 % for inside blades, 28.7 % for outside gloves used for preparation and draping the patient and 14.5 % for light handles within the laminar flow zone [97].

Pulsatile lavage removes between 57 and 87 % of all organisms from wounds [98, 99]. When combined with 0.05 % chlorhexidine its efficacy can be increased to 98 % and was responsible for a 0.45 % infection rate after hip replacement at one unit [100]. A randomised trail of dilute betadine solution irrigation has shown reduction of SSI in spinal surgery [101] and a recent cohort study supports its use in arthroplasty surgery [102].

Body Core Temperature

Peri-operative hypothermia is common during major surgery and causes vasoconstriction resulting in a reduction in subcutaneous tissue perfusion, and an increased risk of infection [103]. Peri-operative hypothermia is associated with increased blood loss, cardiac events, increased transfusion requirements and longer peri-operative hospital stay [104]. Heat loss in theatre is largely conductive and convective, with a small amount of radiated heat. Laminar flow significantly increases convective heat loss in exposed patients, mitigated by active warming.

Warming patients undergoing clean general surgery significantly reduced wound infection from 14 to 5 % [48]. In a further general surgery study, when patients were randomized to either hypothermia or normothermia the trial had to be stopped prematurely due to the profound treatment benefit of normothermia (SSI at 2 weeks: 5.8 % vs. 18.8 %). A similar report of cholecystectomy patients found nearly a six-fold difference in the incidence of wound infection between normothermic and hypothermic patients [105]. The importance of maintaining perioperative normothermia has been recognised in the recent NICE guidelines [106]. However, it is notable that FAW has never been proven to reduce SSIs in orthopaedic implant surgery, and their effect on laminar flow and clean air needs further study [86].

Oxygen Delivery and Fluid Management

Increasing tissue oxygen concentrations has been hypothesised to increase the killing potential of phagocytes and thus decrease infective complications in the perioperative period [107]. Enhancement of tissue oxygen delivery can be achieved via improvement of cardiac output and/or oxygen content of the blood. Increased subcutaneous oxygen concentrations can be achieved by increasing the inspired oxygen concentration intra-operatively (from 30 to 80 %), and by providing supplemental oxygen post-operatively. There are studies supporting the use of supplemental oxygen to reduce wound infections in general surgery, but these have never been extrapolated to arthroplasty surgery [108–110].

Both hypovolaemia and hypervolaemia (oedema) can be detrimental to tissue oxygenation. Current guidance would support optimal tissue oxygenation by maintenance of a normovolaemic state throughout the peri- and early post-operative period by judicious use of intravenous fluids [111, 112].

Anaesthetic Technique

The question of whether regional anaesthesia is superior to general anaesthesia has yet to be adequately assessed, although a recent retrospective population based study found significantly lower 30-day SSI rates in patients undergoing lower limb arthroplasty under a spinal anaesthetic [113]. An RCT examining the potentially beneficial effect of nitrous oxide avoidance failed to show a reduction in SSI. Co-administered anaesthetic and sedative agents may impair immune responses directly, thereby increasing infection [114], and regional anaesthesia may offer particular benefits such as improved tissue oxygen delivery (through vasodilation). Randomised controlled trials are required to address whether choice of agent (such as use of an alpha2 adrenergic versus GABAergic sedative) affects outcome [114, 115]

A recent systematic review and meta-analysis found a significant advantage of haemodynamic goal-directed fluid therapy on surgical site infection rates, based on 3550 patients in 18 RCTs [116].

Anaemia and Blood Transfusion

In a prospective cohort study preoperative anaemia was associated with increased postoperative infections in patients undergoing hip arthroplasty.

This effect was associated with an increase in postoperative blood transfusion [117].

There are no specific recommendations from NICE regarding transfusions. Though it is clear blood loss is primarily a surgical responsibility, regional anaesthetic techniques and attention to perioperative normothermia are associated with reduced blood loss. Transfusion-related immunomodulation is recognised in trauma patients [118], with a 5 % increase risk of infection for every unit of red cells given [119]. A significant increase in infection rates following hip replacement is seen in patients receiving allogeneic RBCs, with higher risk with more units transfused [120]. There is clearly a risk-benefit balance between immunosuppression and enhancing oxygen supply to hypoperfused tissue. If possible, blood transfusion should be avoided intraoperatively [121] and, if anticipated, should be administered at least 48 h prior to surgery to maximise oxygen transportation of transfused blood. Addressing pre-operative anaemia reduces postoperative transfusion requirements [122].

The use of antifibrinolytics, such as tranexamic acid, prevent blood loss following major arthroplasty [123]. Although there is insufficient data to comment on their ability to prevent postoperative infection, they may indirectly reduce the risk by reducing transfusion requirement and improving the wound environment.

Recent evidence suggests that white cell depleted blood reduces infection risk compared to normal blood [124], and red blood cell transfusions in the UK are routinely filtered.

Surgical Factors

Prolonged operating time, reflecting the complexity of surgery or the inexperience of the surgeon, may increase the risk of infection. However, when adjusted for confounding factors such as BMI and diabetes this effect is modest with an increased risk of only 7 % for every additional 15 min [29].

Closed suction drains are a potential entry point of infection, but there is no evidence of any association with wound infection risk [125]. There is also insufficient evidence to recommend that a particular wound dressing is more effective than others in reducing the rates of SSI [126].

Post-operative Period

Thromboembolic Prophylaxis

NICE guidelines state that patients undergoing lower limb joint replacements should have either prophylactic low molecular weight heparin (LMWH) or an orally active direct factor Xa inhibitor for 28 (or 35) days following hip arthroplasty and 14 days following a knee arthroplasty. No increased risk of infection was found with LMWH [127] but prolonged ooze is a recognised risk [128], and each day of prolonged wound drainage increases risk of wound infection by 29–42 % following arthroplasty [128]. Wound-related complications following arthroplasty may increase in patients who receive rivaroxaban, a factor Xa inhibitor, for thromboprophylaxis [129].

Dental Care and Other Procedures

It has been suggested that patients requiring dental care post-arthroplasty should receive prophylactic antibiotics [130]. Other authors argue that there is little evidence to suggest that bacteraemia associated with dental procedures causes prosthetic joint infection [131] – simple tasks, such as brushing teeth and chewing, can produce a greater bacteraemia than one dental procedure and it would be better practice for the surgeon to ensure dentition and oral health are up to standard prior to elective orthopaedic surgery. Currently in the UK, the British Dental Association does not recommend antibiotics. The routine use of amoxicillin antibiotic prophylaxis prior to dental procedures for patients with TJA may not be cost-effective in those where the risk of infection with dental work is low [132].

Table 4.2 summarises the evidence for methods to reduce PJI.

Table 4.2 Methods for reducing surgical site infection in joint replacement

Risk factor	Summary
Patient factors	
Diabetes mellitus	Aggressive glucose control
Rheumatoid arthritis	DMARDs and methotrexate should not be stopped Peri-operative steroids are generally not required Balance the risks and benefits of stopping anti-TNF – stop at 3-5 half lifes pre-operative, restart after wound healing and no evidence of infection Nitrous oxide should be avoided in patients on methotrexate
Obesity	Dietician input to encourage weight loss Adjust peri-operative antibiotic doses appropriately In super-obese consider bariatric surgery prior to surgery
Smoking	Consider a smoking cessation programme
Carrier screening	MRSA and MSSA screening based on local guidelines, and decolonise prior to admission
Pre-operative factors	
Patient preparation	Shower on day of surgery If shaving required, use electric clippers on day of surgery Avoid oil-based skin moisturisers
Antibiotics	Prophylactic antibiotics should be given as early as possible in the anaesthetic room, and continued for 24 h post-operatively (antibiotic type dependent on local guidelines) Administer antibiotics at least 5 min prior to tourniquet inflation If cementation is required, antibiotic-impregnated should be used
Peri-operative factors	
Theatre	Use laminar flow where possible Keep theatre door opening to a minimum
Personnel	Hand wash with antiseptic surgical solution, using a single-use brush or pick for the nails Before subsequent operations hands should be washed with either an alcoholic hand rub or an antiseptic surgical solution Double glove and change gloves regularly Polyprophylene non-woven gowns with adequate mask and hat coverage
Skin preparation	Use an alcohol pre-wash followed by a 2 % chlorhexadine-alcohol scrub solution
Anaesthetic	Maintain normothermia Maintain normovolaemia A higher inspired oxygen concentration peri-operatively and for 6 h post-operative may be of benefit
Drapes	Use of iodine-impregnated incise drapes may be of benefit (in patients without allergy)
Blood transfusion	Optimise pre-operative haemoglobin If possible, transfusion should be avoided intra-operatively and if anticipated should be given more than 48 h prior to surgery Antifibrinolytics may indirectly reduce SSI by reducing the need for transfusion
Post-operative factors	
Dental procedures	Insufficient evidence to recommend the use of prophylactic antibiotics for patients undergoing routine dental procedures following joint replacement
Other	
Surveillance	Initiatives have shown the benefit of collecting and analysing data with appropriate feedback mechanism to prompt changes in practice [133]

Abbreviations: *DMARDs* disease-modifying anti-rheumatic drugs, *TNF* tumour necrosis factor, *MRSA* methicillin-resistant *Staphylococcus aureus*, *MSSA*, methicillin-sensitive *Staphylococcus aureus*, *SSI* surgical site infection

Conclusion

A PJI following routine arthroplasty surgery can have disastrous consequences for the patient and is costly to healthcare providers. Given the wide variety of infection prevention tactics available a team-based approach is essential in order to reduce infection rates. Every possible step must be exercised to reduce contamination of the surgical wound and to optimise the patient's capacity to eradicate any colony forming units entering the wound. Common-sense approaches are required to minimise or correct physiological disturbances and attention should be given to theatre design and etiquette, identification and control of MSSA carriers and the appropriate and timely use of prophylactic antibiotics. It is important to emphasize the need to educate the patient and all members of the healthcare team, and to increase awareness of the importance of their participation in preventive efforts.

References

1. Darouiche RO. Treatment of infections associated with surgical implants. N Engl J Med. 2004;350(14):1422–9 [Review].
2. Edwards C, Counsell A, Boulton C, Moran CG. Early infection after hip fracture surgery: risk factors, costs and outcome. J Bone Joint Surg Br. 2008;90(6):770–7.
3. Bozic KJ, Ries MD. The impact of infection after total hip arthroplasty on hospital and surgeon resource utilization. J Bone Joint Surg Am. 2005;87(8):1746–51. [Research Support, Non-U.S. Gov't].
4. Gurkan I, Wenz JF. Perioperative infection control: an update for patient safety in orthopedic surgery. Orthopedics. 2006;29(4):329–39; quiz 40-1. [Review].
5. Moucha CS, Clyburn T, Evans RP, Prokuski L. Modifiable risk factors for surgical site infection. J Bone Joint Surg Am. 2011;93(4):398–404 [Review].
6. Health-Protection-Agency. Sixth report of the mandatory surveillance of surgical site infection in orthopaedic surgery; 2011. www.hpa.org.uk.
7. Mraovic B, Donghun S, Jacovides C, Parvizi J. Perioperative hyperglycemia and postoperative infection after lower limb arthroplasty. J Diabetes Sci Technol. 2011;5(2):413–8.
8. Komura T, Sakai Y, Honda M, Takamura T, Matsushima K, Kaneko S. CD14+ monocytes are vulnerable and functionally impaired under endoplasmic reticulum stress in patients with type 2 diabetes. Diabetes. 2010;59(3):634–43.
9. Turina M, Fry DE, Polk Jr HC. Acute hyperglycemia and the innate immune system: clinical, cellular, and molecular aspects. Crit Care Med. 2005;33(7):1624–33. [Research Support, Non-U.S. Gov't Review].
10. Golden SH, Peart-Vigilance C, Kao WH, Brancati FL. Perioperative glycemic control and the risk of infectious complications in a cohort of adults with diabetes. Diabetes Care. 1999;22(9):1408–14. [Research Support, Non-U.S. Gov't Research Support, U.S. Gov't, P.H.S.].
11. Ata A, Lee J, Bestle SL, Desemone J, Stain SC. Postoperative hyperglycemia and surgical site infection in general surgery patients. Arch Surg. 2010;145(9):858–64.
12. Rassias AJ, Marrin CA, Arruda J, Whalen PK, Beach M, Yeager MP. Insulin infusion improves neutrophil function in diabetic cardiac surgery patients. Anesth Analg. 1999;88(5):1011–6. [Clinical Trial Randomized Controlled Trial Research Support, U.S. Gov't, P.H.S.].
13. Adams AL, Paxton EW, Wang JQ, Johnson ES, Bayliss EA, Ferrara A, et al. Surgical outcomes of total knee replacement according to diabetes status and glycemic control, 2001 to 2009. J Bone Joint Surg Am. 2013;95(6):481–7.
14. Wicke C, Halliday B, Allen D, Roche NS, Scheuenstuhl H, Spencer MM, et al. Effects of steroids and retinoids on wound healing. Arch Surg. 2000;135(11):1265–70. [Comparative Study].
15. Yong SL, Marik P, Esposito M, Coulthard P. Supplemental perioperative steroids for surgical patients with adrenal insufficiency. Cochrane Database Syst Rev. 2009;(4):CD005367. [Meta-Analysis Review].
16. Luqmani R, Hennell S, Estrach C, Basher D, Birrell F, Bosworth A, et al. British Society for Rheumatology and British Health Professionals in Rheumatology guideline for the management of rheumatoid arthritis (after the first 2 years). Rheumatology (Oxford). 2009;48(4):436–9. [Practice Guideline Research Support, Non-U.S. Gov't].
17. Kameda H, Kanbe K, Sato E, Ueki Y, Saito K, Nagaoka S, et al. Continuation of methotrexate resulted in better clinical and radiographic outcomes than discontinuation upon starting etanercept in patients with rheumatoid arthritis: 52-week results from the JESMR study. J Rheumatol. 2011;38(8):1585–92.
18. Grennan DM, Gray J, Loudon J, Fear S. Methotrexate and early postoperative complications in patients with rheumatoid arthritis undergoing elective orthopaedic surgery. Ann Rheum Dis. 2001;60(3): 214–7. [Clinical Trial Randomized Controlled Trial Research Support, Non-U.S. Gov't].
19. Carpenter MT, West SG, Vogelgesang SA, Casey Jones DE. Postoperative joint infections in rheumatoid arthritis patients on methotrexate therapy. Orthopedics. 1996;19(3):207–10.

20. Sanders RD, Weimann J, Maze M. Biologic effects of nitrous oxide: a mechanistic and toxicologic review. Anesthesiology. 2008;109(4):707–22 [Review].
21. Choy EH, Panayi GS. Cytokine pathways and joint inflammation in rheumatoid arthritis. N Engl J Med. 2001;344(12):907–16. [Research Support, Non-U.S. Gov't Review].
22. Dixon WG, Lunt M, Watson KD, Hyrich KL, Symmons DP. Anti-TNF therapy and the risk of serious post-operative infection: results from the BSR Biologics register (BSRBR). Ann Rheum Dis. 2007;66(Suppl II):118.
23. Bibbo C, Goldberg JW. Infectious and healing complications after elective orthopaedic foot and ankle surgery during tumor necrosis factor-alpha inhibition therapy. Foot Ankle Int. 2004;25(5):331–5. [Clinical Trial Comparative Study Controlled Clinical Trial].
24. Ding T, Ledingham J, Luqmani R, Westlake S, Hyrich K, Lunt M, et al. BSR and BHPR rheumatoid arthritis guidelines on safety of anti-TNF therapies. Rheumatology (Oxford). 2010;49(11):2217–9.
25. Parvizi J, Gehrke T, Chen AF. Proceedings of the international consensus on periprosthetic joint infection. Bone Joint J. 2013;95-B(11):1450–2.
26. Dowsey MM, Choong PF. Early outcomes and complications following joint arthroplasty in obese patients: a review of the published reports. ANZ J Surg. 2008;78(6):439–44 [Review].
27. Jameson SS, Mason JM, Baker PN, Elson DW, Deehan DJ, Reed MR. The impact of body mass index on patient reported outcome measures (PROMs) and complications following primary hip arthroplasty. J Arthroplasty. 2014;29(10):1889–98.
28. Namba RS, Paxton L, Fithian DC, Stone ML. Obesity and perioperative morbidity in total hip and total knee arthroplasty patients. J Arthroplasty. 2005;20(7 Suppl 3):46–50. [Research Support, Non-U.S. Gov't].
29. Namba RS, Inacio MC, Paxton EW. Risk factors associated with surgical site infection in 30,491 primary total hip replacements. J Bone Joint Surg Br. 2012;94(10):1330–8.
30. Fleischmann E, Kurz A, Niedermayr M, Schebesta K, Kimberger O, Sessler DI, et al. Tissue oxygenation in obese and non-obese patients during laparoscopy. Obes Surg. 2005;15(6):813–9. [Research Support, N.I.H., Extramural Research Support, Non-U.S. Gov't Research Support, U.S. Gov't, P.H.S.].
31. Kulkarni A, Jameson SS, James P, Woodcock S, Muller S, Reed MR. Does bariatric surgery prior to lower limb joint replacement reduce complications? Surgeon. 2011;9(1):18–21.
32. Freeman JT, Anderson DJ, Hartwig MG, Sexton DJ. Surgical site infections following bariatric surgery in community hospitals: a weighty concern? Obes Surg. 2011;21:836–40.
33. Kwiatkowski TC, Hanley Jr EN, Ramp WK. Cigarette smoking and its orthopedic consequences. Am J Orthop (Belle Mead NJ). 1996;25(9):590–7 [Review].
34. Moller AM, Villebro N, Pedersen T, Tonnesen H. Effect of preoperative smoking intervention on postoperative complications: a randomised clinical trial. Lancet. 2002;359(9301):114–7. [Clinical Trial Multicenter Study Randomized Controlled Trial Research Support, Non-U.S. Gov't].
35. Moller AM, Pedersen T, Villebro N, Munksgaard A. Effect of smoking on early complications after elective orthopaedic surgery. J Bone Joint Surg Br. 2003;85(2):178–81.
36. Parvizi J, Pawasarat IM, Azzam KA, Joshi A, Hansen EN, Bozic KJ. Periprosthetic joint infection: the economic impact of methicillin-resistant infections. J Arthroplasty. 2010;25(6 Suppl):103–7. [Multicenter Study].
37. Bode LG, Kluytmans JA, Wertheim HF, Bogaers D, Vandenbroucke-Grauls CM, Roosendaal R, et al. Preventing surgical-site infections in nasal carriers of Staphylococcus aureus. N Engl J Med. 2010;362(1):9–17. [Multicenter Study Randomized Controlled Trial Research Support, Non-U.S. Gov't].
38. van Rijen MM, Bode LG, Baak DA, Kluytmans JA, Vos MC. Reduced costs for Staphylococcus aureus carriers treated prophylactically with mupirocin and chlorhexidine in cardiothoracic and orthopaedic surgery. PLoS One. 2012;7(8):e43065.
39. Schmalzried TP, Amstutz HC, Au MK, Dorey FJ. Etiology of deep sepsis in total hip arthroplasty. The significance of hematogenous and recurrent infections. Clin Orthop Relat Res. 1992;280:200–7.
40. Greene KA, Wilde AH, Stulberg BN. Preoperative nutritional status of total joint patients. Relationship to postoperative wound complications. J Arthroplasty. 1991;6(4):321–5.
41. Leaper D, Burman-Roy S, Palanca A, Cullen K, Worster D, Gautam-Aitken E, et al. Prevention and treatment of surgical site infection: summary of NICE guidance. BMJ. 2008;337:a1924. [Research Support, Non-U.S. Gov't].
42. Webster J, Osborne S. Preoperative bathing or showering with skin antiseptics to prevent surgical site infection. Cochrane Database Syst Rev. 2006;(2):CD004985. [Meta-Analysis Review].
43. Jakobsson J, Perlkvist A, Wann-Hansson C. Searching for evidence regarding using preoperative disinfection showers to prevent surgical site infections: a systematic review. Worldviews Evid Based Nurs. 2010;28.
44. Excellence NIfHaC. Surgical site infection: evidence Update June 2013. 2013 [07/05/2015]; Available from: http://www.evidence.nhs.uk/document?ci=http%3A%2F%2Farms.evidence.nhs.uk%2Fresources%2FHub%2F1006598&q=Surgical%20site%20infection%20evidence%20update&ReturnUrl=%2Fsearch%3Fq%3DSurgical%2Bsite%2Binfection%2Bevidence%2Bupdate.
45. Tanner J, Woodings D, Moncaster K. Preoperative hair removal to reduce surgical site infection.

Cochrane Database Syst Rev. 2006;(3):CD004122. [Meta-Analysis Review].
46. van der Horst MW, Wiewel ELVVM, van der Hoeven CWP, Loer SA, Boer C. Preoperative warming reduces the incidence of hypothermia in total hip- and knee replacement surgery under spinal anesthesia. Eur J Anaesthesiol. 2010;27(47):7.
47. Just B, Trevien V, Delva E, Lienhart A. Prevention of intraoperative hypothermia by preoperative skin-surface warming. Anesthesiology. 1993;79(2): 214–8.
48. Melling AC, Ali B, Scott EM, Leaper DJ. Effects of preoperative warming on the incidence of wound infection after clean surgery: a randomised controlled trial. Lancet. 2001;358(9285):876–80. [Clinical Trial Randomized Controlled Trial Research Support, Non-U.S. Gov't].
49. Classen DC, Evans RS, Pestotnik SL, Horn SD, Menlove RL, Burke JP. The timing of prophylactic administration of antibiotics and the risk of surgical-wound infection. N Engl J Med. 1992;326(5):281–6. [Clinical Trial Randomized Controlled Trial Research Support, U.S. Gov't, P.H.S.].
50. Prokuski L, Clyburn TA, Evans RP, Moucha CS. Prophylactic antibiotics in orthopaedic surgery. Instr Course Lect. 2011;60:545–55.
51. Hanssen AD, Osmon DR. Prevention of deep wound infection after total hip arthroplasty: the role of prophylactic antibiotics and clean air technology. Semin Arthroplasty. 1994;5(3):114–21 [Review].
52. AlBuhairan B, Hind D, Hutchinson A. Antibiotic prophylaxis for wound infections in total joint arthroplasty: a systematic review. J Bone Joint Surg Br. 2008;90(7):915–9. [Meta-Analysis Review].
53. Jenkins PJ, Teoh K, Simpson PM, Dave J, Simpson AH, Breusch S. Clostridium difficile in patients undergoing primary hip and knee replacement. J Bone Joint Surg Br. 2010;92(7):994–8.
54. Engesaeter LB, Lie SA, Espehaug B, Furnes O, Vollset SE, Havelin LI. Antibiotic prophylaxis in total hip arthroplasty: effects of antibiotic prophylaxis systemically and in bone cement on the revision rate of 22,170 primary hip replacements followed 0-14 years in the Norwegian Arthroplasty Register. Acta Orthop Scand. 2003;74(6):644–51.
55. Wang J, Zhu C, Cheng T, Peng X, Zhang W, Qin H, et al. A systematic review and meta-analysis of antibiotic-impregnated bone cement use in primary total hip or knee arthroplasty. PLoS One. 2013;8(12), e82745.
56. Hansen EN, Adeli B, Kenyon R, Parvizi J. Routine use of antibiotic laden bone cement for primary total knee arthroplasty: impact on infecting microbial patterns and resistance profiles. J Arthroplasty. 2014;29(6):1123–7.
57. Merollini KM, Crawford RW, Whitehouse SL, Graves N. Surgical site infection prevention following total hip arthroplasty in Australia: a cost-effectiveness analysis. Am J Infect Control. 2013;41(9):803–9.
58. Swoboda SM, Merz C, Kostuik J, Trentler B, Lipsett PA. Does intraoperative blood loss affect antibiotic serum and tissue concentrations? Arch Surg. 1996;131(11):1165–71. discussion 71-2.
59. Mauerhan DR, Nelson CL, Smith DL, Fitzgerald Jr RH, Slama TG, Petty RW, et al. Prophylaxis against infection in total joint arthroplasty. One day of cefuroxime compared with three days of cefazolin. J Bone Joint Surg Am. 1994;76(1):39–45. [Clinical Trial Comparative Study Multicenter Study Randomized Controlled Trial Research Support, Non-U.S. Gov't].
60. Hawn MT, Richman JS, Vick CC, Deierhoi RJ, Graham LA, Henderson WG, et al. Timing of surgical antibiotic prophylaxis and the risk of surgical site infection. JAMA Surg. 2013;148(7):649–57.
61. Bannister GC, Auchincloss JM, Johnson DP, Newman JH. The timing of tourniquet application in relation to prophylactic antibiotic administration. J Bone Joint Surg Br. 1988;70(2):322–4. [Research Support, Non-U.S. Gov't].
62. Challagundla SR, Knox D, Hawkins A, Hamilton D, W V Flynn R, Robertson S, et al. Renal impairment after high-dose flucloxacillin and single-dose gentamicin prophylaxis in patients undergoing elective hip and knee replacement. Nephrol Dial Transplant. 2013;28(3):612–9.
63. Ross AD, Boscainos PJ, Malhas A, Wigderowitz C. Peri-operative renal morbidity secondary to gentamicin and flucloxacillin chemoprophylaxis for hip and knee arthroplasty. Scott Med J. 2013;58(4): 209–12.
64. Bailey O, Torkington MS, Anthony I, Wells J, Blyth M, Jones B. Antibiotic-related acute kidney injury in patients undergoing elective joint replacement. Bone Joint J. 2014;96-B(3):395–8.
65. Craxford S, Bayley E, Needoff M. Antibiotic-associated complications following lower limb arthroplasty: a comparison of two prophylactic regimes. Eur J Orthop Surg Traumatol. 2014;24(4): 539–43.
66. Sewick A, Makani A, Wu C, O'Donnell J, Baldwin KD, Lee GC. Does dual antibiotic prophylaxis better prevent surgical site infections in total joint arthroplasty? Clin Orthop Relat Res. 2012;470(10):2702–7.
67. Sprowson A, Symes T, Khan SK, Oswald T, Reed MR. Changing antibiotic prophylaxis for primary joint arthroplasty affects postoperative complication rates and bacterial spectrum. Surgeon. 2013;11(1):20–4.
68. World Health Organization. Surgical care at the district hopsital. http://www.who.int/surgery/publications/en/SCDH.pdf?ua=1 (date last accessed 18 March 2016).
69. Scaltriti S, Cencetti S, Rovesti S, Marchesi I, Bargellini A, Borella P. Risk factors for particulate and microbial contamination of air in operating theatres. J Hosp Infect. 2007;66(4):320–6. [Research Support, Non-U.S. Gov't].
70. Parienti JJ, Thibon P, Heller R, Le Roux Y, von Theobald P, Bensadoun H, et al. Hand-rubbing

with an aqueous alcoholic solution vs traditional surgical hand-scrubbing and 30-day surgical site infection rates: a randomized equivalence study. JAMA. 2002;288(6):722–7. [Clinical Trial Comparative Study Randomized Controlled Trial Research Support, Non-U.S. Gov't].
71. Tanner J, Swarbrook S, Stuart J. Surgical hand antisepsis to reduce surgical site infection. Cochrane Database Syst Rev. 2008(1):CD004288. [Meta-Analysis Review].
72. Jarral OA, McCormack DJ, Ibrahim S, Shipolini AR. Should surgeons scrub with chlorhexidine or iodine prior to surgery? Interact Cardiovasc Thorac Surg. 2011;12:1017–21.
73. Mahadeva D, Rankin KS, Muller SD. Skin moisturisers and surgical site preparation: a slippery problem? J Hosp Infect. 2007;67(4):386–8. [Letter Research Support, Non-U.S. Gov't].
74. Darouiche RO, Wall Jr MJ, Itani KM, Otterson MF, Webb AL, Carrick MM, et al. Chlorhexidine-alcohol versus povidone-iodine for surgical-site antisepsis. N Engl J Med. 2010;362(1):18–26. [Multicenter Study Randomized Controlled Trial].
75. Raja SG, Rochon M, Jarman JW. Brompton Harefield Infection Score (BHIS): development and validation of a stratification tool for predicting risk of surgical site infection after coronary artery bypass grafting. Int J Surg. 2015;16(Pt A):69–73.
76. U.S.-National-Institutes-of-Health. ClinicalTrials.org. 2015 [16/09/15]; Available from: https://clinicaltrials.gov/ct2/results?term=skin+preparation&Search=Search.
77. Lidwell OM. Air, antibiotics and sepsis in replacement joints. J Hosp Infect. 1988;11 Suppl C:18–40 [Review].
78. Whyte W. The role of clothing and drapes in the operating room. J Hosp Infect. 1988;11 Suppl C:2–17. [Review].
79. Noble WC. Dispersal of skin microorganisms. Br J Dermatol. 1975;93(4):477–85 [Review].
80. Hansen D, Krabs C, Benner D, Brauksiepe A, Popp W. Laminar air flow provides high air quality in the operating field even during real operating conditions, but personal protection seems to be necessary in operations with tissue combustion. Int J Hyg Environ Health. 2005;208(6):455–60.
81. Lidwell OM, Elson RA, Lowbury EJ, Whyte W, Blowers R, Stanley SJ, et al. Ultraclean air and antibiotics for prevention of postoperative infection. A multicenter study of 8,052 joint replacement operations. Acta Orthop Scand. 1987;58(1):4–13. [Clinical Trial Research Support, Non-U.S. Gov't].
82. Brandt C, Hott U, Sohr D, Daschner F, Gastmeier P, Ruden H. Operating room ventilation with laminar airflow shows no protective effect on the surgical site infection rate in orthopedic and abdominal surgery. Ann Surg. 2008;248(5):695–700. [Comment Multicenter Study Research Support, Non-U.S. Gov't].
83. Hooper GJ, Rothwell AG, Frampton C, Wyatt MC. Does the use of laminar flow and space suits reduce early deep infection after total hip and knee replacement?: the ten-year results of the New Zealand Joint Registry. J Bone Joint Surg Br. 2011;93(1):85–90.
84. Zheng H, Barnett AG, Merollini K, Sutton A, Cooper N, Berendt T, et al. Control strategies to prevent total hip replacement-related infections: a systematic review and mixed treatment comparison. BMJ Open. 2014;4(3), e003978.
85. McGovern PD, Reed MR. Forced air warming and ultra-clean ventilation do not mix: an investigation of theatre ventilation, patient warming and joint replacement infection in orthopaedics. J Bone Joint Surg Br. 2011;93(11):1537–44.
86. Wood AM, Moss C, Keenan A, Reed MR, Leaper DJ. Infection control hazards associated with the use of forced-air warming in operating theatres. J Hosp Infect. 2014;88(3):132–40.
87. Demircay E, Unay K, Bilgili MG, Alataca G. Glove perforation in hip and knee arthroplasty. J Orthop Sci. 2010;15(6):790–4.
88. Chan KY, Singh VA, Oun BH, To BH. The rate of glove perforations in orthopaedic procedures: single versus double gloving. A prospective study. Med J Malaysia. 2006;61:3–7 Suppl B.
89. Al-Maiyah M, Bajwa A, Mackenney P, Port A, Gregg PJ, Hill D, et al. Glove perforation and contamination in primary total hip arthroplasty. J Bone Joint Surg Br. 2005;87(4):556–9. [Clinical Trial Randomized Controlled Trial Research Support, Non-U.S. Gov't].
90. Mingoli A, Sapienza P, Sgarzini G, Luciani G, De Angelis G, Modini C, et al. Influence of blunt needles on surgical glove perforation and safety for the surgeon. Am J Surg. 1996;172(5):512–6; discussion 6-7. [Clinical Trial Comparative Study Randomized Controlled Trial].
91. Wright KU, Moran CG, Briggs PJ. Glove perforation during hip arthroplasty. A randomised prospective study of a new taperpoint needle. J Bone Joint Surg Br. 1993;75(6):918–20. [Clinical Trial Comparative Study Randomized Controlled Trial].
92. Tanner J, Parkinson H. Double gloving to reduce surgical cross-infection. Cochrane Database Syst Rev. 2006;(3):CD003087. [Meta-Analysis Review].
93. Newman JB, Bullock M, Goyal R. Comparison of glove donning techniques for the likelihood of gown contamination. An infection control study. Acta Orthop Belg. 2007;73(6):765–71.
94. Aldlyami E, Kulkarni A, Reed MR, Muller SD, Partington PF. Latex-free gloves: safer for whom? J Arthroplasty. 2010;25(1):27–30.
95. Webster J, Alghamdi AA. Use of plastic adhesive drapes during surgery for preventing surgical site infection. Cochrane Database Syst Rev. 2007(4):CD006353. [Meta-Analysis Review].

96. Chiu KY, Lau SK, Fung B, Ng KH, Chow SP. Plastic adhesive drapes and wound infection after hip fracture surgery. Aust N Z J Surg. 1993;63(10):798–801. [Clinical Trial Randomized Controlled Trial].
97. Davis N, Curry A, Gambhir AK, Panigrahi H, Walker CR, Wilkins EG, et al. Intraoperative bacterial contamination in operations for joint replacement. J Bone Joint Surg Br. 1999;81(5):886–9.
98. Hope PG, Kristinsson KG, Norman P, Elson RA. Deep infection of cemented total hip arthroplasties caused by coagulase-negative staphylococci. J Bone Joint Surg Br. 1989;71(5):851–5.
99. Taylor GJ, Leeming JP, Bannister GC. Effect of antiseptics, ultraviolet light and lavage on airborne bacteria in a model wound. J Bone Joint Surg Br. 1993;75(5):724–30.
100. Taylor GJ, Bannister GC, Calder S. Perioperative wound infection in elective orthopaedic surgery. J Hosp Infect. 1990;16(3):241–7.
101. Cheng MT, Chang MC, Wang ST, Yu WK, Liu CL, Chen TH. Efficacy of dilute betadine solution irrigation in the prevention of postoperative infection of spinal surgery. Spine (Phila Pa 1976). 2005;30(15):1689–93.
102. Brown NM, Cipriano CA, Moric M, Sporer SM, Della Valle CJ. Dilute betadine lavage before closure for the prevention of acute postoperative deep periprosthetic joint infection. J Arthroplasty. 2012; 27(1):27–30.
103. Sessler DI, Akca O. Nonpharmacological prevention of surgical wound infections. Clin Infect Dis. 2002;35(11):1397–404. [Research Support, Non-U.S. Gov't Research Support, U.S. Gov't, P.H.S.].
104. Sessler DI. Complications and treatment of mild hypothermia. Anesthesiology. 2001;95(2):531–43. [Research Support, Non-U.S. Gov't Research Support, U.S. Gov't, P.H.S. Review].
105. Flores-Maldonado A, Medina-Escobedo CE, Rios-Rodriguez HM, Fernandez-Dominguez R. Mild perioperative hypothermia and the risk of wound infection. Arch Med Res. 2001;32(3):227–31.
106. https://www.nice.org.uk/guidance/cg65.
107. Babior BM. The respiratory burst of phagocytes. J Clin Invest. 1984;73(3):599–601. [Research Support, Non-U.S. Gov't Research Support, U.S. Gov't, P.H.S. Review].
108. Pryor KO, Fahey 3rd TJ, Lien CA, Goldstein PA. Surgical site infection and the routine use of perioperative hyperoxia in a general surgical population: a randomized controlled trial. JAMA. 2004;291(1):79–87. [Clinical Trial Randomized Controlled Trial Research Support, Non-U.S. Gov't].
109. Belda FJ, Aguilera L, Garcia de la Asuncion J, Alberti J, Vicente R, Ferrandiz L, et al. Supplemental perioperative oxygen and the risk of surgical wound infection: a randomized controlled trial. JAMA. 2005;294(16):2035–42. [Clinical Trial Randomized Controlled Trial Research Support, N.I.H., Extramural Research Support, Non-U.S. Gov't Research Support, U.S. Gov't, P.H.S.].
110. Greif R, Akca O, Horn EP, Kurz A, Sessler DI. Supplemental perioperative oxygen to reduce the incidence of surgical-wound infection. N Engl J Med. 2000;342(3):161–7. [Clinical Trial Randomized Controlled Trial Research Support, Non-U.S. Gov't Research Support, U.S. Gov't, P.H.S.].
111. Arkilic CF, Taguchi A, Sharma N, Ratnaraj J, Sessler DI, Read TE, et al. Supplemental perioperative fluid administration increases tissue oxygen pressure. Surgery. 2003;133(1):49–55. [Clinical Trial Randomized Controlled Trial Research Support, Non-U.S. Gov't Research Support, U.S. Gov't, P.H.S.].
112. Mauermann WJ, Nemergut EC. The anesthesiologist's role in the prevention of surgical site infections. Anesthesiology. 2006;105(2):413–21; quiz 39-40. [Review].
113. Chang CC, Lin HC, Lin HW. Anesthetic management and surgical site infections in total hip or knee replacement: a population-based study. Anesthesiology. 2010;113(2):279–84.
114. Sanders RD, Hussell T, Maze M. Sedation & immunomodulation. Crit Care Clin. 2009;25(3):551–70, ix. [Review].
115. Riker RR, Shehabi Y, Bokesch PM, Ceraso D, Wisemandle W, Koura F, et al. Dexmedetomidine vs midazolam for sedation of critically ill patients: a randomized trial. JAMA. 2009;301(5):489–99. [Comparative Study Multicenter Study Randomized Controlled Trial Research Support, Non-U.S. Gov't].
116. Dalfino L, Giglio MT, Puntillo F, Marucci M, Brienza N. Haemodynamic goal-directed therapy and postoperative infections: earlier is better. A systematic review and meta-analysis. Crit Care. 2011;15(3):R154.
117. Myers E, O'Grady P, Dolan AM. The influence of preclinical anaemia on outcome following total hip replacement. Arch Orthop Trauma Surg. 2004;124(10):699–701.
118. Morales CH, Escobar RM, Villegas MI, Castano A, Trujillo J. Surgical site infection in abdominal trauma patients: risk prediction and performance of the NNIS and SENIC indexes. Can J Surg. 2011;54(1):17–24. [Comparative Study Evaluation Studies].
119. Alexander JW, Solomkin JS, Edwards MJ. Updated recommendations for control of surgical site infections. Ann Surg. 2011;253(6):1082–93 [Review].
120. Steinitz D, Harvey EJ, Leighton RK, Petrie DP. Is homologous blood transfusion a risk factor for infection after hip replacement? Can J Surg. 2001;44(5):355–8. [Clinical Trial].
121. Kendall SJ, Weir J, Aspinall R, Henderson D, Rosson J. Erythrocyte transfusion causes immunosuppression after total hip replacement. Clin Orthopaedics Relat Res. 2000;(381):145–55. [Research Support, Non-U.S. Gov't].
122. Foundation TH. Cutting the need for blood transfusions in knee and hip replacement surgery. 2013 [07/05/2015];

Available from: http://www.health.org.uk/public/cms/75/76/4780/3092/Could%20quality%20be%20cheaper_Airedale%20NHS%20Foundation%20Trust%20case%20study.pdf?realName=52EQeC.pdf.
123. Sukeik M, Alshryda S, Haddad FS, Mason JM. Systematic review and meta-analysis of the use of tranexamic acid in total hip replacement. J Bone Joint Surg Br. 2011;93(1):39–46. [Meta-Analysis Review].
124. Bilgin YM, van de Watering LM, Eijsman L, Versteegh MI, Brand R, van Oers MH, et al. Double-blind, randomized controlled trial on the effect of leukocyte-depleted erythrocyte transfusions in cardiac valve surgery. Circulation. 2004;109(22):2755–60.
125. Cochrane-Library. Wound drains in orthopaedic surgery (surgery on the joints or limbs). 2008 [07/05/2015]; Available from: http://www.cochrane.org/CD001825/MUSKINJ_wound-drains-in-orthopaedic-surgery--surgery-on-the-joints-or-limbs.
126. The-Cochrane-Library. No recommendations regarding type of wound dressing for the prevention of surgical site infection. 2014; Available from: http://www.cochrane.org/CD003091/WOUNDS_no-recommendations-regarding-type-of-wound-dressing-for-the-prevention-of-surgical-site-infection.
127. Jameson SS, Charman S, Reed MR, Gregg PJ, Van der Meulen J. The effect of aspirin and LMWH on venous thromboembolism after hip replacement: a non-randomised comparison in the National Joint Registry. J Bone Joint Surg Br. 2011;93(11):1465–70.
128. Patel VP, Walsh M, Sehgal B, Preston C, DeWal H, Di Cesare PE. Factors associated with prolonged wound drainage after primary total hip and knee arthroplasty. J Bone Joint Surg Am. 2007;89(1):33–8.
129. Jensen CD, Steval A, Partington PF, Reed MR, Muller SD. Return to theatre following total hip and knee replacement, before and after the introduction of rivaroxaban: a retrospective cohort study. J Bone Joint Surg Br. 2011;93(1):91–5.
130. Tong D, Theis JC. Antibiotic prophylaxis and invasive dental treatment in prosthetic joint patients. N Z Med J. 2008;121(1280):45–52.
131. Oswald TF, Gould FK. Dental treatment and prosthetic joints: antibiotics are not the answer! J Bone Joint Surg Br. 2008;90(7):825–6. [Comment Editorial].
132. Slover JD, Phillips MS, Iorio R, Bosco J. Is routine antibiotic prophylaxis cost effective for total joint replacement patients? J Arthroplasty. 2015;30(4):543–6.
133. Frampton L. The value of SSI surveillance. Clin Serv J. 2013:43–6. http://www.icnetplc.com/files/icnetplc/case-study/official_copy_-_the_value_of_ssi_surveillance.docx.pdf.

Who Is at Risk for Periprosthetic Joint Infection?

5

Timothy L. Tan, Michael M. Kheir, and Antonia F. Chen

Abstract

Periprosthetic joint infection (PJI) is one of the most devastating complications after total joint arthroplasty (TJA). The number of TJAs and PJIs is increasing annually, and it is crucial for surgeons to reduce the burden of PJI. In order to effectively do this, an understanding of risk factors for developing PJI is critical for patient selection, instituting preventative measures, and performing preoperative medical risk optimization prior to elective surgery. Unfortunately, even with the absence of risk factors, PJI may still occur. The literature regarding PJI continues to evolve and hundreds of studies and several PJI risk calculators have been generated in the last decade. As we identify new risk factors and enhance our understanding of PJI, it will become increasingly important for surgeons to be cognizant of these risk factors and institute methods to modify them. This chapter aims to succinctly review the current literature regarding preoperative risk factors, including both patient-related risk factors, such as comorbidities and demographics, and surgical factors.

Keywords

Periprosthetic joint infection • Risk factors • Total knee arthroplasty • Total hip arthroplasty • Complications

T.L. Tan, MD • M.M. Kheir, BS
Department of Orthopaedic Surgery, The Rothman Institute of Orthopaedics, Thomas Jefferson University Hospital, Philadelphia, PA, USA
e-mail: timtan00@gmail.com; mikemkheir@gmail.com

A.F. Chen, MD, MBA (✉)
Department of Orthopaedic Surgery, The Rothman Institute of Orthopaedics, Thomas Jefferson University Hospital, 925 Chestnut St., Philadelphia, PA 19107, USA
e-mail: antonia.chen@rothmaninstitute.com

D. Kendoff et al. (eds.), *Periprosthetic Joint Infections: Changing Paradigms*,
DOI 10.1007/978-3-319-30091-7_5

Introduction

The number of patients who receive a total joint arthroplasty (TJA) is growing annually (Fig. 5.1) [1], and now comprises a large population of patients over a broad spectrum of ages. This has led to a surge in both the number and complexity of periprosthetic joint infections (PJIs), a dreaded and costly complication of TJA [2–4]. The burden on the patient and surgeon often includes difficulty diagnosing PJI, variable presentation of PJI post-arthroplasty, and multiple surgical interventions to effectively treat it. Furthermore, PJI places a large economic burden on the institution due to increased need for revision surgeries, as well as insufficient reimbursement for the treatment of these patients. With interest in alleviating the burden of PJI, many studies have been conducted to identify patients who are at greatest risk for developing PJI (Fig. 5.2), based on comorbidities, previous surgeries, and demographic variables (Table 5.1). Understanding the risk factors, especially modifiable risk factors, associated with PJI are essential for patient selection, medical optimization, and prevention of future PJI. Furthermore, preoperative identification of patients at risk for developing PJI is imperative for developing prophylactic strategies that will specifically target these patients.

Because PJI is a relatively uncommon event, large sample sizes are needed to accurately assess the risk factors of PJI. Furthermore, there is considerable overlap in the comorbidities and variability in the literature regarding the definition of PJI, which makes it even more difficult to evaluate risk factors. Thus, this chapter aims to

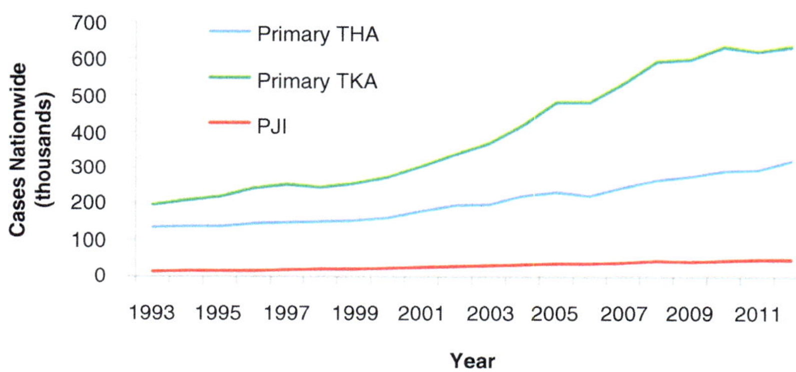

Fig. 5.1 Increasing number of primary TJAs and PJIs obtained from the Healthcare Utilization Project Database [1]

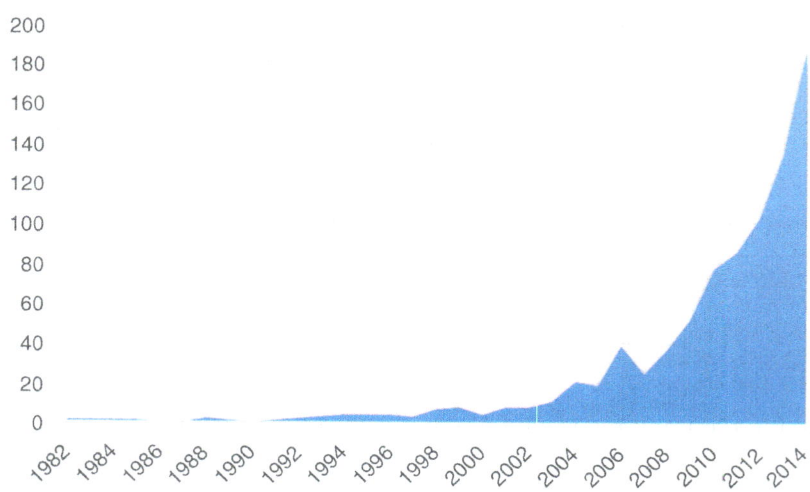

Fig. 5.2 Increasing number of PubMed publications that study PJI each year

Table 5.1 Existing PJI risk calculators

	Bilimoria et al.	Bozic et al.	Berbari et al.
Database	NSQIP	Medicare	Institutional
Number of patients	1414006 (not specific to TJA)	53242	678 TJAs
Components:			
Demographic factors	Age	Age	Female Sex
	Gender	Race	BMI
	Functional status	Height	
		Weight	
		Gender	
		Insurance	
Surgical factors	Emergency case	Operation type (THA or TKA)	Prior operation
	ASA class		Prior arthroplasty
	Wound class		Procedure time
Comorbidities	Steroid use	Alcoholic abuse	Diabetes
	Ascites	Anemia	Immunosuppression
	Systemic sepsis	Cardiac arrhythmia	ASA score
	Ventilator dependence	Cerebrovascular disease	Antibiotic prophylaxis
	Disseminated cancer	COPD	Urinary tract infection
	Diabetes	Chronic liver disease	
	Hypertension	Coagulopathy	
	Previous cardiac event	Congestive heart failure	
	Congestive heart failure	Dementia	
	Dyspnea	Depression	
	Current smoker	Diabetes	
	COPD	Drug Abuse	
	Acute renal failure	Electrolyte disorder	
	BMI	Hemiplegia	
		HIV	
		Hypercholesterolemia	
		Hypertension	
		Ischemic heart disease	
		Lymphoma	
		Malignancy	
		Metastatic Disease	
		Obesity	
		Peptic ulcer disease	
		Peripheral vascular disease	
		Renal disease	
		Rheumatologic disease	
		Urinary tract infection	
		Valvular disease	
		Weight loss	

summarize the accepted risk factors of PJI based on the International Consensus Group definition of PJI [5] and new risk factors and evidence that have been revealed since then. Given the vast number of potential risk factors that exist, we will highlight only preoperative patient-related risk factors and comorbidities. A discussion of risk calculators used as predictive models for PJI will follow.

Review of Individual Factors

In a recent International Consensus Meeting on PJI [5], a committee of orthopaedic infection specialists reached a consensus that the following risk factors for surgical site infection (SSI) and PJI include: history of surgery, poorly controlled diabetes mellitus (glucose >200 mg/L or HbA1C >7 %), malnutrition, morbid obesity (body mass index [BMI] >40 kg/m^2), active liver disease, chronic renal disease, excessive smoking and alcohol consumption, intravenous drug abuse, recent hospitalization, extended stay in a rehabilitation facility, male gender, diagnosis of post-traumatic arthritis, inflammatory arthropathy, prior surgical procedure in the affected joint, and severe immunodeficiency [5]. Since the consensus meeting in 2013, several studies have expanded on this list and have revealed several other contributing factors [6–28]. We will elaborate on the various modifiable (obesity, smoking, alcohol) and non-modifiable (age, gender, race) risk factors and the evidence supporting their association with PJI.

Patient-Related Risk Factors

Obesity

Many studies have demonstrated the influence of obesity ($BMI \geq 30$ kg/m^2) and morbid obesity ($BMI \geq 40$ kg/m^2) on both the rate of complications and the risk of infection [23, 29–33]. In fact, obesity is one of the most universally agreed upon risk factors for infection [5]. While obesity has several associated conditions that may increase the risk of PJI such as diabetes, hypothyroidism, and malnutrition, several studies have demonstrated obesity to be an independent risk factor. Furthermore, this increased risk may also be due to an increase in operative time and a greater need for allogeneic blood transfusions [34]. Obese patients are at an increased risk of wound complications due to poor wound healing and wound dehiscence, which further magnifies the risk. Furthermore, due to increased BMI in these larger patients, prophylactic antibiotics may also be underdosed in this population, which may further augment this risk.

It has been estimated that more than 60 million adults in the United States are classified as obese, representing over one-third of Americans. As the number of obese patients in our country increases [35], the morbidly obese patients we encounter will also likely increase [36] Several recent studies have investigated the outcomes of the morbidly obese and super obese ($BMI \geq 50$ kg/m^2) population with all studies consistently revealing that this population has an increased susceptibility to complications, particularly infection [19, 23, 30, 32]. Jamsem et al. demonstrated that the odds of developing PJI increased to 1.76 (95 % CI: 0.56–5.56) in patients with a BMI between 30 kg/m^2 and 34 kg/m^2, and jumped to 6.41 (95 % CI: 1.67–24.59) in morbidly obese patients [33]. However, the option of optimizing the patient's weight prior to arthroplasty still requires investigation due to conflicting reports in the literature showing that malnutrition can occur in patients who undergo rapid weight loss [10, 11]. Overall, surgeons should be aware of this risk when carefully weighing the risk-benefit analysis of the obese population.

Smoking

Tobacco use is associated with an increased rate of complications and mortality following total hip arthroplasty (THA). Smoking has been linked with an increased risk of infection. Singh et al. found that current smokers undergoing TJA were at an increased risk of developing SSI compared with patients who have never smoked (OR 1.41,

95 % CI: 1.16–1.72) [37]. Similarly, Everhart demonstrated that tobacco abuse was a significant independent risk factor (OR, 2.96; 85 % CI: 1.65–5.11) in a cohort of 1846 TJAs [31]. In addition to infection, smoking has been associated with increased operative time, higher risk of readmission, increased wound complications that may originate from poor tissue oxygenation, and decreased overall implant survivorship, particularly due to aseptic loosening [38, 39]. In a meta-analysis of 21 studies, current smokers demonstrated an increased risk of postoperative complications (RR 1.24, 95 % CI: 1.01–1.54) and death (RR 1.63, 95 % CI: 1.06–2.51) compared to never-smokers [37]. Former smokers had an increased risk of postoperative complications (RR 1.32, 95 % CI: 1.05–1.66) and mortality (RR 1.69, 9 %% CI: 1.08–2.64) when compared to never-smokers.

Several studies have investigated smoking cessation prior to elective surgery and show a reduction in postoperative complications [40–42]. In a randomized controlled trial, Moller et. al. demonstrated a lower complication rate (18 % vs 52 %) and a shorter length of hospital stay in the smoking intervention group compared with the control group [40]. This reduction was particularly significant among wound-related complications and cardiovascular complications. In addition, a meta-analysis of 6 randomized controlled trials demonstrated that smoking cessation prior to surgery decreased overall complications and wound complications with an RR of 0.76 (95 % CI: 0.69–0.84) and 0.73 (95 % CI: 0.61–0.87), respectively [42]. Surgeons should thus be aware of the increased risk of complications in smokers, including infection, and the potential benefits of smoking cessation.

Alcohol Consumption

In addition to the increased risk of PJI in patients with cirrhosis, alcohol alone significantly increased the risk for postoperative infection. In a nationwide database study, Best et. al. demonstrated that alcohol was associated with an increase in both overall in-hospital complications and acute postoperative infections (OR 15.314, range: 14.66 to 15.97, $p<0.001$) [21]. In addition, the authors found that alcohol abusers were nine times more likely to leave the hospital against medical advice and had overall longer inpatient stays. When stratifying by severity of alcohol misuse using a validated alcohol assessment test, several studies showed that the severity of alcohol misuse is directly associated with an increase in the incidence of SSI and other complications [43, 44]. Furthermore, patients with substance abuse are frequently malnourished and have decreased compliance with treatment.

Because of this increased risk of infection, at least four weeks of alcohol cessation is frequently recommended before elective surgery [5]. While the practice of alcohol cessation and intervention programs has not been well-documented in the orthopaedic literature, the surgical literature outside of orthopaedics has suggested that alcohol cessation may reduce the frequency of complications. For example, Tonnesen et al. found that those who quit drinking for more than one month prior to colorectal surgery developed fewer postoperative complications (31 % vs 74 %, $p=0.02$) than those who continued drinking [45].

Drug Abuse

Patients with intravenous (IV) drug abuse have an increased risk of developing PJI and frequently have comorbid conditions such as HIV that may further compound this risk. Lehman et al. and Haberman et al. found infection rates of 25 % and 28.6 %, respectively [46, 47]. In patients with both IV drug abuse and HIV, the PJI rate was 40 %. These findings were confirmed in a large scale national database study of 117903 TKAs (HR 2.08, 95 % CI: 1.17–3.72) [6]. This evidence has led to a recommendation from the International Consensus Meeting that active IV drug users should not be offered elective arthroplasty.

While active drug abusers should not undergo TJA, determining when to undergo TJA following a period of IV drug abstinence may be more difficult to establish. In patients who report drug abstinence to their physician, 18.5 % of patients were still occasional users [48]. Patients with a declared abstinence of less than one year prior to THA were associated with high recurrence rates and septic failure rates. Thus, Wieser et al. suggest at least a one-year period of abstinence from illicit drugs before proceeding with TJA.

Age

While an increase in age is associated with deterioration in the immune system, the influence of age on development of PJI is not as clear. In a large national database study, Kurtz et al. found that age demonstrated a bimodal distribution for PJI risk with 70 to 74 years having the lowest incidence (0.80, 95 % confidence interval [CI]: 0.65–0.96) and those younger than 45 and older than 85 having the highest incidence (1.25, 95 % CI: 0.86–1.65 and 1.01, 95 % CI: 0.69–1.34, respectively) [4]. This bimodal distribution was also confirmed in a large statewide database study. Soohoo et al. demonstrated that patients between 65 and 75 years old had the lowest infection rates while patients older than 75 (odds ratio [OR] 1.28, 95 % CI: 1.09–1.51) and younger than 55 (OR 1.34, 95 % CI: 1.05–1.72) were at an increased risk [49]. In that same database, Meehan et al. found that the risk-adjusted rate of PJI was 1.8 times higher in patients younger than 50 compared with patients 65 years of age or older (95 % CI: 1.33–2.47) [14]. This high prevalence in younger arthroplasty patients may be due to a greater burden of certain comorbid medical conditions such as human immunodeficiency virus (HIV) and hemoglobinopathies that may increase the risk of infection. Several studies have demonstrated that elderly age increases the risk of infection [4, 20, 50, 51], while others have demonstrated no difference [52, 53]. This may occur because of selection bias, as more meticulous medical optimization of elderly patients may be undertaken, especially given the elective nature of TJA. Thus, while there appears to be an association between both youth and older age with PJI, there are many potential confounders that are difficult to account for. Additional studies are needed to explore the mechanism of age with PJI, particularly in younger age groups.

Gender

Hormones and chromosome content have been demonstrated to modulate both the innate and adaptive immune system [25, 54]. Furthermore, there are documented differences in the skin and subcutaneous fat distribution [55, 56] that may account for some of the differences in the PJI rate between males and females. The majority of studies, including our own institutional experience, have demonstrated that males are at an increased susceptibility for PJI. In a large nationwide database representing 10 % of hospital admissions, the PJI rate was 0.81 % (95 % CI: 0.66–0.96) in females and 1.01 % (95 % CI: 0.81–1.22) in males [4]. Bozic et al. demonstrated that female gender was associated with a decreased risk of developing PJI (hazard ratio [HR]=0.55, 95 % CI: 0.30–0.991) [6]. However, while male gender appears to be associated with an increase in the risk of developing PJI, Lubekke revealed that obesity contributes to an elevated risk of PJI in women (relative risk [RR] 16.1, 95 % CI: 3.4–75.7) [57]. This difference was not found in obese and non-obese males. Despite studies demonstrating gender-dependent differences in PJI, other studies have not found any differences in the PJI rate between males and females [29, 50, 51]. Thus, some may not consider male gender a risk factor even though an expert international consensus panel [5] supports male gender as a non-modifiable risk factor for PJI.

Race

Racial disparities in socioeconomic status and immune function [58–61] may influence the differential rate of infection and sepsis across several fields [62–65]. Several studies have demonstrated that complications, including infection, are higher among non-white racial groups [29, 49, 66, 67]. However, the majority of these studies have few patients in the non-white group, and understanding the influence of race on infrequent complications, such as PJI, is difficult. Furthermore, different races were demonstrated to be at different risks for high-risk comorbidities associated with infection. For example, it is well-documented that Native Americans are at an increased risk of developing diabetes and obesity [68, 69]. Additionally, the underlying etiology for TJA may be influenced by race and may thus result in differences in arthroplasty utilization. For example, African Americans are more likely to have sickle cell disease, which is associated with osteonecrosis. Because of these confounding factors, the evidence behind the increased risk of PJI in the non-white population should be interpreted carefully.

Comorbidities

Diabetes Mellitus and Hyperglycemia

Diabetes is associated with an assortment of risk factors for infection and generalized impairment of the immune system, including deficiencies in phagocytosis and neutrophil and lymphocyte dysfunction. The link between hyperglycemia and PJI has been well-established [5, 33]. Dowsey et al. [70] demonstrated an independent OR of 6.87 (95 % CI: 2.42–19.56), while Medicare studies have revealed a crude RR of 1.28 (95 % CI: 1.17–1.40) for total knee arthroplasty (TKA) and 1.36 (95 % CI: 1.27–1.68) for THA [71, 72]. While it is established that diabetes leads to an increased risk of PJI, the influence of the specific characteristics of diabetes is less clear. Several studies have demonstrated that patients with insulin-dependent diabetes (Type 1) are at an increased risk compared with non-insulin-dependent diabetes (Type 2), even though both disease types subject the patient to an increased risk compared to non-diabetics [12, 73, 74]. Using the National Surgical Quality Improvement Program (NSQIP) database, the OR of developing PJI was 1.6 (95 % CI: 1.2–2.0; $p<0.001$) for insulin-dependent diabetics and 1.2 (95 % CI: 1.1–1.4; $p<0.001$) for non-insulin-dependent diabetics when compared with non-diabetics [12].

Furthermore, there is wide variability regarding the optimal lab marker of preoperative glucose level or hemoglobin A1c for predicting complications and PJIs among diabetic TJA candidates. Higher perioperative glucose levels have been associated with an increased risk of PJI. Jamsem et al. demonstrated that patients with higher preoperative glucose levels who underwent TKA were at increased risk for developing PJI [75]. Patients with preoperative blood glucose levels greater than 124 mg/dL demonstrated a 3.3 times increased odds of infection compared with those less than this threshold. Furthermore, Mraovic et. al. demonstrated that PJI patients had higher preoperative and postoperative glucose levels than those without PJI [76]. The authors found that even non-diabetic patients were three times more likely to develop PJI if the postoperative day one glucose levels were high (greater than 140 mg/dL).

However, because glucose levels represent only a single point in time rather than an average, glycosylated hemoglobin A1c levels are frequently used because it represents a three month average of sugar levels. Despite reflecting a longer glycemic control timeframe, Iorio et al., Maradit Kremers et al., and Chrastil et al. found that hemoglobin A1C levels did not correlate with PJI; however, the latter study identified preoperative glucose levels as a much better predictor and suggests targeting this rather than A1c for PJI prevention [53, 57, 58]. However, Harris et. al. was able to demonstrate a relationship between hemoglobin A1c levels and complications and found that the rate of PJI increased linearly rather than surging at a certain threshold [77]. Despite the overwhelming lack of a clear cut-off or optimal preoperative laboratory predictor, almost all studies highlight the importance of glycemic control. Furthermore, the presence of diabetic complications, frequently defined as end-organ damage, has also been demonstrated to influence the risk of PJI. Soohoo et al. found that both uncomplicated and complicated diabetes increased the risk of acute onset PJI by 1.7 (95 % CI: 1.42–2.08) and 3.7 (95 % CI: 2.39–5.74) times, respectively [49].

Malnutrition

Malnutrition has a high prevalence in the arthroplasty population and is frequently comorbid with obesity and diabetes. Several studies have implicated malnutrition as an independent risk factor for PJI. Yi et al. demonstrated that patients with laboratory values suggestive of malnutrition (lymphocyte count <1500 mm^3, serum albumin <3.5 g/dL, or serum transferrin <200 mg/dL) were independently associated with both chronic PJI (OR 2.1, p=0.003) and acute PJI (OR 5.9, p=0.02) following revision TJA. Furthermore, high frequencies of abnormal nutritional parameters were found in both normal and obese patients. Normal-weight patients had a higher frequency of at least one abnormal laboratory value compared with obese patients (51 % vs 32 %, p=0.002). Peersman et. al. revealed that malnutrition increased the risk of PJI in a retrospective review of 6489 TKAs [78]. Font-Vizcarra et al. prospectively investigated 213 patients undergoing TKA and found that malnutrition, as assessed by smaller triceps skin fold levels, was independently associated with PJI; a measurement of 30 mm was associated with a 5 % risk and a 20-mm measurement was associated with a 10 % infection risk [79]. Additionally, Mednick et al. demonstrated that a high preoperative serum albumin level was independently associated with a lower risk for the need for readmission (OR 0.688, 95 % CI: 0.477–0.992) [13].

Rheumatoid Arthritis and Immunosuppression

TJA candidates are frequently immunosuppressed for a variety of reasons, such as osteonecrosis secondary to chronic steroid use, solid organ transplant recipients receiving anti-rejection medications, or patients on disease modifying agents for rheumatologic diseases. While there is difficulty assessing the risk of immunosuppression, as well as a high variability in its definition, most surgeons agree that immunosuppression is a risk factor for developing PJI [5]. Peersman et. al. found immunosuppression to be an important risk factor for SSI in a retrospective review of 6489 TKAs [58]. Furthermore, Berbari et al. found immunosuppression to be a significant contributor (HR 1.96, 95 % CI: 1.4–2.8) to the risk of PJI in their risk model [80].

Several studies have demonstrated that systemic corticosteroid use increases the risk of PJI. Somajaykji et al. found that patients receiving prednisone doses greater than 15 mg/kg a day increased the odds of infection by 21 times (95 % CI: 3.5–127.2) [81]. Additionally, Mednick et al. demonstrated that preoperative corticosteroid use was independently associated with a higher likelihood of hospital readmission (OR 2.928, 95 % CI: 1.731 to 4.953; p<0.001) [13].

In addition to immunosuppression, autoimmune conditions often result in immune dysregulation, which may predispose patients to infection. Rheumatoid arthritis patients have an increased risk of PJI compared to patients undergoing TJA for osteoarthritis, presumably secondary to the use of disease-modifying antirheumatic drugs. In the first year after surgery, rheumatoid arthritis patients have a higher risk of infection compared to osteoarthritis patients, as Jamsem et al. [82] demonstrated an adjusted HR of 1.86 (95 % CI: 1.31–2.63) while Bomgartz [83] demonstrated a 10.3 (95 % CI: 1.31–80.26) times increased odds of infection.

Human Immunodeficiency Virus and Acquired Immunodeficiency Virus

HIV patients frequently require TJA secondary to osteonecrosis. As life expectancy increases due to recent developments in drug therapies, there will continue to be an increase in HIV patients undergoing TJA. Given the severe immune deficits of this disease, HIV has been strongly associated with PJI, despite small sample sizes due to the relative infrequency of this disease. In a large nationwide database of 9275 HIV patients undergoing TJA, there was an increased rate of major complications (OR 1.47, 95 % CI: 1.08–2.00) and wound infections (OR 2.38, 95 % CI: 1.32–4.30) in HIV patients [27]. Capogna et al.

demonstrated that HIV patients were at a 6.2 times increased odds of developing infection [84]. While the rate of PJI has been reported as high as 18.7 % for primary and 36.3 % for revision TJAs, Hicks et al. demonstrated that good survivorship and durable pain relief may still be achievable [85]. Thus, it is important to perform a thorough risk-benefit analysis and optimize HIV patients prior to TJA, in close collaboration with an infectious disease specialist.

It is recommended that suitable candidates for TJA are patients who have a CD4 count greater than 400 cells/ml and with undetectable viral loads. In a study of 31 TJAs in HIV patients, Falakassa suggests that well-controlled HIV patients on highly active antiretroviral therapy with undetectable viral loads and CD4 > 200 possess a risk of developing PJI equivalent to that of the non-HIV population [9]. Future studies with larger cohorts are needed to better elucidate the optimal CD4 thresholds prior to undergoing elective TJA in this group of patients.

Native Septic Joint Arthritis

Prior or current septic arthritis is challenging for the treating orthopaedic surgeon due to extensive bone loss, soft tissue scarring, and increased infection risk. Because of the overall rarity of native septic arthritis, there is little literature regarding the outcomes of these patients. However, the few studies that do exist suggest an increased frequency of complications following TJA, particularly infection, among this patient population. Jerry et al. found an infection rate of 7.7 % in TKA [86]. In THAs after native septic arthritis, Chen et al. [87] demonstrated an infection rate of 14 %, while Jupiter et al. [88] determined a rate of 7.0 %. In addition, Cherney et. al. found that patients undergoing THA with a previous infection without any prosthesis had a failure rate of 37 % [89].

In patients who underwent THA and who had a history of childhood septic hip arthritis, Kim et al. found that all hips with a quiescent period of more than 10 years had no recurrence of infection, while two hips in one patient with a quiescent period of seven years had infection recurrence [90]. However, deferring arthroplasty for such an extensive time is often impractical and the potential benefits of undergoing TJA may far outweigh the increased potential risks. Although the role of inflammatory markers such as erythrocyte sedimentation rate and C-reactive protein remains relatively unknown, the surgeon must ensure that there is no evidence of active infection by performing preoperative aspiration and obtaining cultures. Furthermore, antibiotic laden cement should be used in TJAs containing cement [5]. Future studies are clearly needed to determine the optimal timing of elective TJA following septic arthritis and to elucidate the specific characteristics of septic arthritis that may increase the risk of PJI.

Prior Surgical History and Revision Arthroplasty

A prior surgical procedure has been demonstrated to be an important risk factor for PJI [78]. Although there is scarce literature investigating the association between prior surgery and the development of PJI, revision arthroplasty has been consistently reported to increase the risk of PJI. Everhart et al. and Berbari et al. determined that revision surgery increased the odds of infection by 2.28 (95 % CI: 1.26–3.98) and 2.0 (95 % CI: 1.4–3.0) times, respectively [31, 80]. This may be attributable to prolonged operative time, increased need for transfusion, more frequent wound complications, and higher comorbidities in revision arthroplasty patients. However, even when accounting for these factors, patients with revision surgery remain at an increased risk [80].

Renal Disease

Chronic renal disease has an estimated prevalence of 35 % in diabetics and greater than 40 % in individuals over 60 years of age [91]. Patients with renal disease frequently have several comorbid conditions that may further increase the risk of PJI, such as diabetes or lupus. Several studies have demonstrated that patients with active renal disease, transplantation, and hemodialysis are associated with an increased risk of overall complications, particularly PJI. In Medicare studies, Bozic et al. demonstrated that the relative risk for PJI and 90-day mortality was 1.45 and 3.35 times for THA and 1.46 and 3.80 times in TKA patients, respectively [71, 72]. In patients receiving hemodialysis for end-stage renal disease, Sunday et al. [71] reported a high rate of mortality and infection; 29 % of the patients died from in-hospital complications and 14.5 % died due to sepsis [92]. Sakalkale et al. and Lieberman et al. demonstrated elevated deep infection rates of 13 % and 19 %, respectively [93, 94]. End-stage renal disease is often treated definitively with kidney transplantation, which may pose an even increased risk due to the requirement of immunosuppressive medications. In a large-scale national database, Cavanaugh et al. demonstrated that kidney transplantation increased the risk of SSIs and wound infections, as well as systemic infection, with an adjusted OR of 2.03 and 2.85, respectively [7]. Additionally, patients on dialysis (8.03 %, RR 3.99, $p<0.001$) and with renal transplants (9.09 %, RR 4.517, $p=0.027$) demonstrated an increased risk of developing late infection [95].

Despite the literature supporting renal disease as a significant risk factor for PJI, very few studies have been able to establish a relationship between the severity of kidney disease and PJI [8, 15]. This is significant because the majority of the literature is limited to end-stage renal disease and thus may not account for milder disease. Future studies are needed to determine the relationship and optimal thresholds to assess PJI risk by renal disease severity.

Liver Disease

Recently, several studies have elucidated the role of liver disease in the development of PJI, particularly cirrhosis and hepatitis. Jiang et al. demonstrated that PJIs occurred more frequently in TKA patients with cirrhosis (2.7 % vs 0.8 %; HR 3.4; $p<0.001$) [96]. Cirrhotic patients were also more likely to undergo irrigation and debridement (THA: HR 2.7, TKA: HR 2.5) or resection arthroplasty (THA: HR 5.9, TKA 2.9) than non-cirrhotic patients. While Tiberri et al. [18] and Deleurman et al. [24] found that cirrhosis was a significant risk factor for diabetes, Bozic et al. could not find an association among patients with chronic liver disease in the Medicare population for both TKA (HR 1.08, 95 % CI: 0.84–1.39, $p=0.5285$) and THA (HR 1.02, 95 % CI: 0.69–1.50, $p=0.9333$) [71, 72]. Patients with liver transplant also have an increased risk of developing PJI due to the need for immunosuppressive therapy [7]; Cavanaugh et al. demonstrated an OR of 2.32 in a large nationwide inpatient sample.

Risk Calculators

Several studies have endeavored to develop predictive models that can be tailored to the specific demographics and medical characteristics of each patient (Table 5.1) [80, 97, 98]. Bozic et al. [97] created a risk scoring system that was developed from patients in the Medicare population who were older than 65 years, which was converted into an electronic Smartphone app that was primarily based on comorbidities (29 Elixhauser comorbidities) [99]. Bilimoria et al. created an electronic application to predict surgical complications and SSI based on demographic and surgery-related factors [93]. The risk calculator was based on the National Surgical Quality Improvement Program (NSQIP) database, which included 90-day follow-up for a variety of surgical procedures. However, because the measured variables had to be applicable to general surgery procedures as well, the measured variables did not include specific arthroplasty-related variables such as revision arthroplasty.

Berbari et al. created an institutional model based on 301 PJIs and 316 TJAs as controls that included both preoperative and perioperative variables [80]. Male sex, diabetes, prior operations, previous TJAs, immunosuppression, American Society of Anesthesiologists score, antibiotic prophylaxis, urinary tract infection, and procedure time were all determined to be independent risk factors for infection and were included in the final model.

However, despite the number of currently available predictive models that are primarily based on nationwide databases, there is no universal preoperative risk predictor for PJI that is used in the orthopaedic community. This may be attributable to the limitations of the current models, including the use of a specific population set such as Medicare patients who are older than 65 years old, lack of stratification by procedure, short follow-up time, limited patient-reported information, or a limited patient sample. Therefore, we developed a preoperative risk calculator based on our institutional database of 27117 patients who underwent TJA to identify the at-risk population for PJI and *Staphylococcus aureus* PJI. Our model determined that the significant contributing demographic and surgical factors were BMI, male gender, government insurance (Medicaid, Tricare, and Medicare), revision surgery, knee surgery, and history of orthopaedic surgery. Several comorbidities (Table 5.2) in order of decreasing relative contribution included: drug abuse, coagulopathy, renal failure, psychoses, congestive heart failure, rheumatologic disease, diabetes mellitus, and iron deficiency anemia. While we attempted to create a risk calculator to identify patients at an increased risk of PJI, future studies are needed to discover and implement strategies to prevent PJI in high-risk candidates.

Table 5.2 PJI risk factors at our institution

Comorbidity	Odds ratio	95 % confidence interval
Diabetes	2.00	1.71–2.32
Renal disease	4.63	3.50–6.04
Rheumatic disease	2.41	1.87–3.06
Metastatic	3.85	1.68–7.83
AIDS	6.57	3.53–11.54
Liver disease	3.07	1.91–4.72
Pulmonary circulation disease	1.60	0.95–2.55
Obesity	1.49	1.24–1.79
Weight loss	10.90	4.64–23.70
Electrolyte/fluid	2.81	2.10–3.70
Iron deficiency anemia	1.74	1.48–2.05
Alcohol abuse	2.33	1.13–4.34
Drug abuse	6.53	2.76–13.86
Psychoses	3.18	2.02–4.81
Depression	1.50	1.24–1.81
Smoker	1.43	1.15–1.76

Conclusion

Considerable efforts have been invested into identifying both modifiable and non-modifiable risk factors for PJI. It is crucial that we use this knowledge in the selection and education of patients given the potentially shattering effect PJI has on our patients' quality of life, satisfaction, and overall health. Despite our efforts, we have a poor understanding of several current risk factors; and furthermore, many risk factors likely exist that have yet to be revealed. It is even more crucial to apply our awareness of risk factors into instituting preventative measures in high-risk candidates. Likewise, it is important for the surgeon to continuously work closely with interdisciplinary medical specialists to reduce the risk of PJI after TJA as much as possible. Continued efforts are certainly needed to find novel and effective solutions to minimize the burden of one of the most devastating complications in orthopaedics.

References

1. National HCUP Databases [Internet]. [cited 2015 Mar 15]. Available from: https://www.hcup-us.ahrq.gov/databases.jsp.
2. Kurtz S, Ong K, Lau E, Mowat F, Halpern M. Projections of primary and revision hip and knee arthroplasty in the United States from 2005 to 2030. J Bone Joint Surg Am. 2007;89(4):780–5.
3. Kurtz SM, Lau E, Watson H, Schmier JK, Parvizi J. Economic burden of periprosthetic joint infection in the United States. J Arthroplasty. 2012;27(8 Suppl):61–5.e1.
4. Kurtz SM, Lau E, Schmier J, Ong KL, Zhao K, Parvizi J. Infection burden for hip and knee arthroplasty in the United States. J Arthroplasty. 2008;23(7):984–91.
5. Aggarwal VK, Tischler EH, Lautenbach C, Williams GR, Abboud JA, Altena M, et al. Mitigation and education. J Arthroplasty. 2014;29(2 Suppl):19–25.
6. Bozic KJ, Ward DT, Lau EC, Chan V, Wetters NG, Naziri Q, et al. Risk factors for periprosthetic joint

infection following primary total hip arthroplasty: a case control study. J Arthroplasty. 2014;29(1):154–6.
7. Cavanaugh PK, Chen AF, Rasouli MR, Post ZD, Orozco FR, Ong AC. Total joint arthroplasty in transplant recipients: in-hospital adverse outcomes. J Arthroplasty. 2014;5.
8. Deegan BF, Richard RD, Bowen TR, Perkins RM, Graham JH, Foltzer MA. Impact of chronic kidney disease stage on lower-extremity arthroplasty. Orthopedics. 2014;37(7):e613–8.
9. Falakassa J, Diaz A, Schneiderbauer M. Outcomes of total joint arthroplasty in HIV patients. Iowa Orthop J. 2014;34:102–6.
10. Inacio MCS, Kritz-Silverstein D, Raman R, Macera CA, Nichols JF, Shaffer RA, et al. The impact of preoperative weight loss on incidence of surgical site infection and readmission rates after total joint arthroplastyrrr. J Arthroplasty. 2014;29(3):458–64.e1.
11. Inacio MCS, Paxton EW, Fisher D, Li RA, Barber TC, Singh JA. Bariatric surgery prior to total joint arthroplasty may not provide dramatic improvements in post-arthroplasty surgical outcomes. J Arthroplasty. 2014;29(7):1359–64.
12. Lovecchio F, Beal M, Kwasny M, Manning D. Do patients with insulin-dependent and noninsulin-dependent diabetes have different risks for complications after arthroplasty? Clin Orthop. 2014;472(11):3570–5.
13. Mednick RE, Alvi HM, Krishnan V, Lovecchio F, Manning DW. Factors affecting readmission rates following primary total hip arthroplasty. J Bone Joint Surg Am. 2014;96(14):1201–9.
14. Meehan JP, Danielsen B, Kim SH, Jamali AA, White RH. Younger age is associated with a higher risk of early periprosthetic joint infection and aseptic mechanical failure after total knee arthroplasty. J Bone Joint Surg Am. 2014;96(7):529–35.
15. Miric A, Inacio MCS, Namba RS. The effect of chronic kidney disease on total hip arthroplasty. J Arthroplasty. 2014;29(6):1225–30.
16. Pulos N, McGraw MH, Courtney PM, Lee G-C. Revision THA in obese patients is associated with high re-operation rates at short-term follow-up. J Arthroplasty. 2014;29(9 Suppl):209–13.
17. Ravi B, Croxford R, Hollands S, Paterson JM, Bogoch E, Kreder H, et al. Increased risk of complications following total joint arthroplasty in patients with rheumatoid arthritis. Arthritis Rheumatol Hoboken NJ. 2014;66(2):254–63.
18. Tiberi JV, Hansen V, El-Abbadi N, Bedair H. Increased complication rates after hip and knee arthroplasty in patients with cirrhosis of the liver. Clin Orthop. 2014;472(9):2774–8.
19. Werner BC, Evans CL, Carothers JT, Browne JA. Primary total knee arthroplasty in super-obese patients: dramatically higher postoperative complication rates even compared to revision surgery. J Arthroplasty. 2014;19.
20. Wu C, Qu X, Liu F, Li H, Mao Y, Zhu Z. Risk factors for periprosthetic joint infection after total hip arthroplasty and total knee arthroplasty in Chinese patients. PLoS One. 2014;9(4), e95300.
21. Best MJ, Buller LT, Gosthe RG, Klika AK, Barsoum WK. Alcohol misuse is an independent risk factor for poorer postoperative outcomes following primary total hip and total knee arthroplasty. J Arthroplasty. 2015;30:1293–8.
22. Chrastil J, Anderson MB, Stevens V, Anand R, Peters CL, Pelt CE. Is hemoglobin a1c or perioperative hyperglycemia predictive of periprosthetic joint infection or death following primary total joint arthroplasty? J Arthroplasty. 2015;30:1197–202.
23. D'Apuzzo MR, Novicoff WM, Browne JA. The John Insall Award: Morbid obesity independently impacts complications, mortality, and resource use after TKA. Clin Orthop. 2015;473(1):57–63.
24. Deleuran T, Vilstrup H, Overgaard S, Jepsen P. Cirrhosis patients have increased risk of complications after hip or knee arthroplasty. Acta Orthop. 2015;86(1):108–13.
25. Giefing-Kröll C, Berger P, Lepperdinger G, Grubeck-Loebenstein B. How sex and age affect immune responses, susceptibility to infections, and response to vaccination. Aging Cell. 2015;26.
26. Maradit Kremers H, Lewallen LW, Mabry TM, Berry DJ, Berbari EF, Osmon DR. Diabetes mellitus, hyperglycemia, hemoglobin A1C and the risk of prosthetic joint infections in total hip and knee arthroplasty. J Arthroplasty. 2015;30(3):439–43.
27. Naziri Q, Boylan MR, Issa K, Jones LC, Khanuja HS, Mont MA. Does HIV infection increase the risk of perioperative complications after THA? A nationwide database study. Clin Orthop. 2015;473(2):581–6.
28. Yi PH, Frank RM, Vann E, Sonn KA, Moric M, Della Valle CJ. Is potential malnutrition associated with septic failure and acute infection after revision total joint arthroplasty? Clin Orthop. 2015;473(1):175–82.
29. SooHoo NF, Lieberman JR, Ko CY, Zingmond DS. Factors predicting complication rates following total knee replacement. J Bone Joint Surg Am. 2006;88(3):480–5.
30. McCalden RW, Charron KD, MacDonald SJ, Bourne RB, Naudie DD. Does morbid obesity affect the outcome of total hip replacement?: an analysis of 3290 THRs. J Bone Joint Surg Br. 2011;93(3):321–5.
31. Everhart JS, Altneu E, Calhoun JH. Medical comorbidities are independent preoperative risk factors for surgical infection after total joint arthroplasty. Clin Orthop. 2013;471(10):3112–9.
32. Chee YH, Teoh KH, Sabnis BM, Ballantyne JA, Brenkel IJ. Total hip replacement in morbidly obese patients with osteoarthritis: results of a prospectively matched study. J Bone Joint Surg Br. 2010;92(8):1066–71.
33. Jämsen E, Nevalainen P, Eskelinen A, Huotari K, Kalliovalkama J, Moilanen T. Obesity, diabetes, and preoperative hyperglycemia as predictors of periprosthetic joint infection: a single-center analysis of 7181 primary hip and knee replacements for osteoarthritis. J Bone Joint Surg Am. 2012;94(14), e101.

34. Jibodh SR, Gurkan I, Wenz JF. In-hospital outcome and resource use in hip arthroplasty: influence of body mass. Orthopedics. 2004;27(6):594–601.
35. Ogden CL, Carroll MD, Kit BK, Flegal KM. Prevalence of childhood and adult obesity in the United States, 2011–2012. JAMA. 2014;311(8):806–14.
36. Ogden CL, Carroll MD, Curtin LR, McDowell MA, Tabak CJ, Flegal KM. Prevalence of overweight and obesity in the United States, 1999–2004. JAMA. 2006;295(13):1549–55.
37. Singh JA, Houston TK, Ponce BA, Maddox G, Bishop MJ, Richman J, et al. Smoking as a risk factor for short-term outcomes following primary total hip and total knee replacement in veterans. Arthritis Care Res. 2011;63(10):1365–74.
38. Meldrum RD, Wurtz LD, Feinberg JR, Capello WN. Does smoking affect implant survivorship in total hip arthroplasty? A preliminary retrospective case series. Iowa Orthop J. 2005;25:17–24.
39. Lombardi AV, Berend KR, Adams JB, Jefferson RC, Sneller MA. Smoking may be a harbinger of early failure with ultraporous metal acetabular reconstruction. Clin Orthop. 2013;471(2):486–97.
40. Møller AM, Villebro N, Pedersen T, Tønnesen H. Effect of preoperative smoking intervention on postoperative complications: a randomised clinical trial. Lancet. 2002;359(9301):114–7.
41. Myers K, Hajek P, Hinds C, McRobbie H. Stopping smoking shortly before surgery and postoperative complications: a systematic review and meta-analysis. Arch Intern Med. 2011;171(11):983–9.
42. Mills E, Eyawo O, Lockhart I, Kelly S, Wu P, Ebbert JO. Smoking cessation reduces postoperative complications: a systematic review and meta-analysis. Am J Med. 2011;124(2):144–54.e8.
43. Bradley KA, Rubinsky AD, Sun H, Bryson CL, Bishop MJ, Blough DK, et al. Alcohol screening and risk of postoperative complications in male VA patients undergoing major non-cardiac surgery. J Gen Intern Med. 2011;26(2):162–9.
44. Harris AHS, Reeder R, Ellerbe L, Bradley KA, Rubinsky AD, Giori NJ. Preoperative alcohol screening scores: association with complications in men undergoing total joint arthroplasty. J Bone Joint Surg Am. 2011;93(4):321–7.
45. Tonnesen H, Rosenberg J, Nielsen HJ, Rasmussen V, Hauge C, Pedersen IK, et al. Effect of preoperative abstinence on poor postoperative outcome in alcohol misusers: randomised controlled trial. BMJ. 1999;318(7194):1311–6.
46. Lehman CR, Ries MD, Paiement GD, Davidson AB. Infection after total joint arthroplasty in patients with human immunodeficiency virus or intravenous drug use. J Arthroplasty. 2001;16(3):330–5.
47. Habermann B, Eberhardt C, Kurth AA. Total joint replacement in HIV positive patients. J Infect. 2008;57(1):41–6.
48. Wieser K, Zingg PO, Betz M, Neubauer G, Dora C. Total hip replacement in patients with history of illicit injecting drug use. Arch Orthop Trauma Surg. 2012;132(7):1037–44.
49. Soohoo NF, Farng E, Lieberman JR, Chambers L, Zingmond DS. Factors that predict short-term complication rates after total hip arthroplasty. Clin Orthop. 2010;468(9):2363–71.
50. Ridgeway S, Wilson J, Charlet A, Kafatos G, Pearson A, Coello R. Infection of the surgical site after arthroplasty of the hip. J Bone Joint Surg Br. 2005;87(6):844–50.
51. Dale H, Skråmm I, Løwer HL, Eriksen HM, Espehaug B, Furnes O, et al. Infection after primary hip arthroplasty: a comparison of 3 Norwegian health registers. Acta Orthop. 2011;82(6):646–54.
52. Robertsson O, Knutson K, Lewold S, Lidgren L. The Swedish Knee Arthroplasty Register 1975–1997: an update with special emphasis on 41,223 knees operated on in 1988–1997. Acta Orthop Scand. 2001;72(5):503–13.
53. Pedersen AB, Svendsson JE, Johnsen SP, Riis A, Overgaard S. Risk factors for revision due to infection after primary total hip arthroplasty. A population-based study of 80,756 primary procedures in the Danish Hip Arthroplasty Registry. Acta Orthop. 2010;81(5):542–7.
54. Trigunaite A, Dimo J, Jørgensen TN. Suppressive effects of androgens on the immune system. Cell Immunol. 2015;294:87–94.
55. Man MQ, Xin SJ, Song SP, Cho SY, Zhang XJ, Tu CX, et al. Variation of skin surface pH, sebum content and stratum corneum hydration with age and gender in a large Chinese population. Skin Pharmacol Physiol. 2009;22(4):190–9.
56. Kim M-K, Patel RA, Shinn AH, Choi S-Y, Byun H-J, Huh C-H, et al. Evaluation of gender difference in skin type and pH. J Dermatol Sci. 2006;41(2):153–6.
57. Lübbeke A, Stern R, Garavaglia G, Zurcher L, Hoffmeyer P. Differences in outcomes of obese women and men undergoing primary total hip arthroplasty. Arthritis Rheum. 2007;57(2):327–34.
58. Insaf TZ, Shaw BA, Yucel RM, Chasan-Taber L, Strogatz DS. Lifecourse Socioeconomic Position and Racial Disparities in BMI Trajectories among Black and White Women: Exploring Cohort Effects in the Americans Changing Lives' Study. J Racial Ethn Health Disparities. 2014;1(4):309–18.
59. Thobakgale CF, Ndung'u T. Neutrophil counts in persons of African origin. Curr Opin Hematol. 2014;21(1):50–7.
60. Azab B, Camacho-Rivera M, Taioli E. Average values and racial differences of neutrophil lymphocyte ratio among a nationally representative sample of United States subjects. PLoS One. 2014;9(11), e112361.
61. Wahaidi VY, Dowsett SA, Eckert GJ, Kowolik MJ. Neutrophil response to dental plaque by gender and race. J Dent Res. 2009;88(8):709–14.
62. Barnato AE, Alexander SL, Linde-Zwirble WT, Angus DC. Racial variation in the incidence, care, and outcomes of severe sepsis: analysis of population,

patient, and hospital characteristics. Am J Respir Crit Care Med. 2008;177(3):279–84.
63. Mayr FB, Yende S, Linde-Zwirble WT, Peck-Palmer OM, Barnato AE, Weissfeld LA, et al. Infection rate and acute organ dysfunction risk as explanations for racial differences in severe sepsis. JAMA. 2010;303(24):2495–503.
64. Dombrovskiy VY, Martin AA, Sunderram J, Paz HL. Occurrence and outcomes of sepsis: influence of race. Crit Care Med. 2007;35(3):763–8.
65. Esper AM, Moss M, Lewis CA, Nisbet R, Mannino DM, Martin GS. The role of infection and comorbidity: Factors that influence disparities in sepsis. Crit Care Med. 2006;34(10):2576–82.
66. Mahomed NN, Barrett J, Katz JN, Baron JA, Wright J, Losina E. Epidemiology of total knee replacement in the United States Medicare population. J Bone Joint Surg Am. 2005;87(6):1222–8.
67. Ibrahim SA, Stone RA, Han X, Cohen P, Fine MJ, Henderson WG, et al. Racial/ethnic differences in surgical outcomes in veterans following knee or hip arthroplasty. Arthritis Rheum. 2005;52(10):3143–51.
68. Hutchinson RN, Shin S. Systematic review of health disparities for cardiovascular diseases and associated factors among American Indian and Alaska Native populations. PLoS One. 2014;9(1), e80973.
69. Story M, Evans M, Fabsitz RR, Clay TE, Holy Rock B, Broussard B. The epidemic of obesity in American Indian communities and the need for childhood obesity-prevention programs. Am J Clin Nutr. 1999;69(4 Suppl):747S–54.
70. Dowsey MM, Choong PFM. Obese diabetic patients are at substantial risk for deep infection after primary TKA. Clin Orthop. 2009;467(6):1577–81.
71. Bozic KJ, Lau E, Kurtz S, Ong K, Rubash H, Vail TP, et al. Patient-related risk factors for periprosthetic joint infection and postoperative mortality following total hip arthroplasty in Medicare patients. J Bone Joint Surg Am. 2012;94(9):794–800.
72. Bozic KJ, Lau E, Kurtz S, Ong K, Berry DJ. Patient-related risk factors for postoperative mortality and periprosthetic joint infection in medicare patients undergoing TKA. Clin Orthop. 2012;470(1):130–7.
73. Meding JB, Reddleman K, Keating ME, Klay A, Ritter MA, Faris PM, et al. Total knee replacement in patients with diabetes mellitus. Clin Orthop. 2003;416:208–16.
74. Iorio R, Williams KM, Marcantonio AJ, Specht LM, Tilzey JF, Healy WL. Diabetes mellitus, hemoglobin A1C, and the incidence of total joint arthroplasty infection. J Arthroplasty. 2012;27(5):726–9.e1.
75. Jämsen E, Nevalainen P, Kalliovalkama J, Moilanen T. Preoperative hyperglycemia predicts infected total knee replacement. Eur J Intern Med. 2010;21(3):196–201.
76. Mraovic B, Suh D, Jacovides C, Parvizi J. Perioperative hyperglycemia and postoperative infection after lower limb arthroplasty. J Diabetes Sci Technol. 2011;5(2):412–8.
77. Harris AHS, Bowe TR, Gupta S, Ellerbe LS, Giori NJ. Hemoglobin A1C as a marker for surgical risk in diabetic patients undergoing total joint arthroplasty. J Arthroplasty. 2013;28(8 Suppl):25–9.
78. Peersman G, Laskin R, Davis J, Peterson M. Infection in total knee replacement: a retrospective review of 6489 total knee replacements. Clin Orthop. 2001;392:15–23.
79. Font-Vizcarra L, Lozano L, Ríos J, Forga MT, Soriano A. Preoperative nutritional status and postoperative infection in total knee replacements: a prospective study of 213 patients. Int J Artif Organs. 2011;34(9):876–81.
80. Berbari EF, Osmon DR, Lahr B, Eckel-Passow JE, Tsaras G, Hanssen AD, et al. The Mayo prosthetic joint infection risk score: implication for surgical site infection reporting and risk stratification. Infect Control Hosp Epidemiol. 2012;33(8):774–81.
81. Somayaji R, Barnabe C, Martin L. Risk factors for infection following total joint arthroplasty in rheumatoid arthritis. Open Rheumatol J. 2013;7:119–24.
82. Jämsen E, Huhtala H, Puolakka T, Moilanen T. Risk factors for infection after knee arthroplasty. A register-based analysis of 43,149 cases. J Bone Joint Surg Am. 2009;91(1):38–47.
83. Bongartz T, Halligan CS, Osmon DR, Reinalda MS, Bamlet WR, Crowson CS, et al. Incidence and risk factors of prosthetic joint infection after total hip or knee replacement in patients with rheumatoid arthritis. Arthritis Rheum. 2008;59(12):1713–20.
84. Capogna BM, Lovy A, Blum Y, Kim SJ, Felsen UR, Geller DS. Infection rate following total joint arthroplasty in the HIV population. J Arthroplasty. 2013;28(8):1254–8.
85. Hicks JL, Ribbans WJ, Buzzard B, Kelley SS, Toft L, Torri G, et al. Infected joint replacements in HIV-positive patients with haemophilia. J Bone Joint Surg Br. 2001;83(7):1050–4.
86. Jerry GJ, Rand JA, Ilstrup D. Old sepsis prior to total knee arthroplasty. Clin Orthop. 1988;236:135–40.
87. Chen C-E, Wang J-W, Juhn R-J. Total hip arthroplasty for primary septic arthritis of the hip in adults. Int Orthop. 2008;32(5):573–80.
88. Jupiter JB, Karchmer AW, Lowell JD, Harris WH. Total hip arthroplasty in the treatment of adult hips with current or quiescent sepsis. J Bone Joint Surg Am. 1981;63(2):194–200.
89. Cherney DL, Amstutz HC. Total hip replacement in the previously septic hip. J Bone Joint Surg Am. 1983;65(9):1256–65.
90. Kim Y-H, Oh S-H, Kim J-S. Total hip arthroplasty in adult patients who had childhood infection of the hip. J Bone Joint Surg Am. 2003;85-A(2):198–204.
91. Collins AJ, Foley RN, Chavers B, Gilbertson D, Herzog C, Johansen K, et al. United States Renal Data System 2011 Annual Data Report: Atlas of chronic kidney disease & end-stage renal disease in the United States. Am J Kidney Dis Off J Natl Kidney Found. 2012;59(1 Suppl 1):A7, e1–420.
92. Sunday JM, Guille JT, Torg JS. Complications of joint arthroplasty in patients with end-stage renal disease on hemodialysis. Clin Orthop. 2002;397:350–5.
93. Sakalkale DP, Hozack WJ, Rothman RH. Total hip arthroplasty in patients on long-term renal dialysis. J Arthroplasty. 1999;14(5):571–5.
94. Lieberman JR, Fuchs MD, Haas SB, Garvin KL, Goldstock L, Gupta R, et al. Hip arthroplasty in

patients with chronic renal failure. J Arthroplasty. 1995;10(2):191–5.
95. McCleery MA, Leach WJ, Norwood T. Rates of infection and revision in patients with renal disease undergoing total knee replacement in Scotland. J Bone Joint Surg Br. 2010;92(11):1535–9.
96. Jiang SL, Schairer WW, Bozic KJ. Increased rates of periprosthetic joint infection in patients with cirrhosis undergoing total joint arthroplasty. Clin Orthop. 2014;472(8):2483–91.
97. Bozic KJ, Ong K, Lau E, Berry DJ, Vail TP, Kurtz SM, et al. Estimating risk in Medicare patients with THA: an electronic risk calculator for periprosthetic joint infection and mortality. Clin Orthop. 2013;471(2):574–83.
98. Bilimoria KY, Liu Y, Paruch JL, Zhou L, Kmiecik TE, Ko CY, et al. Development and evaluation of the universal ACS NSQIP surgical risk calculator: a decision aid and informed consent tool for patients and surgeons. J Am Coll Surg. 2013;217(5):833–42.e1–3.
99. Elixhauser A, Steiner C, Harris DR, Coffey RM. Comorbidity measures for use with administrative data. Med Care. 1998;36(1):8–27.

6 Impact of Prior Injections and Surgery on Subsequent Infection Risk

Geert Meermans

Abstract

Several risk factors have been associated with the development of periprosthetic joint infection (PJI). In this chapter the risk of PJI associated with an intra-articular steroid injection prior to joint arthroplasty and the risk of previous surgery of the same joint are reviewed.

Although the data of different studies is conflicting, the risk of developing a PJI in patients who had an intra-articular steroid injection could be twice as high compared with patients who had no injection prior to their joint arthroplasty. The preoperative diagnosis of posttraumatic arthritis and previous open surgery increases the risk of PJI after total joint arthroplasty approximately two to four times. Previous arthroscopic surgery and high tibial osteotomy are possibly not associated with an increased risk of PJI.

All risk factors, including previous intra-articular steroid injections and open surgery, should be discussed preoperatively with the patient and can be used in the stratification of patients for future studies or reporting outcomes.

Keywords

Risk factor • Periprosthetic joint infection • Steroid injection • Previous surgery • Stratification • Joint arthroplasty • Infection • Total hip arthroplasty • Total knee arthroplasty

G. Meermans, MD
Department of Orthopaedics, Bravis Hospital,
Boerhaaveplein 1, Bergen op Zoom 4624VT,
The Netherlands
e-mail: geertmeermans@hotmail.com

D. Kendoff et al. (eds.), *Periprosthetic Joint Infections: Changing Paradigms*,
DOI 10.1007/978-3-319-30091-7_6

Introduction

The incidence of periprosthetic joint infection (PJI) has reduced from 10 % in the first arthroplasties in the late 1960s [1] to 1–2 % in some more recent series of primary arthroplasties [2–4]. Nevertheless, despite this reduction in the rate of infection, the total number of infections remains high due to the increasing number of arthroplasties performed [5–8]. Revision arthroplasty and its possible complications are a considerable burden for patients, health systems, and hospitals. Revision surgery for PJI is associated with longer operating times, more expensive implants, increased blood loss, longer hospital stay, an increase in complications compared with revisions for aseptic loosening, and increases the risk of 1-year mortality [9–13]. Overall, the costs associated with revision arthroplasty because of an infection are two to three times higher than the costs associated with revision for aseptic loosening [9, 10, 12, 14–17].

Many factors are associated with the development of PJI and they include, but are not limited to the risk factors listed in Table 6.1. These risk factors can be patient-related, surgery-related or postoperative [3, 4, 18–28] and can be further categorized as modifiable or nonmodifiable [26, 29]. The data are often based on the results of multivariate analyses and it is not always clear whether the risk factors identified are causally related to PJI, whether they are proxies for the actual causal factors, whether different risk factors act synergistic, or whether there is an interaction with the time since surgery [21].

Appropriate preoperative risk stratification is important for discussing perioperative risks with individual patients and managing modifiable risk factors to reduce postoperative complications [30]. It also facilitates comparing and synthesizing scientific reports. As external regulatory bodies and reporting agencies begin to publish information on hospital and surgeon-specific arthroplasty outcomes it can also be used for risk adjustment and validation of these publicly reported outcomes [21]. Based on the risk factors, high-risk patients can be identified preoperatively which allows diligent monitoring and aggressive treatment when a PJI is suspected [31]. In the future, stratification of patients in a high-risk group may warrant the allocation or prioritizing of the use of emerging technologies to prevent PJI such as vaccines, biofilm disrupting technologies

Table 6.1 Risk factors for periprosthetic joint infection

Active infection
History of previous surgery
Uncontrolled hyperglycemia
Malnutrition
(Morbid) obesity
Smoking
Alcohol consumption
Active renal disease
Active liver disease
Immunosuppression
Intravenous drug abuse
Human immunodeficiency virus infection
Admission from a healthcare facility
Male patients
Age
Subsequent surgery
Urinary tract infection
Rheumatoid arthritis
Long-term stay in a healthcare facility
ASA>2
Operative time
Surgeon and hospital volume
Patients receive public assistance
Increased blood loss
Allogenic blood transfusion
Lack of antibiotic cement
Emergency vs. planned surgery
Postoperative complication
Race
Socioeconomic status
Systemic malignancy
Sickle cell hemoglobinopathies
Hemophilia
Depression
Psychoses
Hip fracture
Postoperative hematoma
Staphylococcus aureus colonizers
Anesthetic management
Persistent wound drainage
Wound-related complications
Distant infection
Cardiovascular complications
Length of stay

or implants with an anti-adhesive surface or coating with antimicrobial substances [32].

The purpose of this chapter is to review the risk of PJI associated with preoperative steroid injection and previous (non-arthroplasty) surgery of the same joint. Much of the information comes from uncontrolled retrospective cohort studies or case-control studies with small sample size and are limited to hip and knee replacement. Because PJI is a relative uncommon complication, well-executed prospective studies examining factors associated with infection after joint replacement and achieving sufficient numbers are difficult to conduct. When referencing this chapter and other resources, these shortcomings of the evidence should be taken into account.

PJI After Steroid Injection

Working Mechanism of Steroids

Steroid injections are frequently used by general practitioners (GP), rheumatologists and orthopaedic surgeons and remain a mainstay of treatment of many causes of joint or soft-tissue pain. Steroids may also be used as to distinguish between pain originating from an arthritic joint and referred pain. In osteoarthritis, inflammation occurs as a reflexive response to mechanical irritation. T-lymphocytes infiltrate the synovial membrane of osteoarthritic joints which results in the release of inflammatory mediators into the synovial fluid.

The aim of intra-articular steroid injections is to provide high concentrations of steroid in the synovial fluid and synovial cells, reducing local inflammation and minimizing plasma concentrations and systemic side effects. The pathways by which injectable steroids mediate symptom relief are not completely understood, and they may differ from the mechanisms associated with systemic steroids. Steroids act by blocking the inflammatory and immune cascade at several levels, including the prostaglandin and cyclo-oxygenase pathways [33, 34]. Through inhibition of these pathways, arachidonic acid production is prevented and hence the formation of prostaglandins, thromboxanes, prostacyclins and leukotrienes is reduced (Fig. 6.1).

Only depot formulations are suitable for intra-articular injections (Table 6.2). These depot formulations tend to remain at the injected site for a long period of time and cause little systemic effects. Compounds with lower solubility may maintain effective synovial levels for a longer time and produce lower systemic levels than compounds with greater solubility. Although some data suggest that decreased solubility correlates

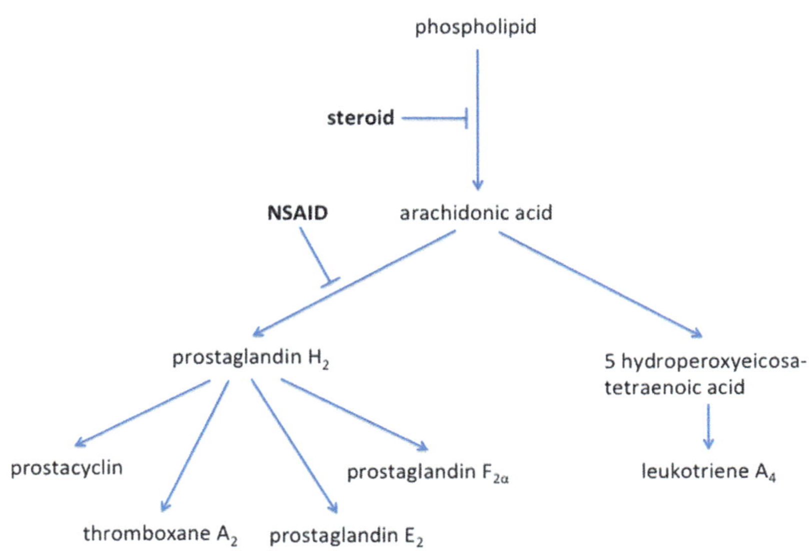

Fig. 6.1 Diagram of the inflammatory cascade, depicting the point of inhibition of steroids and nonsteroidal anti-inflammatory drugs. *NSAID* nonsteroidal anti-inflammatory drugs

Table 6.2 Characteristics of injectable steroids

Compound	Potency (Hydrocortisone equivalent)	Duration
Betamethasone sodium phosphate and betamethasone acetate	25	Long
Cortisone	.08	Short
Dexamethasone sodium phosphate	25	Short
Hydrocortisone acetate	1	Intermediate
Methylprednisolone acetate	5	Intermediate
Prednisolone tebutate	3.5	Intermediate
Triamcinolone acetonide	5	Intermediate
Triamcinolone hexacetonide	5	Long

with a sustained clinical effect, this is not always the case [35, 36].

Side Effects of Steroids

The most common side effects of steroid injections are postinjection flare, facial flushing, and skin or fat atrophy [34, 37–39]. Of the less common side effects, joint sepsis is of the greatest concern, with reported incidences ranging from 1 in 3000 to 1 in 50,000 [40–42]. Current rates may be even lower because of improved sterile technique and the availability of steroid preparations in prefilled syringes which reduces handling. Case reports have also documented the occurrence of tendon ruptures in patients after steroid injections [43]. Although animal studies have suggested that steroid injections may have deleterious effects on articular cartilage, studies in humans have not shown similar results [44–46]. Systemic effects from steroid injections are generally milder than with oral or intravenous formulations. These include osteoporosis, steroid-induced myopathy, suppression of the hypothalamic-pituitary-adrenal axis, increasing hepatic glucose synthesis and antagonizing insulin effects resulting in worsening of preexisting glucose intolerance [38, 39, 47–49].

Primary Total Hip Arthroplasty

An intra-articular steroid injection of the hip can be administered for diagnostic and therapeutic reasons. In conjunction with an intra-articular injection of a long-acting anesthetic, steroids can be used for diagnostic purposes to distinguish intrinsic from extrinsic sources of pain such as that originating in the spine [50–55] with a reported sensitivity of 91.5 %, specificity and positive predictive value of 100 %, and negative predictive value of 84.6 % for response to total hip arthroplasty (THA) [56]. Although steroid injections in the hip were not recommended in the treatment guidelines provided by the American College of Rheumatology for osteoarthritis (OA) of the hip in the past [57], more recent guidelines include steroid injections for the initial management of hip OA [58–60]. They can be helpful in clinical practice when patients with moderate or end-stage OA are not willing or suitable to undergo a THA in the short term or to alleviate inflammatory symptoms that can be associated with mild or moderate OA of the hip joint [61–63].

Patients receiving any form of systemic steroid therapy for greater than 1 week within 1 year before THA have a two-fold increased risk of prosthetic joint infection compared with normal control subjects [18]. Concern regarding the effect of an intra-articular steroid injection on infection rates in subsequent THA was first raised by Kaspar and de V de Beer [64]. In an audit they found a 10 % infection rate in 40 patients who had received an intra-articular steroid infiltration prior to their THA, which was significantly higher than the risk of PJI in a matched group that did not have a steroid injection prior to THA ($p<0.01$). This high prevalence of PJI in patients that had an intra-articular steroid injection prior to THA appears to have been refuted by subsequent studies conducted and although the data is conflicting, none of the studies reproduced infection or revision rates similar to what had been documented by Kaspar and de V de Beer (Table 6.3).

Although most of the subsequent studies did not find an increase in PJI, two other studies did detect an increased risk of infection in patients that had a steroid injection prior to their THA [68, 71]. McIntosh et al. [68] found 3 patients who had a PJI out of a cohort 224 THAs with a prior intra-articular steroid injection (1.3 %). Although this was equivalent to their historic deep infection rate, the deep infection rate in a matched cohort was only 1 out of 224 THAs (0.45 %). Ravi et al. [71] used Cox proportional hazard regression models to determine the relationship between receipt of an intra-articular injection and the risk of infection controlling for Charlson Comorbidity Index, frailty, age, sex, income quintile and surgeon volume. They found an increased risk of PJI with an adjusted hazard ratio of 1.37 ($p=0.03$) for patients who received an injection in the year prior to their THA (56/1691 *versus* 863/35,413). The latter study is definitely the largest study to address this question and adjusts for relevant confounders. Cross-referencing was done using a database including patients that underwent THA and another one including injections performed by a radiologist. The authors were unable to determine what agent was injected into which joint, potentially leading to selection bias.

In an outpatient setting, a great variation of antiseptic technique used during intra-articular steroid injection has been reported [40]. In the three studies that have found an increase in PJI of a THA after an intra-articular steroid injection, the steroid injection was given by a radiologist in the radiology department (see Table 6.3). In the studies that did not find a prior intra-articular steroid injection to increase the risk of PJI, the procedure was done in the vast majority of cases in the operating theatre and always by a member of the surgical team. This could suggest that any breech of sterile technique may be an important factor in the development of PJI after a steroid injection in the hip joint.

Some authors have suggested that an increased risk of PJI could be due to one of the agents injected in the hip joint. However, it is unclear which agent of the injection procedure may be culpable: the arthrography dye, the steroid or its depot vehicle, or the local anesthetic. It has been hypothesized that it may be due to failure of the steroid to dissolve which may cause local immunosuppression at the time of joint arthroplasty [64, 77]. In most studies methylprednisolone acetate was used, so it is unclear whether the steroid compound itself has an influence on the subsequent development of PJI.

Other authors have hypothesized that the time between the steroid injection and subsequent THA could play a role. In the different studies, there was variation in the time between steroid injection and THA which in some cases was more than a year. Hence any potential effect of such timing on infection rates is difficult to establish. McIntosh et al. [68] found that in the patients that had PJI the mean time from injection to THA was 44 days which was much lower than the overall mean time from injection to THA of 112 days. In the study by Meermans et al. [70] the time from injection to THA was 35 days in the patient that had a PJI. However, Kaspar and de V de Beer [64] reported that in their cases, the time interval between injection and THA in those that developed an infection was not statistically different from those with no infection (11.38 months, 95 % confidence interval (CI) 5.6–17.2 months *versus* 10.86 months, 95 % CI 7.2–14.5 months).

Because of the conflicting evidence and the small number of patients included in each study, several meta-analyses were done which are limited due to the heterogeneity of the included studies (Table 6.4). Charalambous et al. [78] found that intra-articular steroid injection had an increased risk ratio on the superficial or deep infection rates of subsequent joint arthroplasty, but this was not statistically significant ($p=0.15$). The difference was bigger in the superficial infection rate, but there is no proposed mechanism that can explain how an injection may increase the risk of superficial infection. McMahon et al. [79]

Table 6.3 Infection rates in patients with an intra-articular steroid injection prior to joint arthroplasty

Joint	Author	Place of admission	Given by	Deep infection		Superfical infection	
				Injected	Control	Injected	Control
Hip	Chitre et al. [65]	Operating theater	Surgeon	0/36 (0 %)	NA	1/36 (2.8 %)	NA
	Croft and Rockwood [66]	Outpatient clinic	Surgeon	0/48 (0 %)	0/48 (0 %)	NR	NR
	Haughton et al. [67]	Operating theater/radiology department	Surgeon/radiologist	4/254 (1.5 %)	14/1063 (1.3 %)	11/254 (4.3 %)	4/1063 (0.4 %)
	Karuppiah et al. [61]	Operating theater	Surgeon	0/128 (0 %)	NA	0/128 (0 %)	NA
	Kaspar and de V de Beer [64]	Radiology department	Radiologist	4/40 (10 %)	0/40 (0 %)	NR	NR
	McIntosh et al. [68]	Radiology department	Radiologist	3/224 (1.3 %)	1/224 (0.4 %)	11/224 (4.9 %)	8/224 (3.6 %)
	McMahon et al. [69]	Operating theater	Surgeon	1/49 (2.0 %)	NA	1/49 (2.0 %)	NA
	Meermans et al. [70]	Operating theater	Surgeon	1/182 (0.5 %)	1/182 (0.5 %)	5/182 (2.7 %)	7/182 (3.8 %)
	Ravi et al. [71]	Radiology department	Radiologist	56/1691 (3.3 %)	863/35,413 (2.4 %)	NR	NR
	Sankar et al. [72]	Operating theater	Surgeon	0/40 (0 %)	NA	1/40 (2.5 %)	NA
	Sreekumar et al. [73]	Radiology department	Surgeon[a]	0/66 (0 %)	1/136 (0.7 %)	0/66 (0 %)	1/136 (0.7 %)
Knee	Desai et al. [74]	Operating theater/outpatient clinic	Surgeon	0/90 (0 %)	0/180 (0 %)	2/90 (2.2 %)	5/180 (2.8 %)
	Horne et al. [75]	Outpatient clinic	Surgeon, rheumatologist, GP	11/81 (13.6 %)	17/166 (10.2 %)	NR	NR
	Joshy et al. [76]	NR	NR	8/17 (47.1 %)	24/47 (51.1 %)	NR	NR
	Papavasiliou et al. [77]	Outpatient clinic	Surgeon, rheumatologist, GP	3/54 (5.6 %)	0/90 (0 %)	12/54 (22.2 %)	10/90 (11.1 %)

Abbreviations: *NR* not reported, *NA* not applicable, *GP* general practitioner
[a]Personal communication

Table 6.4 Meta-analyses of comparative studies of total hip arthroplasty following intra-articular steroid injection

Authors	THA/TKA	Superficial infection	Deep infection
Charalambous et al. [78]	THA and TKA	RR=1.75 (95 % CI 0.76–4.04)	RR=1.87 (95 % CI 0.80–4.35)
	THA	RR=1.91 (95 % CI 0.48–7.56)	RR=1.59 (95 % CI 0.66–3.83
McMahon et al. [79]	THA	OR=1.04 (95 % CI 0.52–2.10)	OR=2.65 (95 % CI 0.79–8.96)
	TKA	OR=0.91 (95 % CI 0.07–11.11)	OR=2.24 (95 % CI 0.08–65.30)
Wang et al. [80]	THA	RD=0.00 (95 % CI −0.03–0.03)	RD=0.00 (95 % CI −0.01–0.02)
	TKA	RD=0.04 (95 % CI −0.12–0.20)	RD=0.02 (95 % CI −0.06–0.11)
Xing et al. [81]	THA and TKA	OR=1.75 (95 % CI 0.74–4.16)	OR=2.13 (95 % CI 1.02–4.45)

THA total hip arthroplasty, *TKA* total knee arthroplasty, *RR* relative risk, *OR* odds ratio, *RD* risk difference

found that patients were twice as likely to develop a PJI if they received an intra-articular steroid injection prior to THA or TKA, but this was not significant (p=0.12 and p=0.64 respectively). In this meta-analysis there was no difference in the risk of superficial infection. Wang et al. [80] also found no significant increase of infection among patients injected with steroid injection prior to the arthroplasty. Xing et al. [81] found that there was a significant effect on the deep infection but not on the superficial infection rates. Although it was not always found to be statistically significant, most meta-analyses agree that the risk of developing a PJI is twice as high in patients who received an intra-articular steroid injection compared with patients who underwent joint arthroplasty without prior injection.

Primary Total Knee Arthroplasty

Because of its easier access, intra-articular steroid injections are more frequently used by orthopaedic surgeons, rheumatologists and general practitioners (GP) for the management of patients with OA in the knee compared with the hip. Steroids are proven to be effective at reducing pain in knee OA, although duration of this treatment is controversial. Some evidence demonstrates that use of steroids decreases pain by roughly one third, as measured by visual analog scale, but provides this benefit for only 1 week [82]. A Cochrane meta-analysis has shown that steroid injections for osteoarthritic knee pain are beneficial at two weeks, with the number needed to treat to give a patient benefit between 1.6 and 3.5 [83]. Although most individual randomised controlled trials included in the study failed to show a clear benefit at 16 and 24 weeks, pooled data showed a significant improvement at 24 weeks [83]. From the limited studies available, triamcinolone appears to be more efficacious than either methylprednisolone or betamethasone [36].

The first study to look at the risk of PJI after intra-articular steroid injection in the knee was done by Papavasiliou et al. [77]. In this retrospective review, the authors found PJI in 3 out of 54 (5.5 %) in patients that had an intra-articular steroid injection prior to their total knee arthroplasty (TKA) compared with 0 out of 90 (0 %) in the non-injected patients (p=0.025). The time from last injection to operation for the three infected cases was 8, 10 and 11 months. There was no statistically significant difference between the two groups for superficial infection.

Another study looking at the effect of intra-articular steroid injection on infection rates after PJI, reported the outcome of 440 TKAs with 1-year follow-up [74]. The authors identified 90 knees in 80 patients from hospital records that had intra-articular steroid injections prior to TKA. A cohort of 180 knees in 170 patients was used as a control group, matched for age, sex and year of operation. There were no cases of PJI in either group. Two cases of superficial infection occurred in the study group and five cases in the control group (p=1). It was noted that for the two infected cases in the study group, steroid injection had been given at 18 months prior to surgery. Of note is that 60 out of 90 knees received steroid injections in the operating room under strict sterile conditions. It has been reported previously that standards of asepsis when injections are not done in the operating room are often poor [40] and therefore the findings of this study cannot be extrapolated to centers where aseptic techniques are less strict. A further limitation of the study is that it did not attempt to identify whether patients in either the study or control groups received steroid injections from outside the Orthopaedic department, potentially leading to selection bias.

In a recent study, Cancienne et al. [84] used a national database and looked at patients that had a TKA within 3 months, 3–6 months or 6–12 months after ipsilateral knee injection. These patients were matched according to age, gender, obesity, smoking status and diabetes with a group of patients that underwent TKA without any prior documented ipsilateral injection. The incidence of infection within 3 and 6 months after surgery was significantly higher in the group of patients that had TKA within 3 months of knee injection compared with the control cohort (138/5313 and 181/5313 versus 181/13,650 and 319/13,650 respectively; $P<0.0001$). There was no significant difference in infection rates in patients who underwent TKA 3–6 months or 6–12 months after ipsilateral knee injection. One of the limitations of this study is that the use of a database does not allow differentiation of the specific type of injection or dosing.

Two case-control studies did not find more patients who had a prior steroid injection in a group of patients with a PJI compared with no PJI. In a retrospective matched case-control study Joshy et al. [76] compared a study group of 32 patients who had TKA complicated by deep infection with a control group of 32 TKA patients selected from a database who did not develop infection. Groups were matched for age, year of operation, American Society of Anesthesia grade and type of arthritis. Exposure of each group to intra-articular steroid injection was determined using hospital notes only. The results showed no significant differences between the numbers of patients who received intra-articular steroid injection in the two groups, leading the authors to conclude that previous steroid injection was not a risk factor for postoperative infection. A more recent retrospective case-control study reported similar findings [75]. Forty patients who either developed postoperative wound infection within 6 months following TKA, or required revision surgery for infection were compared with 352 patients who underwent TKA without postoperative infection. As well as review of hospital records, patients were sent questionnaires asking whether they had ever received a knee injection at any stage prior to TKA, and if so, by which type of practitioner (Orthopaedic surgeon, GP, Rheumatologist). The authors compared 28 infected cases (77.5 % response rate) with 219 patients (69.5 % response rate) who did not develop infection. The average number of injections received prior to surgery was 2.23 (range 1–15), and the mean time of last injection before TKA was 16 months (range 1 month to 45 years). In the control group, it was found that 32 % of patients had received a steroid injection prior to surgery, compared with 39 % in the infected group. The results showed that prior steroid injection was not associated with an increased risk of postoperative infection ($p=0.44$). There was no significant difference in infection rate with regard to whether the GP, Rheumatologist or Orthopaedic surgeon administered the injection. Exposure to steroid injection prior to TKA was identified via the questionnaire only, without attempts to screen Orthopaedic, Rheumatology, or GP records. Therefore, this study is potentially subject to significant recall bias.

Marsland et al. [85] performed a meta-analysis of both retrospective case-control studies and both cohort studies that evaluated the risk of infected TKA in association with pre-operative steroid injection. Due to the small sample size the study rendered as significantly underpowered. One of the major limitations was that there was no apparent attempt by the authors to identify patients given steroid injections in the community, potentially leading to selection bias. The evidence suggesting that patients who receive steroid injections prior to TKA are at increased risk of postoperative infection is weak with no obvious correlation with timing, dosage or frequency of injections. The authors conclude that considering the paucity of data, it is essential that good communication regarding previous steroid treatment exists between GPs, rheumatologists and orthopaedic surgeons when arthroplasty surgery is being considered.

Summary: Steroids and PJI

With regards to the risk of PJI when an intra-articular steroid injection is given prior to joint arthroplasty, the current body of evidence cannot be used to provide clear recommendations and further research is required. Based on different meta-analyses and two large database studies, the risk of developing a PJI could be twice as high in patients who received an intra-articular steroid injection compared with patients who underwent joint arthroplasty without prior injection. Although this difference was not always found to be statistically significant, it might be of clinical relevance. Accurate needle placement is obviously beneficial in both reducing adverse effects and achieving the maximal clinical benefit [86]. When administering steroid injections, it is important to comply with the standards of asepsis to minimize the risk of any breech of sterile technique. In patients that had an intra-articular steroid injection, the surgeon may choose to delay arthroplasty surgery until any residual effects of the steroid injection are thought to have subsided. Caution should be used when planning a THA within 2 months after an intra-articular steroid injection. For TKA after an intra-articular steroid injection, waiting for at least 3 months [84] up to 11 months would be justified [77].

Although several case reports have highlighted the risk of septic arthritis after the intra-articular administration of non-steroids in native joints [87–92], there are no data available on the risk of PJI when injections with compounds other than steroid are given.

PJI After Previous Surgery

Preoperative diagnosis of posttraumatic arthritis with or without prior surgery has consistently been found to be a risk factor for PJI [24, 25, 93–98]. Overall, previous surgery was related to PJI with an odds ratio of 2.1 (95 % CI 0.9–5.0 %) after multivariate regression analysis [94] Potential explanations for this include the complexity of the procedure, prolonged surgical time, low grade infection, and less favorable status of the soft tissue (Fig. 6.2).

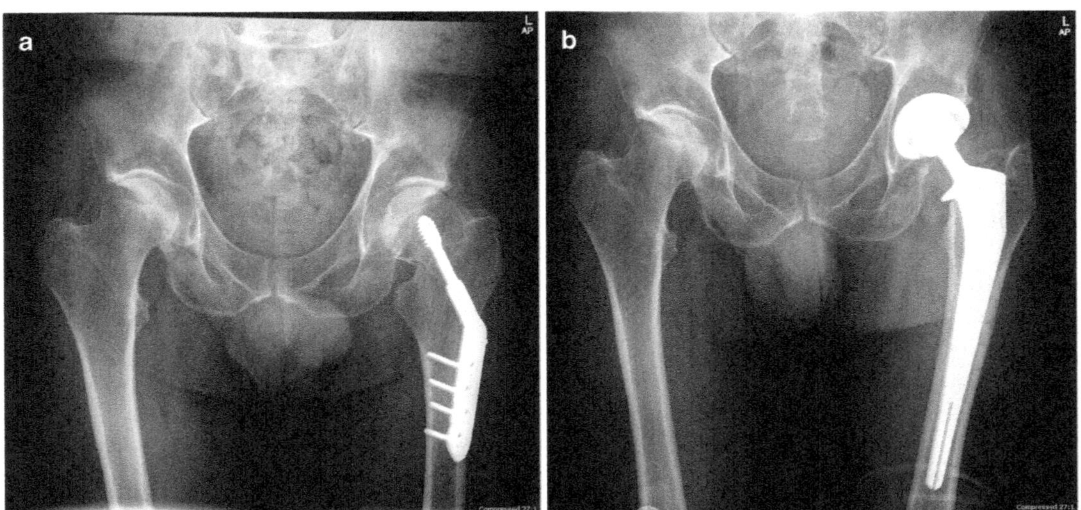

Fig. 6.2 Anteroposterior pelvis radiographs of a 58-year-old man who sustained proximal femoral fracture treated with a sliding hip screw (**a**). The fracture failed to heal and collapsed and he was subsequently treated with a total hip arthroplasty (**b**). Three weeks postoperatively he was readmitted with a periprosthetic joint infection that was successfully treated with open irrigation and debridement

Total Hip Arthroplasty

Depending on the fracture type, internal fixation has been widely accepted as an effective treatment of proximal hip fractures. Nevertheless, treatment of these fractures occasionally fails. This may be due to poor bone quality, the fracture pattern, suboptimal fracture fixation, poor implant position or osteonecrosis [99–101]. The reported overall failure rates with internal fixation are: 3–12 % failure in the internal fixation itself, 2–12 % device penetration, 2–5 % nonunion, and 5–11 % malunion causing varus deformity [102–104]. Failed treatment of hip fractures typically leads to profound functional disability and pain. The two main treatment options for patients who have a proximal hip fracture that has failed after internal fixation are internal fixation of the ununited fracture or salvage treatment with a THA [104–107]. When there is poor bone quality, a damaged femoral head, damaged articular cartilage, or limb-shortening, the chance of achieving a good clinical result is low and THA has been used as a salvage technique [108, 109]. There are a number of specific technical difficulties to successful THA in this setting, including the presence of failed internal fixation devices, bone deformity, bone loss, and poor bone quality. Compared with primary THA, this could lead to an increased complication rate, including PJI, due to possible pre-existing subclinical sepsis, decreased local host resistance because of scarring and reduced vascularity, prolonged operating time and difficulty of surgery.

Fitzgerald et al. [93] found that, excluding the group with miscellaneous diagnoses, the highest incidence of PJI in patients without previous surgery occurred in those with posttraumatic degenerative joint disease. The incidence in infection rates between patients with and without previous surgery was statistically significant: patients with previous surgery had a rate of 2.3 % (23 of 991 hips) and those without a rate of 0.9 % (19 of 2224 hips) ($p=0.001$). Nelson et al. [96] reviewed the results of 711 THAs and found 16 deep infections occurred in the 711 hips for an overall infection rate of 2.3 %. Nine infections developed in the 511 hips that had had no previous surgery, accounting for a rate of 1.8 % and 7 infections occurred in the 200 hips that had had one or more previous operations, accounting for a rate of 3.5 % ($p=0.16$). McKinley et al. [95] compared THA after failed internal fixation versus primary arthroplasty for displaced intracapsular hip fractures. In this retrospective matched control study, there was a superficial infection rate 12 of 107 THAs in the failed fixation group versus 3 of 107 in the primary THA group ($p=0.03$) and deep infection 8 of 107 THAs in the failed fixation group versus 2 of 107 THAs in the primary THA group ($p=0.10$).

Total Knee Arthroplasty

Posttraumatic or secondary osteoarthritis may develop after a fracture around the knee as a result of (1) the alteration of the osseous anatomy leading to altered knee mechanics, (2) cartilage damage as part of the initial injury, or (3) the presence of subchondral implants that may perforate the articular cartilage [110]. Compared with a matched control group and after adjustment for medical comorbidity, tibial plateau fracture repair increased the likelihood of TKA 5.3 times [111]. The TKA rate, however, was fairly low, with only 7.3 % of patients with a tibial plateau fracture having had a TKA by 10 years after fixation. For patients who had a TKA after open reduction internal fixation (ORIF) of the tibial plateau, each year of age older than 16 years at injury conferred an additional risk of eventual TKA of 3.4 %. The vast majority of patients treated with TKA after a previous fracture around the knee have substantial improvement in function and relief of pain. However, the procedure is technically demanding and these patients are at increased risk for perioperative complications and failure [110, 112, 113]. It has been hypothesized that the risk of perioperative complications is increased by previous operations because of poorly planned skin incisions or devitalized tissue planes [114].

In a review of 4171 primary TKAs, the rate of joint infection in patients who had prior knee surgery was 1.4 % compared with 0.3 % in patients without prior surgical intervention ($p=0.007$) [98]. A previous operation on the knee was a significant risk factor for infection, but only for the osteoarthritic knees. In the knees of the patients who had rheumatoid arthritis, an approximately equal percentage of those who did or did not have a previous operation subsequently became infected. Peersman et al. [25] studied a cohort of 6489 TKAs, of which 116 knees became infected and 113 were available for follow up. Each patient with an infected TKA was matched for gender and age with two noninfected TKAs done during the same month. After logistic regression, one of the comorbidities that achieved statistical significance was prior open surgical procedures ($p<0.001$). In another study, a total of 43,149 primary and revision knee arthroplasties, registered in the Finnish Arthroplasty Register, were followed for a median of 3 years of which 387 reoperations were performed because of infection [24]. Cox regression analysis demonstrated that the odds ratio for PJI was 1.86 (95 % CI 1.12–3.11) in patients with secondary OA and 2.4 (95 % CI 1.3–4.2) in patients with posttraumatic OA. Suzuki et al. [97] looked specifically at previous surgery as a risk factor for infection and divided cases of previous operation around the knee joint into two groups: previous arthroscopic surgery and previous non-arthroscopic surgery. In addition, cases of previous non-arthroscopic surgery were divided into previous high tibial osteotomy and previous ORIF groups, and examined accordingly. In the univariate analysis, variables that achieved statistical significance were: previous operation around the knee joint, previous non-arthroscopic surgery, and previous ORIF. Variables not associated with infection included previous arthroscopic surgery and previous high tibial osteotomy. Stepwise logistic regression analysis indicated the predictor of infection was previous ORIF. In addition, remnants of previous internal fixation material were found to be statistically significant related to infection.

Summary: Previous Surgery and PJI

Prolonged surgery, poorly planned skin incisions, devitalized tissue planes, and low blood supply around the scar tissue could be causes of an increase in PJI in patients who had open surgery before their total joint arthroplasty. Although not much literature has been published, at the International Meeting on Periprosthetic Joint Infection there was a strong consensus (94 % agree, 4 % disagree) that a history of previous surgery is a potential risk factor for development of surgical site infection or PJI after elective total joint arthroplasty [115]. The patient's previous surgical history should be documented and a proper evaluation of the local wound environment should be done. Some authors have advocated an infection workup in all patients who have had previous surgery at the site of an upcoming arthroplasty [116]. Others have demonstrated that the retrieval of internal fixation devices and joint arthroplasty can be performed safely as a single stage procedure without significantly increasing the risk of periprosthetic infection [117, 118]. After THA and TKA the risk of PJI can be two to four times higher in patients that had previous (open) surgery. There is some data to suggest that in TKA the risk of PJI is not associated with previous arthroscopic surgery and previous high tibial osteotomy.

Conclusion

Elective arthroplasty needs to be withheld for some patients at extreme risk of PJI, but there is inadequate evidence in the literature as to what the exact threshold for making this decision should be. Based on previous studies, an electronic risk calculator was developed to estimate the risk of PJI which can be used to counsel patients regarding their patient-specific risks of PJI after THA [2]. Some of the risk factors are potentially modifiable and if addressed before surgery may lead to a decrease in the rate of PJI [29].

Prospective studies with meticulous collection of data have problems in achieving sufficient numbers to be effectively statistically powerful. Large registry-based studies often rely on re- admission or re-operation as a surrogate measure of infection and hence miss numerous infections successfully treated conservatively. The findings presented in this chapter are based on retrospective studies with a short follow-up period resulting in significant heterogeneity. Most of the studies covering the subject of this chapter are related to the hip and knee and it is not sure whether these data can be extrapolated to PJI in other joints [119–121].

Until better and more conclusive data is available, orthopaedic surgeons should be aware that previous steroid injection or surgery are potential risk factors for the development of PJI.

Surgeons should remain vigilant for exposure to previous steroid injections, so that a correct sterile technique during injection is maintained at all time and might consider to postpone arthroplasty surgery to reduce the risk of PJI. In patients who had previous open surgery preoperative counseling, management of all modifiable risk factors, diligent monitoring, expeditious diagnosis and treatment are warranted. These implications are minimal in relation to the health and economic burden caused by a possible PJI.

References

1. Charnley J, Eftekhar N. Postoperative infection in total prosthetic replacement arthroplasty of the hip-joint. With special reference to the bacterial content of the air of the operating room. Br J Surg. 1969;56(9):641–9.
2. Bozic KJ, Ong K, Lau E, Berry DJ, Vail TP, Kurtz SM, et al. Estimating risk in Medicare patients with THA: an electronic risk calculator for periprosthetic joint infection and mortality. Clin Orthop Relat Res. 2013;471(2):574–83.
3. Kurtz SM, Ong KL, Lau E, Bozic KJ, Berry D, Parvizi J. Prosthetic joint infection risk after TKA in the Medicare population. Clin Orthop Relat Res. 2010;468(1):52–6.
4. Ong KL, Kurtz SM, Lau E, Bozic KJ, Berry DJ, Parvizi J. Prosthetic joint infection risk after total hip arthroplasty in the Medicare population. J Arthroplasty. 2009;24(6 Suppl):105–9.
5. Kurtz S, Ong K, Lau E, Mowat F, Halpern M. Projections of primary and revision hip and knee arthroplasty in the United States from 2005 to 2030. J Bone Joint Surg Am. 2007;89(4):780–5.
6. Kurtz SM, Ong KL, Lau E, Bozic KJ. Impact of the economic downturn on total joint replacement demand in the United States: updated projections to 2021. J Bone Joint Surg Am. 2014;96(8):624–30.
7. Nemes S, Gordon M, Rogmark C, Rolfson O. Projections of total hip replacement in Sweden from 2013 to 2030. Acta Orthop. 2014;85(3):238–43.
8. Nemes S, Rolfson O, W-Dahl A, Garellick G, Sundberg M, Kärrholm J, et al. Historical view and future demand for knee arthroplasty in Sweden. Acta Orthop. 2015;86:426–31.
9. Assmann G, Kasch R, Maher CG, Hofer A, Barz T, Merk H, et al. Comparison of health care costs between aseptic and two stage septic hip revision. J Arthroplasty. 2014;29(10):1925–31.
10. Bozic KJ, Ries MD. The impact of infection after total hip arthroplasty on hospital and surgeon resource utilization. J Bone Joint Surg Am. 2005;87(8):1746–51.
11. Jafari SM, Coyle C, Mortazavi SM, Sharkey PF, Parvizi J. Revision hip arthroplasty: infection is the most common cause of failure. Clin Orthop Relat Res. 2010;468(8):2046–51.
12. Vanhegan IS, Malik AK, Jayakumar P, Ul Islam S, Haddad FS. A financial analysis of revision hip arthroplasty: the economic burden in relation to the national tariff. J Bone Joint Surg Br. 2012;94(5):619–23.
13. Zmistowski B, Karam JA, Durinka JB, Casper DS, Parvizi J. Periprosthetic joint infection increases the risk of one-year mortality. J Bone Joint Surg Am. 2013;95(24):2177–84.
14. Hebert CK, Williams RE, Levy RS, Barrack RL. Cost of treating an infected total knee replacement. Clin Orthop Relat Res. 1996;331:140–5.
15. Kallala RF, Vanhegan IS, Ibrahim MS, Sarmah S, Haddad FS. Financial analysis of revision knee surgery based on NHS tariffs and hospital costs: does it pay to provide a revision service? Bone Joint J. 2015;97-B(2):197–201.
16. Kapadia BH, McElroy MJ, Issa K, Johnson AJ, Bozic KJ, Mont MA. The economic impact of periprosthetic infections following total knee arthroplasty at a specialized tertiary-care center. J Arthroplasty. 2014;29(5):929–32.
17. Kurtz SM, Lau E, Schmier J, Ong KL, Zhao K, Parvizi J. Infection burden for hip and knee arthroplasty in the United States. J Arthroplasty. 2008;23(7):984–91.
18. Berbari EF, Hanssen AD, Duffy MC, Steckelberg JM, Ilstrup DM, Harmsen WS, et al. Risk factors for prosthetic joint infection: case-control study. Clin Infect Dis. 1998;27(5):1247–54.
19. Bongartz T, Halligan CS, Osmon DR, Reinalda MS, Bamlet WR, Crowson CS, Hanssen AD, Matteson EL. Incidence and risk factors of prosthetic joint infection after total hip or knee replacement in patients with rheumatoid arthritis. Arthritis Rheum. 2008;59(12):1713–20.
20. Bozic KJ, Lau E, Kurtz S, Ong K, Berry DJ. Patient-related risk factors for postoperative mortality and

periprosthetic joint infection in medicare patients undergoing TKA. Clin Orthop Relat Res. 2012;470(1):130–7.
21. Bozic KJ, Lau E, Kurtz S, Ong K, Rubash H, Vail TP, et al. Patient-related risk factors for periprosthetic joint infection and postoperative mortality following total hip arthroplasty in Medicare patients. J Bone Joint Surg Am. 2012;94(9):794–800.
22. Bozic KJ, Ward DT, Lau EC, Chan V, Wetters NG, Naziri Q, Odum S, et al. Risk factors for periprosthetic joint infection following primary total hip arthroplasty: a case control study. J Arthroplasty. 2014;29(1):154–6.
23. Everhart JS, Altneu E, Calhoun JH. Medical comorbidities are independent preoperative risk factors for surgical infection after total joint arthroplasty. Clin Orthop Relat Res. 2013;471(10):3112–9.
24. Jämsen E, Huhtala H, Puolakka T, Moilanen T. Risk factors for infection after knee arthroplasty. A register-based analysis of 43,149 cases. J Bone Joint Surg Am. 2009;91(1):38–47.
25. Peersman G, Laskin R, Davis J, Peterson M. Infection in total knee replacement: a retrospective review of 6489 total knee replacements. Clin Orthop Relat Res. 2001;392:15–23.
26. Pruzansky JS, Bronson MJ, Grelsamer RP, Strauss E, Moucha CS. Prevalence of modifiable surgical site infection risk factors in hip and knee joint arthroplasty patients at an urban academic hospital. J Arthroplasty. 2014;29(2):272–6.
27. Pulido L, Ghanem E, Joshi A, Purtill JJ, Parvizi J. Periprosthetic joint infection: the incidence, timing, and predisposing factors. Clin Orthop Relat Res. 2008;466(7):1710–5.
28. Wu C, Qu X, Liu F, Li H, Mao Y, Zhu Z. Risk factors for periprosthetic joint infection after total hip arthroplasty and total knee arthroplasty in Chinese patients. PLoS One. 2014;9(4):e95300.
29. Maoz G, Phillips M, Bosco J, Slover J, Stachel A, Inneh I, et al. The Otto Aufranc Award: modifiable versus nonmodifiable risk factors for infection after hip arthroplasty. Clin Orthop Relat Res. 2015;473(2):453–9.
30. Møller AM, Villebro N, Pedersen T, Tønnesen H. Effect of preoperative smoking intervention on postoperative complications: a randomised clinical trial. Lancet. 2002;359(9301):114–7.
31. Adeli B, Parvizi J. Strategies for the prevention of periprosthetic joint infection. J Bone Joint Surg Br. 2012;94(11):42–6.
32. Hansen EN, Zmistowski B, Parvizi J. Periprosthetic joint infection: what is on the horizon? Int J Artif Organs. 2012;35(10):935–50.
33. Creamer P. Intra-articular corticosteroid injections in osteoarthritis: do they work and if so, how? Ann Rheum Dis. 1997;56(11):634–6.
34. Pekarek B, Osher L, Buck S, Bowen M. Intra-articular corticosteroid injections: a critical literature review with up-to-date findings. Foot (Edinb). 2011;21(2):66–70.
35. Godwin M, Dawes M. Intra-articular steroid injections for painful knees. Systematic review with meta-analysis. Can Fam Physician. 2004;50:241–8.
36. Pyne D, Ioannou Y, Mootoo R, Bhanji A. Intra-articular steroids in knee osteoarthritis: a comparative study of triamcinolone hexacetonide and methylprednisolone acetate. Clin Rheumatol. 2004;23(2):116–20.
37. Caldwell JR. Intra-articular corticosteroids. Guide to selection and indications for use. Drugs. 1996; 52(4):507–14.
38. Cardone DA, Tallia AF. Joint and soft tissue injection. Am Fam Physician. 2002;66(2):283–8.
39. Cole BJ, Schumacher Jr HR. Injectable corticosteroids in modern practice. J Am Acad Orthop Surg. 2005;13(1):37–46.
40. Charalambous CP, Tryfonidis M, Sadiq S, Hirst P, Paul A. Septic arthritis following intra-articular steroid injection of the knee – a survey of current practice regarding antiseptic technique used during intra-articular steroid injection of the knee. Clin Rheumatol. 2003;22(6):386–90.
41. Chazerain P, Rolland D, Cordonnier C, Ziza JM. Septic hip arthritis after multiple injections into the joint of hyaluronate and glucocorticoid. Rev Rhum Engl Ed. 1999;66(7–9):436.
42. Nallamshetty L, Buchowski JM, Nazarian LA, Narula S, Musto M, Ahn NU, et al. Septic arthritis of the hip following cortisone injection: case report and review of the literature. Clin Imaging. 2003; 27(4):225–8.
43. Smith AG, Kosygan K, Williams H, Newman RJ. Common extensor tendon rupture following corticosteroid injection for lateral tendinosis of the elbow. Br J Sports Med. 1999;33(6):423–4.
44. Huppertz HI, Tschammler A, Horwitz AE, Schwab KO. Intraarticular corticosteroids for chronic arthritis in children: efficacy and effects on cartilage and growth. J Pediatr. 1995;127(2):317–21.
45. Raynauld JP, Buckland-Wright C, Ward R, Choquette D, Haraoui B, Martel-Pelletier J, et al. Safety and efficacy of long-term intraarticular steroid injections in osteoarthritis of the knee: a randomized, double-blind, placebo-controlled trial. Arthritis Rheum. 2003;48(2):370–7.
46. Roberts WN, Babcock EA, Breitbach SA, Owen DS, Irby WR. Corticosteroid injection in rheumatoid arthritis does not increase rate of total joint arthroplasty. J Rheumatol. 1996;23(6):1001–4.
47. Habib GS, Miari W. The effect of intra-articular triamcinolone preparations on blood glucose levels in diabetic patients: a controlled study. J Clin Rheumatol. 2011;17(6):302–5.
48. Habib G, Safia A. The effect of intra-articular injection of betamethasone acetate/betamethasone sodium phosphate on blood glucose levels in controlled diabetic patients with symptomatic osteoarthritis of the knee. Clin Rheumatol. 2009;28(1):85–7.
49. Kallock E, Neher JO, Safranek S. Clinical inquiries. Do intra-articular steroid injections affect glycemic

control in patients with diabetes? J Fam Pract. 2010;59(12):709–10.
50. Brown MD, Gomez-Marin O, Brookfield KF, Li PS. Differential diagnosis of hip disease versus spine disease. Clin Orthop Relat Res. 2004;419:280–4.
51. Crawford RW, Gie GA, Ling RS, Murray DW. Diagnostic value of intra-articular anaesthetic in primary osteoarthritis of the hip. J Bone Joint Surg Br. 1998;80(2):279–81.
52. Faraj AA, Kumaraguru P, Kosygan K. Intra-articular bupivacaine hip injection in differentiation of coxarthrosis from referred thigh pain: a 10 year study. Acta Orthop Belg. 2003;69(6):518–21.
53. Kaspar J, Kaspar S, Orme C, de Beer Jde V. Intra-articular steroid hip injection for osteoarthritis: a survey of orthopedic surgeons in Ontario. Can J Surg. 2005;48(6):461–9.
54. Kleiner JB, Thorne RP, Curd JG. The value of bupivicaine hip injection in the differentiation of coxarthrosis from lower extremity neuropathy. J Rheumatol. 1991;18(3):422–7.
55. Saito J, Ohtori S, Kishida S, Nakamura J, Takeshita M, Shigemura T, et al. Difficulty of diagnosing the origin of lower leg pain in patients with both lumbar spinal stenosis and hip joint osteoarthritis. Spine (Phila Pa 1976). 2012;37(25):2089–93.
56. Deshmukh AJ, Thakur RR, Goyal A, Klein DA, Ranawat AS, Rodriguez JA. Accuracy of diagnostic injection in differentiating source of atypical hip pain. J Arthroplasty. 2010;25(6 Suppl):129–33.
57. Recommendations for the medical management of osteoarthritis of the hip and knee: 2000 update. American College of Rheumatology Subcommittee on Osteoarthritis Guidelines. Arthritis Rheum. 2000;43(9):1905–15.
58. Hochberg MC, Altman RD, April KT, Benkhalti M, Guyatt G, McGowan J, et al. American College of Rheumatology 2012 recommendations for the use of nonpharmacologic and pharmacologic therapies in osteoarthritis of the hand, hip, and knee. Arthritis Care Res (Hoboken). 2012;64(4):465–74.
59. Zhang W, Moskowitz RW, Nuki G, Abramson S, Altman RD, Arden N, et al. OARSI recommendations for the management of hip and knee osteoarthritis, Part II: OARSI evidence-based, expert consensus guidelines. Osteoarthritis Cartilage. 2008;16(2):137–62.
60. Zhang W, Nuki G, Moskowitz RW, Abramson S, Altman RD, Arden NK, et al. OARSI recommendations for the management of hip and knee osteoarthritis: part III: changes in evidence following systematic cumulative update of research published through January 2009. Osteoarthritis Cartilage. 2010;18(4):476–99.
61. Karuppiah SV, Gibson P. The safety of hip injection with corticosteroid in the diagnosis and treatment of osteoarthritis. Hip Int. 2007;17(1):36–9.
62. Lambert RG, Hutchings EJ, Grace MG, Jhangri GS, Conner-Spady B, Maksymowych WP. Steroid injection for osteoarthritis of the hip: a randomized, double-blind, placebo-controlled trial. Arthritis Rheum. 2007;56(7):2278–87.
63. Qvistgaard E, Christensen R, Torp-Pedersen S, Bliddal H. Intra-articular treatment of hip osteoarthritis: a randomized trial of hyaluronic acid, corticosteroid, and isotonic saline. Osteoarthritis Cartilage. 2006;14(2):163–70.
64. Kaspar S, de V de Beer J. Infection in hip arthroplasty after previous injection of steroid. J Bone Joint Surg Br. 2005;87(4):454–7.
65. Chitre AR, Fehily MJ, Bamford DJ. Total hip replacement after intra-articular injection of local anaesthetic and steroid. J Bone Joint Surg Br. 2007;89(2):166–8.
66. Croft S, Rockwood P. Risk of intraarticular steroid injection before total hip arthroplasty. Curr Orthop Pract. 2013;2(24):185–8.
67. Haughton D, Davey C, Sapherson D. Is hip injection safe and effective: the patients perspective? Rheumatology. 2010;1(49 Suppl):65.
68. McIntosh AL, Hanssen AD, Wenger DE, Osmon DR. Recent intraarticular steroid injection may increase infection rates in primary THA. Clin Orthop Relat Res. 2006;451:50–4.
69. McMahon SE, Lovell ME. Total hip arthroplasty after ipsilateral intra-articular steroid injection: 8 years follow up. Acta Orthop Belg. 2012;78(3):333–5.
70. Meermans G, Corten K, Simon JP. Is the infection rate in primary THA increased after steroid injection? Clin Orthop Relat Res. 2012;470(11):3213–9.
71. Ravi B, Escott BG, Wasserstein D, Croxford R, Hollands S, Paterson JM, et al. Intraarticular hip injection and early revision surgery following total hip arthroplasty: a retrospective cohort study. Arthritis Rheumatol. 2015;67(1):162–8.
72. Sankar B, Seneviratne S, Radha S, Rajeev A, Banaszkiewicz P. Safety of total hip replacement following an intra-articular steroid hip injection – an audit. Acta Orthop Belg. 2012;78(2):183–6.
73. Sreekumar R, Venkiteswaran R, Raut V. Infection in primary hip arthroplasty after previous steroid infiltration. Int Orthop. 2007;31(1):125–8.
74. Desai A, Ramankutty S, Board T, Raut V. Does intraarticular steroid infiltration increase the rate of infection in subsequent total knee replacements? Knee. 2009;16(4):262–4.
75. Horne G, Devane P, Davidson A, Adams K, Purdie G. The influence of steroid injections on the incidence of infection following total knee arthroplasty. N Z Med J. 2008;121(1268):U2896.
76. Joshy S, Thomas B, Gogi N, Modi A, Singh BK. Effect of intra-articular steroids on deep infections following total knee arthroplasty. Int Orthop. 2006;30(2):91–3.
77. Papavasiliou AV, Isaac DL, Marimuthu R, Skyrme A, Armitage A. Infection in knee replacements after previous injection of intra-articular steroid. J Bone Joint Surg Br. 2006;88(3):321–3.

78. Charalambous CP, Prodromidis AD, Kwaees TA. Do intra-articular steroid injections increase infection rates in subsequent arthroplasty? A systematic review and meta-analysis of comparative studies. J Arthroplasty. 2014;29(11):2175–80.
79. McMahon SE, LeRoux JA, Smith TO, Hing CB. Total joint arthroplasty following intra-articular steroid injection: a literature review. Acta Orthop Belg. 2013;79(6):672–9.
80. Wang Q, Jiang X, Tian W. Does previous intra-articular steroid injection increase the risk of joint infection following total hip arthroplasty or total knee arthroplasty? A meta-analysis. Med Sci Monit. 2014;20:1878–83.
81. Xing D, Yang Y, Ma X, Ma J, Ma B, Chen Y. Dose intraarticular steroid injection increase the rate of infection in subsequent arthroplasty: grading the evidence through a meta-analysis. J Orthop Surg Res. 2014;9(1):107.
82. Hepper CT, Halvorson JJ, Duncan ST, Gregory AJ, Dunn WR, Spindler KP. The efficacy and duration of intra-articular corticosteroid injection for knee osteoarthritis: a systematic review of level I studies. J Am Acad Orthop Surg. 2009;17(10):638–46.
83. Arroll B, Goodyear-Smith F. Corticosteroid injections for osteoarthritis of the knee: meta-analysis. BMJ. 2004;328(7444):869.
84. Cancienne JM, Werner BC, Luetkemeyer LM, Browne JA. Does timing of previous intra-articular steroid injection affect the post-operative rate of infection in total knee arthroplasty? J Arthroplasty. 2015;30(11):187–82. doi:10.1016/j.arth.2015.05.027.
85. Marsland D, Mumith A, Barlow IW. Systematic review: the safety of intra-articular corticosteroid injection prior to total knee arthroplasty. Knee. 2014;21(1):6–11.
86. Jones A, Regan M, Ledingham J, Pattrick M, Manhire A, Doherty M. Importance of placement of intra-articular steroid injections. BMJ. 1993;307(6915):1329–30.
87. Albert C, Brocq O, Gerard D, Roux C, Euller-Ziegler L. Septic knee arthritis after intra-articular hyaluronate injection. Two case reports. Joint Bone Spine. 2006;73(2):205–7. Epub 2005 Jun 23.
88. Evanich JD, Evanich CJ, Wright MB, Rydlewicz JA. Efficacy of intraarticular hyaluronic acid injections in knee osteoarthritis. Clin Orthop Relat Res. 2001;390:173–81.
89. Morshed S, Huffman GR, Ries MD. Septic arthritis of the hip and intrapelvic abscess following intra-articular injection of hylan G-F 20. A case report. J Bone Joint Surg Am. 2004;86-A(4):823–6.
90. Papanikolaou A, Tzavara V, Chini M, Papatheodorou A. Pyomyositis and septic hip arthritis due to bacteroides fragilis. A case report. Hip Int. 2011;21(4):498–501.
91. Shemesh S, Heller S, Salai M, Velkes S. Septic arthritis of the knee following intraarticular injections in elderly patients: report of six patients. Isr Med Assoc J. 2011;13(12):757–60.
92. Yoong P, Guirguis R, Darrah R, Wijeratna M, Porteous MJ. Evaluation of ultrasound-guided diagnostic local anaesthetic hip joint injection for osteoarthritis. Skeletal Radiol. 2012;41(8):981–5.
93. Fitzgerald Jr RH, Nolan DR, Ilstrup DM, Van Scoy RE, Washington 2nd JA, Coventry MB. Deep wound sepsis following total hip arthroplasty. J Bone Joint Surg Am. 1977;59(7):847–55.
94. Jover-Saénz A, Barcenilla-Gaite F, Torres-Puig-Gros J, Prats-Gispert L, Garrido-Calvo S, Porcel-Pérez JM. Risk factors for total prosthetic joint infection. Case-control study. Med Clin (Barc). 2007;128(13):493–4.
95. McKinley JC, Robinson CM. Treatment of displaced intracapsular hip fractures with total hip arthroplasty: comparison of primary arthroplasty with early salvage arthroplasty after failed internal fixation. J Bone Joint Surg Am. 2002;84-A(11):2010–5.
96. Nelson JP, Glassburn Jr AR, Talbott RD, McElhinney JP. The effect of previous surgery, operating room environment, and preventive antibiotics on postoperative infection following total hip arthroplasty. Clin Orthop Relat Res. 1980;147:167–9.
97. Suzuki G, Saito S, Ishii T, Motojima S, Tokuhashi Y, Ryu J. Previous fracture surgery is a major risk factor of infection after total knee arthroplasty. Knee Surg Sports Traumatol Arthrosc. 2011;19(12):2040–4.
98. Wilson MG, Kelley K, Thornhill TS. Infection as a complication of total knee-replacement arthroplasty. Risk factors and treatment in sixty-seven cases. J Bone Joint Surg Am. 1990;72(6):878–83.
99. Archibeck MJ, Carothers JT, Tripuraneni KR, White Jr RE. Total hip arthroplasty after failed internal fixation of proximal femoral fractures. J Arthroplasty. 2013;28(1):168–71.
100. Haidukewych GJ, Israel TA, Berry DJ. Reverse obliquity fractures of the intertrochanteric region of the femur. J Bone Joint Surg Am. 2001;83-A(5):643–50.
101. Kyle RF, Cabanela ME, Russell TA, Swiontkowski MF, Winquist RA, Zuckerman JD, Schmidt AH, Koval KJ. Fractures of the proximal part of the femur. Instr Course Lect. 1995;44:227–53.
102. Bannister GC, Gibson AG, Ackroyd CE, Newman JH. The fixation and prognosis of trochanteric fractures. A randomized prospective controlled trial. Clin Orthop Relat Res. 1990;254:242–6.
103. Kyle RF, Ellis TJ, Templeman DC. Surgical treatment of intertrochanteric hip fractures with associated femoral neck fractures using a sliding hip screw. J Orthop Trauma. 2005;19(1):1–4.
104. Mariani EM, Rand JA. Nonunion of intertrochanteric fractures of the femur following open reduction and internal fixation. Results of second attempts to gain union. Clin Orthop Relat Res. 1987;218:81–9.

105. Sarathy MP, Madhavan P, Ravichandran KM. Nonunion of intertrochanteric fractures of the femur. Treatment by modified medial displacement and valgus osteotomy. J Bone Joint Surg Br. 1995; 77(1):90–2.
106. Stoffelen D, Haentjens P, Reynders P, Casteleyn PP, Broos P, Opdecam P. Hip arthroplasty for failed internal fixation of intertrochanteric and subtrochanteric fractures in the elderly patient. Acta Orthop Belg. 1994;60 Suppl 1:135–9.
107. Wu CC, Shih CH, Chen WJ, Tai CL. Treatment of cutout of a lag screw of a dynamic hip screw in an intertrochanteric fracture. Arch Orthop Trauma Surg. 1998;117(4–5):193–6.
108. Haentjens P, Casteleyn PP, Opdecam P. Hip arthroplasty for failed internal fixation of intertrochanteric and subtrochanteric fractures in the elderly patient. Arch Orthop Trauma Surg. 1994;113(4):222–7.
109. Kim YH, Oh JH, Koh YG. Salvage of neglected unstable intertrochanteric fracture with cementless porous-coated hemiarthroplasty. Clin Orthop Relat Res. 1992;277:182–7.
110. Saleh KJ, Sherman P, Katkin P, Windsor R, Haas S, Laskin R, Sculco T. Total knee arthroplasty after open reduction and internal fixation of fractures of the tibial plateau: a minimum five-year follow-up study. J Bone Joint Surg Am. 2001;83-A(8):1144–8.
111. Wasserstein D, Henry P, Paterson JM, Kreder HJ, Jenkinson R. Risk of total knee arthroplasty after operatively treated tibial plateau fracture: a matched-population-based cohort study. J Bone Joint Surg Am. 2014;96(2):144–50.
112. Papadopoulos EC, Parvizi J, Lai CH, Lewallen DG. Total knee arthroplasty following prior distal femoral fracture. Knee. 2002;9(4):267–74.
113. Weiss NG, Parvizi J, Trousdale RT, Bryce RD, Lewallen DG. Total knee arthroplasty in patients with a prior fracture of the tibial plateau. J Bone Joint Surg Am. 2003;85-A(2):218–21.
114. Poss R, Thornhill TS, Ewald FC, Thomas WH, Batte NJ, Sledge CB. Factors influencing the incidence and outcome of infection following total joint arthroplasty. Clin Orthop Relat Res. 1984;182:117–26.
115. Aggarwal VK, Tischler EH, Lautenbach C, Williams Jr GR, Abboud JA, Altena M, et al. Mitigation and education. J Arthroplasty. 2014;29(2 Suppl):19–25.
116. Hanssen AD, Osmon DR, Nelson CL. Prevention of deep periprosthetic joint infection. Instr Course Lect. 1997;46:555–67.
117. Klatte TO, Meinicke R, O'Loughlin P, Rueger JM, Gehrke T, Kendoff D. Incidence of bacterial contamination in primary THA and combined hardware removal: analysis of preoperative aspiration and intraoperative biopsies. J Arthroplasty. 2013; 28(9):1677–80.
118. Klatte TO, Schneider MM, Citak M, Oloughlin P, Gebauer M, Rueger M, et al. Infection rates in patients undergoing primary knee arthroplasty with pre-existing orthopaedic fixation-devices. Knee. 2013;20(3):177–80.
119. Kessler B, Sendi P, Graber P, Knupp M, Zwicky L, Hintermann B, Zimmerli W. Risk factors for periprosthetic ankle joint infection: a case-control study. J Bone Joint Surg Am. 2012;94(20):1871–6.
120. Singh JA, Sperling JW, Schleck C, Harmsen W, Cofield RH. Periprosthetic infections after shoulder hemiarthroplasty. J Shoulder Elbow Surg. 2012; 21(10):1304–9.
121. Singh JA, Sperling JW, Schleck C, Harmsen WS, Cofield RH. Periprosthetic infections after total shoulder arthroplasty: a 33-year perspective. J Shoulder Elbow Surg. 2012;21(11):1534–41.

Part III

Diagnosis of Periprosthetic Joint Infection

Diagnosis of Periprosthetic Joint Infections: Traditional Pathways

7

Mohamed Sukeik and Fares S. Haddad

Abstract

Periprosthetic joint infection (PJI) remains a dreaded complication after hip and knee replacement surgery. Therefore, rapid and accurate detection of the causative pathogen is essential to intervene early and control the infection appropriately. The traditional pathway for diagnosing PJIs includes thorough history taking and physical examination, laboratory testing of serum and synovial fluid, various imaging modalities and analysis of intraoperative samples. None of the diagnostic tests available is 100 % sensitive and specific for diagnosing infection. Accordingly, an algorithm of major and minor criteria based on these tests has been devised by the Musculoskeletal Infection Society (MSIS) to aid the diagnosis and treatment.

This chapter aims to summarise the traditional pathway of diagnosing PJI with emphasis on strengths and weaknesses of available tests and strategies implemented to improve the diagnostic yield of those tests. New technologies based on biomarker assays, biofilm targeting and the application of metabolomics are currently underway and will be detailed in the following chapter.

Keywords

Arthroplasty • Biomarkers • Culture • Diagnosis • Hips • Knees • Prosthetic joint infections • Serum • Synovial fluid

M. Sukeik, MD, MRCSEd, PGA (✉)
Department of Trauma and Orthopaedics, The Royal London Hospital, Whitechapel, London E1 1BB, UK
e-mail: msukeik@hotmail.com

F.S. Haddad, BSc, MD(res), MCh, FRCS (Orth)
Department of Trauma and Orthopaedics, University College London Hospitals NHS Trust, London, UK

D. Kendoff et al. (eds.), *Periprosthetic Joint Infections: Changing Paradigms*,
DOI 10.1007/978-3-319-30091-7_7

Introduction

Despite all precautions taken in patient selection and patient optimisation preoperatively, periprosthetic joint infection (PJI) after hip and knee replacements remains an important yet difficult complication to manage. In fact, Sir John Charnley considered stopping hip replacement surgery in the 1960s because of the consequences of PJI [1]. An important factor contributing to the difficulty of managing PJIs is the lack of a test which is 100 % sensitive and specific to diagnose infection. Hence, the huge variations in the approach to managing PJIs and the difficulty comparing strategies and outcomes of infection control. The combination of available tests into an algorithm of major and minor diagnostic criteria by the Musculoskeletal Infection Society has sought to rectify this problem [2]. Further modification of this algorithm by the International Consensus Group (ICG) on PJI has been widely accepted by clinicians, societies and world organisations including the Centers for Disease Control (CDC) (Table 7.1). Nevertheless, identification of the causative organism and its characteristics may not always be feasible. Therefore, a systematic diagnostic approach should be combined with an individualised therapeutic strategy.

This review article aims to summarise the traditional pathway of diagnosing PJI which includes thorough history taking and physical examination, laboratory testing of serum and synovial fluid, various imaging modalities and analysis of intraoperative samples.

History and Physical Examination

A thorough history and physical examination are important to identify the type of PJI encountered and assess patient's risk factors and suitability for surgical treatment. Acute infection according to Tsukayama et al. [3] presents within 4 weeks of the index procedure and is characterised by continuous pain and an erythematous, swollen and fluctuant wound with purulent discharge and occasional wound dehiscence. Systemic symptoms such as fever and chills may also occur. Chronic infection on the other hand, occurs after 4 weeks from the index procedure [3] and is characterised by gradual deterioration of function, persistent pain from the time of the operation and

Table 7.1 Definitions of periprosthetic joint infection

Musculoskeletal Infection Society (MSIS)	Centers for Disease Control (CDC) on PJI
Major criteria:	Major criteria:
1. There is a sinus tract communicating with the prosthesis; or	1. A sinus tract communicating with the joint; or
2. A pathogen is isolated by culture from 2 or more separate tissue or fluid samples obtained from the affected prosthetic joint; or	2. Two positive periprosthetic tissue or fluid cultures with matching organisms; or
Minor criteria:	Minor criteria:
3. When 4 of the following 6 criteria exist:	3. When 3 of the following 5 criteria exist:
(a) Elevated ESR and CRP	(a) CRP >100 mg/L AND ESR >30 mm/h
(b) Elevated synovial WCC	(b) Synovial fluid WCC >10,000 cells/μl OR ++ change on leucocyte esterase strip test of synovial fluid
(c) Elevated synovial polymorphonuclear percentage (PMN%)	(c) Elevated synovial fluid PMN percentage (>90 %)
(d) Presence of purulence in the affected joint	(d) A single positive periprosthetic tissue or fluid culture
(e) Isolation of a microorganism in one culture of periprosthetic tissue or fluid, or	(e) Positive histological analysis of periprosthetic tissue (more than 5 pmns per high power field)
(f) Greater than 5 neutrophils per high-power field in 5 high-power fields observed from histologic analysis of periprosthetic tissue at ×400 magnification	

a draining sinus. Relevant history includes prolonged wound discharge and wound healing after multiple courses of antibiotics. A previous history of infection is also important especially in tuberculosis where reactivation of infection may occur after a prolonged period of quiescence. Haematogenous infection can occur at any time after the index operation [3] and typically involves a prosthesis that has been functioning well for months or years. The most frequent primary seeding site is skin and soft tissue infections [4]. However, other sources of infection may include the urinary, respiratory, and gastrointestinal tract, as well as recent dental work [5]. This type of infection is more likely to occur in immunocompromised patients and hence the importance of carefully assessing this subset of patients for comorbidities such as diabetes, chronic renal impairment, inflammatory arthropathy and malignancies.

Early diagnosis of PJI in a well-fixed implant may allow salvage of the prosthesis using an aggressive early debridement strategy with exchange of modular components, whereas a delay in diagnosis or in the case of chronic infections, a single or staged exchange procedure may be more appropriate to control the infection. In either case, rapid intervention based on thorough assessment has been deemed a primary prognostic factor for infection control as it may prevent biofilm formation by the infecting bacteria [6].

Serological Tests

The white blood cell count (WBC) and polymorphonuclear (PMN) percentage have been found to have a minimal role in routine workup of patients with suspected PJI due to low sensitivity and specificity [7, 8]. However, the C-reactive protein (CRP) and erythrocyte sedimentation rate (ESR) should be used as a screening tool for all patients with suspected infection. The CRP level reaches maximum values within 48 h from surgery and returns to normal within 3 weeks, whereas ESR may remain elevated for months post surgery [6, 9]. Therefore, an elevated CRP is more accurate in identifying infection [10]. A CRP level of >10 mg/L and an ESR level of >30 mm/h correlated with PJI in all total hip arthroplasties (THAs) that were complicated by deep infection in two studies [8, 11]. As a result, authors recommended combining both tests to improve the accuracy of diagnosing infection. It is important though to recognise that ESR and CRP are nonspecific markers of inflammation and that they are frequently elevated in other inflammatory and infectious conditions as well as malignancy, which may cause false-positive results for PJI. Additionally, they are elevated in the early postoperative period after a routine hip or knee replacement. Therefore, Bedair et al. [12] and Yi et al. [13] defined the threshold values for CRP in acute postoperative PJIs of the hip and knee as 93 and 95 mg/L, respectively. Greidanus et al. [14] suggested that both ESR (sensitivity, 0.93; specificity, 0.83; positive likelihood ratio, 5.81; accuracy, 0.86) and CRP (sensitivity, 0.91; specificity, 0.86; positive likelihood ratio, 6.89; accuracy, 0.88) have excellent diagnostic test performance. In a recent study of 320 PJIs, Zajonz et al. [15] showed no differences between hip and knee arthroplasty patients regarding levels of inflammatory markers. Parvizi suggested in a recent study [16] that the best diagnostic strategy after confirming abnormal CRP and ESR levels would be a diagnostic aspiration of the joint. On the other hand, the American Academy of Orthopaedic Surgeons Clinical Practice Guidelines on PJIs [17] suggest that even normal levels of ESR and CRP do not rule out PJI, and that these tests alone should not be relied on for definite exclusion of PJI.

Interleukin-6 (IL-6) and procalcitonin have also been investigated and were initially presented as valuable markers for detecting PJIs [18–20]. However, recent studies showed no superiority of either test over CRP in diagnosing infection [21–23]. Additionally, studies relating to IL6 have been criticised for not accounting for the confounding influence of previous antibiotic use and associated inflammatory conditions on IL-6 performance [18, 19].

Other serum biomarkers elevated in PJI that are under investigation for future application include tumour necrosis factor (TNF)-α, short-chain exocellular lipoteichoic acid, soluble intercellular adhesion molecule-1, and monocyte chemoattractant protein-1 [24].

Synovial Fluid Tests

Hip and knee aspirations are performed using the surgeon's preferred technique. However, a strict aseptic technique is essential to reduce false-positive results and prevent iatrogenic periprosthetic infection. Fluoroscopic guidance is usually utilised for the hip joint but ultrasound-guided hip aspirations have also been reported [25]. Local anaesthetic and contrast material should be avoided due to the potential bactericidal effect and associated false-negative results [26, 27]. Similarly, it is recommended that patients stop any antibiotics for a minimum of 2 weeks prior to obtaining synovial fluid or cultures to avoid false-negative results [28]. The synovial fluid should be sent for microbiologic cultures, WBC count and differentials. Blood culture flasks should be used for the synovial fluid [29], and specialised media are required for suspected atypical infections, such as Lowenstein-Jensen media for mycobacteria [30] or Sabouraud's dextrose agar for fungi [31]. Prolonged culture incubation for 14 days may be required if *P. acnes*, fungi or mycobacterium are suspected [32]. However, cultures for mycobacterium and fungi should not be done routinely as this would not be cost-effective [33]. If the culture results are negative in the setting of elevated synovial and serum markers suggestive of infection, repeat aspiration should be performed prior to surgery or initiation of antimicrobial treatment [34]. The optimal cut-points of synovial WBC count, PMN percentage and serum CRP levels for diagnosing acute and chronic hip and knee PJIs are detailed in Table 7.2 [12, 13, 35].

Leucocyte esterase (LE) testing has recently been added to the minor diagnostic criteria for PJIs used by the ICG/CDC due to the low cost, easy applicability and high sensitivity (80 %) and specificity (100 %) rates reported [36]. However, it is important to remember that the presence of blood in the synovial fluid aspirates, may negatively affect the interpretation of the LE strip but that centrifuging the sample overcomes this problem without affecting the accuracy of the test [37, 38].

Table 7.2 Laboratory threshold values for periprosthetic joint infection of the knee and hip

	Acute		Chronic	
	TKA	THA	TKA	THA
Serum CRP (mg/L)	95	93	10	10
Synovial WBC Count (cells/μL)	27,800	12,800	1100–4000	3000
Synovial PMN Cells (%)	89	89	64–69	80

Abbreviations: *TKA* total knee arthroplasty, *THA* total hip arthroplasty, *CRP* C-reactive protein, *WBC* white blood cell, *PMN* polymorphonuclear

Synovial CRP and IL-6 have also been proposed to improve diagnostic accuracy in PJI. For example, combined measurement of synovial CRP and α-Defensin levels demonstrated a sensitivity of 97 % and a specificity of 100 % for the diagnosis of PJI and correctly diagnosed 99 % of cases as aseptic or infected [39]. However, despite some studies suggesting a superiority of synovial CRP over serum CRP [40, 41], a recent report suggested that synovial CRP does not offer a diagnostic advantage in detection of PJIs [42]. Randau et al. [43] suggested that synovial IL-6 is a more accurate marker than serum WBC and CRP for the detection of PJIs and that combining serum and synovial IL-6, compared with performing each test individually improves the diagnostic yield. Recent studies have also shown that IL-6 has high specificity and accuracy even when patients who were taking antibiotics and those with systemic inflammatory diseases were included [41, 44].

Other synovial biomarkers elevated in PJI which are under investigation for future application include cytokines such as IL-1β, IL-6, IL-8, IL-17, TNF-α, interferon-δ, and vascular endothelial growth factor, human β-defensin-2 (HBD-2) and HBD-3, and cathelicidin LL-37 [24]. New technologies based on synovial fluid biomarker analysis, biofilm targeting and the application of metabolomics are currently underway and will be detailed in the following chapter.

Imaging Modalities

Plain radiographs should be included in any workup for infected joint replacements. However, they are neither sensitive nor specific for detection of infection. Radiographic findings including loosening and osteolysis are common to both septic and aseptic failures. On the other hand, periosteal new bone formation and endosteal scalloping, are more suggestive of infection but are not seen in all cases [8].

Computed tomography (CT) provides detailed analysis of bony structures and may show evidence of soft tissue collections. However, it is limited due to metal artefact, is associated with low sensitivity for detecting PJI and exposes patients to high doses of radiation alongside the significant cost associated with using them [45]. Magnetic resonance imaging (MRI) is also limited due to metal artefact and studies relating to accuracy of metal artefact reduction sequence (MARS) MRIs are limited in the literature [46].

Scintigraphy studies may be helpful when results of serologic tests are falsely elevated due to inflammatory conditions and cultures of synovial fluid are unreliable because of administration of antibiotics or in the case of a dry tap especially if the patient is not planned for surgery [47]. However, the cost of a scan is significant and comparable to that of a CT or MRI scan, the amount of radiation is equivalent to a CT scan, and results can remain positive for as long as one year after a knee or hip arthroplasty due to the increased uptake from the surgery itself. A number of isotopes including Technetium-99 m, Gallium-67 citrate, and Indium-111-labelled WBCs have been used with variable sensitivities and specificities in detecting PJIs. Ouyang et al. [48] reported in a recent systematic review that overall sensitivity and specificity for using triple phase bone scans to detect PJI was 0.83 and specificity was 0.73. However, the sensitivity and specificity for detecting infected arthroplasty of the hip (0.81 and 0.78, respectively) were significantly higher than those of the knee (0.75 and 0.55, respectively; $p<0.05$). A meta-analysis of antigranulocyte scintigraphy with monoclonal antibodies studying PJI in THAs showed sensitivity and specificity of 83 % and 80 %, respectively [49]. On the other hand, sensitivity of Indium-111-labelled white blood cell labelled scans for detecting periprosthetic hip infections has been reported as low as 50 % in the literature [50].

Fluorodeoxyglucose (FDG)-positron emission tomography (FDG-PET) has been investigated over the last decade for a role in diagnosing PJIs. The investigation relies on the fact that inflammatory cells express more glucose transporters, resulting in intracellular accumulation of deoxyglucose which cannot be metabolised by the cell and can be identified by PET imaging. Although a meta-analysis conducted in 2006 by Prandini et al. [51] reported a sensitivity of 94.1 % and a specificity of 87.3 % for detecting PJI, another meta-analysis in 2008 [52] reported the overall diagnostic performance of FDG-PET as moderate to high and warned about heterogeneity of studies available in the literature. Two further studies published over the last 3 years [53, 54] suggested that the role of FDG-PET in diagnosing PJI is still to be determined. It is worth noting as well that this type of imaging is currently only available in tertiary referral centres and that it costs three times the cost of a bone scan or MRI [55].

Intraoperative Assessment

Intraoperative assessment at the time of revision surgery starts with evaluating the tissue appearance and classically performing gram stains of fluid or tissue samples collected. However, it is important to recognise that neither tissue appearance nor gram staining are reliable indicators for ruling in or ruling out infection [8, 56].

Intraoperative frozen sections have been reported as useful methods for detecting PJI in patients planned for revision surgery when other tests have been suggestive but not conclusive of infection [47]. Samples from deep tissues including the interfaces between bone and cement and cement and the implant should be sent for analysis. An experienced pathologist is essential to interpret the results according to the number of

WBCs visualised per high power field. A study of 175 revision arthroplasties recommended using 10 WBCs/high power field as a threshold for diagnosing infection with a sensitivity of 0.84 and specificity of 0.99 [57]. MSIS/CDC guidelines recognise more than 5 PMNs per high power field as a minor diagnostic criterion for PJI [35]. A recent study suggested that at the time of second-stage reimplantation surgery, frozen section is useful in ruling in infection, where the specificity is 94 %; however, there is less utility in ruling out infection, because sensitivity is only 50 % [58]. Intraoperative synovial fluid sampling follows the same principles as preoperative synovial fluid sampling as outlined previously.

Intraoperative cultures are presumed to be the gold standard for identifying PJI. However, they are subject to false-negative and false-positive results [3]. As with joint aspiration, careful technique and withholding antibiotics for at least 2 few weeks preoperatively are essential to reduce false negatives [28]. The definitive diagnosis of PJI is made when the same organism is isolated from at least two intraoperative cultures [35]. However, various studies suggest that three to six samples are collected from superficial, deep and periprosthetic tissues in order to obtain an accurate diagnosis of infection [35, 59, 60]. The explanted component should also be sent to the microbiology lab for sonication as this improves sensitivity of the cultures from 61 to 78 % even with patients who are receiving antibiotic treatment [61]. The incubation period for cultures should be at least 7 days. However, reports published recently suggest prolonging incubation for 14 days as this increases the chances of identifying organisms that otherwise may remain culture negative (26.4 % additional cases were classified as infected at 14 vs. 7 days) [32, 62].

In 10–15 % of cases, despite the presence of clear signs for infection including gross purulence, cultures may still be negative [63]. Possible causes may be inappropriate collection of samples, short incubation duration and the use of antimicrobial therapy prior to samples collection. Interestingly though, Ghanem et al. [64] demonstrated that the administration of preoperative antibiotics to patients with a positive preoperative joint aspirate did not interfere with the isolation of the infecting organism more than when antibiotics were stopped. Therefore, it is paramount to liaise carefully with microbiologists to facilitate rapid and accurate analysis of intraoperative samples.

In conclusion, the combination of various diagnostic tests into the MSIS algorithm has improved consensus and approach to managing PJIs. A paradigm shift towards new technologies based on biomarker assays, biofilm targeting and the application of metabolomics may be the way forward to further improve our ability to diagnose and treat this difficult problem in the future.

References

1. Stockley I. Infected arthoplasty. J Trauma Orthop. 2014;2(3):52–3.
2. Gehrke T, Parvizi J. Proceedings of the international consensus meeting on periprosthetic joint infection. Foreword. J Orthop Res. 2014;32 Suppl 1:S2–3.
3. Tsukayama DT, Estrada R, Gustilo RB. Infection after total hip arthroplasty. A study of the treatment of one hundred and six infections. J Bone Joint Surg Am. 1996;78(4):512–23.
4. Zimmerli W, Moser C. Pathogenesis and treatment concepts of orthopaedic biofilm infections. FEMS Immunol Med Microbiol. 2012;65(2):158–68.
5. Maderazo EG, Judson S, Pasternak H. Late infections of total joint prostheses. A review and recommendations for prevention. Clin Orthop Relat Res. 1988;229:131–42.
6. Moyad TF, Thornhill T, Estok D. Evaluation and management of the infected total hip and knee. Orthopedics. 2008;31(6):581–8; quiz 9–90.
7. Toossi N, Adeli B, Rasouli MR, Huang R, Parvizi J. Serum white blood cell count and differential do not have a role in the diagnosis of periprosthetic joint infection. J Arthroplasty. 2012;27(8 Suppl):51–4.e1.
8. Spangehl MJ, Masri BA, O'Connell JX, Duncan CP. Prospective analysis of preoperative and intraoperative investigations for the diagnosis of infection at the sites of two hundred and two revision total hip arthroplasties. J Bone Joint Surg Am. 1999;81(5):672–83.
9. Shih LY, Wu JJ, Yang DJ. Erythrocyte sedimentation rate and C-reactive protein values in patients with total hip arthroplasty. Clin Orthop Relat Res. 1987;225:238–46.
10. Haaker R, Senge A, Kramer J, Rubenthaler F. Osteomyelitis after endoprostheses. Orthopade. 2004;33(4):431–8.
11. Schinsky MF, Della Valle CJ, Sporer SM, Paprosky WG. Perioperative testing for joint infection in

patients undergoing revision total hip arthroplasty. J Bone Joint Surg Am. 2008;90(9):1869–75.
12. Bedair H, Ting N, Jacovides C, Saxena A, Moric M, Parvizi J, et al. The Mark Coventry Award: diagnosis of early postoperative TKA infection using synovial fluid analysis. Clin Orthop Relat Res. 2011; 469(1):34–40.
13. Yi PH, Cross MB, Moric M, Sporer SM, Berger RA, Della Valle CJ. The 2013 Frank Stinchfield Award: diagnosis of infection in the early postoperative period after total hip arthroplasty. Clin Orthop Relat Res. 2014;472(2):424–9.
14. Greidanus NV, Masri BA, Garbuz DS, Wilson SD, McAlinden MG, Xu M, et al. Use of erythrocyte sedimentation rate and C-reactive protein level to diagnose infection before revision total knee arthroplasty. A prospective evaluation. J Bone Joint Surg Am. 2007;89(7):1409–16.
15. Zajonz D, Wuthe L, Tiepolt S, Brandmeier P, Prietzel T, von Salis-Soglio GF, et al. Diagnostic work-up strategy for periprosthetic joint infections after total hip and knee arthroplasty: a 12-year experience on 320 consecutive cases. Patient Saf Surg. 2015;9:20.
16. Diaz-Ledezma C, Lichstein PM, Dolan JG, Parvizi J. Diagnosis of periprosthetic joint infection in Medicare patients: multicriteria decision analysis. Clin Orthop Relat Res. 2014;472(11):3275–84.
17. Parvizi J, Della Valle CJ. AAOS clinical practice guideline: diagnosis and treatment of periprosthetic joint infections of the hip and knee. J Am Acad Orthop Surg. 2010;18(12):771–2.
18. Berbari E, Mabry T, Tsaras G, Spangehl M, Erwin PJ, Murad MH, et al. Inflammatory blood laboratory levels as markers of prosthetic joint infection: a systematic review and meta-analysis. J Bone Joint Surg Am. 2010;92(11):2102–9.
19. Di Cesare PE, Chang E, Preston CF, Liu CJ. Serum interleukin-6 as a marker of periprosthetic infection following total hip and knee arthroplasty. J Bone Joint Surg Am. 2005;87(9):1921–7.
20. Shaikh MM, Hermans LE, van Laar JM. Is serum procalcitonin measurement a useful addition to a rheumatologist's repertoire? A review of its diagnostic role in systemic inflammatory diseases and joint infections. Rheumatology (Oxford). 2015;54(2):231–40.
21. Glehr M, Friesenbichler J, Hofmann G, Bernhardt GA, Zacherl M, Avian A, et al. Novel biomarkers to detect infection in revision hip and knee arthroplasties. Clin Orthop Relat Res. 2013;471(8):2621–8.
22. Drago L, Vassena C, Dozio E, Corsi MM, De Vecchi E, Mattina R, et al. Procalcitonin, C-reactive protein, interleukin-6, and soluble intercellular adhesion molecule-1 as markers of postoperative orthopaedic joint prosthesis infections. Int J Immunopathol Pharmacol. 2011;24(2):433–40.
23. Yuan K, Li WD, Qiang Y, Cui ZM. Comparison of procalcitonin and C-reactive protein for the diagnosis of periprosthetic joint infection before revision total hip arthroplasty. Surg Infect (Larchmt). 2015;16(2):146–50.
24. Chen A, Fei J, Deirmegian C. Diagnosis of periprosthetic infection: novel developments. J Knee Surg. 2014;27(4):259–65.
25. Battaglia M, Vannini F, Guaraldi F, Rossi G, Biondi F, Sudanese A. Validity of preoperative ultrasound-guided aspiration in the revision of hip prosthesis. Ultrasound Med Biol. 2011;37(12):1977–83.
26. Ali F, Wilkinson JM, Cooper JR, Kerry RM, Hamer AJ, Norman P, et al. Accuracy of joint aspiration for the preoperative diagnosis of infection in total hip arthroplasty. J Arthroplasty. 2006;21(2):221–6.
27. Schmidt RM, Rosenkranz HS. Antimicrobial activity of local anesthetics: lidocaine and procaine. J Infect Dis. 1970;121(6):597–607.
28. Della Valle C, Parvizi J, Bauer TW, DiCesare PE, Evans RP, Segreti J, et al. American Academy of Orthopaedic Surgeons clinical practice guideline on: the diagnosis of periprosthetic joint infections of the hip and knee. J Bone Joint Surg Am. 2011; 93(14):1355–7.
29. Font-Vizcarra L, Garcia S, Martinez-Pastor JC, Sierra JM, Soriano A. Blood culture flasks for culturing synovial fluid in prosthetic joint infections. Clin Orthop Relat Res. 2010;468(8):2238–43.
30. Woods GL. The mycobacteriology laboratory and new diagnostic techniques. Infect Dis Clin North Am. 2002;16(1):127–44.
31. O'Shaughnessy EM, Shea YM, Witebsky FG. Laboratory diagnosis of invasive mycoses. Infect Dis Clin North Am. 2003;17(1):135–58.
32. Schafer P, Fink B, Sandow D, Margull A, Berger I, Frommelt L. Prolonged bacterial culture to identify late periprosthetic joint infection: a promising strategy. Clin Infect Dis. 2008;47(11):1403–9.
33. Tokarski AT, O'Neil J, Deirmengian CA, Ferguson J, Deirmengian GK. The routine use of atypical cultures in presumed aseptic revisions is unnecessary. Clin Orthop Relat Res. 2013;471(10):3171–7.
34. Barrack RL, Jennings RW, Wolfe MW, Bertot AJ. The Coventry Award. The value of preoperative aspiration before total knee revision. Clin Orthop Relat Res. 1997;345:8–16.
35. Parvizi J, Zmistowski B, Berbari EF, Bauer TW, Springer BD, Della Valle CJ, et al. New definition for periprosthetic joint infection: from the Workgroup of the Musculoskeletal Infection Society. Clin Orthop Relat Res. 2011;469(11):2992–4.
36. Parvizi J, Jacovides C, Antoci V, Ghanem E. Diagnosis of periprosthetic joint infection: the utility of a simple yet unappreciated enzyme. J Bone Joint Surg Am. 2011;93(24):2242–8.
37. Aggarwal VK, Tischler E, Ghanem E, Parvizi J. Leukocyte esterase from synovial fluid aspirate: a technical note. J Arthroplasty. 2013;28(1):193–5.
38. Wetters NG, Berend KR, Lombardi AV, Morris MJ, Tucker TL, Della Valle CJ. Leukocyte esterase reagent strips for the rapid diagnosis of periprosthetic joint infection. J Arthroplasty. 2012;27(8 Suppl):8–11.
39. Deirmengian C, Kardos K, Kilmartin P, Cameron A, Schiller K, Parvizi J. Combined measurement of

synovial fluid alpha-Defensin and C-reactive protein levels: highly accurate for diagnosing periprosthetic joint infection. J Bone Joint Surg Am. 2014;96(17):1439–45.
40. Parvizi J, Jacovides C, Adeli B, Jung KA, Hozack WJ, Mark B. Coventry Award: synovial C-reactive protein: a prospective evaluation of a molecular marker for periprosthetic knee joint infection. Clin Orthop Relat Res. 2012;470(1):54–60.
41. Jacovides CL, Parvizi J, Adeli B, Jung KA. Molecular markers for diagnosis of periprosthetic joint infection. J Arthroplasty. 2011;26(6 Suppl):99–103.e1.
42. Tetreault MW, Wetters NG, Moric M, Gross CE, Della Valle CJ. Is synovial C-reactive protein a useful marker for periprosthetic joint infection? Clin Orthop Relat Res. 2014;472(12):3997–4003.
43. Randau TM, Friedrich MJ, Wimmer MD, Reichert B, Kuberra D, Stoffel-Wagner B, et al. Interleukin-6 in serum and in synovial fluid enhances the differentiation between periprosthetic joint infection and aseptic loosening. PLoS One. 2014;9(2), e89045.
44. Deirmengian C, Hallab N, Tarabishy A, Della Valle C, Jacobs JJ, Lonner J, et al. Synovial fluid biomarkers for periprosthetic infection. Clin Orthop Relat Res. 2010;468(8):2017–23.
45. Cyteval C, Hamm V, Sarrabere MP, Lopez FM, Maury P, Taourel P. Painful infection at the site of hip prosthesis: CT imaging. Radiology. 2002;224(2):477–83.
46. Talbot BS, Weinberg EP. MR imaging with metal-suppression sequences for evaluation of total joint arthroplasty. Radiographics. 2015;20:150075.
47. Enayatollahi MA, Parvizi J. Diagnosis of infected total hip arthroplasty. Hip Int. 2015;25(4):294–300.
48. Ouyang Z, Li H, Liu X, Zhai Z, Li X. Prosthesis infection: diagnosis after total joint arthroplasty with three-phase bone scintigraphy. Ann Nucl Med. 2014;28(10):994–1003.
49. Pakos EE, Trikalinos TA, Fotopoulos AD, Ioannidis JP. Prosthesis infection: diagnosis after total joint arthroplasty with antigranulocyte scintigraphy with 99mTc-labeled monoclonal antibodies--a meta-analysis. Radiology. 2007;242(1):101–8.
50. Pill SG, Parvizi J, Tang PH, Garino JP, Nelson C, Zhuang H, et al. Comparison of fluorodeoxyglucose positron emission tomography and (111)indium-white blood cell imaging in the diagnosis of periprosthetic infection of the hip. J Arthroplasty. 2006;21(6 Suppl 2):91–7.
51. Prandini N, Lazzeri E, Rossi B, Erba P, Parisella MG, Signore A. Nuclear medicine imaging of bone infections. Nucl Med Commun. 2006;27(8):633–44.
52. Kwee TC, Kwee RM, Alavi A. FDG-PET for diagnosing prosthetic joint infection: systematic review and metaanalysis. Eur J Nucl Med Mol Imaging. 2008;35(11):2122–32.
53. Brammen L, Palestro C, Sinzinger H. Radionuclide imaging: Past, present and future outlook in the diagnosis of infected prosthetic joints. Hell J Nucl Med. 2015;18 Suppl 1:95–102.
54. Gemmel F, Van den Wyngaert H, Love C, Welling MM, Gemmel P, Palestro CJ. Prosthetic joint infections: radionuclide state-of-the-art imaging. Eur J Nucl Med Mol Imaging. 2012;39(5):892–909.
55. Hsu W, Hearty TM. Radionuclide imaging in the diagnosis and management of orthopaedic disease. J Am Acad Orthop Surg. 2012;20(3):151–9.
56. Della Valle CJ, Zuckerman JD, Di Cesare PE. Periprosthetic sepsis. Clin Orthop Relat Res. 2004;420:26–31.
57. Lonner JH, Desai P, Dicesare PE, Steiner G, Zuckerman JD. The reliability of analysis of intraoperative frozen sections for identifying active infection during revision hip or knee arthroplasty. J Bone Joint Surg Am. 1996;78(10):1553–8.
58. George J, Kwiecien G, Klika AK, Ramanathan D, Bauer TW, Barsoum WK, et al. Are frozen sections and MSIS criteria reliable at the time of reimplantation of two-stage revision arthroplasty? Clin Orthop Relat Res. 2015. [Epub ahead of print].
59. Atkins BL, Athanasou N, Deeks JJ, Crook DW, Simpson H, Peto TE, et al. Prospective evaluation of criteria for microbiological diagnosis of prosthetic-joint infection at revision arthroplasty. The OSIRIS Collaborative Study Group. J Clin Microbiol. 1998;36(10):2932–9.
60. Parvizi J, Azzam K, Ghanem E, Austin MS, Rothman RH. Periprosthetic infection due to resistant staphylococci: serious problems on the horizon. Clin Orthop Relat Res. 2009;467(7):1732–9.
61. Trampuz A, Piper KE, Jacobson MJ, Hanssen AD, Unni KK, Osmon DR, et al. Sonication of removed hip and knee prostheses for diagnosis of infection. N Engl J Med. 2007;357(7):654–63.
62. Larsen LH, Lange J, Xu Y, Schonheyder HC. Optimizing culture methods for diagnosis of prosthetic joint infections: a summary of modifications and improvements reported since 1995. J Med Microbiol. 1995;61(Pt 3):309–16.
63. Parvizi J, Ghanem E, Menashe S, Barrack RL, Bauer TW. Periprosthetic infection: what are the diagnostic challenges? J Bone Joint Surg Am. 2006;88 Suppl 4:138–47.
64. Ghanem E, Parvizi J, Clohisy J, Burnett S, Sharkey PF, Barrack R. Perioperative antibiotics should not be withheld in proven cases of periprosthetic infection. Clin Orthop Relat Res. 2007;461:44–7.

Diagnosis of Periprosthetic Joint Infection: New Technologies and Future Trends

8

Greg Kazarian and Carl Deirmengian

Abstract

Periprosthetic joint infection (PJI) remains a major burden on patients, physicians, and the health care system following joint arthroplasty. There has been extensive research into new and future technologies that could potentially increase the accuracy of diagnosing infection, and improve our ability to identify the infectious agent at the species level. The new generation of diagnostics utilizes traditional molecular and complex new technologies to identify the presence and identity of infectious agents. With respect to molecular diagnostics, the alpha-defensin biomarker assay has demonstrated high levels of sensitivity and specificity in the diagnosis of virulent and non-virulent organisms. Assays based on detecting biofilm antigens have shown promise as well. The advent of new technologies such as matrix-assisted laser desorption ionization time of flight mass spectrometry (MALDI-TOF MS), polymerase chain reaction electrospray ionization mass spectrometry (PCR-ESI/MS), and the application of metabolomics to joint infection, may lead to assays that rivals current standards. With continued improvement and growing acceptance of these new technologies, biomarker assays and MS or PCR based assays have the potential to become the new standards for diagnosing PJI.

G. Kazarian, BA
Rothman Institute/Jefferson, Media, PA, USA

C. Deirmengian, BA, MD (✉)
Department of Orthopaedic Surgery,
Rothman Institute/Jefferson, Lankenau,
26 Springton Pointe Drive, Newton Square, PA
19073, USA

D. Kendoff et al. (eds.), *Periprosthetic Joint Infections: Changing Paradigms*,
DOI 10.1007/978-3-319-30091-7_8

Keywords
Alpha-defensin • Arthroplasty • Biofilm detection • Biomarkers • Broad range PCR • Infection • Knee • MALDI • MALDI-TOF MS • Metabolomics • Molecular diagnostics • Multiplex PCR • PCR • PCR-ESI/MS • PJI • Reverse transcriptase PCR

Despite advances in the detection and treatment of periprosthetic joint infection (PJI), this complication remains a major burden on patients, physicians, and the health care system after joint replacement surgery. New technologies and better treatment algorithms have reduced the incidence of PJI after hip and knee arthroplasty to 0.3 % and 2 %, respectively [1, 2]. Despite the low incidence, the effects of this complication are sufficiently devastating and costly to warrant our continued attention in the fields of diagnosis and treatment.

The timely detection of the presence of infection and the identification of the responsible pathogen are the two most important factors in the diagnosis of PJI. A battery of diagnostic tests for the detection of PJI are now considered part of a traditional work-up, including serological tests (ESR, CRP), synovial fluid tests (WBC count, PMN percentage, culture) and intraoperative tissue tests (histology and tissue culture). These traditional tests have been combined into an algorithm of major and minor criteria for the definition of PJI by the Musculoskeletal Infection Society (MSIS) [3]. However, despite demonstrating their value in the diagnosis of infection over the past few years, they all have shortcomings. Furthermore, a final MSIS criteria-based diagnosis is only available after definitive surgical treatment.

There has been great interest recently in new and future technologies that could potentially increase the accuracy of diagnosing infection, and improve the identification of responsible organisms. Molecular biology in particular, has provided the resources by which research into biomarkers of disease and nucleic acid technologies have become possible.

Molecular Tests

Biomarkers

While methods like cultures and histological tests attempt to directly detect the infectious organism, methods like ESR and CRP detect changes in the host's inflammatory response that may indicate the presence of an infection. The materials and technology necessary to perform systemic blood tests for changes in the body's immune response are readily available at most health care institutions. These tests lack the sensitivity and specificity to act as a reliable diagnostic tool. Other phenomena or diseases, many of which are common to patients who have undergone a joint replacement, can elicit a systemic immune response that mimics infection. For example, autoimmune diseases such as rheumatoid arthritis and systemic infections not affecting the joint of interest may cause elevated levels of inflammatory markers.

Such issues have led to the interest in synovial fluid biomarker-based diagnostics in recent years. While systemic host response markers can have a lower sensitivity and specificity for PJI [4], direct analysis of the synovial fluid offers hope for a more specific marker for infection. Synovial fluid not only contains greater levels of certain biomarkers than blood, but it also is largely unaffected by external causes of inflammation [5, 6]. Therefore, synovial fluid provides a highly concentrated sample from the joint of interest for the analysis of relative changes in biomarker levels and the potential diagnosis of infection.

Early research in this area aimed to identify biomarkers that are elevated in the synovial fluid to differentiate infection from aseptic inflammation. For example, in order to identify differences in genetic transcription between infection and gout, Deirmengian et al. [7] analyzed synovial fluid samples from 7 patients with acute *Staphylococcus aureus* infections of the knee, and 5 samples from patients with acute gout. Genome-wide microarrays were used to identify the up- or down-regulation of genes and genetic pathways. In the infected patients, the interleukin pathway, the tumor necrosis factor pathway, and the anti-bacterial pathway were up-regulated. This proof-of-concept study laid the initial groundwork for the development of more feasible biomarker immunoassays.

Using the up-regulated genes and pathways as a starting point, a second study by Deirmengian et al. [5] initiated the process of converting the microarray data into a viable immunoassay for the diagnosis of joint infection. Of the 124 genes that showed statistically significant differences in the microarray study, 23 biomarkers were selected for analysis based on their involvement in key antimicrobial or inflammatory response pathways. The synovial fluid samples of 51 patients undergoing revision arthroplasty were tested for the 23 potential biomarkers for periprosthetic infection, and results showed that 12 out of the 23 biomarkers demonstrated significantly higher average levels in the synovial fluid of infected versus aseptic patients. The biomarkers interleukin-1b, interleukin-6, and granulocyte colony-stimulating factor were found to have greater specificities and sensitivities than ESR and CRP. Other markers, including interleukin-1a, interleukin-8, interleukin-17, and vascular endothelial growth factor (VEGF) were identified as potentially useful biomarkers in this study as well. Jacovides et al. [8] performed a similar study analyzing 46 proteins as potential predictors of PJI. Five of those proteins were identified as promising markers, three of which matched the publication by Deirmengian et al. [5] (interleukin-6, interleukin-8, and VEGF).

Alpha-Defensin

The initial studies mentioned and research further into the subject led to the identification of alpha-defensin as a highly accurate synovial fluid biomarker for PJI [9]. The alpha-defensin antimicrobial peptide is the body's natural antibiotic, produced by neutrophils upon contact with any pathogen. This represents the innate immune system's most primitive response to a pathogen, allowing for the local buildup of an antimicrobial environment.

Several peer-reviewed clinical studies have demonstrated the high accuracy of the alpha-defensin test [9–13]. Although most previous studies on infection diagnostics have excluded patient populations expected to reduce test performance, the studies on synovial fluid alpha-defensin did not exclude such patients with multiple co-morbidities or those on antibiotics. Deirmengian et al. [11] demonstrated recently that alpha-defensin alone had a sensitivity of 97 % and a specificity of 96 % for PJI among 149 patients tested. The specificity improved to 100 % when also utilizing the synovial fluid CRP to interpret test results. In another study of 57 patients, Bingham et al. [13] reported an alpha-defensin test sensitivity of 100 % and specificity of 95 % for PJI.

In addition to high sensitivity and specificity for PJI, the alpha-defensin test appears to provide equivalent results for both virulent and less virulent organisms. In a study reporting on 244 culture and defensin positive synovial fluid samples [12], the median alpha-defensin level was similar for all organisms and categories of organism causing infection.

Biofilm Detection

Previous studies have demonstrated that certain microbial proteins which are up-regulated during biofilm formation are recognized by the antibody-mediated immune response [14]. One such protein or antigen that is up-regulated during *Staphylococcus aureus* biofilm formation is the MntC (a manganese transporter SACOL0688). Serum immunoglobulin G (IgG) and immunoglobulin A (IgA) antibody levels against a number of antigens were studied in 21 patients with *Staphylococcus aureus* infection and compared to 30 aseptic controls [15]. MntC was the only antigen associated with a 5 fold increase in the initial-to-peak IgG antibody response and a 2 fold increase in IgA antibody response. In a follow-up clinical study, 30 synovial fluid samples from chronically infected PJIs were assessed for the presence of *S. aureus*. Enzyme-linked immunosorbent assays (ELISA) were used to detect host antibody response to MntC in order to determine whether anti-biofilm antibodies could act as a viable diagnostic tool for the identification of *S. aureus* in the synovial fluid. A single sample only produced a positive assay for *S. aureus*. Polymerase chain reaction-based techniques and standard cultures confirmed the presence of *S. aureus* in the sample identified, and the absence of *S. aureus* in all other samples [16].

By conjugating anti-biofilm antibodies to fluorophores, evidence from the literature has shown the ability to use anti-biofilm antibodies to detect and localize *S. aureus* biofilms with high specificity in murine models [16]. With further development, this could become a rapid, sensitive, and inexpensive diagnostic tool in humans for the detection of *S. aureus* and other infectious species.

Bacterial Detection Technologies

MALDI-TOF MS

Matrix-assisted laser desorption ionization time of flight mass spectrometry (MALDI-TOF MS) is a relatively new technology that has shown promise for rapid and cost-effective [17] diagnosis of PJI. In studies analyzing the accuracy of MALDI-TOF MS in detecting species within a bacterial colony, an analysis of 1660 different bacterial isolates demonstrated that MALDI-TOF MS correctly identified 95.4 % of the bacteria; 84.1 % at the species level, and 11.3 % at the genus level [18]. In similar studies using MALDI-TOF MS, van Veen et al. [19] reported correct species identification in 84.8–97.7 % of cases and Bizzini et al. [20] identified the correct species in 93.2 % of cases.

In studies relating to PJI, similar results have also been observed. For example, Peel et al. [21] showed that MALDI-TOF MS performed on cultures isolated from synovial fluid samples of septic and aseptic patients correctly identified the species in 89 % of cases, and the genus in an additional 2 % of cases. The study demonstrated the value of this technique as an ancillary test to help distinguish true positive culture results from false-positives resulting from contamination. Although many of the infectious species accounting for PJI are often the same species that are responsible for culture contamination [22–24], certain species are more likely to cause infection than others. Therefore, the ability to identify the cultured bacteria at a species level may help to differentiate between infectious bacteria and contaminants. In fact, Peel et al. [21] demonstrated that *Staphylococcus aureus* and *Staphylococcus caprae* were always associated with a true infection. On the other hand, *Staphylococcus epidermidis* and *Staphylococcus lugdunensis* were equally likely to be a pathogen or a contaminant and other staphylococci species that were coagulase-negative were more likely to be contaminants. Most streptococcal and *Corynebacterium* pathogens were shown to be pathogens [21]. Therefore, the value of MALDI-TOF MS comes, not through its ability to detect the presence of infection only, but also through its ability to identify pathogens at the species level and characterizing cultured pathogens as true infections or contaminants. More work however, is needed to refine this technique before it can be confidently used as a diagnostic and decision-making tool in the setting of PJI.

PCR

Conventional methods for direct detection of infectious organisms showed less-than-optimal results, with cultures for example failing to reliably confirm or exclude infection. Therefore, methods like polymerase chain reaction (PCR) were introduced to improve the reliability of detecting infection. PCR gained popularity in the 1980s as a rapid method of replicating and sequencing genetic material, giving it widespread use in genetic testing and forensics. In the 1990s,

PCR was applied for the first time in diagnosing PJI [25–28].

As methods for extracting microbial DNA for PCR analysis progressed [29], it became clear that PCR suffered from many of the same drawbacks as previous investigations [30]. As a tool with a strong ability to replicate and magnify nucleic acids, PCR is inherently prone to false positives even in the presence of minute levels of contamination. DNA from noninfectious or even dead bacteria, are also often detected [31]. However, the application of propidium monoazide and ethidium bromide has been introduced to reduce the false positives by removal of DNA derived from cells lacking cell wall integrity [32]. This could prove to be worthy especially in patients who have been treated with antibiotics and still harbor DNA from deceased bacterial cells. However, such treatment is not completely ready for clinical use because they do not fully inhibit the replication of DNA from dead bacterial cells during PCR [33].

The various PCR techniques that have been developed for the detection of PJI are discussed below.

Broad-Range PCR

As opposed to using primers that identify regions of DNA unique to a single species or strain of bacteria, broad-range PCR acts as a universal test for bacterial infection by detecting chromosomal regions that are conserved across most or all bacterial species. Therefore, broad-range PCR is a more sensitive test when the species of the infectious agent is unknown. This increased sensitivity, however, comes with its disadvantages. By using non-specific PCR primers, broad-range PCR increases the false positive results of PCR because it allows for the detection of bacterial species that are not known to cause bacterial infection. Furthermore, as described above, confirming the presence of an infection and the infectious species are important for the subsequent treatment and evisceration of the infectious organism. Due to its non-specific nature, broad-range PCR does not identify the specific species, and further tests to confirm species type can be time-consuming and inaccurate.

Despite these drawbacks, the method has shown some clinical promise. Panousis et al. analyzed a series of 92 consecutive revision knee arthroplasties and demonstrated a sensitivity of 92 % and a specificity of 74 %. The diagnostic value was, however, plagued by high false positives. While the negative predictive value was 98 %, the positive predictive value was only 34 %, leaving Panousis et al. [34] unwilling to confidently endorse this method.

Multiplex PCR

Multiplex PCR is a method that attempts to diminish the high false positive frequency associated with broad-range PCR. While broad-range PCR uses a single set of PCR primers to identify a single universal region of DNA common to all bacteria, multiplex PCR simultaneously uses many sets of PCR primers, each of which is targeted to a DNA region that is unique to the organism being investigated, allowing for the detection of specific bacterial species. By probing only for DNA from species known to cause infections of the joint, this method eliminates many of the false positives associated with broad-range PCR. Additionally, by allowing for the direct detection of both the presence and identity of the pathogen, multiplex PCR represents a vast improvement in turnaround time compared to standard cultures for identifying slow-growing organisms such as *Propionibacterium acnes* [35]. *P. acnes* is a species thought to cause more than one of every three infections after shoulder arthroplasty, and may require roughly 2 weeks to grow on a traditional culture. Because cultures are often not grown for this duration, multiplex PCR offers a method to detect many slow-growing bacteria that would otherwise not be detected by traditional cultures [6].

In a study by Achermann et al. [36] the multiplexing technique was used to analyze 37 cases of PJI. Multiplex PCR using species-specific primers was able to identify the presence and identity in 100 % of the infected samples. Additionally, while the relative sensitivity of cultures in their study dropped by nearly 30 % in cases when the infection was previously treated with antibiotics the sensitivity of multiplex PCR was not changed.

Additionally, PCR using primers for specific regions of DNA can probe specifically for the presence of antibiotic resistance genes [35, 37–39]. For example, Tarkin et al. [39] demonstrated that a rapid, 5 h procedure aimed at detecting the *MecA* gene responsible for methicillin-resistance in MRSA was 97 % sensitive for the presence of infection. Despite other studies showing a slightly lower accuracy for this drug-resistance-gene-specific probing [35], PCR multiplex shows vast improvements over the traditional methods.

Unfortunately, even multiplex PCR is hindered by the balance between sensitivity and specificity. Most reports of highly sensitive tests lack the specificity that would be considered acceptable. Similarly, reports of highly specific multiplex assays generally have a sensitivity that is equivalent to culture techniques. These considerations need to be resolved before a reliable PCR test for PJI is utilized in a clinical setting.

Reverse-Transcriptase PCR

As discussed in the introduction to PCR, methods that rely on the replication of bacterial DNA may unintentionally replicate DNA from dead bacterial cells that result from contamination, or dead cells that remain in the host patient after treatment with antibiotics. Because it is common for patients who are being screened for the presence of infection to be currently using antibiotics or to have used antibiotics in the recent past, it is important to have a diagnostic tool that is insensitive to DNA from dead bacterial cells. Reverse-transcriptase PCR aims to diagnose infection via the detection of RNA rather than DNA. Because RNA is less stable than DNA, it has a shorter half-life and hence more rapidly degrades during a bacterial cell's life and after its death as compared to DNA.

Despite insufficient data to warrant the widespread use of reverse transcriptase PCR for the diagnosis of PJI, the conceptual framework behind this method has been established. In a proof-of-concept experiment, Birmingham at al. [40] demonstrated the strengths of this method in simulated septic synovial fluid. Synovial fluid aspirations were inoculated with bacteria then analyzed using reverse transcriptase PCR to identify bacterial messenger RNA (mRNA). All samples that were inoculated with bacteria were identified as positive for infection, and no false positives were observed. Additionally, Birmingham et al. demonstrated that treatment of synovial fluid with antibiotics to eradicate the infection led to a steady decrease in mRNA concentrations, minimizing the detection of dead or non-viable bacteria by this method and indicating that reverse transcriptase PCR may not yield false positives due to lingering mRNA from dead bacterial cells.

While mRNA is relatively scarce in the cell and few universal bacterial mRNA sequences are known [6], ribosomal RNA (rRNA) is abundant within the cell and has regions of homology across different bacterial species. Even more importantly, rRNA also has regions that are unique to individual species. Therefore, rRNA PCR can be used as both a general screen for infection, as well as a directed probe to identify the species of the infectious organism. Bergin et al. [41] studied the ability of reverse transcriptase PCR to identify bacteria by probing for rRNA. The method was able to identify rRNA in all 6 of the clearly infected patients. There were no false positives amongst the group of 50 uninfected patients. Despite the small sample size of infected patients to make strong conclusions about the sensitivity of reverse transcriptase PCR for rRNA, the elimination of false positives is a large step forward for the use of PCR as a diagnostic tool for PJI.

Similar to Birmingham et al. [40], Bergin et al. [41] found an antibiotic-dependent decrease in the detected levels of rRNA. However, rRNA levels in synovial fluid samples took roughly 1 week to drop below the level of detection after antibiotic treatment, even though these fluid samples showed no growth on cultures. The authors concluded that these samples were "septic but unculturable." If these remaining levels of mRNA are from "septic but unculturable" bacteria rather than remaining rRNA fragments from dead bacterial cells, then reverse transcriptase PCR offers a fantastic method for identifying the presence of a lingering bacterial infection in patients who have been treated with antibiotics, a population in which detection is especially difficult to detect with standard cultures [42].

PCR-ESI/MS

Polymerase chain reaction electrospray ionization mass spectrometry (PCR-ESI/MS) is a technology that couples PCR with electrospray ionization mass spectrometry of fluid from sonicated explanted joint implants. Though the technology is not new [43], its application to the diagnosis of PJI is rather novel [44]. While previous attempts at using this technique for the diagnosis of PJI suffered from low specificities [45], improvements to the technology have yielded about an 81 % sensitivity and 95 % specificity [46]. In addition to its high sensitivity and specificity, this technology allows for the detection of over 3400 bacterial species and four antibiotic resistance markers: bla_{KPC}, *vanA*, *vanB*, and *mecA* [46]. As discussed above, both the presence of infection and the identity of the infectious species, including any genetic variations that confer antibiotic resistance, are highly important in determining the subsequent treatment path. By allowing for the detection and identity of the infectious species, PCR-ESI/MS offers a fantastic opportunity for the rapid and accurate detection of bacterial species.

Metablomics

The field of metablomics involves the study of the chemical fingerprint left behind by cellular and molecular processes [47, 48]. As the byproducts of metabolic processes, metabolites offer insights into the exact nature of the processes that are occurring within the cellular environment being analyzed. Therefore, the study of metabolomics could represent a promising new avenue for the diagnosis of infection. Metabolites specific to the host response to pathogen invasion or specific to the infectious species itself could be identified using the chemometric (profiling) metabolomic method. The quantitative (targeted) method to metablomics could then be used to establish the standard ranges of certain metabolites in septic and aseptic patients. With established baseline levels, metabolite levels from patients suspected to have PJI could be analyzed and compared to the reference standards to diagnose the presence of PJI [6, 49].

More work is needed in the field of metabolomics relative to PJI in order to identify potential metabolites in the synovial fluid, urine, or blood that could be used in the diagnosis of infection. Future work must also focus on methods that decrease the cost and time-commitment demanded by current metabolomics analyses in order to make it a viable method for the diagnosis of PJI.

References

1. Lentino JR. Prosthetic joint infections: bane of orthopedists, challenge for infectious disease specialists. Clin Infect Dis. 2003;36(9):1157–61.
2. Joseph TN, Chen AL, Di Cesare PE. Use of antibiotic-impregnated cement in total joint arthroplasty. J Am Acad Orthop Surg. 2003;11(1):38–47.
3. Parvizi J, Jacovides C, Zmistowski B, Jung KA. Definition of periprosthetic joint infection: is there a consensus? Clin Orthop Relat Res. 2011;469(11): 3022–30.
4. Berbari E, Mabry T, Tsaras G, Spangehl M, Erwin PJ, Murad MH, et al. Inflammatory blood laboratory levels as markers of prosthetic joint infection: a systematic review and meta-analysis. J Bone Joint Surg Am. 2010;92(11):2102–9.
5. Deirmengian C, Hallab N, Tarabishy A, Della Valle C, Jacobs JJ, Lonner J, et al. Synovial fluid biomarkers for periprosthetic infection. Clin Orthop Relat Res. 2010;468(8):2017–23.
6. Choe H, Deirmengian CA, Hickok NJ, Morrison TN, Tuan RS. Molecular diagnostics. J Am Acad Orthop Surg. 2015;23(Suppl):S26–31.
7. Deirmengian C, Lonner JH, Booth Jr RE. The Mark Coventry Award: white blood cell gene expression: a new approach toward the study and diagnosis of infection. Clin Orthop Relat Res. 2005;440:38–44.

8. Jacovides CL, Parvizi J, Adeli B, Jung KA. Molecular markers for diagnosis of periprosthetic joint infection. J Arthroplasty. 2011;26(6 Suppl):99–103.e1.
9. Deirmengian C, Kardos K, Kilmartin P, Cameron A, Schiller K, Parvizi J. Diagnosing periprosthetic joint infection: has the era of the biomarker arrived? Clin Orthop Relat Res. 2014;472(11):3254–62.
10. Deirmengian C, Kardos K, Kilmartin P, Cameron A, Schiller K, Booth Jr RE, et al. The alpha-defensin test for periprosthetic joint infection outperforms the leukocyte esterase test strip. Clin Orthop Relat Res. 2015;473(1):198–203.
11. Deirmengian C, Kardos K, Kilmartin P, Cameron A, Schiller K, Parvizi J. Combined measurement of synovial fluid alpha-Defensin and C-reactive protein levels: highly accurate for diagnosing periprosthetic joint infection. J Bone Joint Surg Am. 2014;96(17):1439–45.
12. Deirmengian C, Kardos K, Kilmartin P, Gulati S, Citrano P, Booth Jr RE. The alpha-defensin test for periprosthetic joint infection responds to a wide spectrum of organisms. Clin Orthop Relat Res. 2015;473(7):2229–35.
13. Bingham J, Clarke H, Spangehl M, Schwartz A, Beauchamp C, Goldberg B. The alpha defensin-1 biomarker assay can be used to evaluate the potentially infected total joint arthroplasty. Clin Orthop Relat Res. 2014;472(12):4006–9.
14. Brady RA, Leid JG, Camper AK, Costerton JW, Shirtliff ME. Identification of Staphylococcus aureus proteins recognized by the antibody-mediated immune response to a biofilm infection. Infect Immun. 2006;74(6):3415–26.
15. den Reijer PM, Lemmens-den Toom N, Kant S, Snijders SV, Boelens H, Tavakol M, et al. Characterization of the humoral immune response during Staphylococcus aureus bacteremia and global gene expression by Staphylococcus aureus in human blood. PLoS One. 2013;8(1):e53391.
16. Parvizi J, Alijanipour P, Barberi EF, Hickok NJ, Phillips KS, Shapiro IM, et al. Novel developments in the prevention, diagnosis, and treatment of periprosthetic joint infections. J Am Acad Orthop Surg. 2015;23(Suppl):S32–43.
17. Lagier JC, Hugon P, Khelaifia S, Fournier PE, La Scola B, Raoult D. The rebirth of culture in microbiology through the example of culturomics to study human gut microbiota. Clin Microbiol Rev. 2015;28(1):237–64.
18. Seng P, Drancourt M, Gouriet F, La Scola B, Fournier PE, Rolain JM, et al. Ongoing revolution in bacteriology: routine identification of bacteria by matrix-assisted laser desorption ionization time-of-flight mass spectrometry. Clin Infect Dis. 2009;49(4):543–51.
19. van Veen SQ, Claas EC, Kuijper EJ. High-throughput identification of bacteria and yeast by matrix-assisted laser desorption ionization-time of flight mass spectrometry in conventional medical microbiology laboratories. J Clin Microbiol. 2010;48(3):900–7.
20. Bizzini A, Durussel C, Bille J, Greub G, Prod'hom G. Performance of matrix-assisted laser desorption ionization-time of flight mass spectrometry for identification of bacterial strains routinely isolated in a clinical microbiology laboratory. J Clin Microbiol. 2010;48(5):1549–54.
21. Peel TN, Cole NC, Dylla BL, Patel R. Matrix-assisted laser desorption ionization time of flight mass spectrometry and diagnostic testing for prosthetic joint infection in the clinical microbiology laboratory. Diagn Microbiol Infect Dis. 2015;81(3):163–8.
22. Parvizi J, Zmistowski B, Berbari EF, Bauer TW, Springer BD, Della Valle CJ, et al. New definition for periprosthetic joint infection: from the Workgroup of the Musculoskeletal Infection Society. Clin Orthop Relat Res. 2011;469(11):2992–4.
23. Osmon DR, Berbari EF, Berendt AR, Lew D, Zimmerli W, Steckelberg JM, et al. Executive summary: diagnosis and management of prosthetic joint infection: clinical practice guidelines by the Infectious Diseases Society of America. Clin Infect Dis. 2013;56(1):1–10.
24. Harris LG, El-Bouri K, Johnston S, Rees E, Frommelt L, Siemssen N, et al. Rapid identification of staphylococci from prosthetic joint infections using MALDI-TOF mass-spectrometry. Int J Artif Organs. 2010;33(9):568–74.
25. Lee AH, Ramanujam T, Ware P, Edelstein PH, Brooks JJ, Freundlich B, et al. Molecular diagnosis of Ureaplasma urealyticum septic arthritis in a patient with hypogammaglobulinemia. Arthritis Rheum. 1992;35(4):443–8.
26. Poole ES, Highton J, Wilkins RJ, Lamont IL. A search for Chlamydia trachomatis in synovial fluids from patients with reactive arthritis using the polymerase chain reaction and antigen detection methods. Br J Rheumatol. 1992;31(1):31–4.
27. Liebling MR, Arkfeld DG, Michelini GA, Nishio MJ, Eng BJ, Jin T, et al. Identification of Neisseria gonorrhoeae in synovial fluid using the polymerase chain reaction. Arthritis Rheum. 1994;37(5):702–9.
28. Nocton JJ, Dressler F, Rutledge BJ, Rys PN, Persing DH, Steere AC. Detection of Borrelia burgdorferi DNA by polymerase chain reaction in synovial fluid from patients with Lyme arthritis. N Engl J Med. 1994;330(4):229–34.
29. Mariani BD, Levine MJ, Booth Jr RE, Tuan RS. Development of a novel, rapid processing protocol for polymerase chain reaction-based detection of bacterial infections in synovial fluids. Mol Biotechnol. 1995;4(3):227–37.
30. Gallo J, Raska M, Dendis M, Florschutz AV, Kolar M. Molecular diagnosis of prosthetic joint infection. A review of evidence. Biomed Pap Med Fac Univ Palacky Olomouc Czech Repub. 2004;148(2):123–9.
31. Choe H, Inaba Y, Kobayashi N, Miyamae Y, Ike H, Fujimaki H, et al. Evaluation of the time period for which real-time polymerase chain reaction detects dead bacteria. Pol J Microbiol. 2014;63(4):393–8.

32. van Frankenhuyzen JK, Trevors JT, Lee H, Flemming CA, Habash MB. Molecular pathogen detection in biosolids with a focus on quantitative PCR using propidium monoazide for viable cell enumeration. J Microbiol Methods. 2011;87(3):263–72.
33. Taylor MJ, Bentham RH, Ross KE. Limitations of using propidium monoazide with qPCR to discriminate between live and dead legionella in biofilm samples. Microbiol Insights. 2014;7:15–24.
34. Panousis K, Grigoris P, Butcher I, Rana B, Reilly JH, Hamblen DL. Poor predictive value of broad-range PCR for the detection of arthroplasty infection in 92 cases. Acta Orthop. 2005;76(3):341–6.
35. Kobayashi N, Inaba Y, Choe H, Aoki C, Ike H, Ishida T, et al. Simultaneous intraoperative detection of methicillin-resistant Staphylococcus and pan-bacterial infection during revision surgery: use of simple DNA release by ultrasonication and real-time polymerase chain reaction. J Bone Joint Surg Am. 2009;91(12):2896–902.
36. Achermann Y, Vogt M, Leunig M, Wust J, Trampuz A. Improved diagnosis of periprosthetic joint infection by multiplex PCR of sonication fluid from removed implants. J Clin Microbiol. 2010;48(4): 1208–14.
37. Choe H, Inaba Y, Kobayashi N, Aoki C, Machida J, Nakamura N, et al. Use of real-time polymerase chain reaction for the diagnosis of infection and differentiation between gram-positive and gram-negative septic arthritis in children. J Pediatr Orthop. 2013;33(3):e28–33.
38. Choe H, Aota Y, Kobayashi N, Nakamura Y, Wakayama Y, Inaba Y, et al. Rapid sensitive molecular diagnosis of pyogenic spinal infections using methicillin-resistant Staphylococcus-specific polymerase chain reaction and 16S ribosomal RNA gene-based universal polymerase chain reaction. Spine J. 2014;14(2):255–62.
39. Tarkin IS, Henry TJ, Fey PI, Iwen PC, Hinrichs SH, Garvin KL. PCR rapidly detects methicillin-resistant staphylococci periprosthetic infection. Clin Orthop Relat Res. 2003;414:89–94.
40. Birmingham P, Helm JM, Manner PA, Tuan RS. Simulated joint infection assessment by rapid detection of live bacteria with real-time reverse transcription polymerase chain reaction. J Bone Joint Surg Am. 2008;90(3):602–8.
41. Bergin PF, Doppelt JD, Hamilton WG, Mirick GE, Jones AE, Sritulanondha S, et al. Detection of periprosthetic infections with use of ribosomal RNA-based polymerase chain reaction. J Bone Joint Surg Am. 2010;92(3):654–63.
42. Barrack RL, Jennings RW, Wolfe MW, Bertot AJ. The Coventry Award. The value of preoperative aspiration before total knee revision. Clin Orthop Relat Res. 1997;345:8–16.
43. Baldwin CD, Howe GB, Sampath R, Blyn LB, Matthews H, Harpin V, et al. Usefulness of multilocus polymerase chain reaction followed by electrospray ionization mass spectrometry to identify a diverse panel of bacterial isolates. Diagn Microbiol Infect Dis. 2009;63(4):403–8.
44. Greenwood-Quaintance KE, Uhl JR, Hanssen AD, Sampath R, Mandrekar JN, Patel R. Diagnosis of prosthetic joint infection by use of PCR-electrospray ionization mass spectrometry. J Clin Microbiol. 2014;52(2):642–9.
45. Jacovides CL, Kreft R, Adeli B, Hozack B, Ehrlich GD, Parvizi J. Successful identification of pathogens by polymerase chain reaction (PCR)-based electron spray ionization time-of-flight mass spectrometry (ESI-TOF-MS) in culture-negative periprosthetic joint infection. J Bone Joint Surg Am. 2012; 94(24):2247–54.
46. Melendez DP, Uhl JR, Greenwood-Quaintance KE, Hanssen AD, Sampath R, Patel R. Detection of prosthetic joint infection by use of PCR-electrospray ionization mass spectrometry applied to synovial fluid. J Clin Microbiol. 2014;52(6):2202–5.
47. Stitt M, Fernie AR. From measurements of metabolites to metabolomics: an 'on the fly' perspective illustrated by recent studies of carbon-nitrogen interactions. Curr Opin Biotechnol. 2003;14(2): 136–44.
48. Fuhrer T, Zamboni N. High-throughput discovery metabolomics. Curr Opin Biotechnol. 2015;31:73–8.
49. Zhang A, Sun H, Wang P, Han Y, Wang X. Modern analytical techniques in metabolomics analysis. Analyst. 2012;137(2):293–300.

Part IV

Local Antibiotic Therapy

Local Antibiotic Therapy: Antibiotic-Loaded Cement

9

Akos Zahar

Abstract

Antibiotic-loaded bone cement is widely used in orthopaedic surgery mainly for fixation of cemented implants in total joint replacement. The prophylactic use in primary and revision arthroplasty is part of the routine antibiotic prophylaxis in addition to the systemic administration. In the treatment of prosthetic joint infection, antibiotic-loaded bone cement is used at the re-implantation of cemented implants at the second stage of two-stage septic exchange, or for fixation of cemented implants at one-stage septic exchange of total joint arthroplasty. But cement is not only a tool of fixation. In two-stage septic exchange, a spacer is inserted after the first-stage surgery where customized antibiotic-loaded bone cement provides high local concentrations of the antimicrobial agent in order to eliminate the bacteria from the infected joint. In direct exchange of the one-stage procedure, it is one of the most important tools to provide effective local concentrations of antibiotics, which allows for direct re-implantation after radical debridement of the infected surgical site. With high local concentrations of antimicrobial agents the recolonization and biofilm formation at the surface of the new implant can be avoided. Industrially manufactured antibiotic-loaded bone cement is preferably used, but hand mixing of additional antibiotics may be required.

Keywords

Antibiotic-loaded bone cement • Antibiotic release • Drug elution • Industrially manufactured antibiotic bone cement • Hand-mixing • Local antibiotic therapy • PMMA

A. Zahar, MD
Prosthetic Joint Infection Center, HELIOS ENDO-Klinik, Hamburg, Germany

Prosthetic Joint Infection Center, Hamburg, Germany
e-mail: akos.zahar@helios-kliniken.de

D. Kendoff et al. (eds.), *Periprosthetic Joint Infections: Changing Paradigms*,
DOI 10.1007/978-3-319-30091-7_9

Introduction

The treatment of prosthetic joint infection (PJI) consists of radical surgical debridement and removal of all foreign material. Supplementary antibiotic therapy ensures the success of the surgical procedure. The treatment of these infections is challenging; therefore, it should be carried out in specialized centres in cooperation with an experienced infectious disease specialist [1]. Antimicrobial therapy can be achieved by systemic use and local application, based upon the recommendation of the infectious disease consultant [2].

Polymetyl-metacrylate (PMMA) bone cement is widely used for fixation of implants at total joint replacement. The cement as a drug delivery system for local antibiotic therapy at prosthetic joint infection is one of the possible treatment options to inhibit biofilm formation on the surface of the implants [2]. Effective bactericidal levels can hardly achieved by systemic administration of antimicrobial agents, but the local use of antibiotics allows for supramaximal dosage and effective killing of bacteria at the site of surgery. Sessile bacteria within the biofilm have an elevated minimal inhibitory concentration (MIC) [3]. Basic research of this topic made it possible to develop prefabricated antibiotic-loaded bone cements that are used in both aseptic and septic revisions. Additional antibiotics can be hand-mixed with these products in order to achieve an individualized anti-infective treatment based upon the microbiological findings [4].

Antibiotic-loaded acrylic bone cement (ALAC) is commonly used for antibiotic delivery during total joint arthroplasty (TJA) for prevention or treatment of periprosthetic joint infection. ALAC is commonly used in two-stage exchange arthroplasty with static and dynamic spacers, beads, rods, and other custom made spacers. The use of commercially available or hand-made ALAC for primary and revision TJA to prevent infection has also been studied. Commonly used antibiotics include gentamicin, tobramycin, and vancomycin powder, and these antibiotics can be used alone or in combination, depending on the organism present. ALAC can be prepared by hand mixing to increase porosity and improve antibiotic elution. Hand-mixed cement is often used in two-stage septic exchange for shaping spacers and beads. Although there are some limitations ALAC is an effective medical implant tool that can be used for treating and preventing PJI [5].

History

Professor H.W. Buchholz, founder of the ENDO-Klinik in Hamburg, started the first investigations in the late 1960s mixing various antibiotics to Palacos R bone cement [6, 7]. He studied the physical, chemical and mechanical characteristics of the modified bone cement and he worked up the samples together with his microbiologist in order to show the antibacterial effect of the new product [7, 8]. Sir J. Charnley from the UK was quite sceptical concerning the antibiotic loading of bone cement and elution of the drug, and wrote: "My dear Buchholz, nothing leaks out of stone." After several investigations at the cement manufacturer's laboratory in Germany about the admixture of antibiotics to bone cement on the mechanical properties, the concerns in terms of poor fixation of the implant were gone [8]. Buchholz and Engelbrecht published their data in 1970 about long elution times of various antibiotics from bone cement [6]. Nowadays the elution characteristics of antibiotics from PMMA bone cement are well known and widely accepted. As late as in 2003, Simplex P with tobramycin became the first cleared antibiotic-impregnated bone cement in the United States approved by the FDA.

Antibiotics

High local levels of antibiotics should be achieved in order to kill the bacteria at the site of surgery and to avoid biofilm formation [2]. The local antibiotic concentration must be above the minimal inhibitory concentration and the minimal bactericidal concentration of the organisms [9]. Not all antibiotics are suitable to be mixed with bone cement. Only substances are used which are highly soluble in water, are heat resistant, which are not destroyed by the polymerization of the cement and are available as powder (and not liquid). At the industrial production of antibiotic-loaded bone cement the antibiotics should be resistant against the sterilization process and should be stable during storage and transportation [10].

In terms of antibacterial effect they have to provide a broad antibacterial spectrum, being very effective against the organisms even at low concentrations, without major side effects for the patient. The most important group of antibiotics that can be mixed with bone cement is aminoglycosides; gentamicin is used in the majority of the cases alone or in combination. Other commercial bone cements may include tobramycin or clindamycin. The combination of gentamycin and clindamycin in revision bone cements has a synergistic bactericidal effect on more than 90 % of the bacteria common to PJI cases. For multiresistant organisms like MRSA vancomycin-loaded cement is available. Vancomycin-loaded bone cement should only be used if pathogens are not sufficiently sensitive towards aminoglycoside antibiotics (e.g., gentamycin) or combinations of aminoglycoside and lincosamide antibiotics (e.g., clindamycin) [10, 11]. The AAOS recommends vancomycin should be reserved for the treatment of serious infections with beta-lactam–resistant organisms or for treatment of infection in patients with life-threatening allergy to beta-lactam antimicrobials. Daptomycin is the next promising candidate for local treatment of bone infection due to its activity against multiresistant Staphylococci [12].

The release of antibiotics from bone cement is a question of the surface and the water solubility [11]. That means, not the thickness of the cement mantle should be enlarged in order to have higher local concentrations, but the area of surface. This can be achieved by small holes or roughened surfaces. A high initial release within the first 24 h is followed by a lower release in the following days, but small amounts of antibiotics are still detectable after several years [10, 13].

The exact behaviour of the antibiotics in combination with PMMA is not predictable by theoretical considerations. For each antibiotic combination and each type of bone cement the elution characteristics are shown in experiments, and these results should be taken into consideration when the individual therapy of PJI is discussed [10, 14].

The concerns about the mechanical strength of the bone cement after adding antibiotics are not without any reason. In fact, the addition of antibiotic powder weakens the bone cement, but proper fixation is still given [13, 15, 16]. The addition of liquid to the PMMA influences the polymerization and the curing of the cement, that's why it is not recommended [10, 13]. When antibiotic powder is mixed to PMMA bone cement by the surgeon, the weight of the powder shouldn't exceed 10 %, which means not more than 4 g of antibiotics with 40 g of PMMA bone cement [10, 13].

The most important antibiotic substances available in industrially manufactured ALAC are shown in Table 9.1.

Carrier for Local Therapy

Vacuum mixing has an effect on the antibiotic release: the porosity of the bone cement facilitates the diffusion, meaning, if the porosity is reduced by vacuum in order to remove the air voids from

Table 9.1 The main antibiotics in industrial manufactured bone cements

Substance	Type of ABX	Characteristics
Gentamycin	Aminoglycoside	Bactericidal, inhibits bacterial protein synthesis
Tobramycin	Aminoglycoside	Bactericidal, inhibits bacterial protein synthesis
Clindamycin	Lincosamide	Bacteriostatic, inhibits bacterial protein synthesis
Vancomycin	Glycopeptide	Bactericidal, inhibits the bacterial cell wall synthesis

the cement matrix, the antibiotic release decreases [13]. That's why we do not recommend vacuum mixing of antibiotic-loaded bone cement in one- or two-staged septic exchange.

Beads showed higher elution characteristics in vivo than the spacers due to their larger surface area; however, a great amount of inter-subject variability was seen for both beads and spacers. The inferior elution properties of spacers emphasize the importance of additional systemic antibiotics for this treatment procedure during the postoperative period. Future studies should clarify whether the dose of antibiotics or length of antibiotic therapy may be reduced in the case of bead implantation, without jeopardizing the control of infection [9].

Hand Mixing of Antibiotics

Industrially manufactured antibiotic-loaded PMMA cements have some clearly defined benefits [11, 14]. Homogenous and reproducible distribution of the antibiotic powder within the dough, reliable release profile and standardized mechanical properties are the main advantages. But there are also some limitations, like resistant organisms against the available antibiotic combinations. Industrially manufactured ALAC products are shown in Table 9.2.

Addition of antibiotics to bone cement by the surgeon or the scrub nurse was recommended by Buchholz, but the method has been criticized, as the mixture might be inhomogeneous and the antibiotic release might be uncontrolled. Manual mixing of antibiotics might result in poorer mechanical properties, which is why industrially manufactured bone cements are preferred [10, 13]. In certain cases hand mixing is the only option to create proper antibiotic mixtures that cover the susceptibility of the organism; these individual cases should be considered as off-label use [10].

Several mixing methods have been studied in the literature. None of the mixing methods had consistently dissimilar homogeneity of antibiotic distribution from the others. Based upon scientific data hand mixed low-dose ALAC is not less homogeneous than commercially premixed formulations [17].

The treatment with a customized antibiotic combination in the bone cement based on the antibiogram can be carried out if no proper industrially manufactured product is available. The antibiotics can be individually adjusted to the susceptibility of the organism and the special requirements of the patient (e.g., allergy).

The effects of the mixing speed of hand-mixed bone cement and the different phases of antibiotic mixing on the elution, mechanical properties, and porosity of antibiotic-loaded bone cement were evaluated. Vancomycin-loaded low viscosity bone cement was prepared at two hand-mixing speeds, normal and high-speed, and with antibiotic addition during three phases (directly mixing with the PMMA powder, in the liquid phase, and in the dough phase). The cumulative antibiotic elution over 15 days in the high-speed group was significantly increased by 24 % compared with the normal-speed group. The delayed antibiotic addition produced significantly

Table 9.2 Industrial manufactured antibiotic-loaded revision bone cements and indications

Manufacturer	Product	Antibiotics	Indication
Biomet	Refobacin revision	1.0 g gentamycin 1.0 g clindamycin	One- or two-stage revision for PJI caused by gentamycin and clindamycin-sensitive bacteria
Heraeus	Copal G+C	1.0 g gentamycin 1.0 g clindamycin	Revision for PJI caused by gentamycin- and clindamycin-sensitive bacteria
	Copal G+V	0.5 g gentamycin 2.0 g vancomycin	Single- or two-stage revision of proven severe PJI by pathogens sensitive to vancomycin (such as MRSA/MRSE)
Stryker	Simplex P with Tobramycin	1.0 g tobramycin	"For the fixation of prostheses to living bone in the second stage of a two-stage revision for total joint arthroplasty"

higher vancomycin elution, but no difference was observed between the liquid and dough phases. Bone cement prepared with high-speed hand mixing and delayed antibiotic addition can exhibit increased antibiotic release [18].

Antibiotic powders used for hand mixing should be commercial preparations or prepared by a designated pharmacy for intravenous use [10]. According to medical law it is the physician's liability to modify the medical product by admixing antibiotics; therefore, it should be well documented and the reasons explained in the patient's file.

Instructions for Hand Mixing of Antibiotics to Bone Cement

The whole procedure must be carried out under sterile conditions in the operating theatre in an accurate way by the surgeon or an experienced scrub nurse. The cement mixing system is used in order to homogenize the cement powder with the antibiotics. The sterile cement mixing system is handled by the scrub nurse (or surgeon), and the antibiotic containers are opened by the unsterile (circulating) nurse with a sterile clamp. Care must be taken with the antibiotic containers, because they are unsterile outside, but sterile inside. Once the container is opened carefully, the powder is spread into a sterile bowl. Now the sterile nurse can homogenize the antibiotic crystals with a proper device. The PMMA cement powder is filled into the cement mixing system without any liquid. Then the antibiotic powder is filled in and the system is closed with the handle. Now the nurse (or surgeon) mixes the powders to achieve a homogenous mixture with an even distribution of the crystals within the cement powder. This is very important in order to take advantage of the elution characteristics of the antibiotics without decreasing the mechanical stability of the cured cement considerably. After homogenization of the powders the mixture is removed from the cement mixing system (into a sterile bowl). Now the preparation is finished, cementing is carried out like always with the liquid first as described in the user's manual of each cementing system. We recommend not using vacuum when mixing the antibiotic-PMMA mixture with the monomer liquid, because small air voids may facilitate the elution of antibiotics by diffusion.

See Figs. 9.1, 9.2, 9.3, 9.4, 9.5, 9.6, 9.7, and 9.8.

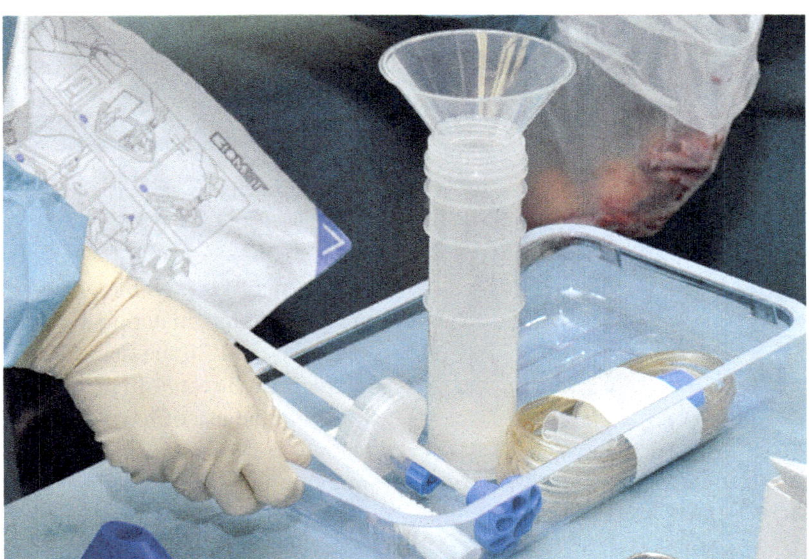

Fig. 9.1 Cement mixing system is prepared; no vacuum is used

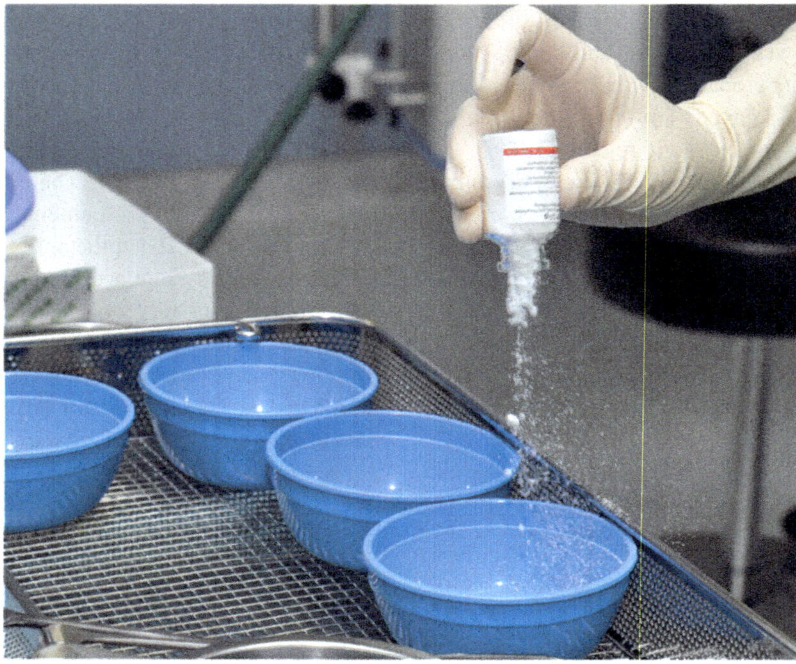

Fig. 9.2 Antibiotic powder is given from the non-sterile side, spread into a sterile bowl

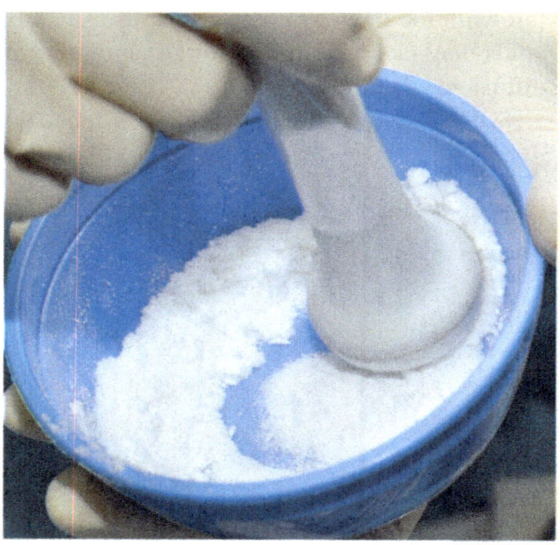

Fig. 9.3 Antibiotic powder is homogenised with a porcelain mortar by the sterile scrub nurse

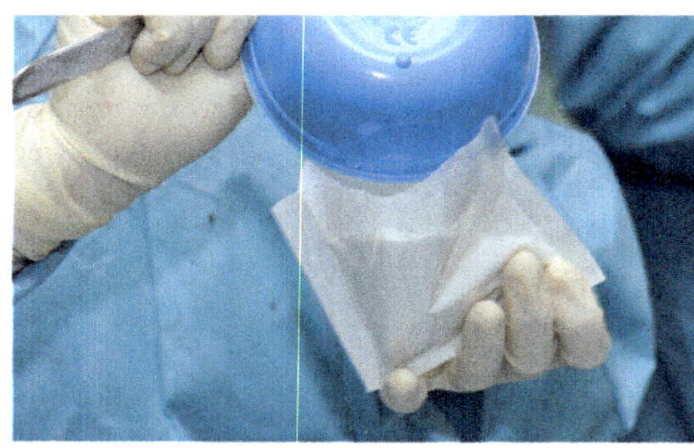

Fig. 9.4 Antibiotics are added to bone cement powder; the original plastic bag is used

Technique with Cemented Implants in One-Stage Septic Exchange

If the microorganism and the susceptibility are known, one-stage septic exchange of the infected implant may be possible. After removal of the infected foreign material, resection of infected bone and soft tissue and following thorough debridement direct re-implantation becomes possible with the use of local antibiotics. One of the treatment options is using cemented implants and antibiotic-loaded bone cement [1].

The special requirements of the one-stage technique consist of individualized antibiotic treatment – both local and systemic – based upon the treatment recommendation of the infectious disease specialist;

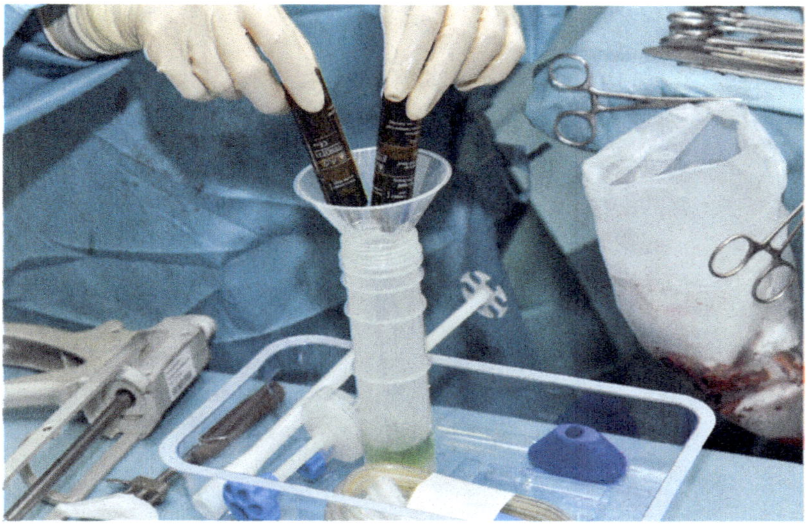

Fig. 9.5 Monomer liquid is filled into the cement mixing system

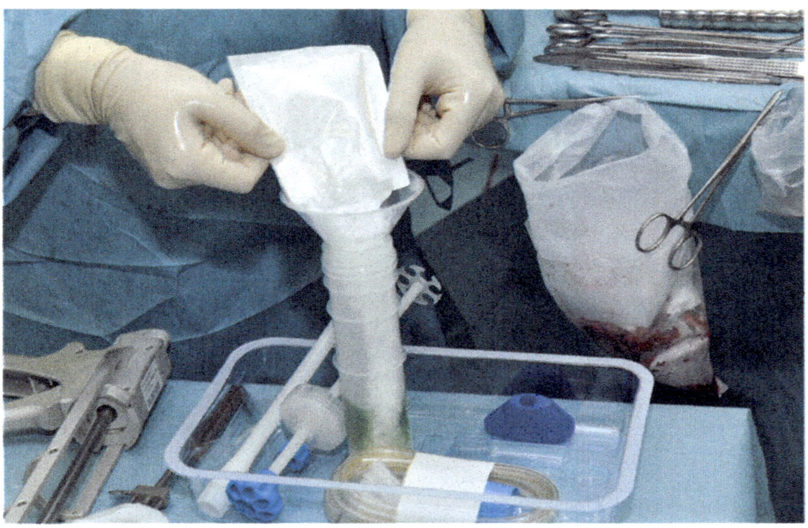

Fig. 9.6 The PMMA-antibiotics mixture is filled in to start the mixing procedure. Working and curing time is measured according to the user's manual of the bone cement

and to create a proper bone stock that allows an optimum of cement penetration. Sclerotic bone may be resected or roughened by high-speed burs in order to open the cancellous bone facilitating the cement interdigitation. The cement mantle shouldn't be very thin; an evenly distributed cement layer is desirable. No metal surface should be uncovered, in exception of the articulating surface. If bone is resected and replaced by the implant (e.g., resection of the proximal femur), a cement mantle is established made out of ALAC. The antibiotics eluted from the cement mantle can treat adjacent bone and soft tissue. A modern cementing technique with pulsatile jet lavage and cement restrictor is used, but vacuum mixing is avoided in order to facilitate the elution from PMMA.

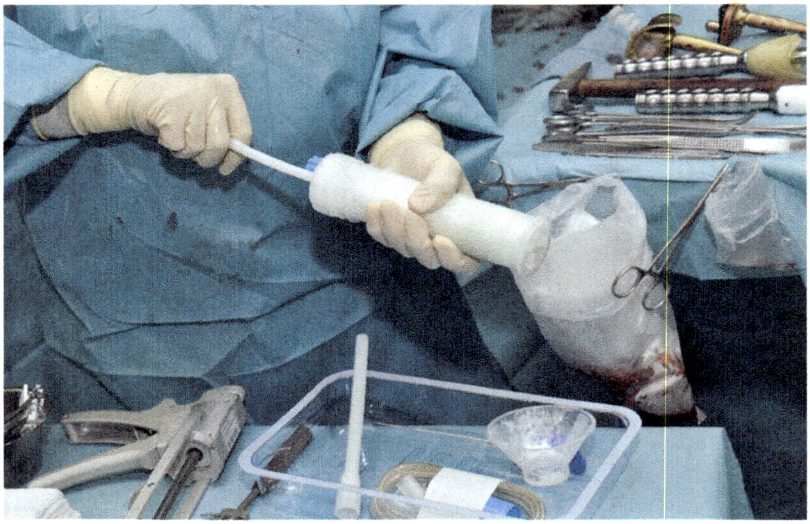

Fig. 9.7 ALAC is mixed without vacuum; instructions of the cement manufacturer are followed. Keep in mind that ALAC has a shorter working time and the proper consistency for cementing is reached earlier as in PMMA without antibiotics

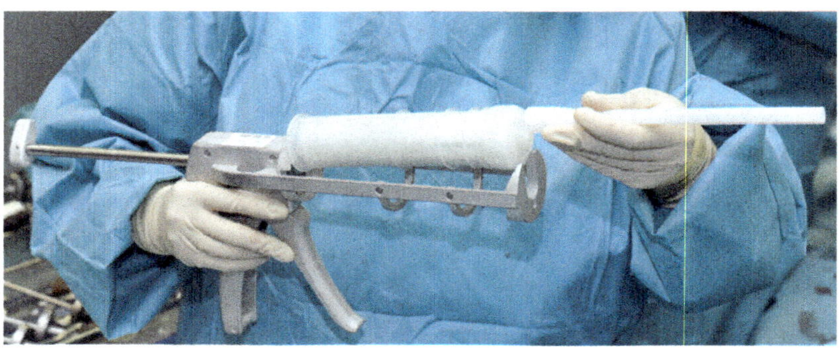

Fig. 9.8 Cement application with the gun. Cement viscosity may be different from PMMA without antibiotics

Antibiotic-Loaded Bone Cement as Spacer

The function of the spacer is to provide effective antibiotic concentrations in the joint after removing the foreign material and a thorough debridement was carried out, and to keep the distance between the two ends of the bones of the infected joint [19]. The lifetime of a spacer is quite short, it is kept in place for several weeks or months. The mechanical strength is obviously a less important issue compared to the cemented implant at one-stage exchange or at re-implantation of the two-stage procedure.

Further expectations towards the ALAC spacer are

- A fair mechanical strength that resists to shear forces when the patient walks on crutches with partial weight bearing,
- Not to irritate the soft tissues, not causing any allergic reaction,
- To provide an acceptable function of the joint for a short interval between first-stage explantation and re-implantation,
- The spacer should be easy to remove without any loss of bone stock.

The spacer usually provides an acceptable function of the joint, at least for a short period of time [19]. It can be static, which means a temporary fusion of the joint or mobile, allowing a range of motion with some limitations. There are some data in the literature showing some considerable benefits of the mobile spacer in the knee, providing not only a better function but also a higher antibiotic elution [20, 21]. Articulating spacers may simplify the surgical exposure at time of re-implantation. If static spacers are used, they should be supplemented by external immobilization, such as a brace or cast, to prevent the joint from instability during the interval between explantation and re-implantation [22].

The spacer may have a higher antibiotic concentration than the ALAC for fixation [23]. An antibiotic concentration up to 20 % can be achieved by hand mixing, which means a maximum of 8 g of antibiotic powder with 40 g of PMMA [10, 13].

The treatment of PJI with methicillin-resistant germs like MRSA/MRSE could be difficult even with the two-stage approach and may be associated with a higher failure rate [21, 24].

There are several advantages of the interim ALAC spacer. It is a modular, custom-made, immediate fit, antibiotic selective, temporary implant that allows the surgeon to reconstruct deficient bone stock safely and effectively using two-stage exchange arthroplasty. It affords the patient rapid pain relief, allows them to mobilize quite quickly while successfully eradicating infection in more than 90 % of hips with severe bone loss, and sets an appropriate soft tissue environment for a second-stage procedure [25].

References

1. Gehrke T, Zahar A, Kendoff D. One-stage exchange: it all began here. Bone Joint J. 2013;95-B(11 Suppl A):77–83.
2. Frommelt L. Principles of systemic antimicrobial therapy in foreign material associated infection in bone tissue, with special focus on periprosthetic infection. Injury. 2006;37 Suppl 2:87–94.
3. Stewart PS, Costerton JW. Antibiotic resistance of bacteria in biofilms. Lancet. 2001;358:135–8.
4. Adams K, Couch L, Cierny G, Calhoun J, Mader JT. In vitro and in vivo evaluation of antibiotic diffusion from antibiotic impregnated polymetylmethacrylate beads. Clin Orthop Relat Res. 1992;278: 244–52.
5. Chen AF, Parvizi J. Antibiotic-loaded bone cement and periprosthetic joint infection. J Long Term Eff Med Implants. 2014;24(2–3):89–97.
6. Buchholz HW, Engelbrecht H. Über die Depotwirkung einiger Antibiotika bei Vermischung mit dem Kunstharz Palacos. Chirurg. 1970;41:511–5.
7. Wahlig H, Buchholz HW. Experimentelle und klinische Untersuchungen zur Freisetzung von Gentamicin aus einem Knochenzement. Chirurg. 1972;43:441–5.
8. Buchholz HW, Elson RA, Lodenkamper H. The infected joint implant. In: McKibbin B, editor. Recent advances in orthopaedics. New York: Churchill Livingstone; 1979. p. 139–61.
9. Anagnostakos K, Wilmes P, Schmitt E, Kelm J. Elution of gentamicin and vancomycin from polymethylmethacrylate beads and hip spacers in vivo. Acta Orthop. 2009;80(2):193–7.
10. Frommelt L. Antibiotic choices in bone surgery – local therapy using antibiotic-loaded bone cement. In: Walenkamp GHIM, editor. Local antibiotics in arthroplasty. State of the art from the interdisciplinary point of view. Stuttgart/New York: Georg Thieme Verlag; 2007. p. 59–64.
11. Kühn KD. PMMA cements. Berlin/Heidelberg: Springer; 2014.
12. Peñalba Arias P, Furustrand Tafin U, Bétrisey B, Vogt S, Trampuz A, Borens O. Activity of bone cement loaded with daptomycin alone or in combination with gentamicin or PEG600 against staphylococcus epidermidis biofilms. Injury. 2015;46(2):249–53.
13. Kühn KD. Antibiotic-loaded bone cements – antibiotic release and influence on mechanical properties. In: Walenkamp GHIM, editor. Local antibiotics in arthroplasty. State of the art from the interdisciplinary point of view. Stuttgart/New York: Georg Thieme Verlag; 2007. p. 47–57.
14. Lewis G. Not all approved antibiotic-loaded PMMA bone cement brands are the same: ranking using the utility materials selection concept. J Mater Sci Mater Med. 2015;26(1):5388.
15. Paz E, Sanz-Ruiz P, Abenojar J, Vaquero-Martín J, Forriol F, Del Real JC. Evaluation of elution and mechanical properties of high-dose antibiotic-loaded bone cement: comparative "In Vitro" study of the influence of vancomycin and cefazolin. J Arthroplasty. 2015;30:1423–9. pii: S0883-5403(15)00164-3.
16. Kühn KD, Ege W, Gopp U. Acrylic bone cements: mechanical and physical properties. Orthop Clin North Am. 2005;29:20–39.
17. McLaren AC, Nugent M, Economopoulos K, Kaul H, Vernon BL, McLemore R. Hand-mixed and premixed antibiotic-loaded bone cement have similar homogeneity. Clin Orthop Relat Res. 2009;467(7):1693–8.

18. Pithankuakul K, Samranvedhya W, Visutipol B, Rojviroj S. The effects of different mixing speeds on the elution and strength of high-dose antibiotic-loaded bone cement created with the hand-mixed technique. J Arthroplasty. 2014;30:858–63. pii: S0883-5403(14) 00916-4.
19. Tsung JD, Rohrsheim JA, Whitehouse SL, Wilson MJ, Howell JR. Management of periprosthetic joint infection after total hip arthroplasty using a custom made articulating spacer (CUMARS); the Exeter experience. J Arthroplasty. 2014;29(9):1813–8. doi: 10.1016.
20. Romanò CL, Gala L, Logoluso N, Romanò D, Drago L. Two-stage revision of septic knee prosthesis with articulating knee spacers yields better infection eradication rate than one-stage or two-stage revision with static spacers. Knee Surg Sports Traumatol Arthrosc. 2012;20(12):2445–53.
21. Munro JT, Garbuz DS, Masri BA, Duncan CP. Articulating antibiotic impregnated spacers in two-stage revision of infected total knee arthroplasty. J Bone Joint Surg Br. 2012;94(11 Suppl A):123–5. doi:10.1302/0301-620X.94B11.30747. Review.
22. Severson EP, Hanssen AD. The infected total knee replacement. In: Norman Scott W, editor. Insall & scott surgery of the knee. 5th ed. Philadelphia: Elsevier Churchill Livingstone; 2012.
23. Sandiford NA, Duncan CP, Garbuz DS, Masri BA. Two-stage management of the infected total hip arthroplasty. Hip Int. 2015;10:308–15. doi:10.5301/hipint.5000265.
24. Leung F, Richards CJ, Garbuz DS, Masri BA, Duncan CP. Two-stage total hip arthroplasty: how often does it control methicillin-resistant infection? Clin Orthop Relat Res. 2011;469(4):1009–15. doi:10.1007/s11999-010-1725-6.
25. Haddad FS, Masri BA, Garbuz DS, Duncan CP. The treatment of the infected hip replacement. The complex case. Clin Orthop Relat Res. 1999;369:144–56. Review.

Local Antibiotic Therapy: Non–cement-based Antibiotic Delivery Methods

10

Moataz El-Husseiny

Abstract

Bone and soft tissue infections are serious problems that can result in significant morbidity that affects patients drastically. Peri-prosthetic infections are difficult to treat and eradicate. Single-stage revision in the form of surgical debridement with retention or exchange of artificial components, or two-stage revision followed by antibiotic administration remain the main stay of treatment. Delivery of antibiotics within the cement mantle has become popular in providing high local levels to treat infection. However, mixing high concentrations of antibiotics to cement affects its porosity and stiffness, thus predisposing loosening at the cement-implant interface. In addition, most drug elution occurs within hours, making it difficult to be above the minimum inhibitory concentration of bacteria until infection is completely treated. This raises the need to develop biodegradable delivery carriers that are able to release high levels of local antibiotics for long periods of time and eventually disintegrate into the system, preventing the need for secondary procedures to remove them. This chapter discusses different systems present that are currently used to treat bone and peri-prosthetic infections. Ongoing research is required to develop these local antibiotics delivery systems to allow them to replace long-term systemic antibiotics with their associated complications and toxicity.

Keywords

Local antibiotics • Delivery systems • Carrier systems • Biodegradable • Collagen sponge • Peri-prosthetic joint infection • Bone graft--based carriers • Protein-based carriers • Synthetic polymers • Local antibiotic microcapsules • Calcium phosphate delivery systems • Drug elution • Local antibiotic fibrin carrier

M. El-Husseiny, MBBCh, MRCS, Dip Sport M, MD (Res)
Department of Orthopaedics and Trauma, Great Ormond Street Hospital, London, UK
e-mail: moatazelhusseiny@gmail.com

D. Kendoff et al. (eds.), *Periprosthetic Joint Infections: Changing Paradigms*,
DOI 10.1007/978-3-319-30091-7_10

Introduction

Peri-prosthetic joint infection remains a devastating complication facing reconstructive surgery. Alexander Fleming was first to observe that locally applied antiseptics decreased bacterial burden, but also failed to sterilize chronically infected wounds. During World War II, Jensen et al. found that thorough debridement, haemostasis, instillation of sulfanilamide crystals followed by primary closure and immobilization, resulted in a reduced infection rate for open fractures [1].

Dombrowski and Dunn, found the use of closed wound irrigation-suction a successful method of delivering high concentrations of antibiotics locally after debridement of infected wounds [2]. Since the early 2000s, increased research into local antibiotic delivery systems paved the way for used of high concentration levels of antibiotics locally, preventing side effects and toxicity of prolonged systemic antibiotics.

Advantages of Local Antibiotic Delivery Methods in Infected Join Replacements

In 2004, Lazzarini et al. [3], considered excision of infected and devascularized tissues, obliteration of dead space, restoration of blood supply and soft tissue coverage, stabilization and reconstruction of the damaged bone, removal of all foreign bodies and systemic antimicrobial therapy were crucial components of the treatment of infected bone and joint replacements. Hanssen et al. [4], argued that in order to achieve therapeutic drug concentration in the affected area, high systemic doses are generally required which can further worsen toxic side effects. In addition, systemic antibiotic treatment may be ineffective in patients with poorly vascularized infected tissues, making the antibiotics unable to breach the glycocalyx or biofilm produced by the infecting bacteria [5].

Recently developed local antibiotic delivery systems also have the advantage of providing the scaffold on which osteoinductive and osteoconductive materials can be placed in addition to local antibiotics [6].

Characteristics of Ideal Local Antibiotic Delivery Method

Scientists have endured to develop the ideal local drug delivery system since antibiotics were discovered. This would produce high antibiotic levels at the site of infection and prevent side effects and toxicity of systemic antibiotics. Sustainability of antibiotic levels and availability above minimum inhibitory concentration (MIC) for bacteria is crucial to allow them to be effective for long period of time until complete eradication of infection. Moreover, antibiotic elution curves including factors that influence elution as local temperature and pH, together with discovery of the most suitable local carrier is still unknown. These materials need to be easily placed, patient friendly and inexpensive. In 2005, Hanssen described the ideal local antibiotic delivery system as one that would "would provide a more efficient delivery of higher levels of antibiotics to the site of infection and yet minimize the risks of systemic toxicity associated with traditional methods of intravenous antibiotics" [7].

Forms of Local Antibiotics Carriers

The simplest way of local antibiotic delivery is powder form. This is done by spraying the antibiotic over the wound area after thorough debridement. Rushton published excellent results for infection eradication and prevention using this method in 1997 [8]. Although this provided short periods of high levels of antibiotics, it potentially resulted in tissue damage.

Irrigation of local antibiotics in liquid form through a closed drainage system was used to provide continuous perfusion to the infected area. This demanded high level of nursing expertise and time to prevent drain blockage and spillage.

Plaster of Paris pellets were used by Santschi and McGarvey in 2003 with gentamicin with excellent results [9]. The main disadvantage was the need of a second stage procedure to remove the pellets as they themselves may act as a foreign body and be a medium for bacterial infection.

In recent years, biodegradable delivery carriers were developed and evaluated for delivery of local antibiotics. Biodegradability means no need for a secondary surgical procedure to remove foreign materials. They also were developed to allow more sustained elution of drugs in order to eradicate infection over a period of weeks. Collagen foam impregnated with gentamicin was used effectively by Ruszczak and Friess [10]. Furthermore, fibrin-sealant biodegradable materials using cephalosporins were developed by Tredwell et al. [11]. However, once collagen foam and fibrin dissolved, no osteoinductive or osteoconductive material was present to provide a structural base for the revision implant.

Cancellous bone and hydroxyapatite blocks containing vancomycin were used by Witso et al. [12] and Shirtliff et al. [13], respectively. In addition to providing base for elution of drugs, they acted as a scaffold on which bone integrated with joint prostheses.

Forms of Antibiotics

In order to select the appropriate antibiotics to treat peri-prosthetic infection, an understanding of bone and soft tissue microbiology is crucial. Peri-prosthetic infection may develop due to haematogenous spread or direct inoculation from surrounding soft tissues. Predisposing factors include environmental factors such as absence of laminar flow theatres, development of methicillin-resistant *Staphylococcus aureus* (MRSA), patient factors as immuno-compromised, diabetic, peripheral vascular disease, patients receiving chemotherapy or corticosteroids, patients with previous open fractures, or at risk patients with recent dental procedures. Normal bone is highly resistant to infection, hence when microbial load reaches critical density, they form a biofilm or glycocalyx that are difficult for antibiotics to penetrate, resulting in chronic infection.

Most common microbes to cause infection in hip and knee arthroplasties are coagulase-negative Staphylococcus, followed by Staphyloccocus aureus [14, 15]. Considering the above criteria, the most acceptable local delivery antibiotics are aminoglycosides. Combination therapy is useful in decreasing toxicity, treating mixed infections and preventing drug resistance. Aminoglycosides are water soluble, allowing diffusion from the carrier, stable at body temperature, active against bone and joint arthroplasty infections. They are released locally at levels exceeding minimum inhibitory concentration for Staphylococcus species. Their stability as compounds makes them suitable to load with any kind of composite. They have a low rate of primary resistance, with a low rate of allergic reaction [16].

The mainstay of choice of antibiotics relies on culture and sensitivity microbiology results. Numerous antibiotics can be used in antibiotic impregnated carriers. Vancomycin and teicoplanin were the most effective antibiotics with overall sensitivity rates of 100 % and 96 %, respectively. Gentamicin combined with vancomycin is the most effective empirical treatment and potentially allow for infected joint arthoplasties to be treated as a one-stage procedure.

Biodegradable Delivery Systems

The main advantage of biodegradable delivery methods over antibiotic loaded cement beads is the avoidance of a secondary procedure to remove the foreign body, that in itself can become a source of infection. In addition, biodegradable carriers may provide structural support to adjacent bone while infection is eradicated and bone remodelling is undertaken. Calhoun and Mader [17] suggest secondary antibiotic release occurs during degradation of the carrier, which would increase antibacterial efficacy.

Biodegradable delivery carriers can be classified into: bone graft-based, protein-based, and synthetic-based materials. Extensive research has been conducted to prolong duration of elution of local antibiotics until infection is overcome. This led to usage of hydrophobic materials the allowed slow release of antibiotics as the materials disintegrated. *In vitro* studies showed drug elution of ciprofloxacin on polylactate carriers up to 350 days [18], and hydroxyapatite carriers were able to elute gentamicin for 90 days [19]. Jia et al. were able to demonstrate Teicoplanin elution on calcium sulfate substrate for 29 days [20]. On the other hand, *in vivo* studies showed drug elution for shorter periods of time in comparison. Stemberger et al. [21] paved the way for the wide use of biodegradable collagen sponge carriers. They showed they were able to elute gentamicin for 56 days in animal models.

Bone Graft–Based Carriers

Bone graft was first used as a local antibiotic carrier in 1986 by McLaren and Miniaci [22]. They used tobramycin on morselized bone graft on rabbit models. They showed that tobramycin was released at a bactericidal level for 3 weeks. Chan et al. used antibiotic impregnated cancellous bone graft in treating infected bone fractures [23]. Although the study group of 36 patients all went to unite, it took 4–5 months to achieve this with the only complication reported as skin rash. They used hydroxyapatite struts with antibiotics aided in local treatment of bone infection in addition to dead space management [24]. The main disadvantage of these implants was the rapid release of antibiotics in a random manner [22]. Calcium sulfate in combination with vancomycin or tobramycin has been used successfully as a local antibiotic delivery system by Gitelis and Brebach [6]. They used 1 g of vancomycin or 1.2 g of tobramycin for every 25 g of calcium sulphate (Fig. 10.1). Rhyu et al. investigated antibiotic-loaded, blood-coated demineralized bone in the treatment of infected bones [25].

Protein-Based Materials

These are natural polymers that are loaded with antibiotics and are used in treatment of bone and soft tissue infections. They include collagen sponge, fibrin-coated, and thrombin-coated substrates. They are not as commonly used as antibiotic loaded bone cement in treatment of periprosthetic infections.

These carriers work on the basis of providing a protein to which local antibiotics bind. These act as physical scaffolds, allowing continuous flow of antibiotics into the circulation. Elution rates are rapid leading to release of all antibiotics in a range from hours to days.

Collagen sponge foam carrier is most widely used worldwide (Fig. 10.2). It is formed of sterile animal skin or tendo-achillis. It derives its popularity from being biocompatible and nontoxic. Following numerous experiments by Rao, they concluded drug elution rates can be modified by changing the porosity of collagen or treating it with chemicals [26]. Moreover, it stimulates osteoblast proliferation, promoting mineralization and production of collagenous callus. Initial *in vitro* studies by Wachol-Drewek et al. suggested antibiotic release from collagen foam took 4 days to complete [27]. When collagen sponge was impregnated with liposome encapsulated antibiotics, the release time increased to 12 days [28]. Their work also showed gentamicin release was superior using collagen sponge compared to polymethycrylate beads. *In vivo* studies by Humphrey et al. [29] showed collagen sponge delivered effective delivery of antibiotics for up to 28 days in rabbit models, and trials undertaken by Kanellakopoulou and Giamarellos-Bourboulis showed they were clinically effective [30]. Further technique refinement and prolongation of drug release are required before they can be recommended as delivery carriers for antibiotics in treatment of joint infections.

Fibrin sealants derived from coagulation proteins have great prospective for delivering antibiotics, growth factors and chemotherapy to targeted sites. They are similar to collagen sponge foams in being biocompatable and nontoxic. They degrade by fibrinolysis within days or weeks [31]. There has been a drive to use them with hip and knee replacements. Antibiotics with hydrophobic characteristics, such as tetracyclines, have shown promising results with fibrin carriers [32]. This is a result of slow release

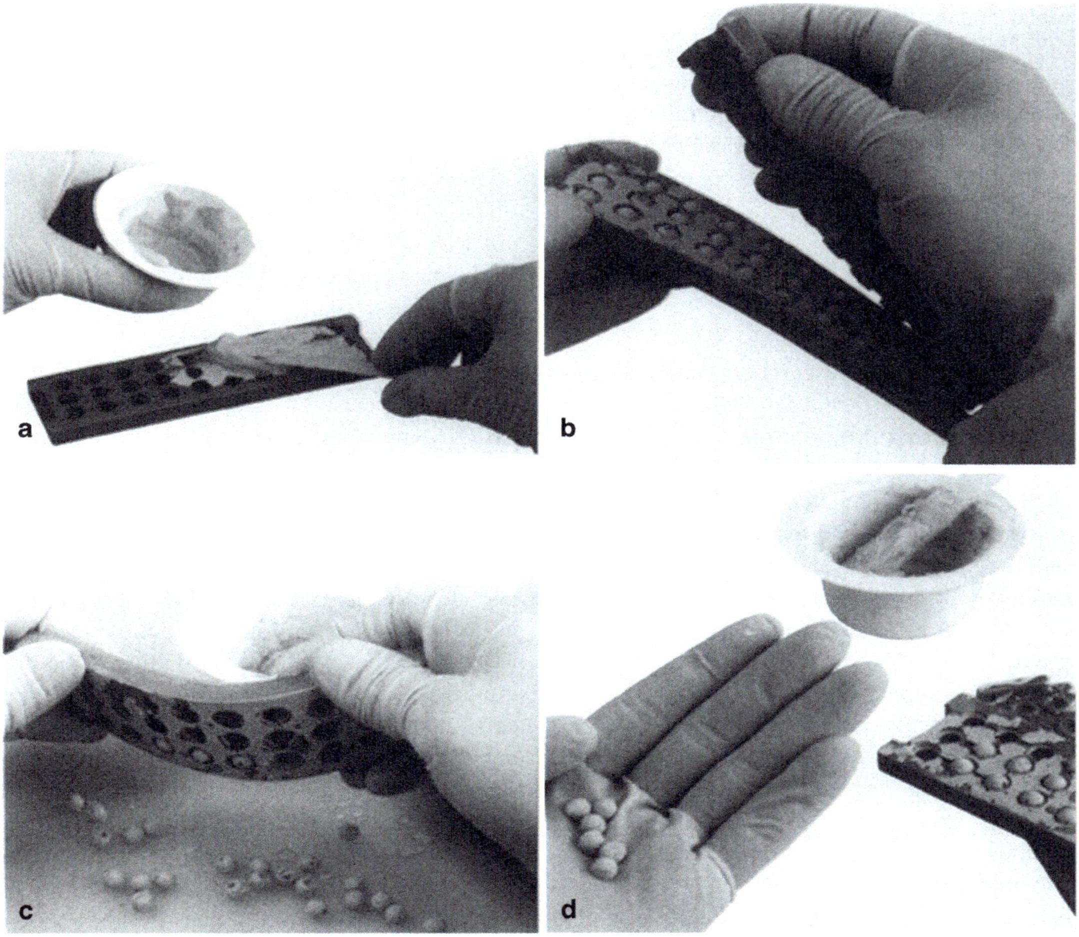

Fig. 10.1 (**a**) Calcium sulphate mixed with antibiotics placed into silicone moulds. (**b**) Mould is opened after 30 min. (**c**) Implants are removed. (**d**) Implants are ready to use (Reprinted with permission from Ref. [6])

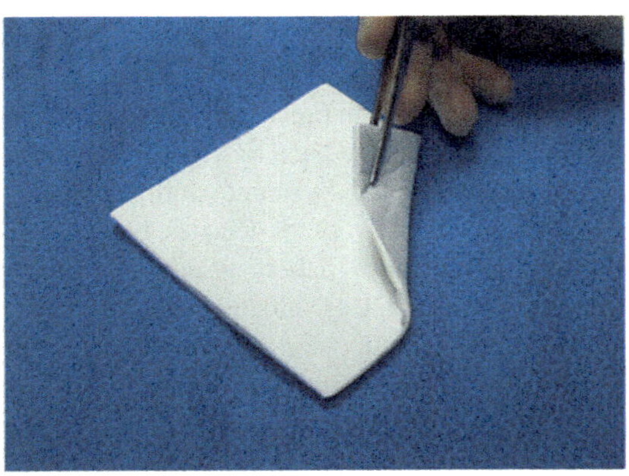

Fig. 10.2 Genatmicin-impregnated collagen fleece from Collatamp® EG, EUSA Pharma, Oxford, United Kingdom

of these antibiotics from fibrin substrate. Cephalosporins and aminoglycosides have shown to be released over 60 days for ciprofloxacin [33] and over 5–7 days for gentamicin [34]. The main drawback was the release of 66 % in the first 2 days.

Initial results from Zilch and Lambiris measured cefotaxime concentrations in serum and wound drainage from 46 patients treated with a fibrin clot mixed with cefotaxime and injected into bone medulla [35]. Serum levels dropped significantly within 12 h, and wound drainage maintained high levels for 3 days. Fibrin sealant carriers provide promising results in delivering local antibiotics used for prophylaxis in joint replacements. Further work is required to ensure the sustained release of drugs from the fibrin clot and the slow degradation of the substrate. In addition, light needs to be shed on the effect of low systemic antibiotics in development and evolution of super micro-organisms with antibiotics resistance.

Synthetic Polymers

Great interest by researchers is present in developing a carrier with better penetration and long lasting drug elution. Synthetic polymers have been widely used in surgery since the 1950s as suture material. Advances in technology have generated more reliable polymers that may be used as carriers [5]. Polyglycolide and polylactide derived polymers were selected for research as a carrier because they undergo gradual controlled degradation and dissolve at physiological pH.

Using different polymers within the construct allows the kinetics of antibiotic release to be modified by altering the geometry of the carrier, selecting copolymers of varying monometric composition, using different polymer crystallinity and molecular weight. Makinen et al. showed high compatibility of wide variety of antibiotics with these polymers and ability to release antibiotics for a long time period in therapeutic concentrations [36]. Polymers of polylactides and polyglycolic acid have been investigated with varying composition ratios [37]. They concluded better stability, delayed decomposition and higher elution concentrations of tobramycin, vancomycin and clindamycin with polymer formed of polylactides and polyglycolic acid with a ratio of 90:10.

Polymers of lactide/glycolide have been suggested as carriers for antibiotics since 1982 due to their biocompatibility, minimum tissue reaction and local inflammatory response [38]. Some studies showed their superiority to parental antibiotics in eradicating infection in animal model [39]. Wei et al. [40] showed that the MIC of antibiotic for the common causative organisms of osteomyelitis was exceeded for 6 weeks in the cortex, the cancellous bone, and in the bone marrow in rabbit models. In addition, majority of the implant material has been absorbed, and bone marrow had returned to a normal state within 9 weeks of implantation.

Development of micro-capsules composed of polylactate shells and containing gentamicin was investigated by Garvin et al. in 1992 [41]. They compressed the micro-capsules and demonstrated that 80 % of antibiotics were released in first 3 weeks. Kanellakopoulou et al. successfully used co-polymers to treat methicillin-resistant Staphylococcus aureus (MRSA) in rabbit models [30]. They showed the peak drug release was reached at 15 days and produced prolonged antibiotic release, and at a higher level.

Synthetic polymers need further evaluation and development if they were to be widely used for treatment of joint and bone infections. They lack the ability of providing structural integrity. This has allowed antibiotic-loaded cement spacers to continue to be used in treatment of periprosthetic infections. However, the use of biodegradable antibiotic-impregnated carriers have grown with recent studies showing single-stage revision hip and knee replacements to be successful in eradicating infections. Currently, there is no polymer that has shown superiority in delivering antibiotics locally.

Conclusion

Micro-organism-specific antibiotic delivery is fundamental in decreasing morbidity and mortality from orthopaedic-related infections. This is also important in preventing the evolution of antibiotic-resistant bacteria, by targeting culture sensitivities. Systemic antibiotics have been used effectively for decades, but development of resistance to these has led to a need for new methods that are able to deliver increased antibiotic levels, for prolonged periods, decreased toxicity, greater efficacy and less patient morbidity. Antibiotic-impregnated cement spacers are currently used successfully to treat periprosthetic infections, but they require a second procedure for removal of the spacer. Single-stage revision total joint replacements rely on thorough debridement, removal of biofilm, exchange of implants and administration of systemic antibiotics for varied periods of time to eradicate infection. There is substantial interest in finding methods of delivering effective doses of antimicrobial drugs locally, both in orthopaedics and other surgical disciplines. Although most of local antibacterial agent contained within a biodegradable system may be eluted, only 25 % is actually released from polymethylmethacrylate cement. In addition, biodegradable materials may add structural support that could be chosen for local drug delivery system in infected joint replacements with significant osteolysis, disintegrating as bone forms – preventing the need for a secondary procedure to remove the carrier and not acting as a source of infection. Much work is still needed in development of biodegradable, bio-compatible materials, the kinetics of antibiotic elution, and further development of current systems before many of these formulations can be used. The sheer diversity of available systems and the lack of suitable trials comparing them *in vivo* make their evaluation difficult. Although collagen foam is currently the most widely used local antibiotic delivery system, the duration of its antibiotic delivery is very short. Other delivery systems have shown greater promise, and those that are able both to stimulate the formation of new bone and provide a scaffold, such as composite antibiotic carriers, are most likely to gain widespread acceptance in the future. Better understanding and development of microcapsules help sustain release of antibiotics, allowing them to be delivered over a prolonged periods of time. There is a wide interest in this field both in preventing and treating joint infections using locally delivered antibiotics, and with further research and development, this will provide a major breakthrough in treatment of such infections.

Acknowledgements The author would like to thank EUSA Pharma for providing the Collatamp sample, and Journal of Orthopaedic Surgery (Hong Kong) for granting permission for re-use of figures.

References

1. Jensen NK, Johnsrud LW, Nelson MC. The local implication of sulfonamide in compound fractures. Surgery. 1939;6:1–12.
2. Dombrowski ET, Dunn AW. Treatment of osteomyelitis by debridement and closed wound irrigation-suction. Clin Orthop Relat Res. 1965;43:215–31.
3. Lazzarini L, Mader JT, Calhoun JH. Osteomyelitis in long bones. J Bone Joint Surg Am. 2004;86-A(10): 2305–18.
4. Hanssen AD. Local antibiotic delivery vehicles in the treatment of musculoskeletal infection. Clin Orthop Relat Res. 2005;437:91–6.
5. El-Husseiny M, Patel S, MacFarlane RJ, Haddad FS. Biodegradable antibiotic delivery systems. J Bone Joint Surg Br. 2011;93(2):151–7.
6. Gitelis S, Brebach GT. The treatment of chronic osteomyelitis with a biodegradable antibiotic-impregnated implant. J Orthop Surg (Hong Kong). 2002;10(1):53–60.
7. Hanssen AD, Osmon DR, Patel R. Local antibiotic delivery systems: where are we and where are we going? Clin Orthop Relat Res. 2005;437:111–4.
8. Rushton N. Applications of local antibiotic therapy. Eur J Surg Suppl. 1997;578:27–30.
9. Santschi EM, McGarvey L. In vitro elution of gentamicin from plaster of Paris beads. Vet Surg. 2003;32(2):128–33.
10. Ruszczak Z, Friess W. Collagen as a carrier for on-site delivery of antibacterial drugs. Adv Drug Deliv Rev. 2003;55(12):1679–98.
11. Tredwell S, Jackson JK, Hamilton D, Lee V, Burt HM. Use of fibrin sealants for the localized, controlled release of cefazolin. Can J Surg. 2006;49(5):347–52.
12. Witso E, Persen L, Loseth K, Benum P, Bergh K. Cancellous bone as an antibiotic carrier. Acta Orthop Scand. 2000;71(1):80–4.
13. Shirtliff ME, Calhoun JH, Mader JT. Experimental osteomyelitis treatment with antibiotic-impregnated hydroxyapatite. Clin Orthop Relat Res. 2002;401:239–47.
14. Nickinson RS, Board TN, Gambhir AK, Porter ML, Kay PR. The microbiology of the infected knee arthroplasty. Int Orthop. 2010;34(4):505–10.
15. Rafiq I, Gambhir AK, Wroblewski BM, Kay PR. The microbiology of infected hip arthroplasty. Int Orthop. 2006;30(6):532–5.
16. Kobayashi H, Shiraki K, Ikada Y. Toxicity test of biodegradable polymers by implantation in rabbit cornea. J Biomed Mater Res. 1992;26(11):1463–76.
17. Calhoun JH, Mader JT. Treatment of osteomyelitis with a biodegradable antibiotic implant. Clin Orthop Relat Res. 1997;341:206–14.
18. Kanellakopoulou K, Kolia M, Anastassiadis A, Korakis T, Giamarellos-Bourboulis EJ, Andreopoulos A, et al. Lactic acid polymers as biodegradable carriers of fluoroquinolones: an in vitro study. Antimicrob Agents Chemother. 1999;43(3):714–6.

19. Shinto Y, Uchida A, Korkusuz F, Araki N, Ono K. Calcium hydroxyapatite ceramic used as a delivery system for antibiotics. J Bone Joint Surg Br. 1992;74(4):600–4.
20. Jia WT, Luo SH, Zhang CQ, Wang JQ. In vitro and in vivo efficacies of teicoplanin-loaded calcium sulfate for treatment of chronic methicillin-resistant staphylococcus aureus osteomyelitis. Antimicrob Agents Chemother. 2010;54(1):170–6.
21. Stemberger A, Grimm H, Bader F, Rahn HD, Ascherl R. Local treatment of bone and soft tissue infections with the collagen-gentamicin sponge. Eur J Surg Suppl. 1997;578:17–26.
22. McLaren AC. Alternative materials to acrylic bone cement for delivery of depot antibiotics in orthopaedic infections. Clin Orthop Relat Res. 2004;427: 101–6.
23. Chan YS, Ueng SW, Wang CJ, Lee SS, Chao EK, Shin CH. Management of small infected tibial defects with antibiotic-impregnated autogenic cancellous bone grafting. J Trauma. 1998;45(4):758–64.
24. Nelson CL. The current status of material used for depot delivery of drugs. Clin Orthop Relat Res. 2004;427:72–8.
25. Rhyu KH, Jung MH, Yoo JJ, Lee MC, Seong SC, Kim HJ. In vitro release of vancomycin from vancomycin-loaded blood coated demineralised bone. Int Orthop. 2003;27(1):53–5.
26. Rao KP. Recent developments of collagen-based materials for medical applications and drug delivery systems. J Biomater Sci Polym Ed. 1995;7(7): 623–45.
27. Wachol-Drewek Z, Pfeiffer M, Scholl E. Comparative investigation of drug delivery of collagen implants saturated in antibiotic solutions and a sponge containing gentamicin. Biomaterials. 1996;17(17):1733–8.
28. Trafny EA, Grzybowski J, Olszowska-Golec M, Antos M, Struzyna J. Anti-pseudomonal activity of collagen sponge with liposomal polymyxin B. Pharmacol Res. 1996;33(1):63–5.
29. Humphrey JS, Mehta S, Seaber AV, Vail TP. Pharmacokinetics of a degradable drug delivery system in bone. Clin Orthop Relat Res. 1998;349:218–24.
30. Kanellakopoulou K, Giamarellos-Bourboulis EJ. Carrier systems for the local delivery of antibiotics in bone infections. Drugs. 2000;59(6):1223–32.
31. Jackson MR. Fibrin sealants in surgical practice: an overview. Am J Surg. 2001;182(2 Suppl):1S–7.
32. Woolverton CJ, Fulton JA, Salstrom SJ, Hayslip J, Haller NA, Wildroudt ML, et al. Tetracycline delivery from fibrin controls peritoneal infection without measurable systemic antibiotic. J Antimicrob Chemother. 2001;48(6):861–7.
33. Tsourvakas S, Hatzigrigoris P, Tsibinos A, Kanellakopoulou K, Giamarellou H, Dounis E. Pharmacokinetic study of fibrin clot-ciprofloxacin complex: an in vitro and in vivo experimental investigation. Arch Orthop Trauma Surg. 1995;114(5):295–7.
34. Kram HB, Bansal M, Timberlake O, Shoemaker WC. Antibacterial effects of fibrin glue-antibiotic mixtures. J Surg Res. 1991;50(2):175–8.
35. Zilch H, Lambiris E. The sustained release of cefotaxim from a fibrin-cefotaxim compound in treatment of osteitis. Pharmacokinetic study and clinical results. Arch Orthop Trauma Surg. 1986;106(1):36–41.
36. Makinen TJ, Veiranto M, Lankinen P, Moritz N, Jalava J, Tormala P, et al. In vitro and in vivo release of ciprofloxacin from osteoconductive bone defect filler. J Antimicrob Chemother. 2005;56(6):1063–8.
37. Bunetel L, Segui A, Cormier M, Langlais F. Comparative study of gentamicin release from normal and low viscosity acrylic bone cement. Clin Pharmacokinet. 1990;19(4):333–40.
38. Thies C. Microcapsules as drug delivery devices. Crit Rev Biomed Eng. 1982;8(4):335–83.
39. Garvin KL, Miyano JA, Robinson D, Giger D, Novak J, Radio S. Polylactide/polyglycolide antibiotic implants in the treatment of osteomyelitis. A canine model. J Bone Joint Surg Am. 1994;76(10):1500–6.
40. Wei G, Kotoura Y, Oka M, Yamamuro T, Wada R, Hyon SH, et al. A bioabsorbable delivery system for antibiotic treatment of osteomyelitis. The use of lactic acid oligomer as a carrier. J Bone Joint Surg Br. 1991;73(2):246–52.
41. Garvin K, Feschuk C. Polylactide-polyglycolide antibiotic implants. Clin Orthop Relat Res. 2005;437:105–10.

Part V

The Hip Joint

Acute Infections: Irrigation and Debridement with Implant Retention

11

Sujith Konan, David A. George, Vaibhav Punjabi, and Fares S. Haddad

Abstract

Prosthetic joint infection (PJI) is a devastating complication for the patient and for the surgeon. Debridement antibiotics and implant retention is an option to manage early presentations of periprosthetic infection. This chapter summarises the current evidence on indications, approach and relevant literature surrounding this treatment option.

Keywords

Early infection • Arthroplasty infection • DAIR • Joint infection • Implant retention • Infection

Introduction

Early onset periprosthetic join infections (PJI) (1–3 months after surgery) are commonly caused by *Staphylococcus aureus* (*S. aureus*) and gram-negative bacilli; being responsible for nearly 60 % of the early onset infections. Polymicrobial infection is also common during this period. Delayed-onset PJI (3 months to 1 or 2 years after surgery) are commonly caused by coagulase-negative staphylococci and enterococci. Late-onset PJI (>1 or 2 years after surgery) are commonly due to hematogenous infection, and *S. aureus* is the predominant microorganism in this group of patients. Culture-negative PJI is encountered in 5–15 % of cases. These are usually in delayed- or late-onset PJI. One option for acute presentations of PJI is irrigation and debridement with implant retention, commonly referred to as a DAIR procedure (debridement, antibiotics, and implant retention).

S. Konan, MBBS, MD, MRCS, FRCS (Tr & Orth)
F.S. Haddad, BSc, MD(res), MCh, FRCS (Orth) (✉)
Department of Trauma and Orthopaedics, University College London Hospitals NHS Trust, London, UK
e-mail: fsh@fareshaddad.co.uk

V. Punjabi, MBBS, MS, FRACS, FA(Ortho)A
Department of Orthopaedics, Princess Grace Hospital, London, UK

D.A. George, MBChB, BmedSc, MRCS (Eng)
Department of Trauma and Orthopaedics, University College Hospitals, London, London, UK

Principles

Successful management of acute PPI using the DAIR technique requires planned surgical and medical intervention. The multidisciplinary team

D. Kendoff et al. (eds.), *Periprosthetic Joint Infections: Changing Paradigms*,
DOI 10.1007/978-3-319-30091-7_11

(MDT) involved in the care of the patient should include the orthopaedic surgeon, infectious disease physician, nursing and allied staff, and the microbiologist.

The goals of treatment are to eradicate the infection, restore pain-free function of the infected joint, and minimize morbidity and mortality for the patient. In order to achieve this, the burden of biofilm has to be decreased such that perioperative antimicrobial therapy can eradicate any remaining infection. It is crucial to identify the responsible microbiological agent, and antibiotics should be withheld until representative samples have been obtained.

The basic surgical principles are to perform an open arthrotomy, explant all exchangeable components while leaving the fixed components in situ, obtain multiple fluid and tissue samples for microbiology, remove any hematoma, debride all necrotic or infected soft tissue, irrigate the joint with large volumes of fluid, and finally replace exchanged modular components. The exchanged components are typically polyethylene liner for knee replacement and the femoral head and acetabular liner for hip replacements. Following irrigation, the joint is closed, typically over a drain [1, 2]. Arthroscopic DAIR procedures may not achieve adequate debridement and does not allow exchange of modular components. Outcomes of DAIR procedure using arthroscopic techniques may be suboptimal [2].

Following debridement, antimicrobial treatment is commenced. Typically, antimicrobials are held prior to surgery to obtain sufficient representative samples for microbiology followed by broad-spectrum antibiotic therapy in the immediate postoperative period. Subsequently, sensitivity testing guides the antibiotic regime. The typical duration of antibiotic regime is 6 weeks or more [1–6]. An exception to this principle would be the patient presenting with systemic sepsis where broad-spectrum antibiotics may have to be commenced before DAIR. Even in this situation, early samples are obtained by means of aspiration when possible before commencing broad spectrum antibiotics.

Indications for DAIR

DAIR reduces the morbidity of extensive surgery required for implant surgery. The overall goal of attempting DAIR should be to select the cohort of patients in whom successful treatment of infection is highly likely. Patients presenting with short duration of symptoms, with a stable implant are ideal candidates for DAIR [7–9].

Early postoperative infections (occurring within the first month) or late acute hematogenous infections (with symptoms for 3 weeks) are most appropriate for this strategy. The presence of radiolucency surrounding the implant does not imply treatment failure, provided the implants are not mechanically loose [3, 10].

With regards to the pathogen, infection with *Staphylococcus* species is associated with a high risk of treatment failure [1–3, 6, 11], likely driven by *S. aureus* [1, 3]. Antimicrobial susceptibility is important, with higher rates of failure for infection with methicillin-resistant *S. aureus* (MRSA) [12], vancomycin-resistant enterococci [12], and fluoroquinolone-resistant gram-negative bacilli.

Host factors such as a high ASA (indicating comorbidity) score [6] or a compromised immune system [9, 13], may also increase the risk of treatment failure.

The presence of an open wound or a sinus, extensive soft tissue compromise and inability to close the wound directly will most likely result in chronic infections, and a staged-exchange may be more appropriate [14]. However, the protocol adopted by the Bone Infection Unit, Nuffield Orthopaedic Centre, Oxford, UK, for candidates for DAIR, includes patients with persistent wound inflammation and sinus discharge. They have demonstrated successful salvage of the prosthesis of 89 % at 1 year, 89 % at 2 years, and 78 % at 3 years [1].

Several studies have reported treatment observations with DAIR procedure. Byren et al. [1] further analyzed this protocol. The treatment failures observed had a mean follow-up of 2.3 years, with more than half the patients had at least one co-morbidity, and 69 % had their primary arthroplasty within 90 days of surgery. Independent risk factors for failure of DAIR (based on multivariate analysis) included infection due to *S. aureus*, methicillin-resistant and methicillin-susceptible strains ($p=0.05$), a previously revised joint ($p=0.008$), and arthroscopic washouts ($p=0.008$). Arthroscopy is more likely to result in poor debridement techniques due to the limited accessibility and views, compared to an open procedure, and limits an exchange of modular components.

A multicenter, observational study undertaken by Lora-Tamayo et al. [13] included cases of PJI over a 7-year period. Following DAIR, the likelihood of failure was increased in patients with immunosuppression ($p=0.013$), complex infections with polymicrobial involvement ($p=0.007$), presence of bacteremia ($p=0.015$), and with a C-reactive protein (CRP) of greater than 100 mg/L at diagnosis ($p=0.021$). Furthermore, patients undergoing two or more debridements were at an increased rate of failure ($p=0.008$). Elsewhere a CRP greater than 220 mg/L ($p=0.01$) has been associated with higher failure rates [15].

According to Lora-Tamayo et al. [13] a non-immunosuppressed patient with a monomicrobial infection and no bacteremia, a CRP of less than 100 mg/L, having undergone only one debridement will have a 77 % chance of a successful outcome at 6 months. A patient with the opposite scenario will have less than 1 % chance of success.

Several other studies have found a strong association between failure and the presence of *S. aureus* [16, 17], and need for a second debridement [15]. Others have not seen this association with the pathogen [18], and Mont et al. concluded a second debridement was protective [19].

Additional factors associated with failure of DAIR have been identified in smaller cohort studies, as well as those confirming the findings of the larger studies. This includes the presence of a sinus tract ($p=0.002$) [3], presence of rheumatoid arthritis ($p=0.03$) [20], immunocompromised [21], erythrocyte sedimentation rate (ESR) at presentation above 60 mm/h ($p=0.005$) [20], coagulase-negative *Staphylococcus* infection ($p=0.002$) [20], in particular highly virulent organisms such as MRSA [17] or polymicrobial infections [22].

Delays to debridement must be avoided [4], with higher failure rates seen when symptoms have been present for more than 7 or 8 days ($p=0.05$, and $p=0.04$ respectively) [3, 20]. Fifty percent failure can be expected if started after 8 weeks of symptoms.

The main difficulty in interpreting the literature and determining the absolute and relative contraindications for undertaking a DAIR is the variability of the medical management and surgical techniques adopted between the Institutes, as well as the criteria used to categorize a PJI [18]. We believe that the decision to attempt a DAIR must be assessed on an individual basis, and the information presented here must be weighed up against previous microbiological and histological findings, as well as the patient's medical status and their choices. A summary of these findings can be found in Table 11.1.

Preoperative Workup

The diagnosis of an infected prosthetic joint is made on clinical grounds supported by pathology results. The preoperative workup for patients with PJI includes haematological and radiological investigations, as outlined in previous chapters.

Table 11.1 Absolute and relative contraindications for undertaking a DAIR in patients presenting with a PJI

Absolute contraindications	Relative contraindications
Loose prosthesis	Sinus tract
Poor soft tissue coverage	*Staphylococcus aureus* (MRSA and MSSA)
Bone cement mantle compromise	Previously revised joint
	Immunosuppression Rheumatoid arthritis
	Polymicrobial involvement
	Presence of bacteremia
	CRP > 100 mg/L
	ESR > 60 mm/h
	Two or more previous debridements
	>3 weeks of symptoms

Imaging investigations like plain radiographs, Magnetic resonance imaging (MRI) and computed tomography (CT) have an indirect role in the workup for PJI for DAIR [23]. Signs of implant loosening, periosteal reaction and bone resorption may indicate compromised prosthetic stability. Radiographic changes, however, lag behind the clinical onset of disease by 1–2 weeks.

Operative Steps

The surgical steps for undertaking a debridement of the infected joint will vary according to the surgeon's preference, and the local Institute's policies. Irrespective of this, it is highly recommended that antibiotics are not commenced before the surgery, or if they have been, they are omitted for a minimum of 48 h beforehand, or longer if possible and clinically safe to do so [1]. This is to increase the chance of identifying a causative pathogen during microbiological sampling of the operative field.

As with all revision surgeries, we advocate the use of the previous skin incision if possible. This avoids multiple unnecessary scars, which may be unappealing to the patient, as well as the heightened risk of necrosis to the skin if the incisions are too close and compromise the vascular supply. Depending upon the original incision, we opt for a midline skin incision and medial parapatella approach to the knee, and a posterior approach to access the hip.

The approach to the joint must adhere to the same principles of the primary procedure, taking care of vital structures and avoiding dissection of neurovascular bundles even in the presence of significant adjacent infection.

During dissection, the presence of infection may be found superficially as soon as the skin is incised, remain deep in the joint, or communicate between the two. If a sinus is present, and a DAIR is still indicated, the tract should be fully excised to a healthy soft tissue envelope. The whole sinus should be sent for microbiological and histological assessment.

Further samples should be sent from all quadrants of the joint, and be correctly labeled during collection, stating whether obtained from a superficial or deep location, medial or lateral compartment of the joint, and whether it involves synovium, soft tissue, or biofilm. If possible, an aspirate of the pus or infected haematoma should be obtained. It is advisable to use separate instruments (forceps, knife, and universal containers) for collecting each sample and placed directly into separate containers for analysis [1].

Once the surgeon is satisfied that a sufficient number of samples have been obtained (we recommend a minimum of five) [24, 25], systemic antibiotics can be administered based upon previous sensitivities obtained from joint aspirations and other systemic samples. All remaining necrotic soft tissue, infected haematoma, and debris adjacent to the prosthesis should be excised to a healthy bleeding base. This is difficult if a tourniquet has been applied during a knee debridement, but is more obvious during a hip debridement.

It is then important to remove all modular components of the prosthesis if possible: tibial insert, acetabular cup insert, and femoral head. Removal of these parts will improve the access to the joint, especially gaining access to the posterior capsule [26], as well as reduce the bioburden of biofilm that may collect beneath these components.

It is then imperative to assess the integrity of the prosthesis, which can be done by gently taping the prosthesis with a universal explant, inline with its axis. If it remains firmly fixed and mechanically sound the procedure can continue as previously planned, and any mobile components should be replaced as appropriate. Smooth polished tapered cemented femoral stems may be easily exchanged without breaching the cement mantle. However, should the implant be loose on examination, proceeding with implant retention is no longer viable. A staged procedure may then be planned, and the instruments and implants of this should be on hand if such a predicament should occur.

Prior to closure, it is necessary to undertake a thorough irrigation of the wound, with a combination of large volumes of warm pulsatile lavaged saline (0.9 % sodium chloride), combined with aqueous chlorhexidine or povidine-iodine. We close the wound in a similar manner as that of a primary procedure, and use a drain that is removed after 24–48 h depending upon the output.

Post-operatively the intraoperative antibiotics are continued intravenously until the results of the samples taken during the procedure are known. If the pathogen has altered, the antibiotics must be amended to reflect this, and continued for a variable period. As previously stated, arthroscopy has no role in DAIR. It is associated with high rates of recurrence [1] due to poor access to the whole infected field, compromising the debridement.

Postsurgical Management and Discussion

Routine mobilisation is encouraged after DAIR procedure while closely monitoring wound healing. Monitoring the trend for serum inflammatory markers ESR and CRP may be beneficial to document.

Following DAIR patients are commenced on appropriate antibiotic management based on the isolated organism and sensitivities. The choice and duration of antibiotics is variable, but in majority of cases 2–6 weeks of intravenous choice is chosen, followed by oral antibiotics for 3–6 months.

Combination Therapy for DAIR in Staphylococcal PPI

Using rifampicin combination therapy increases success rate for DAIR in the presence of staphylococcus infection [13, 19, 27, 28]. However, it is important to monitor susceptibility to rifampicin and to look for drug interactins with other treatment agents [29]. For both *S. aureus* and coagulase-negative staphylococci, rifampin is typically given with an intravenous agent, most commonly a-lactam or glycopeptide, for the initial 2–6 weeks. This is followed by continued rifampin combined with a fluoroquinolone to complete either a 6-month (knee) or a 3-month (hip) total duration of rifampin combination therapy [7].

Using combination of fluoroquinolone with rifampin even during the initial phase of therapy [13, 14, 30] is supported by the International Consensus Meeting documents [7, 14]. When rifampin cannot be administered, the initial period of intravenous antimicrobials should be at least 4 weeks. Among intravenous agents, cefazolin or antistaphylococcal penicillins are preferred over vancomycin for treatment of infection with methicillin-susceptible *S. aureus* (MSSA) [31].

The treatment of PPI due to MRSA is challenging. The options for combination therapy include fusidic acid [15, 32], trimethoprim-sulfamethoxazole and minocycline [29]. Vancomycin remains the preferred intravenous antimicrobial for PPI due to MRSA, while daptomycin may be an option [33]. The addition of rifampin may be more effective than daptomycin monotherapy and may prevent the emergence of daptomycin resistance [34–36]. Linezolid is a suitable oral alternative. Its prolonged use of linezolid is limited by bone marrow suppression and close monitoring of complete blood counts is recommended [37, 38].

Management after treatment failure. Patients who fail a DAIR procedure typically ultimately undergo a two-stage arthroplasty exchange [6]. Another option for treatment of ongoing infection after a DAIR procedure is repeated debridement followed by chronic antimicrobial therapy. Unfortunately, the likelihood of success for a repeated DAIR procedure after prior failure is low.

Conclusion

Historically, the treatment success rate varies depending on DAIR, one stage or two stage revision arthroplasty. The reported success rate of DAIR varies between 31 and 82 %. These results report infections due to a variety of microorganisms, host factors and treatment protocols. Recent studies using a combination therapy of fluoroquinolone with rifampicin for *S. aureus* PJI have reported improved success rate from 62 to 75 %. However, this remains inferior to results of 87 % success rate after one-stage revision arthroplasty; and 87–100 % success rate after two-stage revision arthroplasty.

References

1. Byren I, Bejon P, Atkins BL, Angus B, Masters S, McLardy-Smith P, et al. One hundred and twelve infected arthroplasties treated with 'DAIR' (debridement, antibiotics and implant retention): antibiotic duration and outcome. J Antimicrob Chemother. 2009;63(6):1264–71.
2. Koyonos L, Zmistowski B, Della Valle CJ, Parvizi J. Infection control rate of irrigation and debridement for periprosthetic joint infection. Clin Orthop. 2011;469(11):3043–8.
3. Marculescu CE, Berbari EF, Hanssen AD, Steckelberg JM, Harmsen SW, Mandrekar JN, et al. Outcome of prosthetic joint infections treated with debridement and retention of components. Clin Infect Dis. 2006;42(4):471–8.
4. Brandt CM, Sistrunk WW, Duffy MC, Hanssen AD, Steckelberg JM, Ilstrup DM, et al. Staphylococcus aureus prosthetic joint infection treated with debridement and prosthesis retention. Clin Infect Dis. 1997;24(5):914–9.
5. El Helou OC, Berbari EF, Lahr BD, Eckel-Passow JE, Razonable RR, Sia IG, et al. Efficacy and safety of rifampin containing regimen for staphylococcal prosthetic joint infections treated with debridement and retention. Eur J Clin Microbiol Infect Dis. 2010;29(8):961–7.
6. Azzam KA, Seeley M, Ghanem E, Austin MS, Purtill JJ, Parvizi J. Irrigation and debridement in the management of prosthetic joint infection: traditional indications revisited. J Arthroplasty. 2010;25(7): 1022–7.
7. Osmon DR, Berbari EF, Berendt AR, Lew D, Zimmerli W, Steckelberg JM, et al. Diagnosis and management of prosthetic joint infection: clinical practice guidelines by the Infectious Diseases Society of America. Clin Infect Dis. 2013;56(1):e1–25.
8. Leone S, Borrè S, Monforte A, Mordente G, Petrosillo N, Signore A, et al. Consensus document on controversial issues in the diagnosis and treatment of prosthetic joint infections. Int J Infect Dis. 2010;14:S67–77.
9. Silva M, Tharani R, Schmalzried TP. Results of direct exchange or debridement of the infected total knee arthroplasty. Clin Orthop. 2002;404:125–31.
10. Crockarell Jr JR, Hanssen AD, Osmon DR, Morrey BF. Treatment of infection with debridement and retention of the components following hip arthroplasty. J Bone Joint Surg Series A. 1998;80(9):1306–13.
11. Konigsberg BS, Valle CJ, Ting NT, Qiu F, Sporer SM. Acute hematogenous infection following total hip and knee arthroplasty. J Arthroplasty. 2013;29:469–72.
12. Soriano A, García S, Bori G, Almela M, Gallart X, Macule F, et al. Treatment of acute post-surgical infection of joint arthroplasty. Clin Microbiol Infect. 2006;12(9):930–3.
13. Lora-Tamayo J, Murillo O, Iribarren JA, Soriano A, Sánchez-Somolinos M, Baraia-Etxaburu JM, et al. A large multicenter study of methicillin-susceptible and methicillin-resistant staphylococcus aureus prosthetic joint infections managed with implant retention. Clin Infect Dis. 2013;56(2):182–94.
14. Parvizi J, Gehrke T, Chen AF. Proceedings of the international consensus on periprosthetic joint infection. Bone Joint J. 2013;95 B(11):1450–2.
15. Aboltins CA, Page MA, Buising KL, Jenney AW, Daffy JR, Choong PF, et al. Treatment of staphylococcal prosthetic joint infections with debridement, prosthesis retention and oral rifampicin and fusidic acid. Clin Microbiol Infect. 2007;13(6):586–91.
16. Deirmengian C, Greenbaum J, Stern J, Braffman M, Lotke PA, Booth Jr RE, et al. Open debridement of acute gram-positive infections after total knee arthroplasty. Clin Orthop. 2003;416:129–34.
17. Zmistowski B, Fedorka CJ, Sheehan E, Deirmengian G, Austin MS, Parvizi J. Prosthetic joint infection caused by gram-negative organisms. J Arthroplasty. 2011;26 Suppl 6:104–8.
18. Cobo J, Miguel LG, Euba G, Rodríguez D, García-Lechuz JM, Riera M, et al. Early prosthetic joint infection: outcomes with debridement and implant retention followed by antibiotic therapy. Clin Microbiol Infect. 2011;17(11):1632–7.
19. Mont MA, Waldman B, Banerjee C, Pacheco IH, Hungerford DS. Multiple irrigation, debridement, and retention of components in infected total knee arthroplasty. J Arthroplasty. 1997;12(4):426–33.
20. Kuiper JWP, Van DB, Van DS, Nolte PA, Colen S. 2-stage revision recommended for treatment of fungal hip and knee prosthetic joint infections. Acta Orthop. 2013;84(6):517–23.
21. Peel TN, Cheng AC, Choong PFM, Buising KL. Early onset prosthetic hip and knee joint infection: treatment and outcomes in Victoria, Australia. J Hosp Infect. 2012;82(4):248–53.
22. Westberg M, Grøgaard B, Snorrason F. Early prosthetic joint infections treated with debridement and implant retention. Acta Orthop. 2012;83(3):227–32.
23. Vilchez F, Martínez-Pastor JC, García-Ramiro S, Bori G, Maculé F, Sierra J, et al. Outcome and predictors of treatment failure in early post-surgical prosthetic joint infections due to staphylococcus aureus treated with debridement. Clin Microbiol Infect. 2011;17(3): 439–44.
24. Fink B, Makowiak C, Fuerst M, Berger I, Schäfer P, Frommelt L. The value of synovial biopsy, joint aspiration and C-reactive protein in the diagnosis of late peri-prosthetic infection of total knee replacements. J Bone Joint Surg Series B. 2008;90(7):874–8.

25. Spangehl MJ, Masri BA, O'Connell JX, Duncan CP. Prospective analysis of preoperative and intraoperative investigations for the diagnosis of infection at the sites of two hundred and two revision total hip arthroplasties. J Bone Joint Surg Series A. 1999;81(5):672–83.
26. Tsukayama DT, Estrada R, Gustilo RB. Infection after total hip arthroplasty: a study of the treatment of one hundred and six infections. J Bone Joint Surg Series A. 1996;78(4):512–23.
27. Zimmerli W, Widmer AF, Blatter M, Frei R, Ochsner PE. Role of rifampin for treatment of orthopedic implant-related staphylococcal infections: a randomized controlled trial. J Am Med Assoc. 1998;279(19):1537–41.
28. Widmer AF, Gaechter A, Ochsner PE, Zimmerli W. Antimicrobial treatment of orthopedic implant-related infections with rifampin combinations. Clin Infect Dis. 1992;14(6):1251–3.
29. Forrest GN, Tamura K. Rifampin combination therapy for nonmycobacterial infections. Clin Microbiol Rev. 2010;23(1):14–34.
30. Barberán J, Aguilar L, Carroquino G, Giménez MJ, Sánchez B, Martínez D, et al. Conservative treatment of staphylococcal prosthetic joint infections in elderly patients. Am J Med. 2006;119(11):993. e7-993.e10.
31. Tice AD, Hoaglund PA, Shoultz DA. Outcomes of osteomyelitis among patients treated with outpatient parenteral antimicrobial therapy. Am J Med. 2003;114(9):723–8.
32. Siddiqui MM, Lo NN, Ab Rahman S, Chin PL, Chia SL, Yeo SJ. Two-year outcome of early deep MRSA infections after primary total knee arthroplasty: a joint registry review. J Arthroplasty. 2013;28(1):44–8.
33. Byren I, Rege S, Campanaro E, Yankelev S, Anastasiou D, Kuropatkin G, et al. Randomized controlled trial of the safety and efficacy of daptomycin versus standard-of-care therapy for management of patients with osteomyelitis associated with prosthetic devices undergoing two-stage revision arthroplasty. Antimicrob Agents Chemother. 2012;56(11):5626–32.
34. John AK, Baldoni D, Haschke M, Rentsch K, Schaerli P, Zimmerli W, et al. Efficacy of daptomycin in implant-associated infection due to methicillin-resistant staphylococcus aureus: importance of combination with rifampin. Antimicrob Agents Chemother. 2009;53(7):2719–24.
35. Garrigós C, Murillo O, Euba G, Verdaguer R, Tubau F, Cabellos C, et al. Efficacy of usual and high doses of daptomycin in combination with rifampin versus alternative therapies in experimental foreign-body infection by methicillin-resistant staphylococcus aureus. Antimicrob Agents Chemother. 2010;54(12):5251–6.
36. Saleh-Mghir A, Muller-Serieys C, Dinh A, Massias L, Crémieux AC. Adjunctive rifampin is crucial to optimizing daptomycin efficacy against rabbit prosthetic joint infection due to methicillin-resistant staphylococcus aureus. Antimicrob Agents Chemother. 2011;55(10):4589–93.
37. Nguyen S, Pasquet A, Legout L, Beltrand E, Dubreuil L, Migaud H, et al. Efficacy and tolerance of rifampicin-linezolid compared with rifampicin-cotrimoxazole combinations in prolonged oral therapy for bone and joint infections. Clin Microbiol Infect. 2009;15(12):1163–9.
38. Bassetti M, Vitale F, Melica G, Righi E, Di Biagio A, Molfetta L, et al. Linezolid in the treatment of gram-positive prosthetic joint infections. J Antimicrob Chemother. 2005;55(3):387–90.

One-Stage Approach with Cement 12

Daniel Kendoff, Akos Zahar, and Thorsten Gehrke

Abstract

The one-stage approach including mixed topical antibiotics to cement has been established in the ENDO Klinik Hamburg in the early 1970s. Based on the obligatory preoperative aspiration and knowledge of the infecting bacteria, a individualized antibiotic regime can be tailored to each patient, based on topical antibiotics with the cement and systemic application postoperatively. Surgically, our approach really needs an aggressive debridement of all infected hardware, bone and soft tissues during the single stage. In general this procedure offers certain obvious advantages. This mainly includes the need for only one operation, shorter hospitalization, reduced systemic antibiotic treatment. The key to success is based on the well-defined and detailed intra-hospital infrastructure and cooperation of surgeons and microbiologists.

Keywords

One-stage • Antibiotic-loaded cement • Single-stage revision • Topical antibiotics

Introduction

Management of periprosthetic joint infections (PJI) after hip arthroplasty remains a challenge to any arthroplasty surgeon. The therapeutic goal in either one- or more stage revisions of PJI is in general defined by the complete eradication of the infection and further maintenance of the joint function.

While it has been accepted worldwide that the treatment of a late chronic infection should be obtained by a two- or even more staged revision

D. Kendoff, MD, PhD (✉)
Department of Orthopaedics and Trauma, Helios Klinikum Berlin Buch, Berlin, Germany
e-mail: daniel.kendoff@helios-kliniken.de

A. Zahar, MD • T. Gehrke, MD
Department of Orthopedic Surgery, Helios ENDO-Klinik, Hamburg, Germany

D. Kendoff et al. (eds.), *Periprosthetic Joint Infections: Changing Paradigms*,
DOI 10.1007/978-3-319-30091-7_12

technique, a distinct single-stage revision approach in infected total hip arthroplasty has shown comparable results within the last 30 years in our own clinical set-up [1–4].

Generally, both revision techniques should be available depending on the clinical status of the patient, the local set-up and the surgeon's expertise. In the most frequently used clinical scenarios, an implant removal is followed by 6 weeks of systemic antibiotic treatment and delayed re-implantation of a new prosthesis, cemented or cementless. The introduction of antibiotic-impregnated spacers in hip revisions seemed to improve the functional outcome of the more-staged approach and has gained increasing popularity [5, 6].

However, looking carefully at the current available literature and guidelines for the treatment of infected THA, there is no clear evidence that a two- or more stage procedure has a clearly higher success rate than a one-stage approach. Although postulated in a larger number of relevant articles describing the two-stage technique as the gold standard in infection eradication, most of the herein mentioned recommendations, e.g., duration of antibiotic treatment, static vs. mobile spacer, interval of spacer retention, cemented vs. uncemented implant fixation, are based on level IV to III evidence studies or even expert opinions, rather than on prospective randomized or comparative data.

In our opinion, a distinct one-stage exchange offers certain advantages with a comparative success rate of infection eradication. Obvious further advantages are mainly based on need for only one operative procedure and short interval of intravenous antibiotics, reduced hospitalization time and overall costs [4, 7, 8].

In order to fulfill a one-stage approach with the aforementioned potential success rate, there are obligatory pre-, peri- and postoperative details that need to be meticulously respected. The following text describes the experience at the authors' institution and the management strategies of our one-stage approach in PJI, with a strict cemented pathway. Emphasis is given to all detailed requirements that provide the basis for a high clinical success rate.

Early Infections/Acute PJI

We aggressively treat an acute infected THA (<3 weeks or less 3 weeks onset of symptoms) still with a local irrigation and debridement (I&D), soft tissue revision and lavage, and polyethylene liner exchange, including preservation of the initially implanted prosthesis. Systemic antibiotics in this scenario are adapted to the algorithm described by Zimmerli et al. [9]. Any failed I&D will undergo an elective complete exchange (usually one stage), and no further I&D attempts are carried out. Any defined late infection (>3 weeks), however, should always be treated with a definite complete implant removal.

Diagnosis

We refer to Chap. 7 to highlight the importance of mandatory preoperative aspiration before every planned one-stage septic exchange. Currently, the diagnosis of PJI in our clinic is in line with the Consensus Meeting from Philadelphia 2013 [10].

Joint Aspiration

A mandatory and most relevant preoperative diagnostic test needed in any case of a planned one-stage exchange is based on the joint aspiration with an exact identification of the bacteria! The presence of a positive bacterial culture and respective antibiogram is essential for the one-stage procedure. Specific antibiotic-loaded acrylic cement (ALAC) is based on this diagnostic tool, in order to achieve a high topic antibiotic elution directly at the surgical side [11–14].

This absolute strict aspiration-based diagnostic algorithm became standard for every planned THA revision in our clinic, including all late or early aseptic loosening cases. Furthermore, we expanded this regime on all cases of unclear pain or malfunction after primary or revision THA, based on an own performed aspiration study, showing that between 4 and 7 % of all our patients initially planned for an aseptic THA revision had evidence of a subtle low-grade infection in the past [15].

Indications

Very few arguments against a one-stage approach exist; consequently, we are able to fulfill 85 % of all infected THA cases in this technique. The absolute mandatory infrastructural requirement is based on the clear evidence of the bacteria in combination with a distinct patient-specific plan for the following topical and systemic antibiotic treatment.

Contraindications

We defined the following criteria to deviate from our one-stage approach to a two-stage procedure:

- Failure of ≥2 previous one-staged procedures, and infection spreading to the nerve-vessel bundle
- Unclear preoperative bacteria specification
- Non-availability of appropriate antibiotics
- High antibiotic resistance

Preoperative Preparation and Planning

Again, we would like to highlight the absolute mandatory presence of a positive bacterial culture and antibiogram for the one-stage procedure. The proposed cemented fixation using ALAC is considered to be the treatment of choice in order to achieve a high topical therapeutic level of antibiotic elution from the cement [13, 14].

Future-oriented approaches might also include antibiotic local implant or silver coatings alternatives for a one-stage approach as well. In addition there have been reports using a non-cemented technique, which also will be described further in later chapters of this book [16, 17].

The principal success of a one-stage approach does not only depend on the removal of all hardware material (including cement and restrictors) in combination with the ALAC. It also includes a very aggressive and complete debridement of any infected soft tissues and bone material. This includes a full removal of the anterior and posterior capsule of the hip joint.

Surgical Preparation

Implants and Cement

- The surgeon should be aware of the implant in situ and be familiar with its removal and disassembly. Occasionally, the use of implant-specific instrumentation becomes necessary.
- Inadequate bone stock, possible intraoperative complications such as acetabular/femoral fractures, perforations of the cortex, osseous windows and disintegration must be taken into consideration when choosing an appropriate implant.
- Proximal femoral replacements, usually modular ones, may have to be chosen in patients with significant bone deficiency and persistent osteomyelitis of the femur. Bone loss is usually significantly more extensive than radiographically evident. However, the potential need for total femoral replacement implants needs to be considered relatively rarely.
- ALAC with additional antibiotics in powder form to be added intraoperatively is necessary in our cemented technique. Invariably at least two to three mixes of cement (80–120 g) including large mixing systems and appropriate cement guns are required. In patients with a narrow diaphysis, extra-narrow nozzles allow for appropriate retrograde cementing technique.
- Knowledge about possible type of ALAC used at primary implantation, as resistance to the previously used AB must be expected.
- Often industrially pre-manufactured ALAC cement may even be appropriate. Currently, companies offer more variability of pre-mixed antibiotics to the cement, as e.g.,vancomycin or gentamycin. This, however, is also influenced by country-specific regulations (U.S. vs. Europe vs. Asia).
- As mentioned above, for the success of any one-stage cemented procedure, the antibiogram for the final topic cement impregnation is absolute mandatory.

Operative Technique

Skin Incision and Debridement

- Old scars in the line of the skin incision should be excised. The prior incision from the last operative approach should be used.
- Fistulae should be integrated into the skin incision and radically excised to the joint capsule.
- All non-bleeding tissues and related bone need to be excised radically. In cases with severe and long ongoing history of osteomyelitis of the proximal bone formation, a complete resection of this area is suggested. A complete removal of all hardware includes the implant itself as well as distinct removal of all materials, including cables, wires and cement and possible cement stoppers.
- Biopsy material, preferably five to six samples, should be taken as a routine measure from all relevant areas of the operation site for combined microbiological/cultures and histological evaluation [18, 19]. Only afterwards the defined antibiotics should be administered systemically.

Implant Removal and Completion of Debridement

- Removing cemented implants often might be easier to remove and less invasive than removing ingrown cementless components (Fig. 12.1).
- In cases of well-fixed uncemented components, cortical windows are required to gain access to the interface. High-speed burrs and curved saw blades can aid the removal.
- Narrow straight osteotomes with symmetrically coned blades should remove all accessible bone cement that can be removed without causing further loss of bone stock. Removal of cement stoppers can be time-consuming; a distinct drilling technique can help here (Fig. 12.2).
- A full range of narrow and wide osteotomes of various thicknesses should be available
- Extraction of the implant necessitates special or universal extraction instruments, if available. Otherwise, general punches are required.

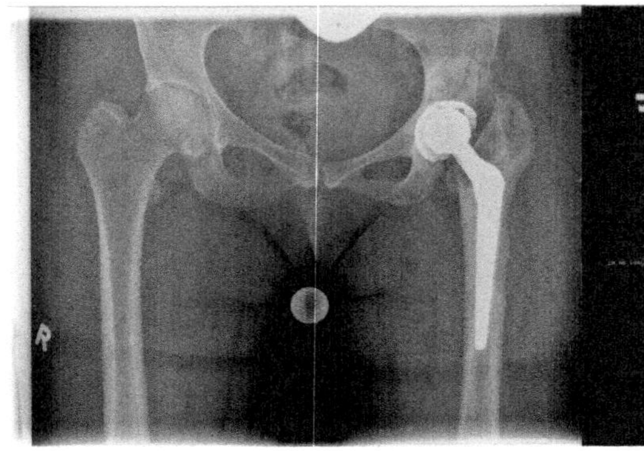

Fig. 12.1 Ingrown cementless total hip implants with secondary subsidence usually need extensive work to remove

- Special curved chisels, long rongeurs, curetting instruments, long drills and cement taps are used to remove the cement (Fig. 12.3). In the hip joint retrograde chisels can be of relevant help in many cases.
- General debridement of bone and suspicious soft tissues must be as radical as possible. It must include all areas of osteolysis and non-viable bone.
- Finalisation of the aggressive debridement often exceeds the amount of resected materials in a two-stage approach.
- We recommend the general use of pulsatile lavage throughout the procedure, however, after all implant removal and completed debridement; the intramedullary canals are packed with polymeric biguanid-hydrochlorid (polyhexanid)–soaked swabs.
- The complete team now re-scrubs, while new instruments are used for re-implantation.
- A second dose of antibiotics is given after 1.5 h of operating time or if blood loss at this point exceeds 1 L.

Reimplantation

- Inadequate bone stock may require the use of allografts, although ideally this should be avoided. We even prefer to fill large defects with ALAC, and do not favour the use of allograft (Fig. 12.4).
- Alternatively, the use of tantalum-based acetabular wedges or jumbo cups have been

Fig. 12.2 (a) Drilling of a plug. (b) Stepwise drilling of the cement plug. (c) Utilizing a centralizer. (d) Final extraction with corcscrew driver. (e) The femoral antecurvation must be respected by drill placement and approach to prevent "via falsa" attempts

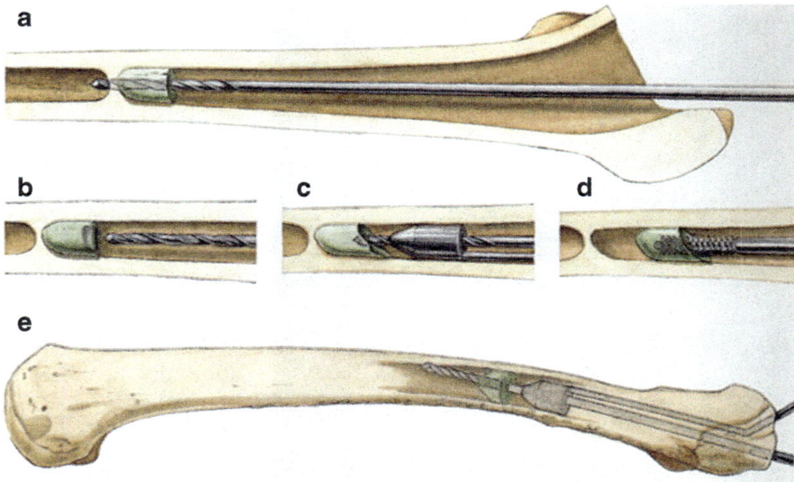

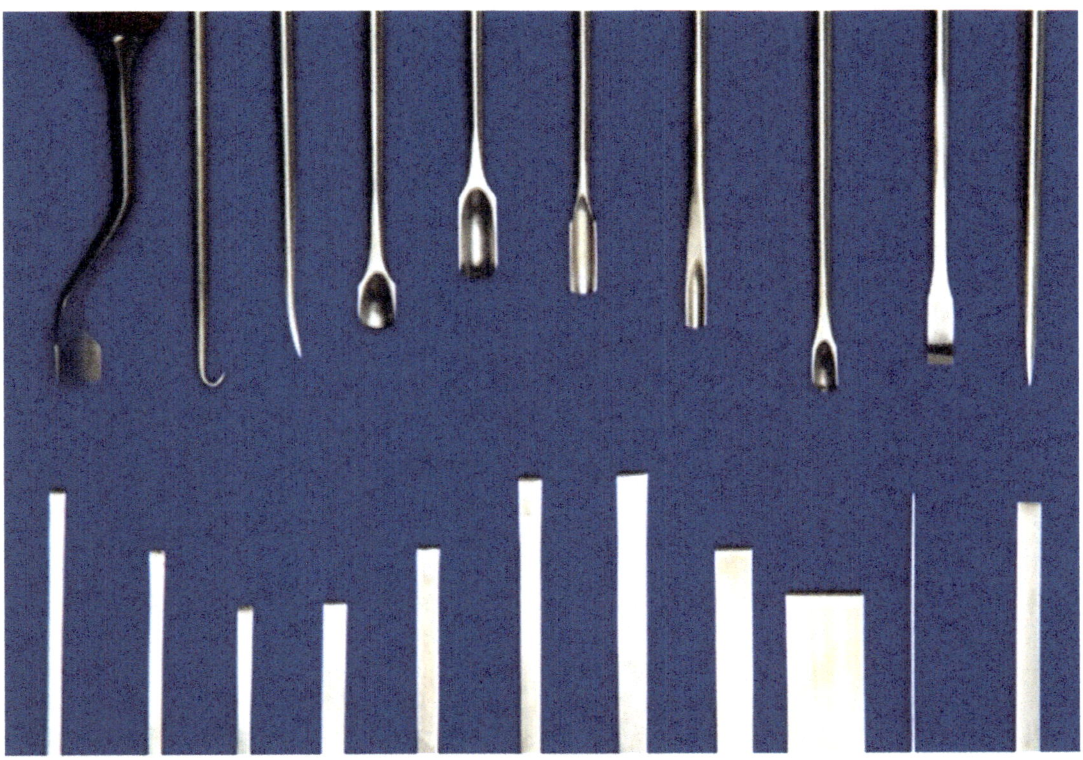

Fig. 12.3 Endofemoral removal of cement needs special instruments such as long curved chissels, rongeurs, etc

implemented in our regular clinical use for some years now [20]. Variations of depth and width of those augments allow for a proper reconstruction of the resulting bone loss, including an excellent biocompatibility and related stiffness and cellular structure. Consequently, a combined fixation of the cement with the prosthesis and tantalum

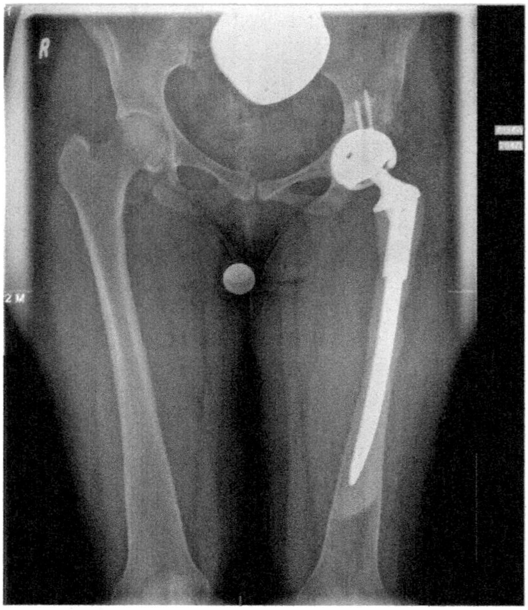

Fig. 12.4 A larger proximal femur defect after severe infection filled with cement and additional cement coverage of the implant

augment becomes possible. In addition, it has been postulated that tantalum should have antibacterial potential in total joint replacement; this, however, has not yet been proven clinically in larger series [21]. Furthermore, we do include quite often the use of dual-mobility cups in cases of abductor muscle absence or necessary removal of the proximal femur (Fig. 12.5a, b).

- The antibiotic-loaded cement is prepared in the meantime, while it is mandatory to fulfil the following criteria:
  - Appropriate antibiotic (antibiogram, adequate elusion characteristics)
  - Bactericidal (exception clindamycin)
  - Powder form (never use liquid antibiotic)
  - Maximum addition of 10 % PMMA powder, to ensure biomechanical stability.
- Antibiotics (e.g., vancomycin) might change the polymerisation behaviour of the cement, causing acceleration of cement curing.
- Generally, current principles of modern cementing techniques should be applied, including retrograde filling, cement stopper and pressurization.

Postoperative Antibiotics

Associated postoperative systemic antibiotic administration is usually followed for 10–14 days (exception: streptococci). Whereas a prolonged administration of intravenous antibiotics for 6 weeks is common in the two-stage approach, the rational for this prolongation has not been 100 % clarified in studies. To the contrary, there is evidence about possible relevant systemic and organ-specific complications after any prolonged antibiotic administration [8, 9].

Postoperative Care and Rehabilitation

The related hospitalisation time postoperatively ranges from 12 to 20 days (mean 14) in our set-up. The physiotherapeutic approach in any one stage cannot be generalised. Due to the variety of soft tissue and bone damage and the extent of infection, in most cases an individual plan is developed. However, we recommend an early and aggressive mobilisation within the first days postoperatively. Weight bearing should then be adapted to the intraoperative findings and substance defects. In quite a larger number of patients, the adequate bone stock and relative low soft tissue involvement allows an immediate mobilisation under full weight bearing, which is another advantage of the cemented technique (Fig. 12.6a, b).

Postoperative Complications

Persistence or recurrence of infection remains the most relevant complication in the one-stage technique. As failures rates with a two-stage exchange have been described as between 9 and 20 % in non-resistant bacteria, our unpublished data show comparative results after 8–10 years of follow-up, using the one-stage approach (unpublished data) [22–25]. Consequently, we discuss at the time of patient's consent a possible risk of recurrent or new infection of about 10–20 %.

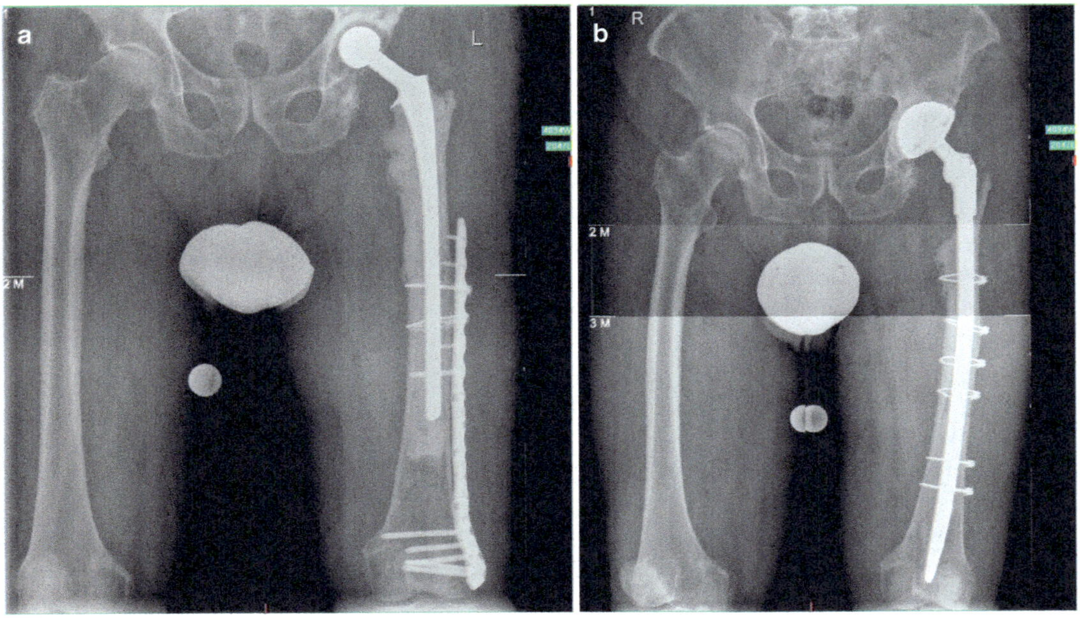

Fig. 12.5 (**a**) PJI after long cemented stem revision, postoperative distal femur fracture and secondary plate osteosynthesis. (**b**) Dual-mobility cup in combination with long-stemmed proximal femoral replacement and absence of abductor muscles

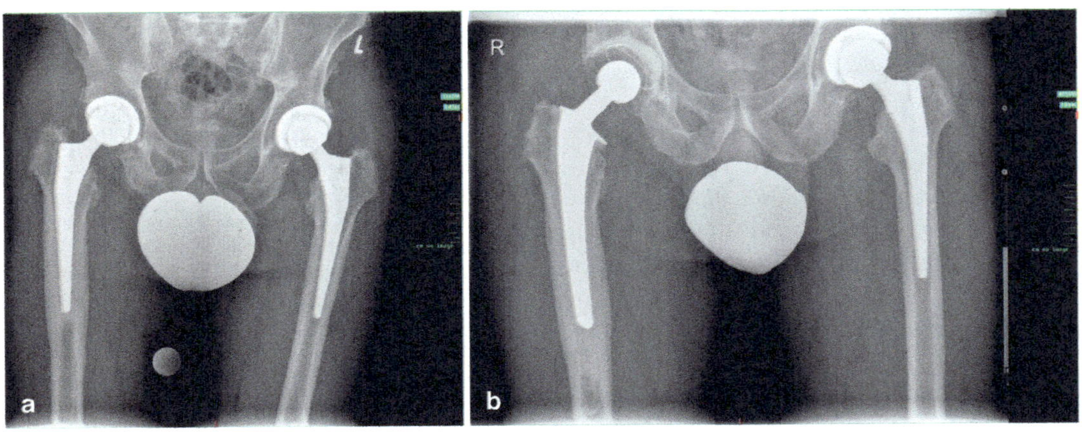

Fig. 12.6 (**a**) Primary infection of right uncemented THA. (**b**) Fully cemented one-stage revision allows for immediate postoperative full weight bearing

Although we are unable to present general comparative data evaluating the functional outcome between a two- vs. one-stage approach, we truly believe that neither any articulating spacer nor girdle stone situation of the hip joint will result in better functional outcome.

We consider the risk for direct damage to the sciatic nerve and main vessels as relatively low for an experienced surgeon, even in such an extended aggressive debridement, and relatively comparable to a two-stage exchange. The general risk of intra- and postoperative fractures should also be comparable to the two- or more stage exchange.

Outcome

The two-stage approach has become the most used technique worldwide, with a reported re-infection rate of between 9 and 20 % [22–25]. Although advocated as the "gold standard," we established and followed the aforementioned one-stage approach in our clinic for over 35 years in over 8 % of all our infected THA patients.

Accordingly, far more studies have been published about the two- or more-stage revision technique. Very few studies or case series evaluating the one-stage exchange are currently available [1–4, 8, 16, 26, 27].

Although most reports are from or with our institution, some international experience exists, with comparable high success rates between 90 and 75 %, in either hip or knee infections [8, 16, 26–29].

Besides obvious surgical benefits, by eliminating a second major operative procedure, further major advantage arises from the relevantly reduced duration of postoperative systemic antibiotics. This rarely lasts for more than 14 days in our current set-up.

Summary

A distinct one-stage infected TJA approach is still very rarely used within the orthopaedic society. From our perspective, the one-stage revision offers certain obvious advantages. This mainly includes the need for only one operation, shorter hospitalization, reduced systemic antibiotic treatment, lower overall cost and relatively high patient satisfaction. The key to success is based on the well-defined and detailed intra-hospital infrastructure, including a meticulous preoperative aspiration regime, planning, aggressive intraoperative surgical approach and postoperative specific patient care.

References

1. Kordelle J, Frommelt L, Kluber D, Seemann K. Results of one-stage endoprosthesis revision in periprosthetic infection cause by methicillin-resistant Staphylococcus aureus. Z Orthop Ihre Grenzgeb. 2000;138(3):240–4.
2. Siegel A, Frommelt L, Runde W. Therapy of bacterial knee joint infection by radical synovectomy and implantation of a cemented stabilized knee joint endoprosthesis. Chirurg. 2000;71(11):1385–91.
3. Steinbrink K, Frommelt L. Treatment of periprosthetic infection of the hip using one-stage exchange surgery. Orthopade. 1995;24(4):335–43.
4. Schmitz HC, Schwantes B, Kendoff D. One-stage revision of knee endoprosthesis due to periprosthetic infection and Klippel-Trenaunay syndrome. Orthopade. 2011;40(7):624–6, 628–9.
5. Biring GS, Kostamo T, Garbuz DS, Masri BA, Duncan CP. Two-stage revision arthroplasty of the hip for infection using an interim articulated prostalac hip spacer: a 10- to 15-year follow-up study. J Bone Joint Surg Br. 2009;91(11):1431–7.
6. Masri BA, Duncan CP, Beauchamp CP. Long-term elution of antibiotics from bone-cement: an in vivo study using the prosthesis of antibiotic-loaded acrylic cement (PROSTALAC) system. J Arthroplasty. 1998;13(3):331–8.
7. Buechel FF. The infected total knee arthroplasty: just when you thought it was over. J Arthroplasty. 2004;19(4 Suppl 1):51–5.
8. Buechel FF, Femino FP, D'Alessio J. Primary exchange revision arthroplasty for infected total knee replacement: a long-term study. Am J Orthop (Belle Mead NJ). 2004;33(4):190–8; discussion 198.
9. Zimmerli W, Trampuz A, Ochsner PE. Prosthetic-joint infections. N Engl J Med. 2004;351(16):1645–54.
10. Parvizi P, Gehrke T, editors. Proceedings of the international consensus meeting on periprosthetic joint infection. Towson: Data Trace Publishing Company; 2013.
11. Hanssen AD, Spangehl MJ. Practical applications of antibiotic-loaded bone cement for treatment of infected joint replacements. Clin Orthop Relat Res. 2004;427:79–85.
12. Trampuz A, Osmon DR, Hanssen AD, Steckelberg JM, Patel R. Molecular and antibiofilm approaches to prosthetic joint infection. Clin Orthop Relat Res. 2003;414:69–88.
13. Wahlig H, Dingeldein E, Buchholz HW, Buchholz M, Bachmann F. Pharmacokinetic study of gentamicin-loaded cement in total hip replacements. Comparative effects of varying dosage. J Bone Joint Surg Br. 1984;66(2):175–9.

14. Fink B, Vogt S, Reinsch M, Buchner H. Sufficient release of antibiotic by a spacer 6 weeks after implantation in two-stage revision of infected hip prostheses. Clin Orthop Relat Res. 2011;469(11):3141–7.
15. Kordelle J, Klett R, Stahl U, Hossain H, Schleicher I, Haas H. Infection diagnosis after knee-TEP-implantation. Z Orthop Ihre Grenzgeb. 2004;142(3):337–43.
16. Winkler H. Rationale for one stage exchange of infected hip replacement using uncemented implants and antibiotic impregnated bone graft. Int J Med Sci. 2009;6(5):247–52.
17. Zeller V, Lhotellier L, Marmor S, Leclerc P, Krain A, Graff W, et al. One-stage exchange arthroplasty for chronic periprosthetic hip infection: results of a large prospective cohort study. J Bone Joint Surg Am. 2014;96(1):e1.
18. Schafer P, Fink B, Sandow D, Margull A, Berger I, Frommelt L. Prolonged bacterial culture to identify late periprosthetic joint infection: a promising strategy. Clin Infect Dis. 2008;47(11):1403–9.
19. Fink B, Makowiak C, Fuerst M, Berger I, Schafer P, Frommelt L. The value of synovial biopsy, joint aspiration and C-reactive protein in the diagnosis of late peri-prosthetic infection of total knee replacements. J Bone Joint Surg Br. 2008;90(7):874–8.
20. Klatte TO, Kendoff D, Sabihi R, Kamath AF, Rueger JM, Gehrke T. Tantalum acetabular augments in one-stage exchange of infected total hip arthroplasty: a case-control study. J Arthroplasty. 2014;29(7):1443–8.
21. Tokarski AT, Novack TA, Parvizi J. Is tantalum protective against infection in revision total hip arthroplasty? Bone Joint J. 2015;97-B(1):45–9.
22. Azzam K, McHale K, Austin M, Purtill JJ, Parvizi J. Outcome of a second two-stage reimplantation for periprosthetic knee infection. Clin Orthop Relat Res. 2009;467(7):1706–14.
23. Goldman RT, Scuderi GR, Insall JN. 2-stage reimplantation for infected total knee replacement. Clin Orthop Relat Res. 1996;331:118–24.
24. Haleem AA, Berry DJ, Hanssen AD. Mid-term to long-term followup of two-stage reimplantation for infected total knee arthroplasty. Clin Orthop Relat Res. 2004;428:35–9.
25. Kilgus DJ, Howe DJ, Strang A. Results of periprosthetic hip and knee infections caused by resistant bacteria. Clin Orthop Relat Res. 2002;404:116–24.
26. Parkinson RW, Kay PR, Rawal A. A case for one-stage revision in infected total knee arthroplasty? Knee. 2011;18(1):1–4.
27. Silva M, Tharani R, Schmalzried TP. Results of direct exchange or debridement of the infected total knee arthroplasty. Clin Orthop Relat Res. 2002;404:125–31.
28. Lu H, Kou B, Lin J. One-stage reimplantation for the salvage of total knee arthroplasty complicated by infection. Zhonghua Wai Ke Za Zhi. 1997;35(8):456–8.
29. Selmon GP, Slater RN, Shepperd JA, Wright EP. Successful 1-stage exchange total knee arthroplasty for fungal infection. J Arthroplasty. 1998;13(1):114–5.

Infections of the Hip Joint: One-Stage Approach Without Cement

13

Heinz Winkler and Peter Haiden

Abstract

Problems with infection of a total hip replacement (THR) derive from the presence of biofilms with inherent resistance to usual antibiotic treatment and bone defects resulting from infection-induced osteolysis. Discussions on the choice of treatment mainly focus on the chance of eradicating the infection in either one or more stages. The advantages of only one operation regarding patients' satisfaction, functional results and economical burden are evident. However, the fear of re-infection usually leads surgeons to multiple-stage procedures, mostly using antibiotic-loaded spacers in the interval. Antibiotic concentrations eluted from spacers have no effect on biofilms and might be associated with a high rate of complications like breakage or dislocation.

One-stage revisions so far were mostly with cemented prostheses admixing antibiotics to the cement. Cemented revisions show several disadvantages: the addition of antibiotics to cement reduces its biomechanical properties with inferior long-term results compared to uncemented techniques. Efficient cementing techniques result in tight bonding with the underlying bone, making eventual removal time-consuming and possibly associated with further damage to the osseous structures. Uncemented implants appear more advantageous but are at risk of becoming colonized by eventually remaining biofilm fragments, requiring local application of antibiotics. Uncemented prostheses can be removed as easily as spacers in case of failure and may be left in place in case of success.

H. Winkler, MD (✉)
Osteitis Zentrum, Privatklinik Döbling, Heiligenstaedter, Strasse 57-63A-1190, Wien, Austria
e-mail: h-winkler@aon.at

P. Haiden, MD
Department of Traumatology, Landesklinikum Korneuburg, Wiener Ring 3–5, A-2100 Korneuburg, Austria

D. Kendoff et al. (eds.), *Periprosthetic Joint Infections: Changing Paradigms*,
DOI 10.1007/978-3-319-30091-7_13

Allograft bone may be impregnated with high loads of antibiotics using special impregnation techniques, resulting in an antibiotic bone compound (ABC). ABC provides local concentrations exceeding those of cement by more than a 100-fold and efficient release is prolonged for several weeks. The same time it is most likely to restore bone stock, which usually is compromised after removal of an infected endoprosthesis. Effective local antimicrobial concentrations in combination with radical debridement may be suitable for eradicating infection with a single operation in the majority of cases.

Based on these considerations a new protocol for one-stage exchange of infected TJR has been established in our institution. Bone defects are filled with ABC, uncemented implants are fixed in original healthy bone. With ABC, providing a sustained antibiotic release with biofilm-active concentrations, microscopical remnants of biofilm may be eliminated. Results indicate an overall success rate of more than 90 % with one operation, without any adverse side effects. Incorporation of allografts appears as after grafting with unimpregnated bone, in the radiographic follow-up. One-stage revision using ABC together with uncemented implants should be at least comparably safe as multiple-stage procedures, offering clear advantages for the quality of life of patients as well as from economic standpoints.

Keywords
Infection • Biofilm • MBEC • Revision THR • One-stage • Two-stage • Antibiotic • Cement • Cementless • Implant • Local antibiotic treatment • Bone defect • Allograft • Processing • Purification • Grafting • Quality of life

The Problem of Periprosthetic Joint Infection

Prosthetic joint infection (PJI) still is the most feared complication in total hip replacement (THR). It meanwhile is generally accepted that systemic antibiotic therapy may be appropriate for suppressing clinical symptoms but is insufficient for eradicating infection. At least chronic or delayed infections require complete removal of the prosthesis and all other materials, such as cement and restrictors. Re-implantation may be performed in one or more stages, whereas two-stage revision still is considered the gold standard. However, there is no evidence-based reason for that assumption. The benefits of a single-stage procedure are obvious, as outlined in Chap. 12, but the fear of re-infection usually leads surgeons to multiple-stage procedures, mostly using antibiotic-loaded spacers in the interval [1–6].

The Biofilm Issue

The traditional conceptions of infection deal with freely floating planktonic bacteria invading a host organism. It has been more than 30 years since William Costerton elucidated the reasons for resistance against conventional antimicrobial therapies in device-related infections [7]. Bacteria may change from the familiar planktonic forms into phenotypically different sessile forms after adhesion to dead surfaces. The surfaces of poorly vascularized bone and implants act as substratum for attachment of pathogens that immediately start producing a protecting extracellular matrix, the glycocalix, forming the organized community of a biofilm [8, 9]. It is already well accepted that biofilm-embedded bacteria do not show growth in traditional cultures and require much higher concentrations of antibiotics for elimination than their planktonic forms. Meanwhile, several reasons for that specific behaviour have been cleared but did not yet find full awareness in the orthopaedic world: Antimicrobial molecules must diffuse through the biofilm matrix in order to inactivate the encased cells. The extracellular polymeric substances present a diffusion barrier for these molecules by influencing either the rate of transport of the molecule to the biofilm interior or the reaction of the antimicrobial material with the matrix material. The delay in penetration allows bacteria in deeper layers to react to the attack by slowing or even ceasing their growth, adopting a dormant state. Biofilm-associated cells grow significantly more slowly than planktonic cells and, as a result, only extremely high concentrations of antimicrobial agents may affect them.

In late or chronic PJI our most obstinate opponents therefore are not the familiar planktonic pathogens but their phenotypically different sessile forms and we need to adjust our strategies to their typical behaviour. When dealing with chronic infections the well-established parameter MIC loses its relevance since it describes the susceptibility only of planktonic pathogens. For the sessile phenotypes, the Minimum Biofilm Eradicating Concentration (MBEC) should be the basis of treatment; however, we still lack detailed information on the MBEC of most pathogens. Radical debridement still is a prerequisite for success; it may remove the predominant amount of bacteria, but even after a perfect debridement some microscopical colonies released from the biofilm during manipulation may remain at site, able to colonize poorly vascularised or dead surfaces. It is already clear that antibiotic levels reached by systemic antibiosis or local therapy with established carriers cannot be effective in eliminating remaining biofilm clusters. Biofilm-embedded pathogens require up to 1000-fold concentrations for elimination [10] and as such usually are inaccessible for systemic antibiotic therapy as well as for antibiotics released from PMMA [11].

Antibiotic-Loaded Cement and Spacers

One-stage revisions so far have been associated with cemented prostheses admixing antibiotics to the cement. Cemented revisions show several disadvantages: the addition of antibiotics to cement reduces its biomechanical properties; inferior long-term results compared to uncemented techniques must be expected [12]. Efficient cementing techniques will result in tight bonding with the underlying bone, making eventual removal time-consuming and possibly associated with further damage to the osseous structures.

For improving functional results after implant removal, antibiotic loaded spacers have become widely used. However, spacers are foreign bodies themselves and in addition show a surface ideal for biofilm attachment. In both applications the released AB-concentrations may be sufficient for eliminating planktonic bacteria but are far below MBEC. Therefore, it is not surprising that spacers explanted at the second stage, even when antibiotic-loaded, show a high rate of contamination: more than one-third [13–15] are covered with biofilms at explantation, and up to 90 % in experimental settings [16], showing that a spacer cannot be considered an effective tool against biofilms. A spacer by definition is unstable, not fully loadable and is associated with a high rate of complications like breakage or dislocation. Spacers are likely to increase defects by erosion due to instability (Fig. 13.1) and need to be removed. The only justification of a spacer is that it can be removed more easily than a fully cemented prosthesis during the second stage. The same advantage is provided by an uncemented prosthesis – should it come to a re-infection – avoiding the disadvantages of instability and fragility and providing a definite solution in case of successful infection control. In addition all disadvantages of cemented revisions may be avoided by using an uncemented implant as a "potentially permanent spacer". Still such implants are at risk of becoming colonized by

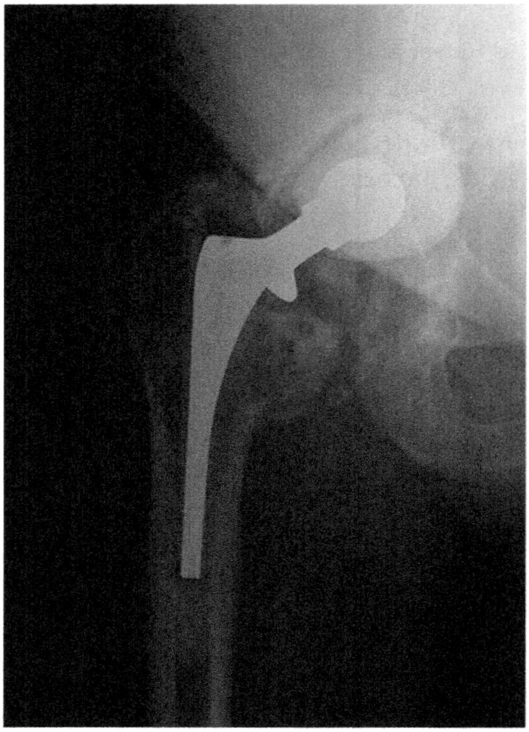

Fig. 13.1 Spacer after infected THR, second attempt: no influence on infection with *S. epidermidis* (methicillin-resistant) and *Mycoplasma hominis* with ongoing fistulation. Massive bone defect at the acetabular site due to erosion by spacer

eventually remaining biofilm fragments. To overcome that risk adequate concentrations of antibiotics should be provided locally. which requires new forms of antibiotic carriers.

Antibiotic Delivery

The idea of increasing AB concentrations at the infection site by delivering antibiotics by a local drug delivery system is not new. Buchholz et al. were the first to mix antibiotics and polymethylmethacrylate (PMMA) for creating a local carrier [17], introducing one-stage revision as a routine protocol in infected THR. His successors in the Endo-Klinik have followed the one-stage approach for over 30 years and in 85 % of infected TJR patients with rates of success between 75 and 90 % [18]. However, most of the antibiotic mixed into the cement does not get released. In fact, between 90 and 95 % of the antibiotic remains trapped in the cement leaving antibiotic-loaded cement ineffective as an anti-biofilm tool.

For reaching MBEC higher concentrations are needed that are only feasible by local application. Few antibiotics have been identified to meet criteria for local application, whereas glycopeptides (vancomycin) and aminoglycosides seem to be the most widely evaluated ones. Both show an inferior tissue penetration compared with other antibiotics, which has been considered a disadvantage in systemic administration. In local application the disadvantage turns into an advantage, since vice versa there is also very slow resorption and penetration from the bone into the vascular system. Both show the least cytotoxic effect of all commonly used antibiotics [19] and are not likely to cause systemic side effects after local application [20]. The carrier should provide for high initial levels to penetrate remaining biofilms rapidly and consequently keep the concentrations above the critical level (which in the case of vancomycin may be estimated to be between 200 and 500 mg/l) for a minimum of 72 h.

The Issue of Bone Defects

After removal of an infected prosthesis bone defects always are present to some extent. Dead space management (DSM) and reconstruction may be favourably performed with cancellous bone that can become incorporated into the original bone structure. Bone taken from the patient's own body has been considered preferable; however, the availability of autologous bone is limited and harvesting leaves another surgical site possibly causing additional morbidity. Allogeneic bone (from a different human donor) has been used to overcome this drawback, leading to comparable results [21]. Grafting defects with allogeneic bone has been used with good success, both with impacted morselized bone and with structural grafts [22, 23]. Defects may be repaired in a biological way in order to restore the original bone stock, creating more advantageous conditions in case of another revision and improving long-term results in case of success. However, fresh allograft bone is dead material, filled with necrotic marrow and fat that may elicit antigenic reaction and inflammation, thus being an ideal substrate for bacterial colonisation. Its use in infected sites, therefore, has been obsolete. Removing fat and marrow should lower the risk of infection markedly but still leaves dead surfaces likely to be a substrate for biofilm formation. Covering the surfaces with adequate antibiotics may create a barrier against bacterial contamination that performs favourably in the second stage of two-stage THR-revisions [24].

Consequences for an Effective Therapy

In clinical practice of treatment of bone infection the only possibility presently available is precise surgical debridement in combination with provision of sufficiently high concentrations of established antibiotics. In order to eradicate microbial pathogens completely basic requirements need to be followed which may be summarized as the "5d" rule:

1. DETECT: Detect habitats of sessile microbes as exactly as possible.
2. DIMINISH: Drastically diminish their number by removing all identified dead material as radically as possible;
3. DISRUPT: Disturb the community live of eventual remaining biofilm colonies by mechanically disrupting their established structures as thoroughly as possible;
4. DEAD SPACE MANAGEMENT: Avoid re-establishment of colonisation grounds by filling dead space with inaccessible material as completely as possible;
5. DECONTAMINATE: Decontaminate the site by eliminating remaining biofilm fragments using antimicrobial substances in local concentrations as high and as consistent as possible.

While items 1–4 have been covered by diligent application of established surgical rules, item 5 so far was not attainable, which lead to the development of new carrier systems.

Antibiotic Bone Compound (ABC)

When loading bone grafts with antibiotics, it turned out that their storage capability for antibiotics exceeds that of PMMA by far. Especially when using highly purified cancellous bone as a carrier local concentrations of up to 20,000 mg/l can be released with vancomycin and up to 13,000 mg/l with tobramycin [25]. A new technique has been developed to reproducibly impregnate bone with antibiotics. Bone of human origin, harvested from either living or deceased donors according to European Union legislation, is highly purified using supercritical carbon dioxide (sCO2) [26]. This kind of treatment removes all lipids and possibly antigenic parts of the bone, leaving the pure matrix intact. Beside that it is a validated method for virus inactivation [27]. The bone is loaded with antibiotics in a proprietary technique [25]. The standardized impregnation technique grants uniform antibiotic content of either 1 g vancomycin per 10 cc or 480 mg tobramycin per 10 cc of cancellous bone, respectively. Vancomycin covers almost all gram-positive germs, tobramycin the majority of the gram-negative spectrum. The storage capacities and pharmacological kinetics of the resulting antibiotic bone compound (ABC, Fig. 13.2) are more advantageous than the ones of antibiotic-loaded cement. Due to the special impregnation technique the antibiotics are eluted with sustained release. Higher local antibiotic concentration and longer-lasting antimicrobial activity are achieved, more favourable than with any other available carrier (Fig. 13.3). Concentrations in the immediate surroundings reach levels more than 1000 times the levels reachable with systemic antibiotic therapy. Release of the antibiotic is completed after several weeks and therefore is not likely to create resistances. With this kind of impregnation the whole amount of loaded antibiotic is available for antimicrobial activity and the activity remains beyond the MBEC of relevant pathogens for weeks. These capacities make them attractive as a tool for local therapy and allow using uncemented implants simultaneously.

Method

Our protocol shows distinct differences from previous algorithms [28]; the changes in indications, preoperative planning and technical execution are mainly resulting from the increasing knowledge on the behaviour of biofilm-embedded bacteria. Biological restoration of bone stock has been the second aim of developing a new approach. Resistant bacteria like MRSA, draining sinuses, duration of infection or other features indicated in the known protocols have no influence in the choice of our method. There are very few contraindications against a one-stage procedure in the described technique: patients in bad general condition due to the infection (septicaemia) primarily are salvaged by removing the implants and radical debridement; re-implantation is only performed after the patient has recovered sufficiently (no defined time frame).

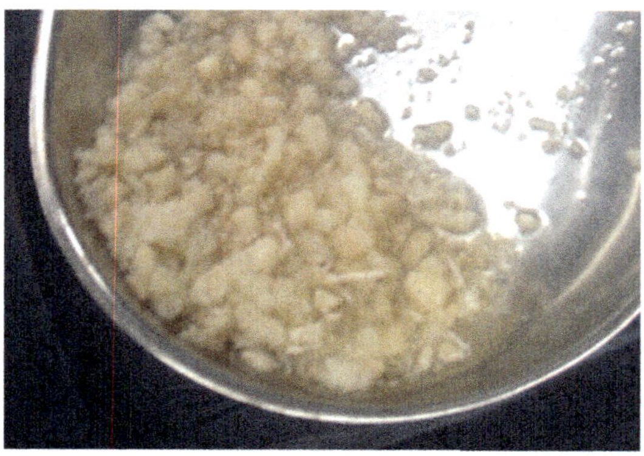

Fig. 13.2 Antibiotic-impregnated cancellous bone allograft (ABC), morsellized, hydrated

Surgical Technique

Diagnosis and evaluation of the given conditions follows the recommendations as outlined in Chap. 7. We always use the same access as has been used at the foregoing surgery. Fistulas on the way are excised and followed down to the implant. All infected tissue found during preparation is removed immediately. The access is enlarged stepwise until a sufficient exposition of the joint is provided. Loose implants are removed, and firmly attached ones are undermined using thin chisels, whereas care is taken to save own bone as much as possible. Remaining cement, all granulation and infected tissue adherent to bone are removed carefully together with radical synovectomy. Debridement is followed by extensive cleaning using pulsed pressurized saline for lavage.

As soon as the site is considered to be clean the wound is closed provisionally. Instruments and drapings are removed, and the team is

AB loaded bone graft versus
AB loaded cement

AB carrier (vancomycin)	Purified bone graft	PMMA cement
Storage capacity/ 10 cc	1 g	0.1g
Availability	> 90 %	< 10%
Release 1 day	10,000–20,000 mg/	40–400 mg/l
Release 6 day	60–130 mg/l	subinhibitory traces
Release 100 day	0	subinhibitory traces

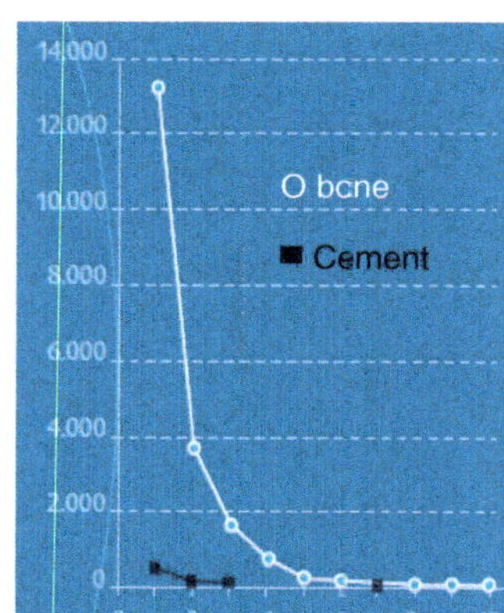

Fig. 13.3 Comparison between kinetics. Initial local concentrations of antibiotic-loaded bone graft (ABC) exceed the ones of antibiotic-loaded cement by more than 1000-fold

changing gowns and gloves. After new washing and draping the procedure commences with new instruments. The extent of bone deficiencies is examined and preparation of the surfaces is performed as in usual revision THR, saving the original bone as much as possible. On the acetabular side hemispherical reamers are used for creating a sufficient contact with own bone at the rim. Remaining osseous cavities and deficiencies are filled with morsellized antibiotic-impregnated bone (Fig. 13.4a) using a modified impaction grafting technique [29]. Final smoothing of the surface is performed with reverse reaming. In cases with minor osseous defects (Paprosky I [30]) a standard uncemented hemispherical cup is implanted, eventually additionally stabilized with one or two screws. When there are major defects (Paprosky II–III) we now use revision cups of modular design with fins and a caudal hook. The design allows reconstruction of both medial (see Fig. 13.4) and lateral (Fig. 13.5) defects and also perform favourably in combination with structural allografts, should they become necessary (Fig. 13.6). Care is taken that the implant surface is as rough as possible, providing high

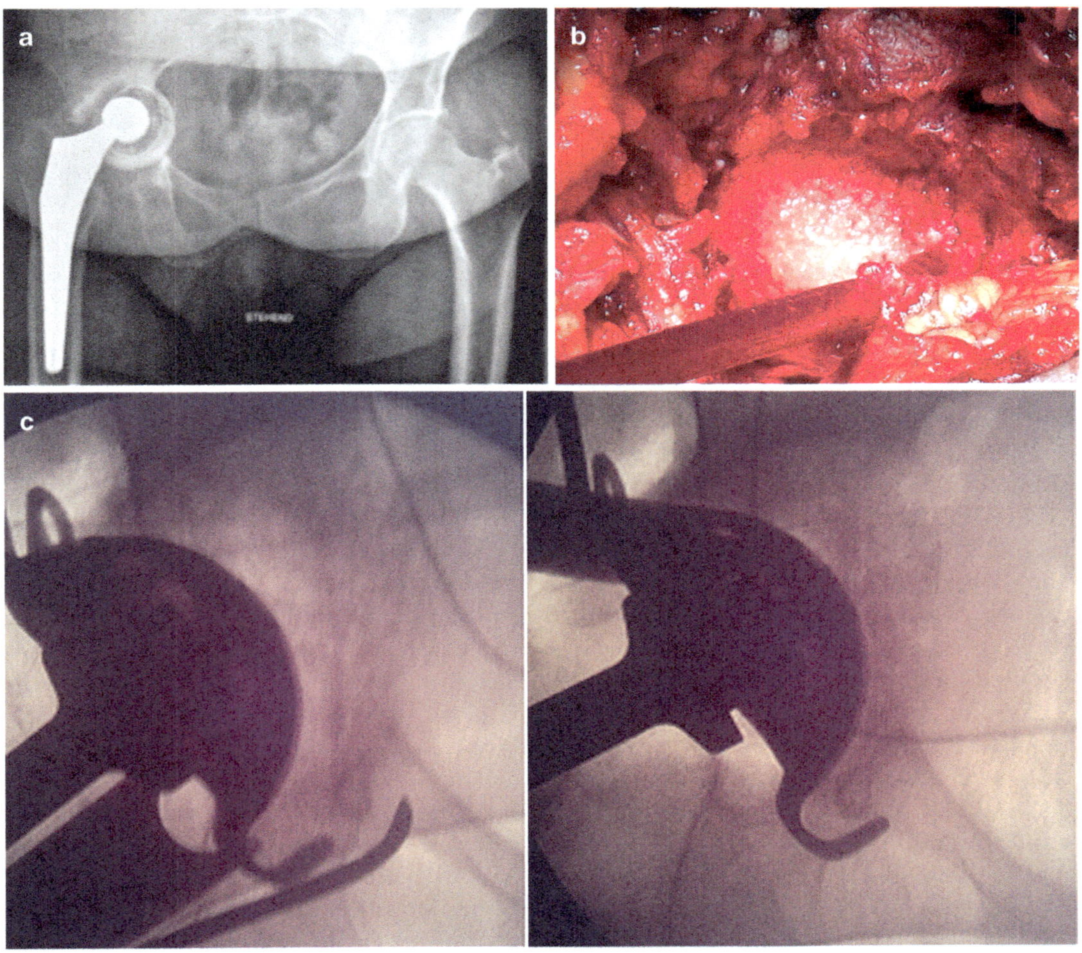

Fig. 13.4 (**a**) Female, 64 years old, chronic infection with *S. aureus* (MSSA), *S. epidermidis* (MRSE) and enterocci. Medial acetabular defect. (**b**) Impaction grafting. (**c**) Intraoperative fluoroscopy. (**d**) Radiograph postoperatively. (**e**) Radiograph 2 years postoperatively

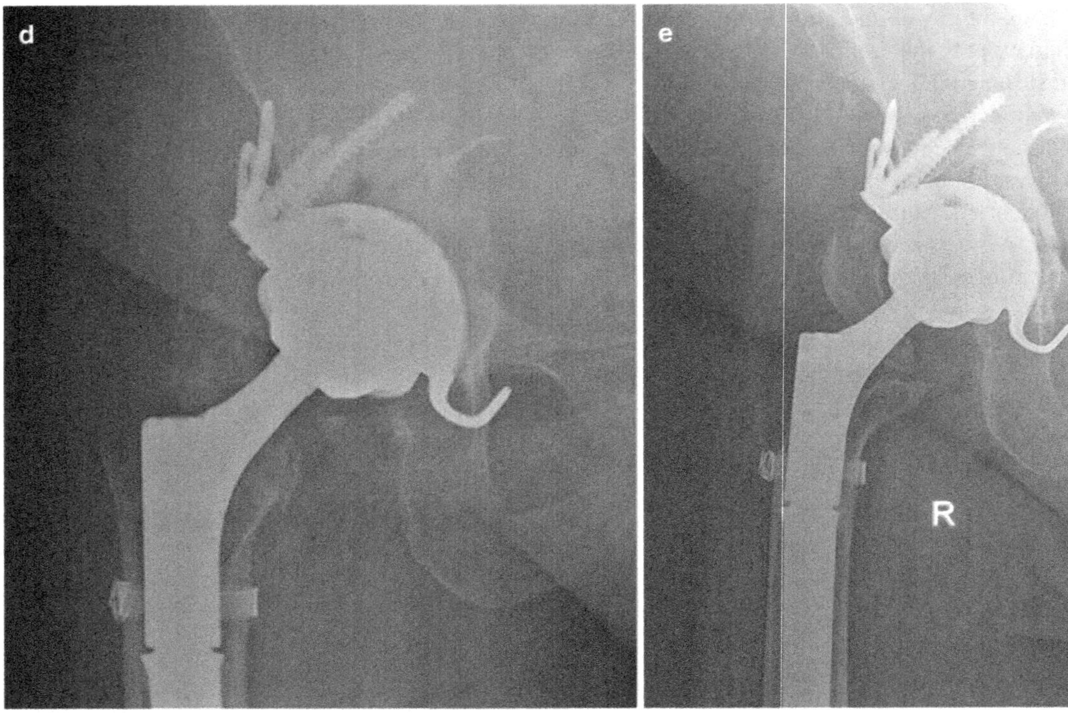

Fig. 13.4 (continued)

friction with own bone. The correct centre of rotation should always be restored. On the femoral side we prefer using stems with rectangular diameter as long as the diaphysis is intact (Paprosky I–II). The design offers the advantage of firm anchorage in original bone at the medial and lateral side while being covered with antibiotic-releasing allograft at the less loaded anterior and posterior sides (see Fig. 13.6). In type III defects modular stems with longitudinal ribs are used for distal fixation (see Figs. 13.4 and 13.5). The medullary cavity is prepared with rasps of adequate size for good contact with cortical bone. ABC then is inserted stepwise and dispersed by re-rasping using the respective oscillating rasp or the reamer of last size by reverse reaming, respectively (see Fig. 13.4a.). After completion of the reconstruction the original prosthesis is inserted. The construction shows primary stability being predominantly anchored in own healthy bone, enabling immediate partial weight bearing. After final rinsing the wound is closed and drained as in conventional arthroplasty. The method is easy to perform in cases with only cavitary osseous defects, in cases with major segmental defects special techniques need to be applied, occasionally requiring structural allografts (see Fig. 13.6).

Postoperative Care

Systemic antibiotic therapy follows the results of preoperative cultures; if no pathogen could be identified, a second-generation cephalosporine is administered as a routine. The choice of antibiotics is adjusted to the result of intraoperative cultures as soon as they are available. Intravenous antibiotics are discontinued after complete wound healing and normalization of CRP, which usually is the case after 12 days. Drains are left in place usually for 3 days. All patients are mobilized from the first postoperative day with partial weight bearing using two crutches. Intensive physiotherapy is performed consequently. On the twelfth postoperative day

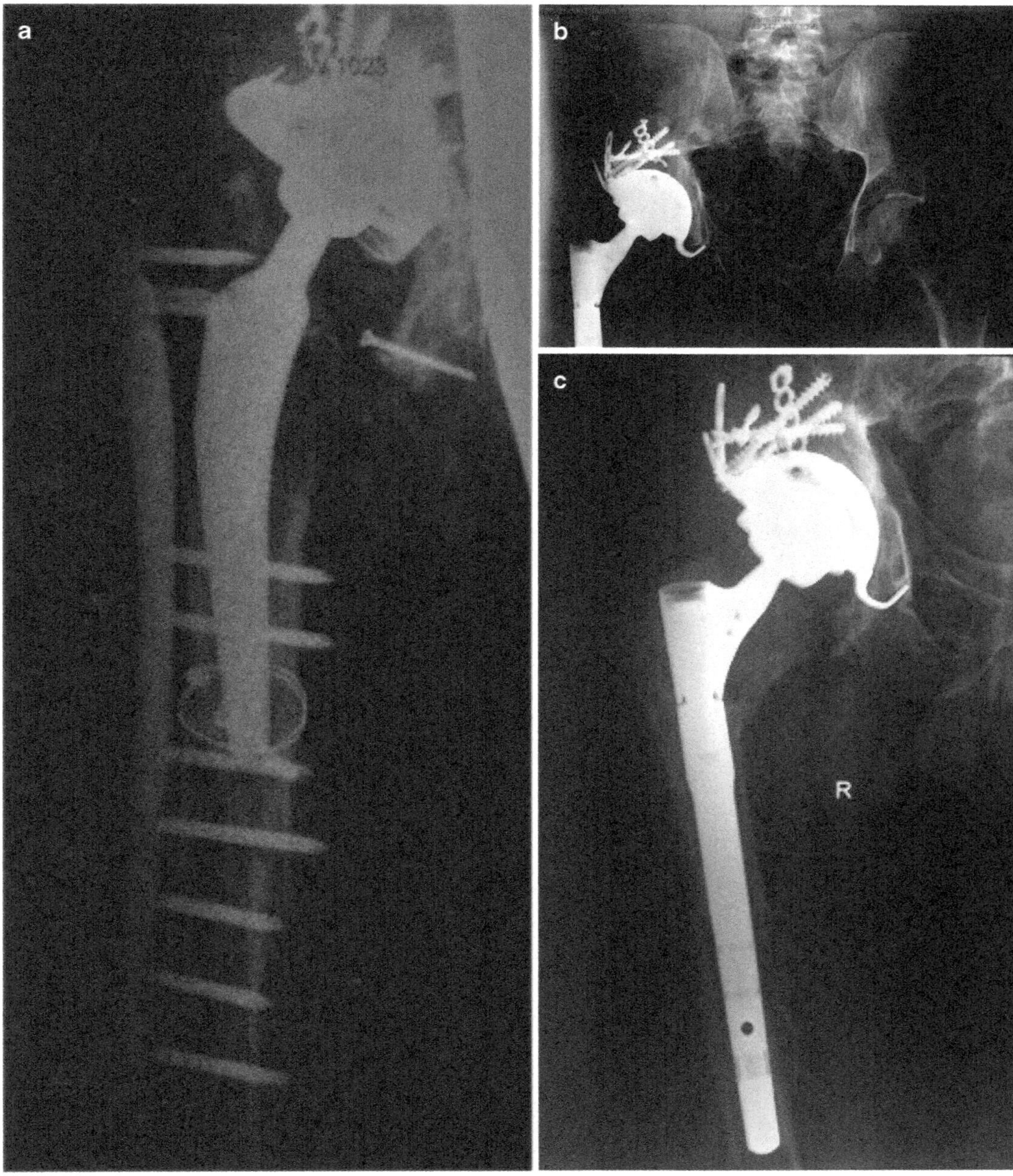

Fig. 13.5 (**a**) Male, 43 years old, polytrauma, infection, five revisions, MSSE+MRSE, supero-lateral defect, pseudarthrosis femur. (**b**) Radiograph postoperatively. Restoration of center of rotation. Modular stem passing fracture site. (**c**) Two years postoperatively

stitches are removed and the patient is dismissed to home care, continuing with active exercises and appropriate oral antibiotic medication. Six weeks after surgery the patient is followed clinically and radiologically; when there are no conspicuous features and no changes of implant position, full weight bearing is encouraged and antibiotics are discontinued. Further follow-ups are scheduled 3 months, 6 months and 12 months postoperatively.

Complications and Outcome

The results of our first series were published in 2008 [31]. In brief there were 37 one-stage revisions, of which three required further revision because of recurrent infection. Two of the recurrences could be revised successfully using the same technique again, and one was converted to a resection arthroplasty. No more infections or loosenings have been observed since then. Meanwhile 54 hips additionally were followed for a minimum of 2 years. Three of these patients have died of causes not related to infection. In those there were six recurrences of infection, two of them associated with loosening of the cup and one with loosening of the stem. In two otherwise bland hips loosening of the cup was found, one hip showed recurrent dislocation and one patient suffered a periprosthetic fracture. All of them were revised successfully with no sign of infection being present at the time of re-revision. There has been no case of loosening of the femoral component so far.

It is remarkable that in our series we found only one case of recurrence with gram-positives, which are the most prevalent pathogens in orthopaedic surgery. There was one persisting infection with MRSE and no case of recurrence with MRSA. Four out of six recurrences were caused by gram-negatives (2× Pseudomonas, Klebsiella, Enterobacter) and one by Mycoplasma (see Fig. 13.6).

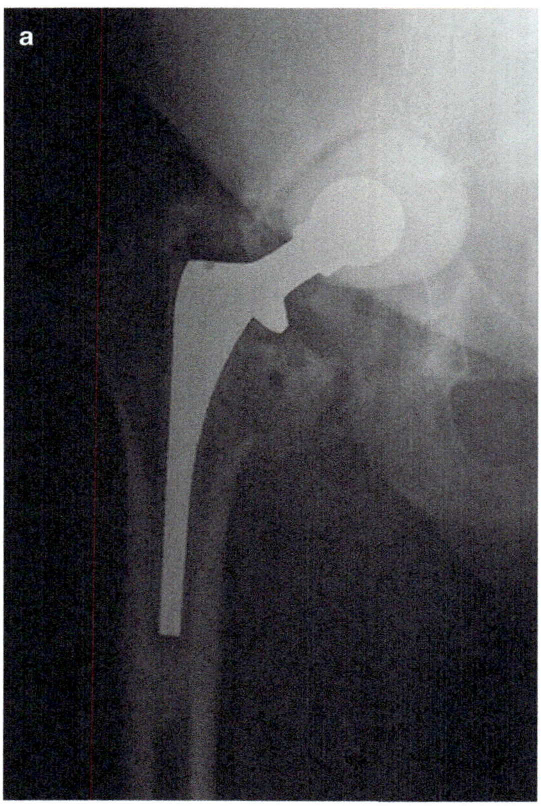

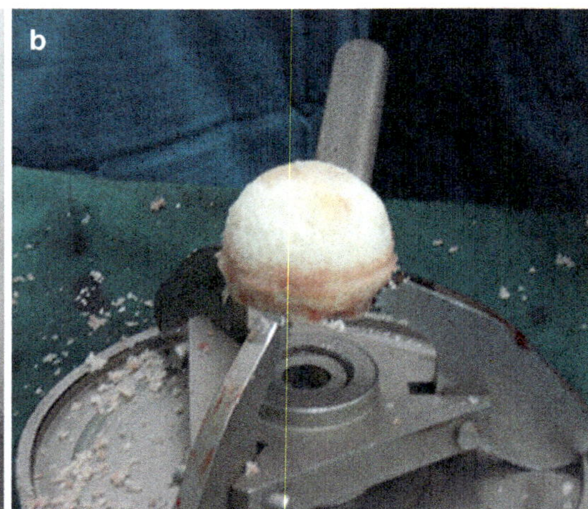

Fig. 13.6 (**a**) Same patient as Fig. 13.1. Acetabular defect involved complete anterior column and medial floor. Impaction not feasible. Good femoral bone stock. (**b**) Structural allograft, thoroughly purified by supercrit CO2, impregnated with 6 g vancomycin ("home made"). (**c**) Radiograph postoperatively. Acetabular reconstruction with shaped structural allograft + morsellised chips + modular cup. Femoral side supplied with standard stem, fixed in original bone medially and laterally. (**d**) Radiograph 1 year postoperatively. Moderate condensation of acetabular reconstruction with cranial migration but stable fixation of cup and stem. No growth of bacteria but persistent infection with *Mycoplasma hominis*. Draining sinus. Re-revision pending

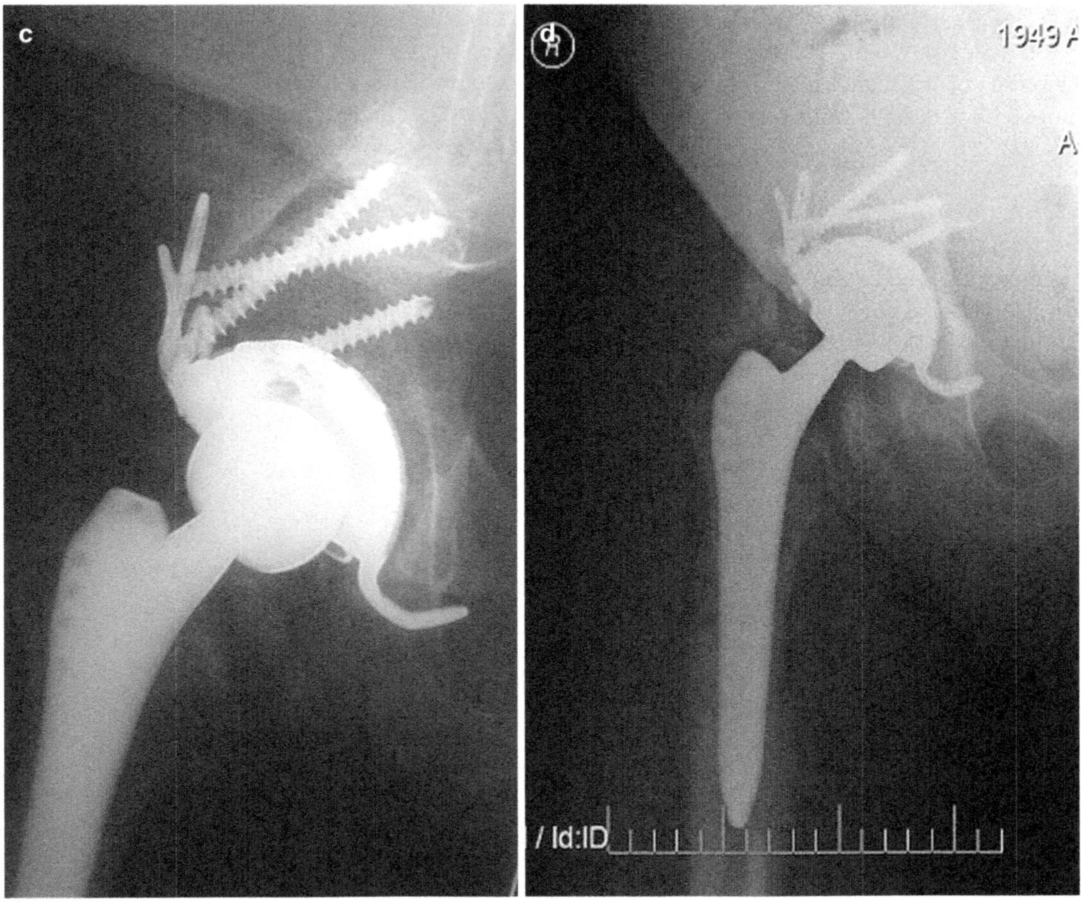

Fig. 13.6 (continued)

Developments and Future Aspects

Cleaning and impregnation of the allograft bone in the beginning has been performed inside the hospital, using established techniques of bone banking like defatting with ether and alcohol. Since 2008 the bone has been cleaned with sCO2, granting improved purification of the matrix. Impregnation with vancomycin or tobramycin, respectively, since 2010 is performed according to standardized pharmaceutical-like procedures (GMP). Errors and variability in purity or antibiotic content therefore can be excluded.

We always try to get cultures from aspirated fluid or tissue from the depth of a draining sinus before revision. In the beginnings of our technique we chose the locally applied antibiotics according to the results of the preoperative cultures. Today preoperative cultures only direct the choice of concomitant systemic antibiotic therapy. Especially in cases with previous infect related surgery we now consider infections as being multimicrobial, irrespective of culture results, and routinely use a combination of vancomycin and tobramycin locally. Sonication of explanted endoprostheses [32] mostly confirms our assumption. We take care of using 90 cc of ABC as a minimum in every septic revision. There are still not enough cases to draw a final conclusion but in our protocol there seems to be another change of paradigm regarding "difficult to treat pathogens": biofilms of gram-negatives, mycoplasma and fungi (in knees and infected osteosynthesis) seem to be more persistent than biofilms of the feared multiply-resistant staphylococci and deserve further attention.

Summary

Antibiotic-loaded bone graft seems to provide sufficient local antibiosis for protection against colonisation of uncemented implants, the eluted amounts of antibiotics are likely to eliminate even biofilm remnants. Dead space management is more complete and defects may be reconstructed efficiently. Incorporation of allograft appears as after grafting with unimpregnated bone grafts. Uncemented implants may be considered as a "potentially permanent spacer" that may be removed easily in case of failure and kept in place in case of success (Fig. 13.7). One-stage revision THR using ABC together with uncemented implants should be at least as

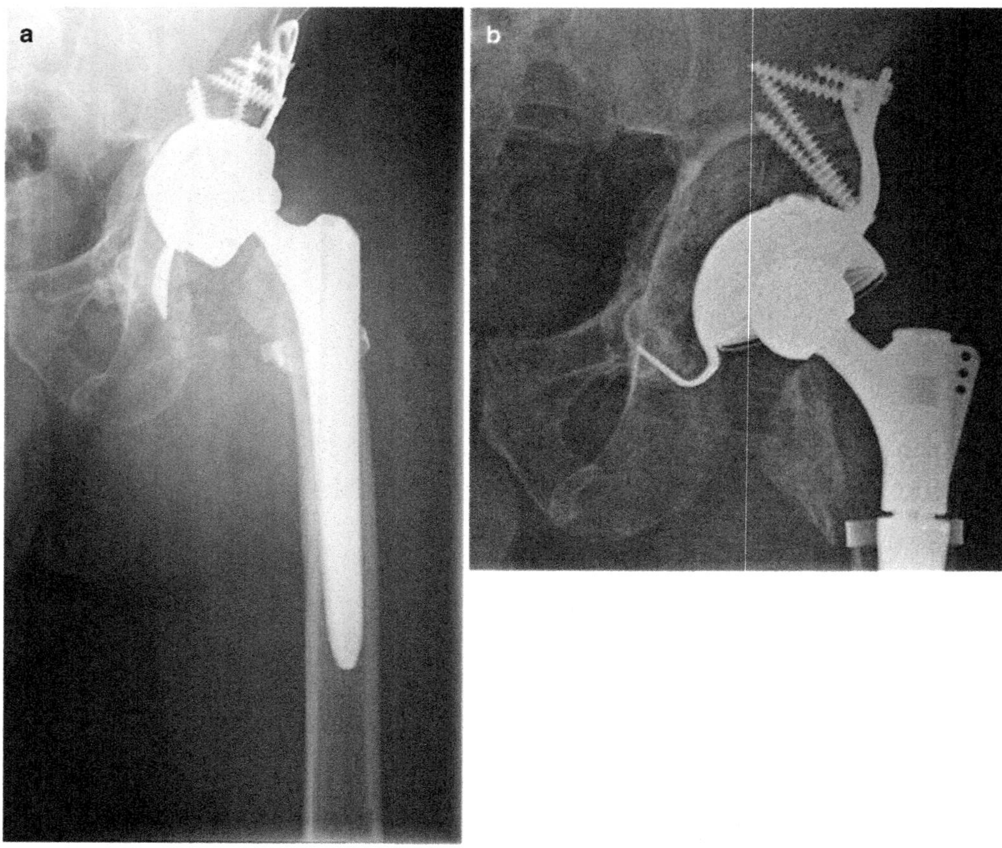

Fig. 13.7 (**a**) Male, 53 years: 1991 pelvic fracture, osteosynthesis, infection, two revisions, implant removal, suction-irrigation-drainage, necrosis femoral head. 1993 THR, 1994 draining sinus, **MRSA**. 1994–2013 13 revisions (2× two-stage exchange). 2013 massive acetabular defect, draining sinus, MRSA. (**b**) 2013: complete removal of implants, radical debridement. Reconstruction of acetabular defects + restoration of centre of rotation with 110 cc ABC (=11 g vancomycin locally) + impaction + modular cup. Intraoperative femoral fracture during removal of well fixed stem, exchange to modular stem. Two weeks teicoplanin + 4 weeks fucidic acid. Preoperatively the patient was informed that surgery is aiming at elimination of infection with implants to be considered as "potentielly permanent spacer". Hospital stay 2 weeks, full weight bearing after 6 weeks. (**c**) Three months postoperatively: Breakage of the caudal hook with partial resorption of the graft and dislocation of the cup. No sign of infection. (**d**) Re-revision 6 months postoperatively: remaining graft completely incorporated. Exchange of cup, minor grafting, well incorporated stem left in place. Cultures + sonication no bacterial growth. No sign of infection. Hospital stay 7 days, full weight bearing after 6 weeks

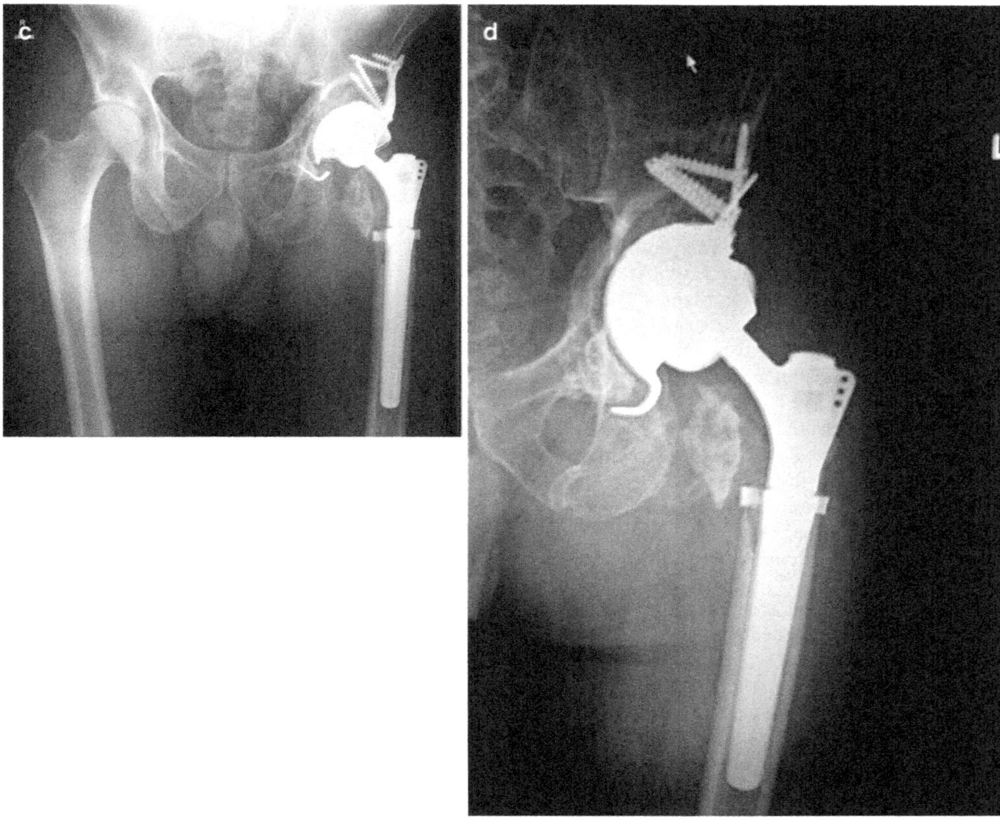

Fig. 13.7 (continued)

comparably safe as multiple-stage procedures, avoiding second-stage-revisions in the majority of cases and taking advantage of the obvious benefits for patients and economy. Although the results of the new protocol seem very promising we never can have certainty of having cured infection. Assuming that recurrence may occur within an unknown period of time it should be the responsibility of the surgeon to provide for a treatment reducing the burden for the patient to an absolute minimum. In this sense it should be agreed that treatments should be kept as short and as pain-free as possible. Long hospital stays should be avoided the same as treatments associated with prolonged periods of pain and/or reduced mobility. The described protocol seems to be in conformance with these principles. Our series indicates an overall rate of infection control of more than 90 % with one operation [31, 33], without any adverse side effects. These numbers are comparable with published data, both regarding traditional one stage and multiple stage procedures, but avoiding the indicated disadvantages of established approaches. The method is refined continuously and hope of further improving the results seems to be justified.

References

1. Kuiper JW, Vos SJ, Saouti R, Vergroesen DA, Graat HC, Debets-Ossenkopp YJ, et al. Prosthetic joint-associated infections treated with DAIR (debridement, antibiotics, irrigation, and retention): analysis of risk factors and local antibiotic carriers in 91 patients. Acta Orthop. 2013;84(4):380–6.
2. Beswick AD, Elvers KT, Smith AJ, Gooberman-Hill R, Lovering A, Blom AW. What is the evidence base to guide surgical treatment of infected hip prostheses? systematic review of longitudinal studies in unselected patients. BMC Med. 2012;10:18 [Meta-Analysis Research Support, Non-U.S. Gov't Review].

3. McKenna PB, O'Shea K, Masterson EL. Two-stage revision of infected hip arthroplasty using a shortened post-operative course of antibiotics. Arch Orthop Trauma Surg. 2008;129:489–94.
4. Puhto AP, Puhto T, Syrjala H. Short-course antibiotics for prosthetic joint infections treated with prosthesis retention. Clin Microbiol Infect. 2012;18(11): 1143–8.
5. Bozic KJ, Ries MD. The impact of infection after total hip arthroplasty on hospital and surgeon resource utilization. J Bone Joint Surg Am. 2005;87(8):1746–51.
6. Wolf CF, Gu NY, Doctor JN, Manner PA, Leopold SS. Comparison of one and two-stage revision of total hip arthroplasty complicated by infection: a Markov expected-utility decision analysis. J Bone Joint Surg Am. 2011;93(7):631–9.
7. Costerton JW, Stewart PS, Greenberg EP. Bacterial biofilms: a common cause of persistent infections. Science. 1999;284(5418):1318–22.
8. Gristina AG, Costerton JW. Bacterial adherence to biomaterials and tissue. The significance of its role in clinical sepsis. J Bone Joint Surg Am. 1985; 67(2):264–73.
9. Costerton JW. Biofilm theory can guide the treatment of device-related orthopaedic infections. Clin Orthop Relat Res. 2005;437:7–11.
10. Saginur R, Stdenis M, Ferris W, Aaron SD, Chan F, Lee C, et al. Multiple combination bactericidal testing of staphylococcal biofilms from implant-associated infections. Antimicrob Agents Chemother. 2006; 50(1):55–61.
11. van de Belt H, Neut D, Schenk W, van Horn JR, van der Mei HC, Busscher HJ. Infection of orthopedic implants and the use of antibiotic-loaded bone cements. A review. Acta Orthop Scand. 2001; 72(6):557–71.
12. Lie SA, Havelin LI, Furnes ON, Engesaeter LB, Vollset SE. Failure rates for 4762 revision total hip arthroplasties in the Norwegian Arthroplasty Register. J Bone Joint Surg Br. 2004;86(4):504–9.
13. Cabo J, Euba G, Saborido A, Gonzalez-Panisello M, Dominguez MA, Agullo JL, et al. Clinical outcome and microbiological findings using antibiotic-loaded spacers in two-stage revision of prosthetic joint infections. J Infect. 2011;67:82–4.
14. Nelson CL, Jones RB, Wingert NC, Foltzer M, Bowen TR. Sonication of antibiotic spacers predicts failure during two-stage revision for prosthetic knee and hip infections. Clin Orthop Relat Res. 2014;472(7): 2208–14.
15. Sorli L, Puig L, Torres-Claramunt R, Gonzalez A, Alier A, Knobel H, et al. The relationship between microbiology results in the second of a two-stage exchange procedure using cement spacers and the outcome after revision total joint replacement for infection: the use of sonication to aid bacteriological analysis. J Bone Joint Surg Br. 2012;94(2):249–53.
16. Neut D, van De Belt H, Stokroos I, van Horn JR, van Der Mei HC, Busscher HJ. Biomaterial-associated infection of gentamicin-loaded PMMA beads in orthopaedic revision surgery. J Antimicrob Chemother. 2001;47(6):885–91.
17. Buchholz HW, Engelbrecht H. Depot effects of various antibiotics mixed with Palacos resins. Chirurg. 1970;41(11):511–5.
18. Gehrke T, Zahar A, Kendoff D. One-stage exchange: it all began here. Bone Joint J. 2013;95-B(11 Supple A):77–83.
19. Edin ML, Miclau T, Lester GE, Lindsey RW, Dahners LE. Effect of cefazolin and vancomycin on osteoblasts in vitro. Clin Orthop Relat Res. 1996;333: 245–51.
20. Buttaro MA, Gimenez MI, Greco G, Barcan L, Piccaluga F. High active local levels of vancomycin without nephrotoxicity released from impacted bone allografts in 20 revision hip arthroplasties. Acta Orthop. 2005;76(3):336–40.
21. Hazlett JW. The use of cancellous bone grafts in the treatment of subacute and chronic osteomyelitis. J Bone Joint Surg Br. 1954;36-B(4):584–90.
22. Ammon P, Stockley I. Allograft bone in two-stage revision of the hip for infection. Is it safe? J Bone Joint Surg Br. 2004;86(7):962–5.
23. Hsieh PH, Shih CH, Chang YH, Lee MS, Yang WE, Shih HN. Treatment of deep infection of the hip associated with massive bone loss: two-stage revision with an antibiotic-loaded interim cement prosthesis followed by reconstruction with allograft. J Bone Joint Surg Br. 2005;87-B(6):770–5.
24. Buttaro MA, Pusso R, Piccaluga F. Vancomycin-supplemented impacted bone allografts in infected hip arthroplasty. Two-stage revision results. J Bone Joint Surg Br. 2005;87(3):314–9.
25. Winkler H, Janata O, Berger C, Wein W, Georgopoulos A. In vitro release of vancomycin and tobramycin from impregnated human and bovine bone grafts. J Antimicrob Chemother. 2000;46(3):423–8.
26. Fages J, Marty A, Delga C, Condoret JS, Combes D, Frayssinet P. Use of supercritical CO2 for bone delipidation. Biomaterials. 1994;15(9):650–6.
27. Fages J, Poirier B, Barbier Y, Frayssinet P, Joffret ML, Majewski W, et al. Viral inactivation of human bone tissue using supercritical fluid extraction. ASAIO J. 1998;44(4):289–93.
28. Zimmerli W, Trampuz A, Ochsner PE. Prosthetic-joint infections. N Engl J Med. 2004;351(16): 1645–54.
29. Ibrahim MS, Raja S, Haddad FS. Acetabular impaction bone grafting in total hip replacement. Bone Joint J. 2013;95-B(11 Suppl A):98–102 [Review].
30. Paprosky WG, Perona PG, Lawrence JM. Acetabular defect classification and surgical reconstruction in revision arthroplasty. A 6-year follow-up evaluation. J Arthroplasty. 1994;9(1):33–44.

31. Winkler H, Stoiber A, Kaudela K, Winter F, Menschik F. One stage uncemented revision of infected total hip replacement using cancellous allograft bone impregnated with antibiotics. J Bone Joint Surg Br. 2008;90-B(12):1580–4.
32. Trampuz A, Piper KE, Jacobson MJ, Hanssen AD, Unni KK, Osmon DR, et al. Sonication of removed hip and knee prostheses for diagnosis of infection. N Engl J Med. 2007;357(7):654–63.
33. Winkler H, Kaudela K, Stoiber A, Menschik F. Bone grafts impregnated with antibiotics as a tool for treating infected implants in orthopedic surgery – one stage revision results. Cell Tissue Bank. 2006;7(4):319–23.

Late Infections: Two-Stage Traditional Solution

14

Tim Harrison and Ian Stockley

Abstract

Two-stage revision surgery for infection reliably produces good results and is the only safe method for treating chronic infection where the infecting organism or it's sensitivities are not fully known. The areas of controversy in two stage surgery include the duration between stages, whether to use a spacer or cement beads and the use of systemic antibiotics. This chapter presents our approach to two stage revision surgery which focuses on radical surgical debridement and the delivery of high concentrations of local antibiotics.

Keywords

Two-stage • Revision • Infection • Hip • Antibiotic cement • Antibiotics

Introduction

The incidence of periprosthetic joint infection (PJI) varies from hospital to hospital but is typically reported as 1–2 % following primary arthroplasty and significantly higher following revision surgery [1–3, 8, 13]. It is a devastating complication for both patient and surgeon in terms of associated morbidity, effect on quality of life and cost to both the patient and institution [4–6]. Decisions on management must take into account the individual patient, duration of infection, the infecting organism and the surgeons' experience. Although strategies such as debridement and implant retention, single-stage revision and long-term antibiotic suppression can be utilised in specific circumstances, only two-stage revision surgery can reliably produce good results in the majority of cases. Despite this, the success of a two-stage approach still requires expertise in diagnosis, surgical planning, microbiological input and surgical technique. We believe the key to successful eradication of infection is radical debridement of all infected tissue and foreign material along with the local delivery of high

T. Harrison, FRCS (Tr & Orth), MBBS, BSc
I. Stockley, MB, ChB, MD, FRCS (✉)
Orthopaedic Department, Northern General Hospital, Sheffield, UK
e-mail: ian.stockley@sth.nhs.uk

D. Kendoff et al. (eds.), *Periprosthetic Joint Infections: Changing Paradigms*,
DOI 10.1007/978-3-319-30091-7_14

dose targeted antibiotics [7]. In this chapter we will focus on our experience and strategy in the two stage management of prosthetic joint infection.

Indications

Although a two-stage solution can be utilised in the majority of situations, we will consider debridement and implant retention for acute infections (less than 2–4 weeks) and single-stage revisions in patients where the infecting organism and its sensitivities are known. For all other cases, if the patient is deemed safe from an anaesthetic perspective and willing to undergo surgery, a two-stage solution is indicated.

Patient Assessment

PJI is often under-diagnosed and therefore one should have a high index of suspicion in all cases of unexplained pain or early implant failure following hip arthroplasty surgery as the majority of patients do well [8]. The assessment of a patient with a suspected PJI starts with a thorough history of all their previous surgery including their recovery and any complications in the postoperative period, irrespective of how minor they may seem. Where possible it is ideal to have access to the previous clinic and operation notes. Examination should focus on the site and health of previous scars, sinuses and surrounding soft tissues (Fig. 14.1).

It is important at this stage, to gauge the patients understanding and expectations of what the diagnosis and subsequent management of PJI entails. Beyond the eradication of infection, the successful treatment of a patient with PJI requires the patient to be well informed with regards to the surgery, timing, length of treatment and the likely outcome including the implications of failure to eradicate the infection.

In addition to plain radiological imaging (and comparison with previous films) and blood markers (CRP, ESR and FBC), patients should undergo aseptic aspiration of the joint either in the operating theatre or by designated musculoskeletal radiologists according to an agreed protocol in the radiology department [9]. We have previously shown that the results for diagnosing infection by aspiration are no different if the investigation is performed in the operating theatre or in the radiology department [10]. In our institution a musculoskeletal radiologist, under image guidance, aspirates the majority of patients; a stab incision and small retractor are used to ensure that the needle does not pass through the skin, risking potential contamination. Samples are incubated in broth for 14 days and reviewed by a microbiologist with a specialist interest in PJI.

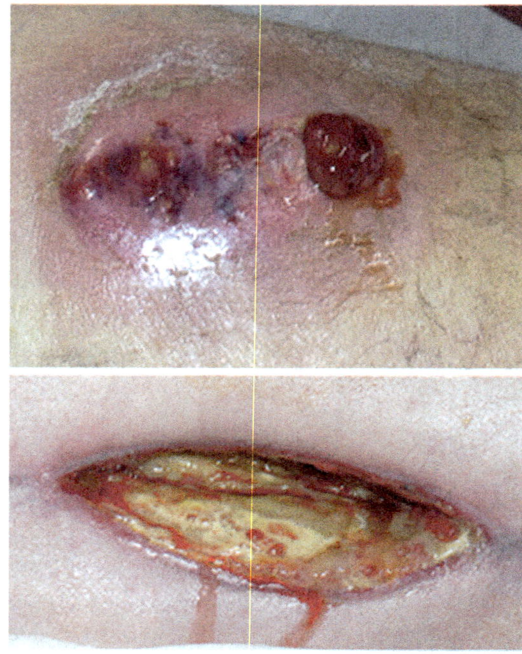

Fig. 14.1 Sinuses and scars with underlying infected implants

Planning

Infected revision cases often end up being more complex than initially expected, so thorough planning is essential to avoid unnecessary complications and ensure success.

All patients require an anaesthetic assessment and should have blood cross-matched, as the use of cell salvage is contraindicated in infected cases. Ideally, they should be booked onto an elective list with a plan to spend the first postoperative night in the critical care department. A significant proportion will require inotropic support in the immediate postoperative period (partly due to the septic load from debrided infected tissue), and all need close monitoring of their fluid balance to ensure haemodynamic stability.

Imaging should consist of a minimum of an AP pelvis along with an AP and lateral of the affected hip to include the tip of the stem and cement if present. Judet views and CT scans can be used to gauge bone stock and pelvic continuity, but this tends to be more accurately assessed 'real time' intraoperatively during the first-stage debridement. This often allows for a much more accurate planning in readiness for the second-stage reconstruction.

Knowledge of the specific implants currently in situ is essential to ensure that all the necessary kit is available in order to make extraction as easy as possible during the first stage. It is important to try and avoid iatrogenic bone damage and loss.

All cases should ideally be discussed preoperatively at a multi-disciplinary meeting that includes surgical colleagues, microbiologists and senior theatre staff. This provides a forum to discuss and evaluate the surgical plan, ensure the necessary equipment will be available on the day and review the joint aspirate microbiology. The microbiologist should be able to advise on the appropriate use, dose and duration of antibiotics and or antifungals for prophylaxis, local and or systemic therapeutic therapy. We believe high-dose local antibiotic therapy is much more beneficial than systemic therapy in the two-stage regime [7, 15, 28]. The use of additional antibiotics that may be added to the bone cement need to be discussed at this stage, as dosage is of paramount importance. In our experience, the requirement for plastic surgical input has been rare but in some cases, especially those who have undergone multiple previous operations and have numerous scars or tethered skin, it maybe required.

First-Stage Procedure

The first-stage procedure is the key to successful eradication of infection in a two-stage strategy. The aim is to radically debride all the infected or nonviable tissue, thereby removing all macroscopic infection, then ensure high-level local delivery of antibiotic via a depot, whether that be cement beads or a cement spacer to eradicate any residual bacteria.

Ideally, the case should be undertaken on a planned, elective list, with the expectation that the patient will go to the critical care department for close monitoring post operatively. Occasionally, when a patient is critically ill with sepsis, a first-stage procedure has to be performed as a life-saving procedure as a matter of urgency.

Systemic antibiotics should be withheld until deep tissue samples have been taken, even if a previous aspirate has had a positive growth.

When the scar of a previous incision is used, we prefer to excise the scar as well as any sinus tracts (Fig. 14.2). We also extend the incision, usually distally, to formally identify normal anatomy and tissue planes, as we find this helps the dissection through the scarred and infected region. It also helps with subsequent closure of the wound. Upon entering the joint, a minimum of five deep tissue specimens should be taken, all with clean instruments for microbiological assessment. The samples should be taken before there is any disturbance of cement in case any elution of antibiotic from the cement affects bacterial viability [11]. After this, systemic prophylactic antibiotics can be given (in our practice this is currently flucloxacillin and gentamicin unless advised differently by the microbiologist).

There are many different surgical techniques available for removing the existing prostheses. It is essential to remove all foreign material, be that a broken screw, cement restrictor, wire and cement if present. If it is possible to remove the femoral cement from the 'top' using osteotomes, drills and taps, thereby leaving an intact femur, this is desirable but should not be done at the expense of an incomplete debridement of the cement. We do not use ultrasonic cement removal tools to aid removal of well-fixed cement as we

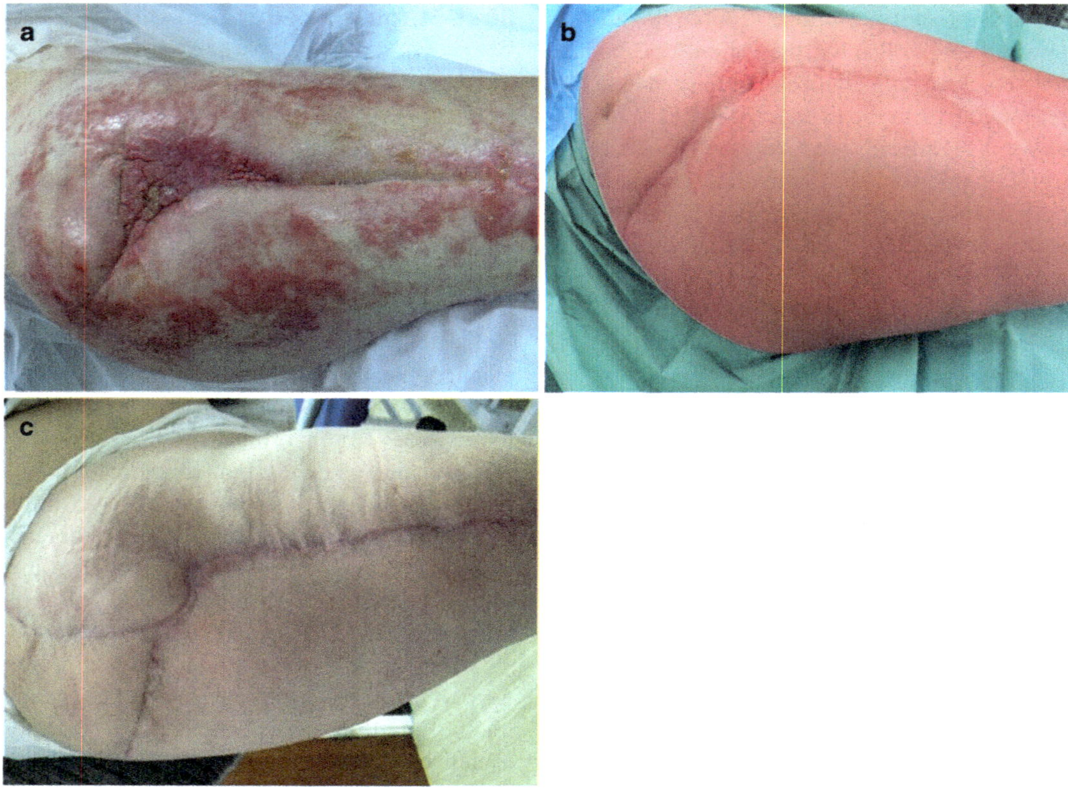

Fig. 14.2 The progress of the patient's skin and scar from (**a**) pre-first stage, (**b**) pre-second stage to (**c**) post-second stage

have concerns that some residual cement is often missed, especially distally, and this is only fully appreciated on the postoperative film. We have a low threshold for the use of an extended trochanteric osteotomy to access the canal and ensure complete removal of all the cement. If there is significant involvement of the proximal femur by infection and the bone appears dead and avascular, then this should also be resected. No compromise should be made if the tissues do not appear healthy. In this situation a trochanteric slide can be performed, prior to resection to maintain the integrity of the abductor/vastus lateralis complex.

On the acetabular side preservation of healthy bone is important for later reconstruction; we use an explant device for uncemented cups and for well-fixed cemented components we ream out the polyethylene cup and use cement chisels to remove the underlying cement.

Once the implants have been removed and dead bone resected or reamed to expose healthy bleeding bone, attention is again turned to the soft tissues. All nonviable or infected tissue should be removed exposing healthy, bleeding compliant tissue (Fig. 14.3).

Throughout the procedure and especially after debridement, all tissues are continually irrigated with aqueous chlorhexidine 0.05 % both to remove debris and for its antiseptic properties.

Once debridement is complete, a final assessment of available bone stock and soft tissue integrity should be made to help plan the subsequent second stage reconstruction.

Various options are available for the delivery of antibiotic from cement including beads, static spacers and articulating spacers. Antibiotic-loaded methylmethacrylate has been shown to give higher concentrations of antibiotics locally than that what can be achieved by intravenous

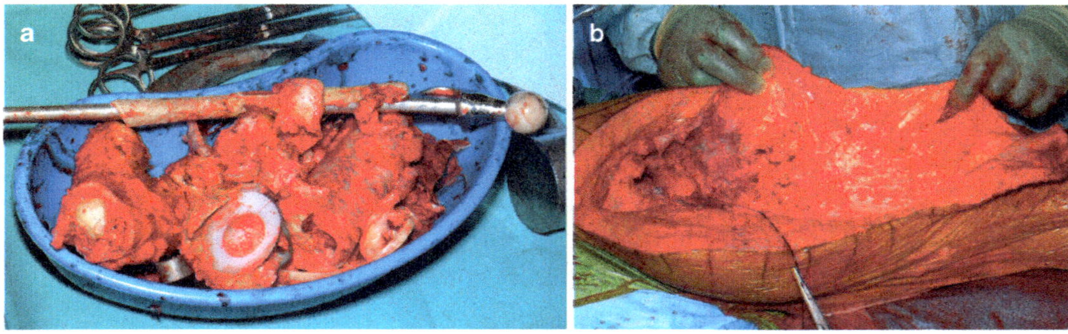

Fig. 14.3 (**a**) Removal of all infected bone and implant material including the scar and sinus. (**b**) Healthy bleeding compliant tissue after radical debridement

administration [12, 13]. Elution from cement beads has been shown to achieve local concentrations of antibiotics up to 17 times higher than that found after intravenous administration without the toxic side effects of the commonly used intravenous antibiotics [14]. Articulating spacers have potential advantages in terms of mobilisation for the patient by maintaining joint mobility and preventing stiffness (though this is less of a problem in the hip than in the knee and most of the published literature refers to articulating spacers in the knee) [16–18]. On the other hand, the use of beads and static spacers may offer an advantage by not promoting movement such that the soft tissues are allowed to rest as well as delivering the higher doses of antibiotic [19]. Articulating spacers require adequate host bone in order to hold the spacer in place. Many of the patients we see have compromised bone stock (often both femoral and acetabular) and often have required an ETO to remove all the existing femoral cement/implant. In these situations the use of an articulating cement spacer becomes less practical and often impossible.

The addition of high doses of antibiotic to the cement can weaken its structural properties, a potential problem with articulating spacers as they can fracture but not a problem with beads [20, 21]. Beads also have a much higher surface area than articulating spacers and hence release a greater amount of antibiotic [19]. A potential additional advantage of using beads, especially in the femoral canal, is that in our experience they appear to facilitate the formation of a new endosteal-like surface, unlike solid spacers, which in our hands tend to leave a rather sclerotic canal.

The exact antibiotic cocktail to add to the cement will depend on the culture and antibiotic sensitivity pattern from the aspirate, but in the absence of a known pathogen we routinely add vancomycin to bone cement containing gentamicin since this covers the majority of common pathogens. Up to 8 g of dry antibiotic powder can be added to a 40-g mix of cement powder before it significantly affects the ability of the cement to 'cure,' but the structural properties are significantly altered after addition of 4.5 g [13]. In our practice, we usually add 2 g of vancomycin to a 40-g mix of cement already containing 1 g of gentamicin [7]. Cement is hand-mixed, without a vacuum, with a spatula in a bowl, as the aim is to produce an optimal antibiotic delivery system and not a cement of structural integrity with low porosity [22]. The cement is then used to form small (<1 cm) biconcave discs and held on an 18-gauge braided wire for form chains (Fig. 14.4). The biconcave discs have the optimal shape in terms of ratio of volume to surface area for the elution of antibiotic [23, 24]. The bead chains from a single 40-g mix are usually sufficient in volume to pack the joint space, acetabulum and femoral canal.

The wound should be carefully closed in layers and any dead space eliminated. Drains are not recommended as they simply remove the eluted antibiotic.

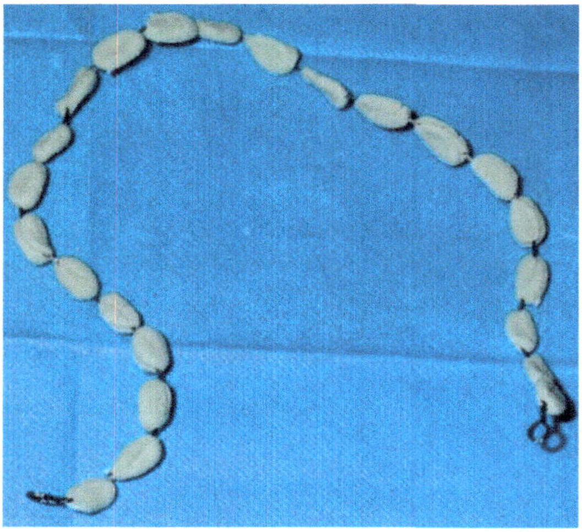

Fig. 14.4 Cement beads

Postoperative Phase

The patient should ideally spend the first 24 h in a critical care unit and only be discharged to the general ward once physiologically stable. We recommend a minimum of 2–3 days of bed rest to allow the soft tissues to settle and help the wound heal by primary intention. These patients have had a massive soft tissue insult, the tissues have been traumatised, they are swollen and they need to rest. When the wound is dry, the patient can start to mobilise, weight bearing as able on crutches or a frame under the supervision of a physiotherapist.

In cases where a positive pre-operative aspirate has allowed targeted antibiotics to be added to the cement beads we don't believe there is any benefit in additional systemic antibiotic therapy post operatively as the beads themselves are delivering high local concentrations of antibiotic [7]. If the 14-day culture of the deep tissue samples reveals an additional infecting organism not previously identified in the aspirate then one could consider an additional course of antibiotic therapy. In our experience this is not necessary, as the mainstay of treatment has been the radical debridement. Antibiotics obviously play an important role, but we regard their usage as being secondary in the management of PJI. We accept this view is not shared by all clinicians; some rely heavily on intravenous antibiotics, either in combination with local antibiotics in the bone cement or in isolation.

Interval Phase

The main purpose of the interval phase is to allow the patient and the soft tissues to recover from the septic insult. Long periods of systemic antibiotics are not required, as the surgical debridement and high-dose local antibiotic elution have treated the infection [7, 28].

The duration of the interval phase can vary greatly depending on the patient's soft tissue recovery following the first stage procedure. We try and aim for a second-stage reconstruction after a period of some 8–12 weeks [25, 26]. Simply prolonging the period with a pseudarthrosis makes subsequent surgery more difficult and a probable worse functional outcome. In the majority of cases, the soft tissue swelling has resolved by 2–3 months, the wound has healed and inflammatory markers such as the erythrocyte sedimentation rate (ESR) and C-reactive protein (CRP) have fallen from their high presurgery levels. If the soft tissues have not settled and the ESR and CRP remain elevated, a repeat first-stage procedure should be performed as opposed to second-stage reimplantation.

Second-Stage Procedure

The cases should be re-discussed in an MDT planning meeting and the reconstructive plan (noted in the operative notes from the first stage) reviewed. The second-stage operation should be regarded as an aseptic procedure, and the most appropriate method of reconstruction for the particular patient's needs should be used. The results of the deep tissue specimens from the first stage should also be reviewed and a plan made in conjunction with the microbiologist as to which antibiotic to add to the cement, if a cemented reconstruction is to be utilised. The dose of antibiotic for the cement will not be as high as that used in the first stage, as the reconstruction is now deemed aseptic and it is important not to adversely affect the mechanical properties of the cement.

At the time of surgery prophylactic antibiotics should again be withheld until deep tissue specimens have been taken for microbiological analysis. An advantage of a two-stage over a one-stage strategy is that it allows for a second debridement of tissues and this second debridement, although not as radical, should be as meticulous as the first-stage debridement.

In the postoperative period, our experience would suggest there is no need for systemic antibiotic therapy, as the reconstruction was planned as an aseptic procedure; however, in many other centres patients will receive a further course of systemic antibiotics. There is debate about what should happen if cultures from the second-stage procedure come back positive. We see little point in prescribing antibiotics as the specimens were taken prior to the second debridement and our experience suggests positive second-stage culture results have had no bearing on the final outcome.

Follow-Up

Regular follow-up of these patients is essential, especially for the first 12–18 months as any recurrence of infection will usually occur within this period [7, 27]. In addition, these patients often need encouragement and support as the recovery after such surgery can be slow and they must be encouraged to be patient and understand that the primary aim is to be infection free and functional recovery will come with time.

Figure 14.5 demonstrates a series of x-rays of a patient who underwent a two-stage procedure after an attempt to eradicate infection at another hospital was not successful.

Results of Two-Stage Revision Surgery and the Role of Systemic Antibiotic Therapy

There are numerous reports in the literature on the outcome of a two-stage strategy and most report a successful eradication in about 90 % of patients [29]. Most authors stress the importance of the surgical debridement, but the two areas of controversy are the time interval between stages and the use or duration of systemic antibiotics.

The time interval between stages will often depend on the individual patient, their soft tissues and their clinical response to the first stage. A time interval of 6–12 weeks is usually appropriate to allow the soft tissues to settle. One study looking at longer intervals (after 20 weeks) compared to shorter intervals (within 6 weeks) demonstrated higher rates on re-infection in those patients who had a longer interval between stages [26].

In terms of the systemic antibiotic regimen there is little consensus in the literature. Many studies use 6 weeks of antibiotics (either IV or IV then oral), although there is no good basic science to justify this duration. Several studies have achieved almost identical success with much shorter regimens ranging from no postoperative antibiotics to 14 days of antibiotics. At the 3rd Sheffield Orthopaedic/Microbiology meeting in 2010, the results of the surgical treatment of prosthetic hip infection from three well-recognised units; Oxford (Gundle), Hamburg (Schwantes) and Sheffield (Stockley), were presented (Table 14.1). Gundle and Stockley reported on their respective two-stage series, and Schwantes on single-stage surgery. Despite different systemic antibiotic regimes and the use or a two-stage or single-stage strategy, the results with respect to the eradication of infection were very similar. Hsieh compared a standard 4–6-week course of systemic antibiotics between stages with a short 1-week course and also achieved very similar outcomes with respect to infection control [30]. These very consistent results across the studies would suggest that the use of or duration of systemic antibiotic is not essential or

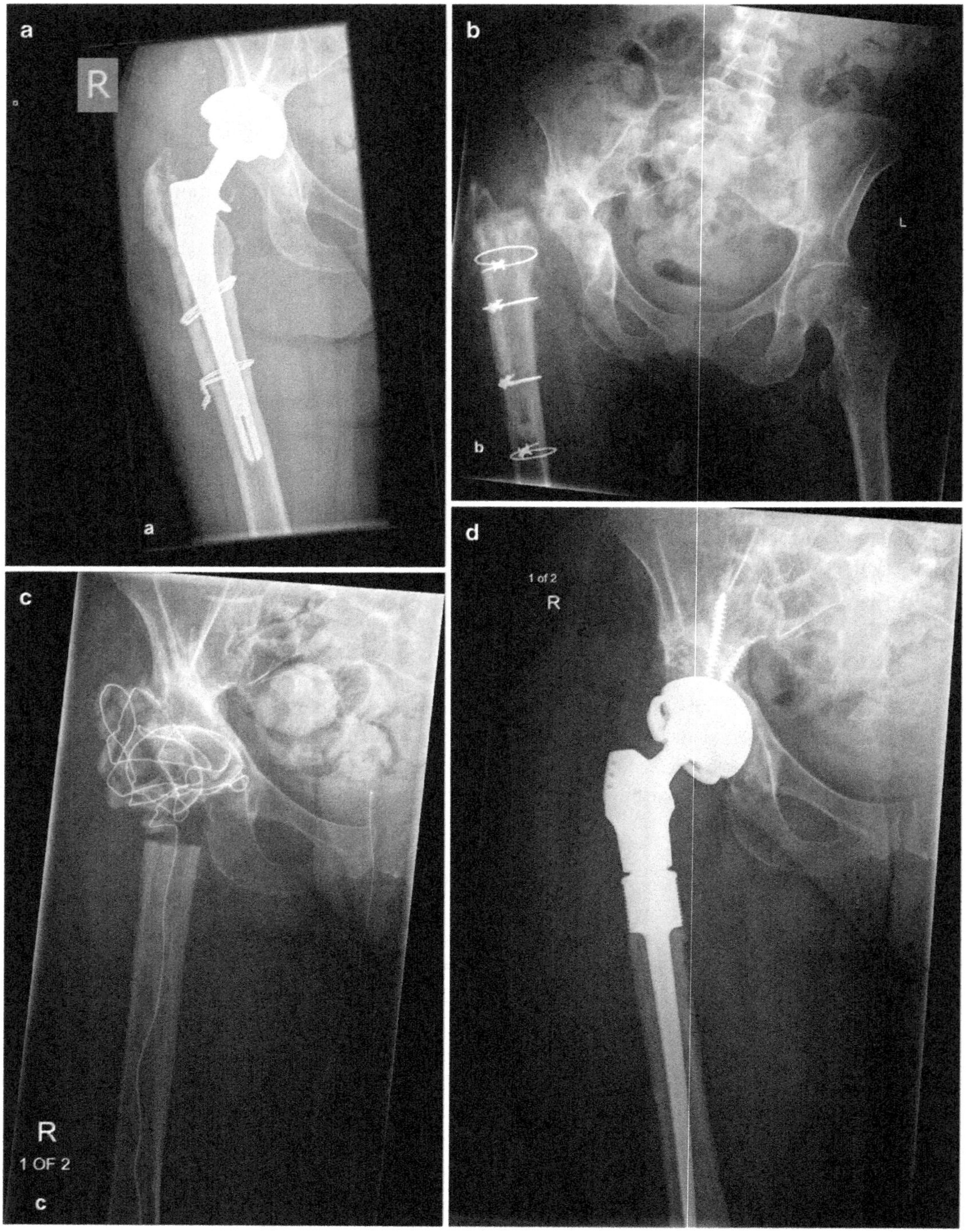

Fig. 14.5 (**a**) Original infected implant, (**b**) upon presentation to our unit, (**c**) after first stage, (**d**) after successful second stage

Table 14.1 Results of two stage revisions with different antibiotic regimens

Centre	Number of patients	Duration of follow-up	Stages	Antibiotic-loaded bone cement used	Antibiotic regimen	Success rate (%)
Sheffield	114	6.1 years	Two	Yes	Prophylactic antibiotics only. No systemic antibiotics between stages	88
Oxford	152	5.8 years	Two	Yes	Prolonged courses of systemic antibiotics after both stages	89
Hamburg	105	6.5 years	Single	Yes	10–12 days	88

potentially relevant; the success of a two-stage strategy and that of a single-stage procedure is due to the common principles that all studies embrace, namely radical surgical debridement and delivery of local antibiotic via antibiotic eluting cement.

Summary

A two-stage revision strategy provides reliably good outcomes and is the only safe option when the nature of the infecting organism is not fully known. The keys to success are the use of a multidisciplinary approach, radical surgical debridement of all infected or nonviable tissue and delivery of high-dose local antibiotics (with or without systemic antibiotics).

References

1. Kurtz SM, Ong KL, Lau E, Bozic KJ, Berry D, Parvizi J. Prosthetic joint infection risk after TKA in the Medicare population. Clin Orthop Relat Res. 2010;468(1):52–6.
2. Ong KL, Kurtz SM, Lau E, Bozic KJ, Berry DJ, Parvizi J. Prosthetic joint infection risk after total hip arthroplasty in the Medicare population. J Arthroplasty. 2009;24(6 Suppl):105–9.
3. Hanssen AD, Rand JA. Evaluation and treatment of infection at the site of a total hip or knee arthroplasty. Instr Course Lect. 1999;48:111–22.
4. Kapadia BH, McElroy MJ, Issa K, Johnson AJ, Bozic KJ, Mont MA. The economic impact of periprosthetic infections following total knee arthroplasty at a specialized tertiary-care center. J Arthroplasty. 2014;29(5):929–32.
5. Kallala RF, Vanhegan IS, Ibrahim MS, Sarmah S, Haddad FS. Financial analysis of revision knee surgery based on NHS tariffs and hospital costs: does it pay to provide a revision service? Bone Joint J. 2015;97-B(2):197–201.
6. Klouche S, Sariali E, Mamoudy P. Total hip arthroplasty revision due to infection: a cost analysis approach. Orthop Traumatol Surg Res. 2010;96(2):124–32.
7. Stockley I, Mockford BJ, Hoad-Reddick A, Norman P. The use of two-stage exchange arthroplasty with depot antibiotics in the absence of long-term antibiotic therapy in infected total hip replacement. J Bone Joint Surg Br. 2008;90(2):145–8.
8. Osmon DR, Berbari EF, Berendt AR, Lew D, Zimmerli W, Steckelberg JM, Rao N, Hanssen A, Wilson WR, Infectious Diseases Society of America. Diagnosis and management of prosthetic joint infection: clinical practice guidelines by the Infectious Diseases Society of America. Clin Infect Dis. 2013;56(1):e1–25.
9. Spangehl MJ, Masri BA, O'Connell JX, Duncan CP. Prospective analysis of preoperative and intraoperative investigations for the diagnosis of infection at the sites of two hundred and two revision total hip arthroplasties. J Bone Joint Surg Am. 1999;81(5):672–83.
10. Ali F, Wilkinson JM, Cooper JR, Kerry RM, Hamer AJ, Norman P, Stockley I. Accuracy of joint aspiration for the preoperative diagnosis of infection in total hip arthroplasty. J Arthroplasty. 2006;21(2):221–6.
11. Powles JW, Spencer RF, Lovering AM. Gentamicin release from old cement during revision hip arthroplasty. J Bone Joint Surg Br. 1998;80(4):607–10.
12. Henry SL, Seligson D, Mangino P, Popham GJ. Antibiotic-impregnated beads. Part I: bead implantation versus systemic therapy. Orthop Rev. 1991;20(3):242–7.
13. Cui Q, Mihalko WM, Shields JS, Ries M, Saleh KJ. Antibiotic-impregnated cement spacers for the treatment of infection associated with total hip or knee arthroplasty. J Bone Joint Surg Am. 2007;89(4):871–82.

14. Salvati EA, Callaghan JJ, Brause BD, Klein RF, Small RD. Reimplantation in infection. Elution of gentamicin from cement and beads. Clin Orthop Relat Res. 1986;207:83–93.
15. Whittaker JP, Warren RE, Jones RS, Gregson PA. Is prolonged systemic antibiotic treatment essential in two-stage revision hip replacement for chronic gram-positive infection? J Bone Joint Surg Br. 2009; 91(1):44–51.
16. Toms AD, Davidson D, Masri BA, Duncan CP. The management of peri-prosthetic infection in total joint arthroplasty. J Bone Joint Surg Br. 2006;88(2):149–55.
17. Hsieh PH, Shih CH, Chang YH, Lee MS, Shih HN, Yang WE. Two-stage revision hip arthroplasty for infection: comparison between the interim use of antibiotic-loaded cement beads and a spacer prosthesis. J Bone Joint Surg Am. 2004;86-A(9):1989–97.
18. Biring GS, Kostamo T, Garbuz DS, Masri BA, Duncan CP. Two-stage revision arthroplasty of the hip for infection using an interim articulated prostalac hip spacer: a 10- to 15-year follow-up study. J Bone Joint Surg Br. 2009;91(11):1431–7.
19. Anagnostakos K, Wilmes P, Schmitt E, Kelm J. Elution of gentamicin and vancomycin from polymethylmethacrylate beads and hip spacers in vivo. Acta Orthop. 2009;80(2):193–7.
20. Duncan CP, Masri BA. The role of antibiotic-loaded cement in the treatment of an infection after a hip replacement. Instr Course Lect. 1995;44:305–13.
21. Hanssen AD, Spangehl MJ. Practical applications of antibiotic-loaded bone cement for treatment of infected joint replacements. Clin Orthop Relat Res. 2004;427:79–85.
22. Kuechle DK, Landon GC, Musher DM, Noble PC. Elution of vancomycin, daptomycin, and amikacin from acrylic bone cement. Clin Orthop Relat Res. 1991;264:302–8.
23. Walenkamp G. Small PMMA beads improve gentamicin release. Acta Orthop Scand. 1989;60(6): 668–9.
24. Seeley SK, Seeley JV, Telehowski P, Martin S, Tavakoli M, Colton SL, Larson B, Forrester P, Atkinson PJ. Volume and surface area study of tobramycin-polymethylmethacrylate beads. Clin Orthop Relat Res. 2004;420:298–303.
25. Lieberman JR, Callaway GH, Salvati EA, Pellicci PM, Brause BD. Treatment of the infected total hip arthroplasty with a two-stage reimplantation protocol. Clin Orthop Relat Res. 1994;301:205–12.
26. Colyer RA, Capello WN. Surgical treatment of the infected hip implant. Two-stage reimplantation with a one-month interval. Clin Orthop Relat Res. 1994;298:75–9.
27. Lynch M, Esser MP, Shelley P, Wroblewski BM. Deep infection in Charnley low-friction arthroplasty. Comparison of plain and gentamicin-loaded cement. J Bone Joint Surg Br. 1987;69(3):355–60.
28. McKenna PB, O'Shea K, Masterson EL. Two-stage revision of infected hip arthroplasty using a shortened post-operative course of antibiotics. Arch Orthop Trauma Surg. 2009;129(4):489–94.
29. Zimmerli W, Trampuz A, Ochsner PE. Prosthetic-joint infections. N Engl J Med. 2004;351:1645–54.
30. Hsieh PH, Huang KC, Lee PC, Lee MS. Two-stage revision of infected hip arthroplasty using an antibiotic-loaded spacer: retrospective comparison between short-term and prolonged antibiotic therapy. J Antimicrob Chemother. 2009;64(2):392–7.

Management of Periprosthetic Infection Following Hip Arthroplasty in Two Stages Using an Articulating Antibiotic-Loaded Spacer

15

N. Amir Sandiford, Donald Garbuz, Bassam Masri, and Clive P. Duncan

Abstract

Periprosthetic joint infection (PJI) is one of the most serious potential complications following total hip arthroplasty (THA). Despite significant advances in our understanding of the pathophysiology of infection and its diagnosis, the incidence remains relatively unchanged over the last decade. Surgical management of PJI can be challenging; therefore, the surgeon needs to be aware of the management options available as well as the effectiveness of these options.

Two-stage reconstruction is considered by many surgeons to be the gold standard for management of the infected THA. This chapter reviews the options for two-stage management of the infected PJI affecting the hip. It focuses on the role of articulating spacers and presents an evidence-based and contemporary overview of their role in the modern management of patients with an infected total hip arthroplasty.

Keywords

Periprosthetic joint infection (PJI) • Infected • Hip • Arthroplasty • Articulating • Spacers • Management • Surgery

Introduction

Periprosthetic joint infection (PJI) is one of the most serious complications that can follow joint replacement. Fifty years ago Charnley was able to reduce the risk of this occurring from 9.5 to 0.5 % using clear air systems and occlusive surgical gowns [1]. Since then, despite the significant improvements which have been made in arthroplasty surgery, the incidence of infection has

N.A. Sandiford, MSc, FRCS (Trauma/Orth)
D. Garbuz, MD, MHSc, FRCS(C) • B. Masri, MD, FRCS(C)
Department of Orthopaedics, The University of British Columbia, Vancouver, BC, Canada

C.P. Duncan, MB, MSc, FRCSC (✉)
Department of Orthopaedics, University of British Columbia, Vancouver General and University Hospitals, Vancouver, BC, Canada
e-mail: cpduncan@gmail.com

D. Kendoff et al. (eds.), *Periprosthetic Joint Infections: Changing Paradigms*,
DOI 10.1007/978-3-319-30091-7_15

remained essentially unchanged. The reported incidence of PJI varies from 0.3 to 2.9 % following total hip arthroplasty [2, 3].

National joint registries around the World indicate that PJI accounts for 12–14.5 % of revision THA procedures [4–7]. Infection is associated with increased morbidity and mortality within the first year post surgery, prolonged hospitalisation and impairment of physical and psychological function of the patient. Management of PJI is resource-intensive and expensive for the treating institution and the community at large [8]. The aim of management is to fully eradicate the infection and to restore a pain-free, stable and functional hip.

Revision in two stages, with delayed reimplantation, is widely favoured [9], but the single stage approach, in selected cases is gaining increasing attention and favour [10–15]. The two-stage procedure involves removal of the implants, acrylic cement if it was used, and necrotic tissue, along with careful debridement and lavage. There follows a period of treatment with antibiotic, followed by restaging to rule out persisting infection and the revision replacement. Insall demonstrated the importance of removing all foreign material (implant +/– cement) and using antibiotics for definitive management in 1983 [16].

Two stage procedures without the use of an interim spacer have been associated with the development of joint contractures, risk of instability, stiffness, pain, difficulty with mobilisation, and ultimately, technical difficulties during reconstruction [17]. The purpose of a spacer is to maintain leg length, stability and motion of the affected joint, to facilitate mobilization and rehabilitation of the patient between stages, to also maintain soft tissue pliability and planes, while delivering a very high dose of antimicrobial to the effective joint space [10, 17, 19].

This chapter presents the results of two-stage revision with the use of interim articulating spacers in the management of PJI complicating total hip arthroplasty.

Diagnosis of PJI

The Musculoskeletal Infection Society (MSIS) has recently published diagnostic criteria which are required for making the diagnosis of PJI. The inclusion of biomarkers has significantly improved the sensitivity and specificity of diagnostic tests [20]. The classification system proposed by Toms et al. [22] is commonly used and provides a guide to management [21–26].

As the diagnosis and classification of PJI will be dealt with elsewhere in this text, we will focus on two-stage revision with articulating spacers in this chapter.

The Rationale for Two-Stage Reconstruction

Single-stage revision has been used in Europe since the 1970s. Carlsson reported a 75.5 % success rate at 2–6-year follow-up of patients infected with a single organism with this technique in 1978 [11]. Buchholz et al. [13] reported 77 % success with the one-stage procedure at 5-year follow-up.

In all major studies in which single-stage reconstruction has been used, patients have been very carefully selected. The successful results of single-stage reconstruction have been achieved in healthy, immune-competent patients with favourable soft tissue envelope who present with an acute infection caused by a known organism which is sensitive to first-line antibiotics [22–27]. Also, traditionally, a single-stage exchange has relied on the use of antibiotic cement for fixation, hence the use of cemented implants.

One-stage revision is contraindicated in patients who are clinically septic, where an organism is not identified, the presence of a sinus tract and if nonviable soft tissue which might require flap reconstruction is present. It is therefore difficult to directly compare published results for one- and two-stage reconstruction.

Spacers

Several types and designs of spacers are used in the modern management of PJI complicating total hip arthroplasty. These can be broadly classified as non articulating (static) or articulating. Articulating spacers are further classified based on the articulating surfaces, i.e., metal on polyethylene, cement on polyethylene, cement on cement and cement on bone (unipolar monoblock)

Static Spacers

Static spacers act as a reservoir for the local delivery of high-dose antibiotics. They consist of a block of PMMA cement bridging the joint space. Although they deliver antibiotics, they can result in limitation of joint motion, which can result in soft tissue contractures, and loss of bone stock due to erosion of bone at its mobile interface with the rough surface of the spacer [10]. Such restriction of mobility has been associated with difficulty during surgical exposure at the second stage [28–30]. Static devices have also been associated with increased blood loss and transfusion requirements during the second stage when compared to mobile spacers [31]. Reinfection rates with the use of static spacers have been shown to be similar to those of mobile spacers, however. They are used more commonly in the knee.

This chapter will focus on the role of articulating spacers in revision total hip arthroplasty.

Articulating Spacers for Revision THA

Articulating spacers which are used for revision THA can be broadly categorised into two main designs based on their bearing surfaces. In the first group the head of the prosthesis (which is made of cement) articulates with the native acetabulum. These are made from cement and have the overall shape of a monopolar hemiarthroplasty. They are often constructed from cement with reinforcing rods to minimise the risk of fracture. The second group consists of a femoral component coated in PMMA cement articulating with a polyethylene acetabular component which has been inserted with cement. When inserted this design has the physical appearance of a poorly cemented hip arthroplasty.

The all-cement varieties can be handmade, custom-moulded or prefabricated. Handmade spacers are relatively simple to make, they are economical, and the amount and type of antibiotics incorporated can be customised for the infecting organism. Infection eradication rates of 88–100 % have been reported by several authors [33–35]. Barrack [35] used Rush pins to reinforce their design. Other authors have created endoskeletons using Ender nails and K-wires in order to minimise the risk of fracture during weight bearing in the interval period and during stem removal at the second stage [33, 35, 36].

Potential drawbacks with this design include inconsistencies in the geometry which can affect the degree of femoral stability and potentially predispose to dislocation [3].

Custom-moulded spacers bear several similarities to hand-moulded designs in that they are structurally similar to hemiarthroplasty prostheses and consist of a cement mantle often surrounding a metal endoskeleton. They have more predictable shapes and reproducible sizes and the antibiotics which are added can be tailored to the infecting species. The main drawback of this type of spacer is that the sizes are limited by the sizes of the moulds. For this reason the risk of dislocation [31, 34] is present. Infection eradication rates of 96–100 % have been obtained with the use of this design, however.

Prefabricated spacers (e.g., Spacer G, Tecres, Verona, Italy) (Fig. 15.1) are offered by a variety of manufacturers. Success rates of >90 % have been reported with this design by several authors [37–39]. Potential issues with this type include limitations in size as for custom-moulded spacers but also the antibiotic content is determined by

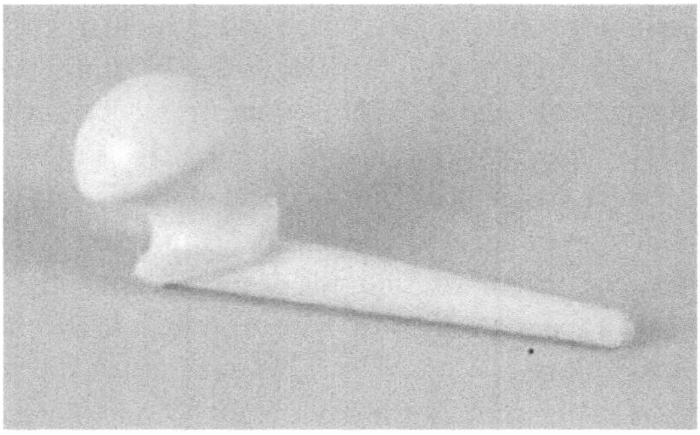

Fig. 15.1 An example of a prefabricated spacer (Spacer G, Tecres, Verona, Italy) (Author photograph)

the manufacturer. Some authors have attempted to address this by drilling holes into the spacer which are then filled with antibiotic-impregnated cement prepared by the surgeon [39]. The effect of this practice on elution characteristics as well as the mechanical strength of the spacer are unknown.

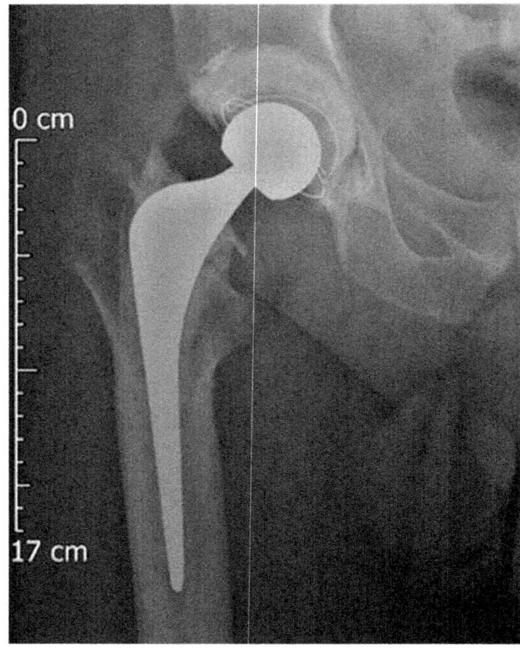

Fig. 15.2 The custom-made articulating spacer (CUMARS). This design consists of an Exeter stem which is covered with antibiotic-loaded PMMA cement to the neck and a cemented acetabular component

Metal on Polyethylene Hip Spacers

Several designs of MOP spacers have been described in the literature. They all include the use of a femoral component coated with cement and coupled with a cemented polyethylene socket. Hofmann et al. [18] re-sterilised the explanted femoral component and reinserted it with antibiotic loaded cement. They reported 94 % eradication rate at 76-month follow-up using this technique along with improved function, maintenance of soft tissue tension and bone stock. Etienne et al. [40] used a new low-demand femoral stem and a polyethylene acetabular component. Three of 31 patients had recurrent infection with this technique. Tsung et al. [41] reported excellent results using the Exeter universal stem for their custom spacer (Fig. 15.2). Their functional results were so encouraging that 44 % of patients opted to delay the second stage as they were asymptomatic.

Romano et al. [42] and Etienne et al. [40] both reported dislocation with the use of this design. The issue has been addressed in several ways. Evans [30] recommended constrained liners. Kuzyk et al. [3] used a custom-moulded cement shelf fixed to the ilium with cancellous screws to act as a superior restraint to dislocation.

The prosthesis of antibiotic-loaded acrylic cement (PROSTALAC) (Depuy, Warsaw, IN, USA) articulating hip spacer has been the most represented MOP design in contemporary literature and was the precursor to most articulated designs currently available. This device has been routinely used by the senior authors since 1986. It consists of a low-demand femoral component with a modular 32-mm head which is snap-fitted into a simple 42-mm (OD) polyethylene acetabular component. Tobramycin (3.6 g/40 g of cement) and vancomycin (1.5 g/40 g of cement) are added (Figs. 15.3, 15.4, and 15.5).

Younger et al. [43] found significant improvement in pain and functional scores at a mean 47 months follow-up with the use of the PROSTALAC device in 30 patients with significant proximal femoral bone loss. Ninety-six percent of patients remained infection-free at final follow-up. No difference in infection control

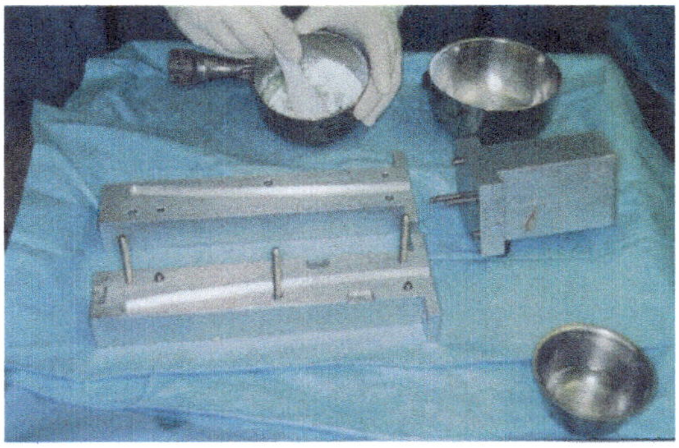

Fig. 15.3 The molds for making the PROSTALAC femoral component

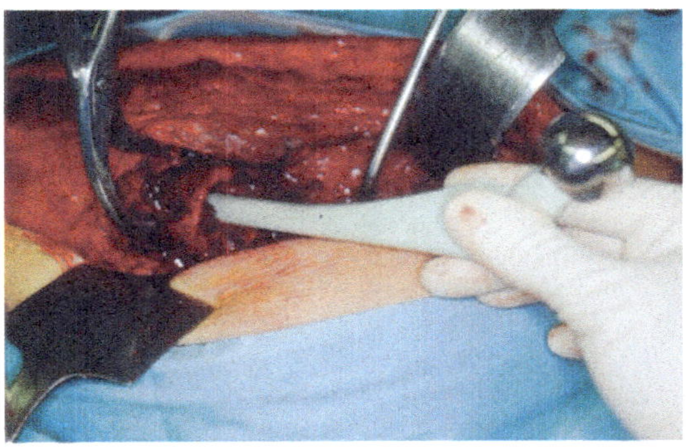

Fig. 15.4 The PROSTALAC stem prior to insertion. Note the stem is coated with cement almost to the head-neck junction

rates, functional outcome or complication rates were found between the cement on cement and metal on polyethylene types. Masri et al. [44] reported three failures in 29 patients treated with this technique at a minimum 2 years post surgery. Infections recurred in two patients with insulin-dependent diabetes mellitus and one who was receiving high-dose steroid therapy.

Biring et al. [45] reviewed 99 patients at an average of 12 years post surgery. They found that improvement in patient-reported outcome measures noted in the early stages was maintained and infection was successfully treated in 89 % of patients. Seven of the eleven patients who had recurrent infections responded to a second two-stage procedure which led to a final success rate of 96 % for the long-term resolution of infection. To our knowledge these are the longest term

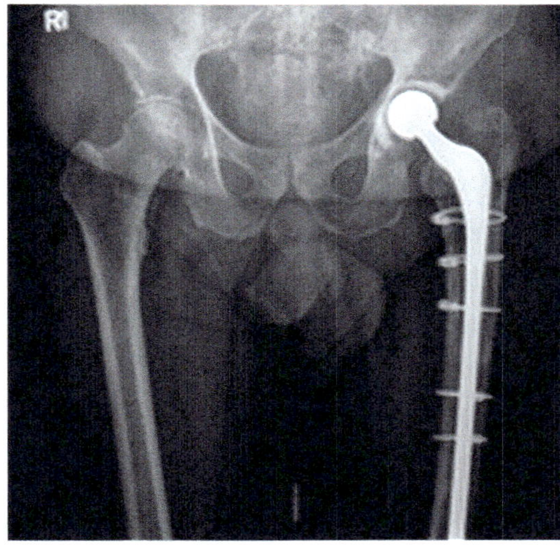

Fig. 15.5 Postoperative radiograph of a long-stemmed PROSTALAC component

results which have been published examining the success of articulating spacers.

Comparative studies have been difficult to perform due to the differences in design and antibiotic content- similar to devices used to manage PJI in the knee. What has been shown is that patients treated with an antibiotic loaded spacer have lower infection recurrence rates [46]. Results of the different designs reported in the literature are presented in Table 15.1.

Complications of Mobile Spacers

Fractures have been described with use of cement on cement knee spacers [32]. Several authors have reported fractures [31, 47] and dislocations [10, 31, 47] (Fig. 15.6) as the major complications associated with mobile hip spacers.

Jung and colleagues [47] reviewed 88 articulating custom moulded spacers used for two-stage revision THA procedures. They encountered 17 % dislocations, 13.6 % femoral fractures and five cases (6 %) of nephrotoxicity. The incidence of dislocations, femoral fractures and nephrotoxicity in this series are higher than those experienced by the senior authors, but they do emphasize that implantation of a mobile

Table 15.1 Composition and results of spacers used for management of the infected total hip arthroplasty

Type of spacer	Author	N	Reinfection rate (%)	Follow up (months)	Antibiotics	Type of cement used
Static	Haddad [58]	50	8	68	–	–
	Hsieh [31]	70	1.4	57	–	–
Mobile						
Handmade[a]	Barrack [35]	12	0	60	–	–
	Leunig [59]	12	1	27	Gentamicin 05 g/40 g cement	Palacos R, (Zimmer, Warsaw, IN)
	Younger [43]	15	1	47	Tobramycin 3.6 g/ vancomycin 1.0 g/40 g cement	Palacos R
Molded[a]	Durbhakula [28]	24	8	33	Tobramycin 2.4 g/ vancomycin 1.0 g/40 g cement	Palacos R
Prefabricated[a]	Bertazzoni Minelli [39]	20	15	33	Gentamicin 1.9 g/100 g cement vancomycin 1.0 g/40 g cement	Cemex, (Tecres, Verona, Italy)
Metal on polyethylene designs	Evans [30]	23	4.3	Minimum 24	Tobramyici 4.6 g/ vancomycin 4.0 g/40 g cement	Palacos R
	Younger [43]	15	0	47	Tobramyici 3.6 g/ vancomycin 1.0 g/40 g cement	Palacos R
	Masri [44]	29	10.3	47	Tobramycin 3.6 g/ vancomycin 1.5 g/40 g cement	Palacos R
	Hofmann [18]	27	6	76	Tobramycin 4.8 g	Simplex P (Stryker, Mahwah, NJ)
	Biring [45]	99	11	60	Tobramycin 3.6 g/ vancomycin 1.0 g/40 g cement	Palacos R
	Tsung [41]	76	15.8	79	–	Simplex P and Palacos R

Abbreviation: *g* grams

[a]Prostheses resembling monopolar hemiarthroplasty stems with a bearing surface made of cement

hip spacer does carry potential risks which need to be discussed with the patient.

Factors Affecting the Results of Spacers

Spacers have structural, functional and therapeutic roles. From the structural and functional perspectives they hold the soft tissues out to optimal length and facilitate movement and load bearing during the interval period.

From a therapeutic perspective they act as a local depot for antibiotics. The type of cement, method used for mixing, as well as the choice of antibiotic, its thermal stability and interaction with other antibiotics incorporated in the spacer, are important factors.

The ideal antibiotic should be thermostable, bactericidal at low concentrations and water-soluble with minimal risk of renal or hepatotoxicity [10, 48]. Addition of antibiotics in liquid form has been shown to reduce the compressive and tensile strength of PMMA cement by 49 %

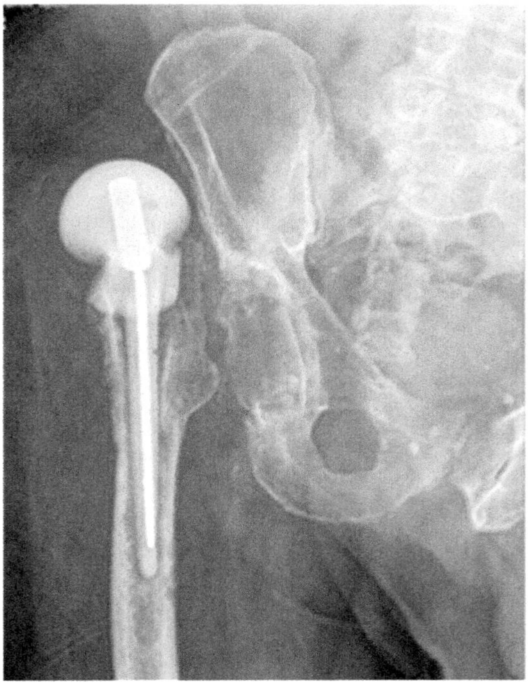

Fig. 15.6 A dislocated mobile hip spacer

and 46 %, respectively [49]. Antibiotics which are to be added should therefore be available in powder form, have low serum albumin binding capacity and be thermostable. Spacers have been shown to produce higher local concentrations of antibiotics than can be achieved via systemic administration. This can be achieved with minimal increase in serum and urine levels of the drug thus minimising the risk of systemic toxicity [25, 40].

The most commonly used agents are gentamicin, tobramycin and vancomycin [10, 32], although if the organism is identified and sensitivities known then it is logical to tailor the agent(s) used. This is important as up to 41–66 % staphylococci isolated from infected joints have been found to be resistant to gentamicin and tobramycin at the usual concentrations obtained via parenteral administration [50]. However, at the very high local levels achieved by antibiotic loaded cement, these antibiotics may be effective. Combining antibiotics can alter the elution characteristics and joint fluid concentration of each drug [32]. The combination of 3.6 g of tobramycin and 1.5 g of vancomycin/40 g of PMMA cement has been shown to facilitate release of the vancomycin (so called passive opportunism) [51]. Penner et al. [52] suggested that as one antibiotic dissolves and elutes, the resultant increased porosity of the PMMA facilities release of the other antibiotics.

Elution characteristics have also been shown to be influenced by surface area and porosity of the cement [10]. The type of cement and mixing methods can influence this. Stevens et al. [53] reported better eluting characteristics for tobramycin when used with Palacos (Zimmer, Warsaw, IN, USA) compared to Simplex (Stryker, Warsaw, IN, USA) cement. The local concentration of antibiotics achieved is influenced by the initial dose incorporated into the spacer.

Commercially available cements contain low doses of antibiotics and, by themselves, are not suitable for use in two-stage reconstructions [32]. Most antibiotic elution occurs within the first 24 h [39, 54] and levels remain elevated at up to 4 months post insertion. Mixing technique also influences elution characteristics. Hand mixing without a vacuum results in greater porosity and increased antibiotic elution [55, 56].

In our practice a multidisciplinary approach is adopted in the management of these challenging cases. All patients are seen by the infections disease team. Our choice of intravenous antibiotics during the interval period as well as the need for any further antibiotics are guided by the microbiologist with whom we liaise closely. The antibiotics are added intraoperatively to cement in powder form and hand mixed.

Summary of Results

Two-stage revision is a widely accepted standard for the management of PJI. Static and articulating spacers can be used in the hip. Infection control rates seem identical with both techniques. Mobility in the interval period, maintenance of periarticular soft tissue length and tension and ultimately surgical access at the second stage seem to be improved with the use of articulating spacers. The current literature suggests that metal on polyethylene spacers provide significant pain relief, acceptable levels of function and high levels of patient satisfaction based on Patient Reported Outcome Measures. The longest term results, mainly based on the PROSTALAC spacers, suggest that relief of infection and functional improvement are maintained in the long term.

The choice of antibiotic should be guided by sensitivity of the organism. At least 3.6 g of antibiotic should be added per 40 g of cement. The surgeon should be familiar with the chosen antibiotic's elution characteristics and mixing should be done by hand to increase porosity of the cement as suggested by Clyburn and Qui [57].

Conclusion

Articulating spacers provide a viable option for management of patients undergoing two-stage revision arthroplasty for infection. They enable the patients to bear weight, allow functional movements of the joint and facilitate operative exposure during the second stage. Careful consideration must be given to the choice of antibiotics and preparation of the spacer.

References

1. Charnley J. A clean-air operating enclosure. Br J Surg. 1964;51:202–5.
2. Kurtz S, Ong K, Lau E, Mowat F, Halpern M. Projections of primary and revision hip and knee arthroplasty in the United States from 2005 to 2030. J Bone Joint Surg Am. 2007;89(4):780–5.
3. Kuzyk PR, Dhotar HS, Sternheim A, Gross AE, Safir O, Backstein D. Two-stage revision arthroplasty for management of chronic periprosthetic hip and knee infection: techniques, controversies, and outcomes. J Am Acad Orthop Surg. 2014;22(3):153–64. doi:10.5435/JAAOS-22-03-153. Review.
4. https://www.njrcentre.org.uk/njrcentre/Portals/0/Documents/England/Reports/11th_annual_report/NJR%2011th%20Annual%20Report%202014.pdf. Page 83. Accessed 7 Sep 2014.
5. https://secure.cihi.ca/free_products/CJRR%20 2014%20Annual%20Report_EN-web.pdf. Page 48. Accessed 7 Sep 2014.
6. http://www.shpr.se/Libraries/Documents/AnnualReport_2012_Eng_WEB.sflb.ashx. Page 42. Accessed 7 Sep 2014.
7. https://aoanjrr.dmac.adelaide.edu.au/presentations-2014.
8. Zmistowski B, Karam JA, Durinka JB, Casper DS, Parvizi J. Periprosthetic joint infection increases the risk of one-year mortality. J Bone Joint Surg Am. 2013;95(24):2177–84.
9. Hanssen AD. Local antibiotic delivery vehicles in the treatment of musculoskeletal infection. Clin Orthop Relat Res. 2005;437:91–6. Review.
10. Cui Q, Mihalko WM, Shields JS, Ries M, Saleh KJ. Antibiotic-impregnated cement spacers for the treatment of infection associated with total hip or knee arthroplasty. J Bone Joint Surg Am. 2007;89(4):871–82. Review.
11. Carlsson AS, Josefsson G, Lindberg L. Revision with gentamicin-impregnated cement for deep infections in total hip arthroplasties. J Bone Joint Surg Am. 1978;60(8):1059–64.
12. Oussedik SI, Dodd MB, Haddad FS. Outcomes of revision total hip replacement for infection after grading according to a standard protocol. J Bone Joint Surg Br. 2010;92(9):1222–6.
13. Buchholz HW, Elson RA, Engelbrecht E, Lodenkämper H, Röttger J, Siegel A. Management of deep infection of total hip replacement. J Bone Joint Surg Br. 1981;63-B(3):342–53.
14. Raut VV, Orth MS, Orth MC, Siney PD, Wroblewski BM. One stage revision arthroplasty of the hip for deep gram negative infection. Int Orthop. 1996; 20(1):12–4.
15. Callaghan JJ, Katz RP, Johnston RC. One-stage revision surgery of the infected hip. A minimum 10-year followup study. Clin Orthop Relat Res. 1999;369: 139–43.
16. Insall JN, Thompson FM, Brause BD. Two-stage reimplantation for the salvage of infected total knee arthroplasty. J Bone Joint Surg Am. 1983;65(8):1087–98.
17. Haddad FS, Masri BA, Campbell D, McGraw RW, Beauchamp CP, Duncan CP. The PROSTALAC functional spacer in two-stage revision for infected knee replacements. Prosthesis of antibiotic-loaded acrylic cement. J Bone Joint Surg Br. 2000;82(6):807–12.
18. Hofmann AA, Goldberg TD, Tanner AM, Cook TM. Ten-year experience using an articulating antibiotic cement hip spacer for the treatment of chronically infected total hip. J Arthroplasty. 2005;20(7):874–9.
19. Hanssen AD, Rand JA. Evaluation and treatment of infection at the site of a total hip or knee arthroplasty. Instr Course Lect. 1999;48:111–22. Review.
20. Parvizi J, Zmistowski B, Berbari EF, Bauer TW, Springer BD, Della Valle CJ, et al. New definition for periprosthetic joint infection: from the Workgroup of the Musculoskeletal Infection Society. Clin Orthop Relat Res. 2011;469(11):2992–4.
21. Fitzgerald Jr RH, Nolan DR, Ilstrup DM, Van Scoy RE, Washington 2nd JA, Coventry MB. Deep wound sepsis following total hip arthroplasty. J Bone Joint Surg Am. 1977;59(7):847–55.
22. Toms AD, Davidson D, Masri BA, Duncan CP. The management of peri-prosthetic infection in total joint arthroplasty. J B one Joint Surg Br. 2006;88(2): 149–55.

23. Tsukayama DT, Estrada R, Gustilo RB. Infection after total hip arthroplasty. A study of the treatment of one hundred and six infections. J Bone Joint Surg Am. 1996;78(4):512–23.
24. Joseph TN, Chen AL, Di Cesare PE. Use of antibiotic-impregnated cement in total joint arthroplasty. J Am Acad Orthop Surg. 2003;11:38–47.
25. Hanssen AD, Spangehl MJ. Treatment of the infected hip replacement. Clin Orthop Relat Res. 2004;420: 63–71.
26. Atkins BL, Athanasou N, Deeks JJ, Crook DW, Simpson H, Peto TE, et al. Prospective evaluation of criteria for microbiological diagnosis of prosthetic-joint infection at revision arthroplasty. The OSIRIS Collaborative Study Group. J Clin Microbiol. 1998;36:2932–9.
27. Gulhane S, Vanhegan IS, Haddad FS. Single stage revision: regaining momentum. J Bone Joint Surg Br. 2012;94(11 Suppl A):120–2.
28. Durbhakula SM, Czajka J, Fuchs MD, Uhl RL. Spacer endoprosthesis for the treatment of infected total hip arthroplasty. J Arthroplasty. 2004;19:760–7.
29. Scharfenberger A, Clark M, Lavoie G, Scharfenberger A, Clark M, Lavoie G, et al. Treatment of an infected total hip replacement with the PROSTALAC system. Part 2: health-related quality of life and function with the PROSTALAC implant in situ. Can J Surg. 2007;50(1):29–33.
30. Evans RP. Successful treatment of total hip and knee infection with articulating antibiotic components: a modified treatment method. Clin Orthop Relat Res. 2004;427:37–46.
31. Hsieh PH, Shih CH, Chang YH, Lee MS, Shih HN, Yang WE. Two-stage revision hip arthroplasty for infection: comparison between the interim use of antibiotic-loaded cement beads and a spacer prosthesis. J Bone Joint Surg Am. 2004;86-A(9):1989–97.
32. Jacobs C, Christensen CP, Berend ME. Static and mobile antibiotic-impregnated cement spacers for the management of prosthetic joint infection. J Am Acad Orthop Surg. 2009;17(6):356–68. Review.
33. Takahira N, Itoman M, Higashi K, Uchiyama K, Miyabe M, Naruse K. Treatment outcome of two-stage revision total hip arthroplasty for infected hip arthroplasty using antibiotic-impregnated cement spacer. J Orthop Sci. 2003;8(1):26–31.
34. Yamamoto K, Miyagawa N, Masaoka T, Katori Y, Shishido T, Imakiire A. Clinical effectiveness of antibiotic-impregnated cement spacers for the treatment of infected implants of the hip joint. J Orthop Sci. 2003;8(6):823–8.
35. Barrack RL. Rush pin technique for temporary antibiotic-impregnated cement prosthesis for infected total hip arthroplasty. J Arthroplasty. 2002;17(5): 600–3.
36. Koo KH, Yang JW, Cho SH, Song HR, Park HB, Ha YC, et al. Impregnation of vancomycin, gentamicin, and cefotaxime in a cement spacer for two-stage cementless reconstruction in infected total hip arthroplasty. J Arthroplasty. 2001;16(7):882–92.
37. Pattyn C, De Geest T, Ackerman P, Audenaert E. Preformed gentamicin spacers in two-stage revision hip arthroplasty: functional results and complications. Int Orthop. 2011;35(10):1471–6. doi:10.1007/s00264-010-1172-8. PubMed PMID: 21116817, PubMed Central PMCID: PMC3174299, Epub 2010 Nov 30.
38. D'Angelo F, Negri L, Binda T, Zatti G, Cherubino P. The use of a preformed spacer in two-stage revision of infected hip arthroplasties. Musculoskelet Surg. 2011;95(2):115–20. doi:10.1007/s12306-011-0128-5. Epub 2011 Apr 9.
39. Bertazzoni Minelli E, Benini A, Magnan B, Bartolozzi P. Release of gentamicin and vancomycin from temporary human hip spacers in two-stage revision of infected arthroplasty. J Antimicrob Chemother. 2004;53(2):329–34. Epub 2003 Dec 19. PubMed.
40. Etienne G, Waldman B, Rajadhyaksha AD, Ragland PS, Mont MA. Use of a functional temporary prosthesis in a two-stage approach to infection at the site of a total hip arthroplasty. J Bone Joint Surg Am. 2003;85-A Suppl 4:94–6.
41. Tsung JD, Rohrsheim JA, Whitehouse SL, Wilson MJ, Howell JR. Management of periprosthetic joint infection after total hip arthroplasty using a custom made articulating spacer (CUMARS); the Exeter experience. J Arthroplasty. 2014;29(9): 1813–8. doi:10.1016/j.arth.2014.04.013. Epub 2014 Apr 18.
42. Romanò CL, Romanò D, Albisetti A, Meani E. Preformed antibiotic-loaded cement spacers for two-stage revision of infected total hip arthroplasty. Long-term results. Hip Int. 2012;22 Suppl 8:S46–53. doi:10.5301/HIP.2012.9570.
43. Younger AS, Duncan CP, Masri BA. Treatment of infection associated with segmental bone loss in the proximal part of the femur in two stages with use of an antibiotic-loaded interval prosthesis. J Bone Joint Surg Am. 1998;80(1):60–9.
44. Masri BA, Panagiotopoulos KP, Greidanus NV, Garbuz DS, Duncan CP. Cementless two-stage exchange arthroplasty for infection after total hip arthroplasty. J Arthroplasty. 2007;22(1):72–8.
45. Biring GS, Kostamo T, Garbuz DS, Masri BA, Duncan CP. Two-stage revision arthroplasty of the hip for infection using an interim articulated prostalac hip spacer: a 10- to 15-year follow-up study. J Bone Joint Surg Br. 2009;91(11):1431–7. doi:10.1302/0301-620X.91B11.22026.
46. Nelson CL, Evans RP, Blaha JD, Calhoun J, Henry SL, Patzakis MJ. A comparison of gentamicin-impregnated polymethylmethacrylate bead implantation to conventional parenteral antibiotic therapy in infected total hip and knee arthroplasty. Clin Orthop Relat Res. 1993;295:96–101.
47. Jung J, Schmid NV, Kelm J, Schmitt E, Anagnostakos K. Complications after spacer implantation in the treatment of hip joint infections. Int J Med Sci. 2009;6(5):265–73. PubMed PMID: 19834592, PubMed Central PMCID: PMC2755123.

48. Jiranek WA, Hanssen AD, Greenwald AS. Antibiotic-loaded bone cement for infection prophylaxis in total joint replacement. J Bone Joint Surg Am. 2006;88(11):2487–500. Review.
49. Seldes RM, Winiarsky R, Jordan LC, Baldini T, Brause B, Zodda F, et al. Liquid gentamicin in bone cement: a laboratory study of a potentially more cost-effective cement spacer. J Bone Joint Surg Am. 2005;87:268–72.
50. Anguita-Alonso P, Rouse MS, Piper KE, Jacofsky DJ, Osmon DR, Patel R. Comparative study of antimicrobial release kinetics from polymethylmethacrylate. Clin Orthop Relat Res. 2006;445:239–44.
51. Masri BA, Duncan CP, Beauchamp CP. Long-term elution of antibiotics from bone-cement: an in vivo study using the prosthesis of antibiotic-loaded acrylic cement (PROSTALAC) system. J Arthroplasty. 1998;13(3):331–8.
52. Penner MJ, Masri BA, Duncan CP. Elution characteristics of vancomycin and tobramycin combined in acrylic bone-cement. J Arthroplasty. 1996;11(8):939–44.
53. Stevens CM, Tetsworth KD, Calhoun JH, Mader JT. An articulated antibiotic spacer used for infected total knee arthroplasty: a comparative in vitro elution study of simplex and palacos bone cements. J Orthop Res. 2005;23:27–33.
54. Seyral P, Zannier A, Argenson JN, Raoult D. The release in vitro of vancomycin and tobramycin from acrylic bone cement. J Antimicrob Chemother. 1994;33(2):337–9.
55. Postak PD, Greenwald AS. Assuring cement fixation: all mixing systems are not the same. Proc Am Acad Orthop Surg. 2003;4:656.
56. Davies JP, Harris WH. Effect of hand mixing tobramycin on the fatigue strength of simplex P. J Biomed Mater Res. 1991;25(11):1409–14.
57. http://www.aaos.org/news/bulletin/may07/clinical7.asp.
58. Haddad FS, Muirhead-Allwood SK, Manktelow AR, Bacarese-Hamilton I. Two-stage uncemented revision hip arthroplasty for infection. J Bone Joint Surg Br. 2000;82(5):689–94.
59. Leunig M, Chosa E, Speck M, Ganz R. A cement spacer for two-stage revision of infected implants of the hip joint. Int Orthop. 1998;22(4):209–14. PubMed PMID: 9795805, PubMed Central PMCID: PMC3619609.

Late Infections: Algorithm Approach

16

Sujith Konan and Fares S. Haddad

Abstract

Late infections in a well-functioning joint pose a significant diagnostic and treatment challenge to the surgeon. Periprosthetic joint infection (PJI) is associated with significant morbidity to the patient and tremendous economic burden to the treating organisation. The aim of treating PJI is to eradicate infection, achieve a pain-free, functional joint and minimise morbidity. A systematic evidence-based approach will help realise this goal. This chapter summarises an algorithmic approach to management of late PJI.

Keywords

Late infection • Two-stage • Single-stage • Infection algorithm • Implant infection

Introduction

Arthoplasty has revolutionised the management of the arthritic joint. Several advances in arthroplasty have ensured continued improvement in patient outcomes. Literature [1] looking at the projected incidence of arthroplasty in the United States of America suggest that there will be a 174 % increase in the incidence of total hip arthroplasty (THA) and a 673 % increase in the incidence of total knee arthroplasty (TKA) by 2030. The incidence of complications from joint arthroplasty is relatively low. However, with the rising prevalence of joint arthropasties worldwide, the burden of complications is high. It is estimated that approximately 6 % of primary implants require revision after 5 years and 12 % after 10 years [2].

Periprosthetic joint infections (PJI) are a common cause for revision surgery and pose considerable challenge at several levels. Infection is the commonest cause of early revision of TKA and the third most common of THA. The 5-year

S. Konan, MBBS, MD(res), MRCS, FRCS (Tr & Orth)
F.S. Haddad, BSc, MD(res), MCh, FRCS (Orth) (✉)
Department of Trauma and Orthopaedics,
University College London Hospitals NHS Trust,
London, UK
e-mail: sujithkonan@yahoo.co.uk;
fsh@fareshaddad.co.uk

D. Kendoff et al. (eds.), *Periprosthetic Joint Infections: Changing Paradigms*,
DOI 10.1007/978-3-319-30091-7_16

mortality after revision arthroplasty for infection is higher than revision for aseptic loosening [3]. For the patient, dealing with PJI is a source of significant physical morbidity and psychosocial distress and they can pose serious financial burden for healthcare systems.

The management of PJI must involve multiple strategies starting with patient selection and modifying some of the predisposing risk factors. Care must be taken during surgery and during the early postoperative phase to reduce the risk of seeding the joint with organisms. However, despite all these efforts, there may be late presentations of PJI, and this needs to be approached in a systematic evidence-based manner so as to achieve successful outcome for the patient and reduce the economic burden of managing PJI.

Prevention

A single revision surgery for PJI is higher than the cost of revision for non-infectious reasons. The higher costs may be due to need for prolonged procedure, higher blood loss, increased need for bone allograft, and higher complications [4]. Added to this there are the indirect individual and societal costs of the prolonged treatment required for PJI. Prevention may hence be the most cost-effective strategy for dealing with the high economic burden of PJI. The strategies for prevention of PJI should focus on optimising host factors as well as perioperative surgical factors.

The immunocompromised host presenting for total joint arthroplasty presents a unique challenge and all measures to optimise the patients' perioperative care is essential for optimal outcome. Composite risk scores such as the National Nosocomial Infections Surveillance (NNIS) System surgical score (length of the surgical procedure, the American Society of Anesthesiologists (ASA) preoperative assessment score, and surgical wound classification for each procedure) correlate with increased odds of infection [5]. An elevated ASA score, suggesting high perioperative comorbidities, has also been associated with an increased risk of infection [6–9].

In the presence of global immunosuppression including rheumatoid arthritis, systemic immunosuppression, diabetes mellitus, chronic kidney disease, and malignancy the risk of PJI is as high as 2.2-fold [9].

Inflammatory arthritis as well as the **medications** used for their management are associated with a higher risk of infection [10, 11]. The International Consensus Group has published practice guidelines for discontinuing anti-rheumatoid medications prior to joint arthroplasty [12]. It may be safe to continue nonbiologic disease-modifying antirheumatic drugs (DMARDs) through joint arthroplasty [13, 14], methotrexate may be withheld when there is concern for wound healing problems. It is recommended to withhold tumor necrosis factor alpha inhibitors around the time of arthroplasty surgery or revision [15, 16]. In practice, the management of biologic and nonbiologic DMARDs during joint arthroplasty or PJI treatment is varied and should be individualized, in consultation with the treating rheumatologist.

Glycemic control in the perioperative period essential to decrease the risk of PJI, especially in diabetics [8, 17–20]. Perioperative hyperglycemia may be a better marker of control than Haemoglobin A1c [8]. Postopertaive blood glucose should be maintained between 110 and 180 g/dL and standard diabetic algorithm to maintain strict control of blood glucose in the peri-operative phase can be beneficial [17, 21].

High and low **body weight (BMI)** have been associated with an increased risk of infection [6, 8, 17, 18, 20–22]. Optimising the patients weight by education, counselling, dietician review and or surgical intervention seems to be beneficial approach to reduce the risk of PJI.

Perioperative infection at a distant site, including the urinary or respiratory tract, is associated with an increased risk of PJI [6, 18]. Presence of symptomatic urinary tract infection or urinary tract obstruction and WBC count greater than 10,000 cells/ML should prompt delaying surgery until after treatment [23, 24].

There is also some **selected evidence** to recommend the possible role of smoking [18], antecedent bacteremia (during the previous year) [25], antecedent septic arthritis of the index joint [5], postoperative surgical site hematoma, superficial surgical site infection, wound drainage, and wound dehiscence [5, 6, 25] in the development of PJI. Care to avoid prolonged procedure duration [5, 26, 27], and allogeneic blood transfusion [5, 6, 28, 29] may also be beneficial in avoiding PJI.

Preoperative **screen for staphylococcus skin flora** and decolonisation [30, 31] and perioperative antimicrobial prophylaxis [32, 33] reduces the risk of surgical site infection, which is a well-established risk factor for subsequent PJI [5, 6, 25].

Antibiotic Prophylaxis

Evidence from rigorous case-control studies suggests that there is no increased risk of PJI following either low- or high-risk dental procedures [9]. Furthermore, antimicrobial prophylaxis given before dental procedures does not decrease the risk of subsequent PJI [9]. Antimicrobial prophylaxis is also not indicated for prevention of PJI in patients undergoing urologic or endoscopic gastrointestinal procedures. However, given the heterogenous nature of these procedures, the decision to provide prophylaxis should be made on an individual basis.

Diagnosing PJI

It is essential to understand that no test for PJI has 100 % diagnostic accuracy and the treating surgeon must correlate the clinical and radiographic presentation with a combination of serum blood tests, synovial fluid analysis, microbiological and histopathological evaluation of periprosthetic tissue and intraoperative inspection to reach a definitive diagnosis.

Diagnosis should begin with a **high index of suspicion** for new onset of pain or symptoms in well-functioning joints. Plain radiographs may identify osteolysis or early signs of implant failure and should be promptly investigated further for PJI.

Serum Blood Tests

Serum blood tests such as peripheral blood ESR and CRP remain the most widely used next step for the diagnosis of PJI. Both these tests are widely available, inexpensive, and have a rapid turnaround time in laboratories. The results should be interpreted with caution due to their relative lack of specificity. The sensitivity and specificity values for CRP are approximately 88 and 74 %, respectively; while that of ESR is slightly lower at 75 and 70 %, respectively [34]. The combined ESR and CRP tests are 96 % sensitive for ruling out PJI, but the specificity of this combination is as low as 56 % [35]. The role of interleukin-6 and procalcitonin in routine clinical practice for diagnosing infection remains to be established.

Advanced Imaging Modalities

Advanced imaging modalities such as three-phase bone scintigraphy, radioactive. 111In labelled autologous leukocytes scan, [18F] Fluoro-2-deoxyglucose positron emission tomography (FDG-PET) may be used as a part of the diagnostic algorithm at this point. However, they require expert interpretation and are limited by availability and high costs. When available they have high sensitivity and specificity [12, 36, 37], but their routine use is not recommended and indications have to be individualised in the light of clinical presentation.

Synovial Fluid Analysis

In the presence of high clinical suspicion and elevated peripheral blood ESR and or CRP, the clinician should plan synovial fluid analysis. This provides a synovial fluid white cell count with differential cell count, specimen for culture and possibility of analysing other synovial fluid markers.

Synovial Fluid White Cell Count and Differential

A white cell count of 3000 cells/microL and 80 % differential has been set as the threshold for diagnosis of chronic infections, by the International Consensus Group [12]. It is important to note that failed metal-on-metal hip arthroplasties can give a falsely elevated synovial fluid cell count when using automated cell counters. This can be overcome by manually counting cell numbers.

Synovial Fluid Culture

Synovial fluid should be directly into blood culture bottles [38], and antibiotics should be withheld at least 2 weeks [39, 40] prior to aspiration, whenever possible. The pooled sensitivity of synovial fluid culture is 72 % and a specificity as high as 95 % [41]. Cultures also help establish the organism, virulence and sensitivities that help plan subsequent treatment algorithm.

Novel Synovial Fluid Markers

The role of synovial fluid ESR, CRP, leucocyte esterase and antimicrobial peptides continue to be researched. Synovial fluid leucocyte esterase remains the most widely studied and can be measured using commercially available colorimetric strips. It has been included as supporting criteria for diagnosis of PJI in the International Consensus Meeting definition of PJI [42].

Synovial fluid analysis is an excellent adjuvant to establish PJI and guide further treatment. If aspirate fails to yield fluid despite a second repeated attempt, the surgeon should formulate a working diagnosis based on the presentation and peripheral blood markers. The advanced imaging modalities discussed above are helpful in this scenario. In our practice a MDT approach is used to decide the best practice at this point. Where there is a high clinical, laboratory or radiological suspicion of infection, the working diagnosis should be PJI until proven otherwise.

Periprosthetic Tissue Biopsy

Testing periprosthetic tissue provides valuable information in microbiological diagnosis and workup of PJI. Where an opportunity is available to obtain pre-operative samples such as when arthroscopic assessment or washout of the joint is conducted, tissue biopsy is recommended. However, routine attempt at pre-operative tissue biopsy is not necessary due to lack of demonstrated superiority over aspiration and the additional expense and possible complications of the involved procedure [43].

Routine use of **gram staining** is not recommended due to poor sensitivity [44]. However, frozen section may have some role [30], especially when performed by skilled pathologist and finding of 5–10 neutrophils per high power field is considered consistent with PJI [45].

Tissue culture remains the gold standard for diagnosis despite false-positive and false-negative results. Whenever possible multiple samples should be obtained (three to five) to aid interpretation [12]. A threshold of two to three positive specimens yielding indistinguishable microorganisms has been recommended to improve sensitivity [30, 46].

Histological Analysis of Periprosthetic Tissue

Acute inflammation, evidenced by neutrophilic infiltrate on fixed or frozen tissue, is suggestive of PJI. Acute inflammation, defined as the presence of at least five neutrophils per high-powered field, in at least five separate microscopic fields [24], has been included in the recent consensus definitions for PJI [42].

Sonication of Removed Prosthetic Component

Sonication of the prosthesis is used to dislodge the biofilm and the associated bacteria from the surface of the implant. With this approach, low-frequency ultrasound waves pass through liquid surrounding the prosthesis, creating areas of high and low pressure [47]. Microscopic bubbles are formed during the low-pressure stage and collapse during the high-pressure stage, releasing energy and liberating bacteria from the surface of the implant. The fluid surrounding the implant can used for culture or analysis. Vortexing of the prosthesis alone may be a viable alternative in laboratories in which sonication is not available [48]. Several studies have demonstrated a higher sensitivity for culture of sonication fluid (62–94 %) than periprosthetic tissue (54–88 %) [46, 49–54].

PCR Testing

Synovial fluid aspirate, periprosthetic tissue or sonicate fluid may be subject to molecular diagnosis to amplify genetic material and improve microbilogical diagnosis of PJI [49]. This technique has shown increased sensitivity in patients who had received antibiotics within 14 days before implant removal. Results have to carefully interpreted with due consideration for possibility of false positive results.

Treatment

The goals of managing late PJI treatment are to eradicate the infection, restore pain-free function of the joint, and minimize patient morbidity and mortality. This may be achieved using several techniques, and the latter are often guided by patient and microbiological factors (Fig. 16.1).

MDT Approach

We have published on our multidisciplinary team approach for diagnosis and management of periprosthetic infection [55]. The multidisciplinary team included microbiologists, infectious disease specialists, orthopaedic surgeons, radiologists, physiotherapists and physicians who review all patients, and their management is discussed at every stage in their pathway. The outcome of aspiration and biopsy is used to isolate the micro-organism and determine its antibiotic sensitivity and the most appropriate antibiotics for the first stage. Multiple tissue samples are sent at the time of this operation and helped to determine the type and duration of antibiotic treatment in the interval period, and the antibiotic cover required for the second stage.

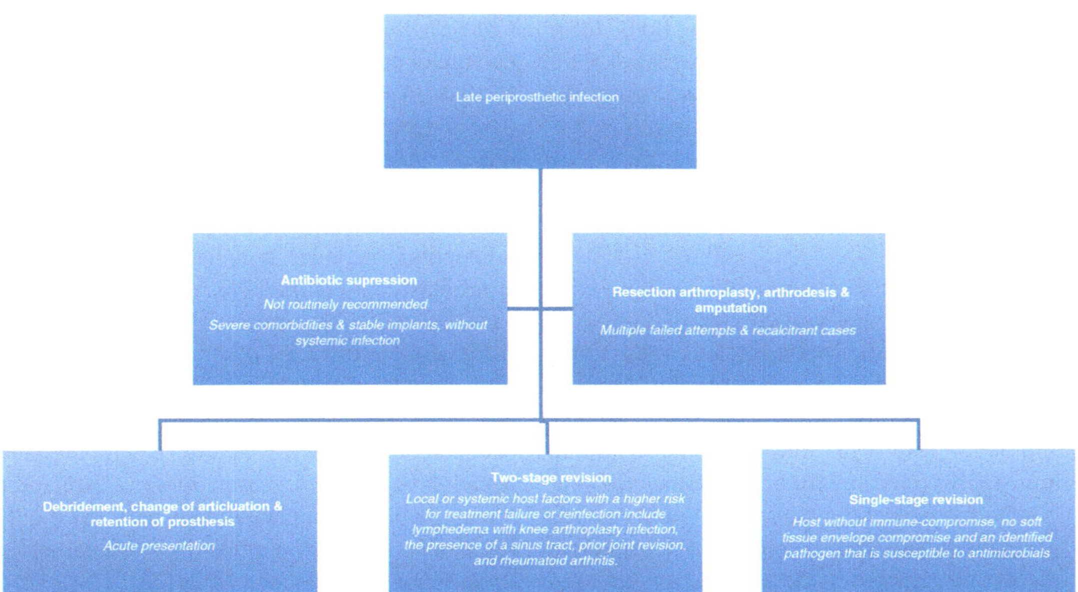

Fig. 16.1 Guide to treatment options in late periprosthetic infection

Debridement and Implant Retention (DAIR)

Late acute (<3 weeks) haematogenous infections, may be suitable for debridement and modular exchange with implant retention if the implants are not loose. The attraction of implant retention is the presumed lower morbidity to the patient of non-removal of well-fixed implants. The success rate of this technique is low when infection has been present for more 3 weeks, if a sinus tract is present or an arthroscopic debridement was undertaken for knee PJI [56]. As the success of this technique is dependent on debridement, it must be meticulous, and all infected-looking material must be removed. Adding local antibiotic-impregnated cement beads can be added to achieve high-dose local antibiotic delivery [57]. The treatment success rate of DAIR reported in the literature ranges from 31 to 82 % depending on the type of infections and the nature of microorganisms [56, 58–61].

Revision Arthroplasty

Debate continues worldwide over the ideal revision technique for PJI, with enthusiast demonstrating comparable results with both these approaches [62–67]. In our centre we have demonstrated successful results achieved using the single stage technique.

Two-Stage Revision

One approach for treatment of late PJI is a two-stage revision with a variable length course of high-dose antibiotics between the stages (traditionally 4–6 weeks). A cement spacer impregnated with antibiotic can be used to produce high local levels of antibiotic and maintain limb stability and length between the two procedures [68]. Vancomycin is commonly added for gram positive infections and tobramycin for gram-negative infections. Articulating spacers have been used to limit the functional deficit following multiple procedures and to avoid extended periods of compromised joint function. They also make revision surgery technically easier and have shown superior results to static spacers [69]. So-called "poorly cemented" cheaper prostheses are increasingly used in some centres as a stable temporary joint replacement to permit near full function, whilst providing all the benefits of local antibiotic therapy of cement spacers and reducing the risks of spacer fracture. In the knee, the removed components can be sterilised and loosely cemented to act as articulating spacers with excellent infection eradication and obvious cost benefits [70, 71].

The timing of reimplantion in a two-stage revision should be based on clinical evaluation, assessment of peripheral blood ESR and CRP and repeat synovial aspiration where possible. The use of inflammatory markers has not been found to be prognostic; despite no evidence of residual infection at time of revision, an elevated ESR and CRP were found in 50 and 20 % of cases, respectively [72]. There is some evidence that repeat synovial aspiration prior to second stage revision in the knee is beneficial in reducing the failure rate [73], if positive sampling is treated with repeat debridement and a second parenteral course of antibiotics.

Risk factors for treatment failure following two-stage arthroplasty exchange can be host-related factors, pathogen-related factors, or treatment-related factors. Local or systemic host factors with a higher risk for treatment failure or reinfection include lymphedema with knee arthroplasty infection [74], the presence of a sinus tract [75, 76], prior joint revision [77], and rheumatoid arthritis [77].

Reimplantation within 2 weeks of resection has a low likelihood of success, particularly in patients infected with *S. aureus* or aerobic gram-negative bacilli [78]. Furthermore, a structured protocol where reimplantation is performed only if cultures are negative prior to the second-stage surgery may improve outcomes [73].

One-Stage Revision

Proposed advantages one stage revision include lower morbidity, shorter overall hospital stay, lower cost and less interference with patients quality of life [79, 80]. Results from European centres using cemented revision components suggest more than 90 % eradication of infection [79]. Some of the criteria associated with successful single stage include host without immune compromise, no soft tissue envelope compromise and an identified pathogen that is susceptible to antimicrobials available orally and in PMMA [81, 82] (60, 352 t). The pooled results for single stage revisions showed an overall infection free rate of 82 % [83].

Antimicrobial Treatment Alone

Nonsurgical management of PJI is not recommended. It should be considered only for those who are unable to undergo even a single surgical procedure (e.g., due to multiple comorbidities) or are unwilling to undergo surgery and who have a well-fixed prosthesis and infection with microorganisms that are susceptible to oral antibiotics. Such a strategy is likely to be more successful in those with early rather than delayed or chronic infection [84].

The optimal antimicrobial treatment program with a nonsurgical strategy is unknown. Typically, patients are given 4–6 weeks of pathogen-directed intravenous or highly bioavailable oral antimicrobials, based on antimicrobial susceptibilities determined by joint aspirate culture. This may be given as combination therapy with rifampin [84]. Many patients will ultimately be placed on prolonged or indefinite oral antimicrobial suppression. The choice of the suppressive antimicrobial must take into account toxicity, oral bioavailability, cost, and frequency of administration, drug interactions, and the need for ongoing therapeutic monitoring.

Resection Arthroplasty, Arthrodesis, and Amputation

These are reserved for frail patient with recalcitrant infection, who is not suitable for reconstruction, or those with failed treatment with repeated revisions.

Surgical Technique for Revision THA

The following section describes the surgical technique we use in our institution for infected revision arthroplasty [85].

The skin is prepared twice with 3 M™ DuraPrep™ solution, containing iodine povacrylex and isopropyl alcohol. Drapes are applied in a regular fashion, the previous incision is marked, and a 3 M™ Ioban™ antimicrobial incision drape is then placed directly on the skin. We do not routinely inflate the tourniquet for the knee joint at this stage, as our experience has shown that this minimizes tourniquet-related adverse effects.

In all hip arthroplasty patients, we use a posterior approach. A midline incision and medial parapatella approach is used in knee arthroplasty, utilising the previous incision scar when possible. Following adequate exposure, a thorough synovectomy is undertaken, and all inflamed tissue is debrided and excised using a combination of curettage, knife and surgical diathermy whilst maintaining haemostatsis.

Both superficial and deep samples of any fluid, infected tissue, bone or tissue between implant-cement or implant-bone interfaces are sent for aerobic, anaerobic and extended microbiology cultures. Five samples are adequate but must be representative of the entire surgical field, as the isolation of an indistinguishable microorganism from three or more independent specimens has been shown to be highly predictive of infection (sensitivity 65 %; specificity 99.6 %), except unusual virulent species where a single growth is significant. Histological samples are only sent if there is suspicion within the joint tissue, that macroscopically appears unusual for infection (the procedure will continue as previously planned, except in extreme circumstances).

Microbe-specific antibiotics, based on previous sensitivities or empirically chosen following discussions with the microbiologists, are now administered.

Specifically designed or generic instruments are used to explant the prosthesis, taking care to avoid any inadvertent bone loss. In the presence of florid infection, implants may be loose and easy to extract. Once the implant has been removed, further debridement will be required of the distal femoral and tibial shafts, or of the acetabulum and proximal femoral shaft, to remove necrotic tissue or biofilm.

Following debridement, the wound is irrigated with 12 l of warm 0.9 % saline via pulsatile lavage, followed by a 50:50 mix of 100 mL of 3 % hydrogen peroxide and 100 mls of sterile water solution. Hydrogen peroxide is used for its chemical debriding characteristics, as it has been shown to be relatively ineffective at reducing bacterial count. A further 0.9 % saline irrigation removes the hydrogen peroxide from the surgical field, which is then irrigated with 200 mL of 10 % aqueous povidone-iodine (1 % available iodine) although more dilute concentrations have shown some benefit. Povidone-iodine is known to have bactericidal activity without adversely effecting wound healing, but there is controversy over possible cytotoxic effects to host tissues.

The same concentration of povidone-iodine is used to soak cotton-gauze, which is then packed within the wound, and skin edges approximated temporarily with a continuous 1-vicryl. This is covered with an antimicrobial incision drape to maintain wound sterility.

The drapes are discarded and the operative team descrubs with the wound protected by the antimicrobial incision drape. The next step depends on whether a single-stage or two-stage revision is planned. For a two-stage revision, an antibiotic-loaded cement spacer, either dynamic or static, is inserted after changing drapes and equipment.

The spacer usually contained 3 g of vancomycin and 2 g of gentamicin per 40 g sachet of Palacos R cement (Schering Plough Ltd, Labo nv, Belgium), unless otherwise indicated.

For a single-stage revision, the team then prepares for the second half of the procedure by rescrubbing and opening new sterile instruments. None of the previously used instruments are reused at this stage. The surgical field is re-draped and the skin and the antimicrobial incision drape overlying the wound is prepped using 3 M™ DuraPrep™ solution.

The sterile wound drape is then removed, together with the sutures and gauze. The wound is irrigated further with 200 mL of 10 % aqueous povidone-iodine, followed by 1 l of pulsatile lavaged 0.9 % saline.

The femur and tibia, or acetabulum, are prepared for the insertion of the new prostheses, which may require antibiotic-laden acrylic cement or tantalum cones if there has been significant bone loss.

During the cementing of the components, we add 2 g of vancomycin per 40 g of Simplex P bone cement, which does not compromise tensile or compressive strength of the cement. In high-risk patients, higher doses of antibiotics such as 6–8 g of antibiotic per 40 g of cement have been shown to be systemically safe and effective. The cement is hand mixed with vacuum, but once fully mixed the powdered vancomycin is added and mixed by hand without vacuum to improve antibiotic elution.

Alternatively, if the components are uncemented, autogenic cancellous bone graft may be used with 3.64 % vancomycin per weight of bone graft. Powdered vancomycin can be placed upon the prosthetic stems, or as pellets on the surgical site before closure. The antibiotic choice may vary depending upon microbiology sensitivities.

The tourniquet is only inflated during cementing of knee arthroplasty to improve haemostasis and cement-bone interface, and remains inflated until the end of the procedure.

Prior to closure, further irrigation is undertaken with 1 l of 0.9 % sodium chloride. Drains may be inserted to prevent early postoperative haematoma formation, but removed within the first 24 h to allow high local concentrations of antibiotics. A meticulous closure is established with 2/0 VICRYL™ suture to the fascial and subcutaneous layer, and 3/0 MONOCRYL™ as a continuous subcuticular suture. A sterile Mepore® absorbent dressing is then applied, with compression obtained by a layer of folded cotton gauze and Mefix® for THEA, or wool and bandage for TKEA.

Conclusion

Late presentation of PJI can be a devastating complication to the patient and can pose a huge economic burden to the treating organisation. We have presented here an evidence-based algorithmic approach to prevention, diagnosis and treatment of PJI. In our opinion, measures to prevent PJI remain the key strategy for future and perhaps the most cost-effective. New-onset pain or symptoms in a well-functioning joint should raise the suspicion of infection. A thorough history and examination followed by serum ESR, CRP and synovial aspirate helps to confirm diagnosis in most cases. Several new imaging modalities as well as biomarkers are available as adjunctive tools to aid diagnosis. Treatment should be tailored to individual patients, taking into consideration host and microbiological factors.

References

1. Kurtz S, Ong K, Lau E, Mowat F, Halpern M. Projections of primary and revision hip and knee arthroplasty in the united states from 2005 to 2030. J Bone Joint Surg Series A. 2007;89(4):780–5.
2. Labek G, Thaler M, Janda W, Agreiter M, Stöckl B. Revision rates after total joint replacement: cumulative results from worldwide joint register datasets. J Bone Joint Surg Series B. 2011;93B(3):293–7.
3. Zmistowski B, Karam JA, Durinka JB, Casper DS, Parvizi J. Periprosthetic joint infection increases the risk of one-year mortality. J Bone Joint Surg Series A. 2013;95(24):2177–84.
4. Vanhegan IS, Malik AK, Jayakumar P, Ul Islam S, Haddad FS. A financial analysis of revision hip arthroplasty. J Bone Joint Surg Series B. 2012;94B(5):619–23.
5. Berbari EF, Hanssen AD, Duffy MC, Steckelberg JM, Ilstrup DM, Harmsen WS, et al. Risk factors for prosthetic joint infection: case-control study. Clin Infect Dis. 1998;27(5):1247–54.
6. Pulido L, Ghanem E, Joshi A, Purtill JJ, Parvizi J. Periprosthetic joint infection: the incidence, timing, and predisposing factors. Clin Orthop. 2008; 466(7):1710–5.
7. Namba RS, Inacio MCS, Paxton EW. Risk factors associated with surgical site infection in 30 491 primary total hip replacements. J Bone Joint Surg Series B. 2012;94B(10):1330–8.
8. Namba RS, Inacio MCS, Paxton EW. Risk factors associated with deep surgical site infections after primary total knee arthroplasty: an analysis of 56,216 knees. J Bone Joint Surg Series A. 2013;95(9):775–82.
9. Berbari EF, Osmon DR, Carr A, Hanssen AD, Baddour LM, Greene D, et al. Dental procedures as risk factors for prosthetic hip or knee infection: a hospital-based prospective case-control study. Clin Infect Dis. 2010;50(1):8–16.
10. Pandey R, Berendt AR, Athanasou NA. Histological and microbiological findings in non-infected and infected revision arthroplasty tissues. Arch Orthop Trauma Surg. 2000;120(10):570–4.
11. Cipriano CA, Brown NM, Michael AM, Moric M, Sporer SM, Della Valle CJ. Serum and synovial fluid analysis for diagnosing chronic periprosthetic infection in patients with inflammatory arthritis. J Bone Joint Surg Series A. 2012;94(7):594–600.
12. Parvizi J, Zmistowski B, Berbari EF, Bauer TW, Springer BD, Della Valle CJ, et al. New definition for periprosthetic joint infection: from the workgroup of the musculoskeletal infection society. Clin Orthop. 2011;469(11):2992–4.
13. Tanaka N, Sakahashi H, Sato E, Hirose K, Ishima T, Ishii S. Examination of the risk of continuous leflunomide treatment on the incidence of infectious complications after joint arthroplasty in patients with rheumatoid arthritis. J Clin Rheumatol. 2003;9(2): 115–8.
14. Grennan DM, Gray J, Loudon J, Fear S. Methotrexate and early postoperative complications in patients with rheumatoid arthritis undergoing elective orthopaedic surgery. Ann Rheum Dis. 2001;60(3):214–7.
15. Ding T, Ledingham J, Luqmani R, Westlake S, Hyrich K, Lunt M, et al. BSR and BHPR rheumatoid arthritis guidelines on safety of anti-TNF therapies. Rheumatology. 2010;49(11):2217–9.
16. Saag KG, Teng GG, Patkar NM, Anuntiyo J, Finney C, Curtis JR, et al. American College of Rheumatology 2008 recommendations for the use of nonbiologic and biologic disease-modifying antirheumatic drugs in rheumatoid arthritis. Arthritis Care Res. 2008;59(6): 762–84.
17. Malinzak RA, Ritter MA, Berend ME, Meding JB, Olberding EM, Davis KE. Morbidly obese, diabetic, younger, and unilateral joint arthroplasty patients have elevated total joint arthroplasty infection rates. J Arthroplasty. 2009;24(6):84–8.
18. Peersman G, Laskin R, Davis J, Peterson M. The insall award paper: infection in total knee replacement: a retrospective review of 6489 total knee replacements. Clin Orthop. 2001;392:15–23.
19. Dowsey MM, Choong PFM. Obesity is a major risk factor for prosthetic infection after primary hip arthroplasty. Clin Orthop. 2008;466(1):153–8.

20. Cazanave C, Greenwood-Quaintance KE, Hanssen AD, Karau MJ, Schmidt SM, Gomez Urena EO, et al. Rapid molecular microbiologic diagnosis of prosthetic joint infection. J Clin Microbiol. 2013;51(7):2280–7.
21. Dowsey MM, Choong PFM. Obese diabetic patients are at substantial risk for deep infection after primary TKA. Clin Orthop. 2009;467(6):1577–81.
22. Berbari EF, Osmon DR, Lahr B, Eckel-Passow JE, Tsaras G, Hanssen AD, et al. The Mayo prosthetic joint infection risk score: implication for surgical site infection reporting and risk stratification. Infect Control Hosp Epidemiol. 2012;33(8):774–81.
23. Fehring TK, McAlister Jr JA. Frozen histologic section as a guide to sepsis in revision joint arthroplasty. Clin Orthop. 1994;304:229–37.
24. Feldman DS, Lonner JH, Desai P, Zuckerman JD. The role of intraoperative frozen sections in revision total joint arthroplasty. J Bone Joint Surg Series A. 1995;77(12):1807–13.
25. Aslam S, Reitman C, Darouiche RO. Risk factors for subsequent diagnosis of prosthetic joint infection. Infect Control Hosp Epidemiol. 2010;31(3):298–301.
26. Fitzgerald Jr RH, Nolan DR, Ilstrup DM, Van Scoy RE, Washington II JA, Coventry MB. Deep wound sepsis following total hip arthroplasty. J Bone Joint Surg Series A. 1977;59(7):847–55.
27. Ong KL, Kurtz SM, Lau E, Bozic KJ, Berry DJ, Parvizi J. Prosthetic joint infection risk after total hip arthroplasty in the medicare population. J Arthroplasty. 2009;24(6):105–9.
28. Innerhofer P, Klingler A, Klimmer C, Fries D, Nussbaumer W. Risk for postoperative infection after transfusion of white blood cell-filtered allogeneic or autologous blood components in orthopedic patients undergoing primary arthroplasty. Transfusion. 2005;45(1):103–10.
29. Rosencher N, Kerkkamp HE, Macheras G, Munuera LM, Menichella G, Barton DM, et al. Orthopedic Surgery Transfusion Hemoglobin European Overview (OSTHEO) study: blood management in elective knee and hip arthroplasty in Europe. Transfusion. 2003;43(4):459–69.
30. Schäfer P, Fink B, Sandow D, Margull A, Berger I, Frommelt L. Prolonged bacterial culture to identify late periprosthetic joint infection: a promising strategy. Clin Infect Dis. 2008;47(11):1403–9.
31. Ghanem E, Parvizi J, Clohisy J, Burnett S, Sharkey PF, Barrack R. Perioperative antibiotics should not be withheld in proven cases of periprosthetic infection. Clin Orthop. 2007;461:44–7.
32. Hill C, Mazas F, Flamant R, Evrard J. Prophylactic cefazolin versus placebo in total hip replacement: report of a multicentre double-blind randomised trial. Lancet. 1981;317(8224):795–7.
33. AlBuhairn B, Hind D, Hutchinson A. Antibiotic prophylaxis for wound infections in total joint arthroplasty: a systematic review. J Bone Joint Surg Series B. 2008;90(7):915–9.
34. Berbari E, Mabry T, Tsaras G, Spangehl M, Erwin PJ, Murad MH, et al. Inflammatory blood laboratory levels as markers of prosthetic joint infection: a systematic review and meta-analysis. J Bone Joint Surg Series A. 2010;92(11):2102–9.
35. Austin MS, Ghanem E, Joshi A, Lindsay A, Parvizi J. A simple, cost-effective screening protocol to rule out periprosthetic infection. J Arthroplasty. 2008;23(1):65–8.
36. Kwee TC, Kwee RM, Alavi A. FDG-PET for diagnosing prosthetic joint infection: systematic review and meta-analysis. Eur J Nucl Med Mol Imaging. 2008;35(11):2122–32.
37. Teller RE, Christie MJ, Martin W, Nance EP, Haas DW. Sequential indium-labeled leukocyte and bone scans to diagnose prosthetic joint infection. Clin Orthop. 2000;373:241–7.
38. Hughes JG, Vetter EA, Patel R, Schleck CD, Harmsen S, Turgeant LT, et al. Culture with BACTEC Peds Plus/F bottle compared with conventional methods for detection of bacteria in synovial fluid. J Clin Microbiol. 2001;39(12):4468–71.
39. Ali F, Wilkinson JM, Cooper JR, Kerry RM, Hamer AJ, Norman P, Stockley I. Accuracy of joint aspiration for the preoperative diagnosis of infection in total hip arthroplasty. J Arthroplasty. 2006;21(2):221–6.
40. Roberts P, Walters AJ, McMinn DJW. Diagnosing infection in hip replacements. The use of fine-needle aspiration and radiometric culture. J Bone Joint Surg Series B. 1992;74(2):265–9.
41. Parvizi J, Jacovides C, Zmistowski B, Jung KA. Definition of periprosthetic joint infection: is there a consensus? Clin Orthop. 2011;469(11):3022–30.
42. Parvizi J, Gehrke T, Chen AF. Proceedings of the international consensus on periprosthetic joint infection. Bone Joint J. 2013;95B(11):1450–2.
43. Parvizi J, Heller S, Berend KR, Della Valle CJ, Springer BD. Periprosthetic joint infection: the algorithmic approach and emerging evidence. Instr Course Lect. 2015;64:51–60.
44. Mirra JM, Marder RA, Amstutz HC. The pathology of failed total joint arthroplasty. Clin Orthop. 1982;170:175–83.
45. Padgett DE, Silverman A, Sachjowicz F, Simpson RB, Rosenberg AG, Galante JO. Efficacy of intraoperative cultures obtained during revision total hip arthroplasty. J Arthroplasty. 1995;10(4):420–6.
46. Trampuz A, Piper KE, Jacobson MJ, Hanssen AD, Unni KK, Osmon DR, et al. Sonication of removed hip and knee prostheses for diagnosis of infection. N Engl J Med. 2007;357(7):654–63.
47. Trampuz A, Osmon DR, Hanssen AD, Steckelberg JM, Patel R. Molecular and antibiofilm approaches to prosthetic joint infection. Clin Orthop. 2003;414:69–88.
48. Kobayashi H, Oethinger M, Tuohy MJ, Procop GW, Bauer TW. Improved detection of biofilm-formative bacteria by vortexing and sonication: a pilot study. Clin Orthop. 2009;467(5):1360–4.

49. Achermann Y, Vogt M, Leunig M, Wüst J, Trampuz A. Improved diagnosis of periprosthetic joint infection by multiplex PCR of sonication fluid from removed implants. J Clin Microbiol. 2010;48(4):1208–14.
50. Bori G, Muñoz-Mahamud E, Garcia S, Mallofre C, Gallart X, Bosch J, et al. Interface membrane is the best sample for histological study to diagnose prosthetic joint infection. Mod Pathol. 2011;24(4):579–84.
51. Esteban J, Gomez-Barrena E, Cordero J, Martín-de-Hijas NZ, Kinnari TJ, Fernandez-Roblas R. Evaluation of quantitative analysis of cultures from sonicated retrieved orthopedic implants in diagnosis of orthopedic infection. J Clin Microbiol. 2008;46(2):488–92.
52. Holinka J, Bauer L, Hirschl AM, Graninger W, Windhager R, Presterl E. Sonication cultures of explanted components as an add-on test to routinely conducted microbiological diagnostics improve pathogen detection. J Orthop Res. 2011;29(4):617–22.
53. Piper KE, Jacobson MJ, Cofield RH, Sperling JW, Sanchez-Sotelo J, Osmon DR, et al. Microbiologic diagnosis of prosthetic shoulder infection by use of implant sonication. J Clin Microbiol. 2009;47(6):1878–84.
54. Vergidis P, Greenwood-Quaintance KE, Sanchez-Sotelo J, Morrey BF, Steinmann SP, Karau MJ, et al. Implant sonication for the diagnosis of prosthetic elbow infection. J Shoulder Elbow Surg. 2011;20(8):1275–81.
55. Ibrahim MS, Raja S, Khan MA, Haddad FS. A multidisciplinary team approach to twostage revision for the infected hip replacement: a minimum five-year follow-up study. Bone Joint J. 2014;96B(10):1312–8.
56. Marculescu CE, Berbari EF, Hanssen AD, Steckelberg JM, Harmsen SW, Mandrekar JN, et al. Outcome of prosthetic joint infections treated with debridement and retention of components. Clin Infect Dis. 2006;42(4):471–8.
57. Wininger DA, Fass RJ. Antibiotic-impregnated cement and beads for orthopedic infections. Antimicrob Agents Chemother. 1996;40(12):2675–9.
58. Cobo J, Miguel LG, Euba G, Rodríguez D, García-Lechuz JM, Riera M, et al. Early prosthetic joint infection: outcomes with debridement and implant retention followed by antibiotic therapy. Clin Microbiol Infect. 2011;17(11):1632–7.
59. Konigsberg BS, Valle CJ, Ting NT, Qiu F, Sporer SM. Acute hematogenous infection following total hip and knee arthroplasty. J Arthroplasty. 2014;29(3):469–72.
60. Koyonos L, Zmistowski B, Della Valle CJ, Parvizi J. Infection control rate of irrigation and debridement for periprosthetic joint infection. Clin Orthop. 2011;469(11):3043–8.
61. Mont MA, Waldman B, Banerjee C, Pacheco IH, Hungerford DS. Multiple irrigation, debridement, and retention of components in infected total knee arthroplasty. J Arthroplasty. 1997;12(4):426–33.
62. Deirmengian C, Hallab N, Tarabishy A, Della Valle C, Jacobs JJ, Lonner J, et al. Synovial fluid biomarkers for periprosthetic infection. Clin Orthop. 2010;468(8):2017–23.
63. Azzam KA, Seeley M, Ghanem E, Austin MS, Purtill JJ, Parvizi J. Irrigation and debridement in the management of prosthetic joint infection: traditional indications revisited. J Arthroplasty. 2010;25(7):1022–7.
64. Greidanus NV, Masri BA, Garbuz DS, Wilson SD, McAlinden MG, Xu M, et al. Use of erythrocyte sedimentation rate and C-reactive protein level to diagnose infection before revision total knee arthroplasty: a prospective evaluation. J Bone Joint Surg Series A. 2007;89(7):1409–16.
65. Odum SM, Fehring TK, Lombardi AV, Zmistowski BM, Brown NM, Luna JT, et al. Irrigation and debridement for periprosthetic infections: does the organism matter? J Arthroplasty. 2011;26:114–8.
66. Parvizi J, Jacovides C, Adeli B, Jung KA, Hozack WJ, Mark B. Coventry award. Clin Orthop. 2012;470(1):54–60.
67. Sherrell JC, Fehring TK, Odum S, Hansen E, Zmistowski B, Dennos A, et al. The Chitranjan Ranawat award: fate of two-stage reimplantation after failed irrigation and debridement for periprosthetic knee infection. Clin Orthop. 2011;469(1):18–25.
68. Evans RP. Successful treatment of total hip and knee infection with articulating antibiotic components: a modified treatment method. Clin Orthop. 2004;427:37–46.
69. Romanò CL, Gala L, Logoluso N, Romanò D, Drago L. Two-stage revision of septic knee prosthesis with articulating knee spacers yields better infection eradication rate than one-stage or two-stage revision with static spacers. Knee Surg Sports Traumatol Arthrosc. 2012;20(12):2445–53.
70. Lee JK, Choi CH. Two-stage reimplantation in infected total knee arthroplasty using a re-sterilized tibial polyethylene insert and femoral component. J Arthroplasty. 2012;27(9):1701–1706.e1.
71. Hofmann AA, Kane KR, Tkach TK, Plaster RL, Camargo MP. Treatment of infected total knee arthroplasty using an articulating spacer. Clin Orthop. 1995;321:45–54.
72. Kusuma SK, Ward J, Jacofsky M, Sporer SM, Della Valle CJ. What is the role of serological testing between stages of two-stage reconstruction of the infected prosthetic knee? Clin Orthop. 2011;469(4):1002–8.
73. Mont MA, Waldman BJ, Hungerford DS. Evaluation of preoperative cultures before second-stage reimplantation of a total knee prosthesis complicated by infection. A comparison-group study. J Bone Joint Surg Series A. 2000;82(11):1552–7.
74. Kubista B, Hartzler RU, Wood CM, Osmon DR, Hanssen AD, Lewallen DG. Reinfection after two-stage revision for periprosthetic infection of total knee arthroplasty. Int Orthop. 2012;36(1):65–71.

75. Betsch BY, Eggli S, Siebenrock KA, Täuber MG, Mühlemann K. Treatment of joint prosthesis infection in accordance with current recommendations improves outcome. Clin Infect Dis. 2008;46(8):1221–6.
76. Mortazavi SMJ, Vegari D, Ho A, Zmistowski B, Parvizi J. Two-stage exchange arthroplasty for infected total knee arthroplasty: predictors of failure. Clin Orthop. 2011;469(11):3049–54.
77. Hirakawa K, Stulberg BN, Wilde AH, Bauer TW, Secic M. Results of 2-stage reimplantation for infected total knee arthroplasty. J Arthroplasty. 1998;13(1):22–8.
78. Rand JA, Bryan RS. Reimplantation for the salvage of an infected total knee arthroplasty. J Bone Joint Surg Series A. 1983;65(8):1081–6.
79. Gehrke T, Zahar A, Kendoff D. One-stage exchange: it all began here. Bone Joint J. 2013;95B(11):77–83.
80. Sia IG, Berbari EF, Karchmer AW. Prosthetic joint infections. Infect Dis Clin North Am. 2005;19(4):885–914.
81. Osmon DR, Berbari EF, Berendt AR, Lew D, Zimmerli W, Steckelberg JM, et al. Diagnosis and management of prosthetic joint infection: clinical practice guidelines by the Infectious Diseases Society of America. Clin Infect Dis. 2013;56(1):e1–25.
82. Leone S, Borrè S, Monforte A, Mordente G, Petrosillo N, Signore A, et al. Consensus document on controversial issues in the diagnosis and treatment of prosthetic joint infections. Int J Infect Dis. 2010;14: S67–77.
83. Cordero-Ampuero J, González-Fernández E, Martínez-Vélez D, Esteban J. Are antibiotics necessary in hip arthroplasty with asymptomatic bacteriuria? Seeding risk with/without treatment. Clin Orthop. 2013;471(12):3822–9.
84. Pavoni GL, Giannella M, Falcone M, Scorzolini L, Liberatore M, Carlesimo B, et al. Conservative medical therapy of prosthetic joint infections: Retrospective analysis of an 8-year experience. Clin Microbiol Infect. 2004;10(9):831–7.
85. George DA, Konan S, Haddad FS. Single-stage hip and knee exchange for periprosthetic joint infection. J Arthroplasty. 2015;30(12):2264–70.

Late Infections of the Hip Joint: Resection Arthroplasty and Other Solutions

17

Kevin L. Garvin, Beau S. Konigsberg, and Curtis W. Hartman

Abstract

Resection arthroplasty is an acceptable treatment option for an infected hip prosthesis. The operation was described in the literature as a treatment for other pathologic hip conditions long before arthroplasty was a common procedure. It gained popularity as a treatment for infected hip prostheses shortly thereafter and was considered a more necessary intervention before the proliferation of antibiotics and reconstruction implants and techniques available today. The historical perspective, surgical technique, current indications and results are described in this chapter. Also, alternatives to resection arthroplasty, other than hip joint reconstruction, are discussed, including chronic antibiotic suppression with component retention and amputation.

Keywords

Resection arthroplasty • Girdlestone • Failed total hip arthroplasty • Late infections • Indications • Results • Alternatives • Prosthetic infection • Amputation

Historical Perspective

What began as a primary treatment for acute pyogenic arthritis of the hip is most often used now as a salvage operation for patients whose prosthetic joint has become infected and failed reimplantation. In the mid 1800s, Anthony White described femoral head and neck resection for septic arthritis. In 1921 Robert Jones described resection of the femoral head to treat hip ankylosis; and just two years later Girdlestone described resection of the proximal femur as well as the

K.L. Garvin, MD (✉) • B.S. Konigsberg, MD
C.W. Hartman, MD
Department of Orthopaedic Surgery and Rehabilitation, University of Nebraska Medical Center, Omaha, NE, USA
e-mail: kgarvin@unmc.edu

D. Kendoff et al. (eds.), *Periprosthetic Joint Infections: Changing Paradigms*,
DOI 10.1007/978-3-319-30091-7_17

lateral portion of the acetabulum for treatment of the advanced hip infection, particularly tuberculosis [1]. The indications gradually expanded to include the surgical procedure as a primary treatment for osteoarthritis, femoral neck non-unions, muscle spasticity of the hip, neuropathy, acetabular protrusio and other conditions associated with hip destruction. Contemporary resection arthroplasty of the hip is commonly and perhaps inaccurately used synonymously with the procedure described by Girdlestone. Girdlestone did popularize the surgical treatment of hip disease, first describing excision arthroplasty for treating tuberculosis hips in 1928. He later described the operation for severe infections of the hip and stated they were rare in times of peace [1]. As antibiotics were still unavailable, surgical treatment, debridement and drainage for these infections was paramount. The principles of surgical treatment included wide surgical exposure, excision of infected and necrotic tissue (including a large mass of muscle tissue), and leaving the surgical wound packed with Vaseline gauze. Patients were subsequently immobilized for several weeks, often in a hip spica cast. Girdlestone described the surgery for patients with articulating as well as ankylosed joints. He justified the excision of a "large mass of muscle" because the hip joint would either be ankylosed or a pseudoarthrosis and neither type of joint relied on the muscle that he resected.

Although the procedure was life-saving in the early part of the twentieth century, the current role of resection arthroplasty has changed significantly. Bourne et al. provided a six-year follow-up study including 33 Girdlestone arthroplasties performed to salvage the hip after a prosthetic joint infection [2]. The operation effectively relieved the pain of 91 % of the patients and controlled infection in 97 % of the patients. The procedure did not perform as effectively for restoration of function, with only 42 % of the patients satisfied with their functional ability. Eighty-five percent of the patients required a walking aid and three were confined to a bed or wheelchair as non-ambulators. Despite the functional limitations, most (79 %) were satisfied. Currently, resection arthroplasty is performed for patients who, because of medical illness or other reasons, are not candidates for reimplantation of their prosthetic joint. The purpose of this chapter is to provide contemporary information on the indications and results of resection arthroplasty of the hip and other types of salvage procedures for prosthetic joint infection.

Indications

The most common indications for resection arthroplasty include prosthetic joint infection, persistent or recurrent infection after a one- or two-stage reimplantation and rarely aseptic loosening in medically infirm patients. The primary goal of treatment of a prosthetic joint infection is eradication of the infection. The majority of patients are successfully managed as their infection is cleared and they have a successful reimplantation of the prosthesis either in one or two stages. However, a small percent of patients are not candidates for reimplantation of the prosthetic joint. Reimplantation of the prosthesis for a patient with a prosthetic joint infection may not be performed for a number of reasons including patient refusal, poor health, resistant organisms, absent bone or soft tissue compromising the reconstruction or any combination of the above factors (Table 17.1).

The varying number or percent of patients from one study to another may also reflect the surgeon's bias to either recommend or not recommend prosthetic joint reimplantation. Malcolm

Table 17.1 Contemporary indications for resection arthroplasty

Prosthetic joint infection
Medically infirm patients
Patients who refuse further surgery
Chronic infection with resistant pathogens
Severe loss of bone and/or soft tissue
Aseptic loosening
Medically infirm patients
Patients who refuse further surgery
Severe loss of bone and/or soft tissue
Any combination of the above factors

et al. evaluated their experience with resection arthroplasty as indicated for patients with aseptic compared to septic failure of the hip. Overall their patients were older with a mean age of 70.5 (standard deviation = 12.3). Parvizi et al. evaluated patients after total hip arthroplasty and determined those who suffered major complications were approximately eight years older than patients with no complications (P = 0.0001) [3]. The patients also had more comorbidities than patients who had primary joint replacement. The results with regard to complications, reoperations and the risk of death were similar between the two groups [4]. Berend et al. identified 202 patients (205 hips) who were treated for a prosthetic joint infection and then an anticipated two-stage reimplantation [5]. Fourteen of the patients died before reimplantation and two were not reimplanted because of medical comorbidities. Thus, 16 patients, or 8 %, had a resection arthroplasty as their definitive procedure. The percent of prosthetic joint infections treated by resection arthroplasty in their series was similar to others [6, 7].

Rarely would a patient choose resection arthroplasty over a one- or two-stage reimplantation, given the likelihood of significant limb length discrepancies, need for walking aids and potential for persistent pain, as well as the social and psychological burden. However, for elderly patients that already rely on walking aids or are wheelchair-bound, have compromised immune systems or a limited life expectancy, resection arthroplasty may be the best option.

Alternatives to the resection arthroplasty would include preserving the joint and treating the patient with chronic antibiotic suppression, a prosthesis with antibiotic laden polymethyl methacrylate (PROSTALAC) or amputation.

Surgical Technique

Girdlestone's original technique included first a lateral approach to the hip via a transverse skin incision [1]. Next, gluteal muscles were resected from the ilium proximal to the acetabulum through transverse deep incisions, and then the superolateral rim of the acetabulum was resected. The proximal femur was then resected, the greater trochanter was removed first, then the femoral neck osteotomy was made at the intertrochanteric ridge and the femoral head and neck were removed.

The original technique described by Girdlestone, unfortunately, does not allow for functional hip stability due to removal of the abductor musculature. Many modifications have therefore been made over the years to retain the greater trochanter and abductors to provide better hip stability and function with resection. Preserving the abductor musculature and proximal bone also allows for possible future hip replacement and joint stability. Girdlestone described removing the lateral rim of the acetabulum as well to prevent bony impingement from the resected femur; however, if future reconstruction with total hip replacement is a possibility, it should be retained. Some authors have recommended soft tissue interposition between the acetabulum and the remaining femur in order to facilitate a pseudoarthrosis, but others have reported good results without this [8, 9]. A complete synovectomy, in addition to removal of all components and extensive irrigation should be performed routinely. An extended trochanteric osteotomy is often utilized to facilitate femoral stem and cement removal and to prevent femoral shaft fracture, but may lead to trochanteric non-union. Postoperatively, patients were originally placed in skeletal traction for 3–6 weeks followed by limited weight bearing for 6–8 months to try to limit leg shortening and external rotation contracture, but this doesn't show evidence in the literature to provide any functional or subjective difference.

Results of Resection Arthroplasty

The results of resection arthroplasty for a prosthetic joint infection are exceptionally good when they are measured by the eradication of infection for the patients. The primary goal of resection arthroplasty for an infected total hip arthroplasty (THA) is eradication of infection for pain relief

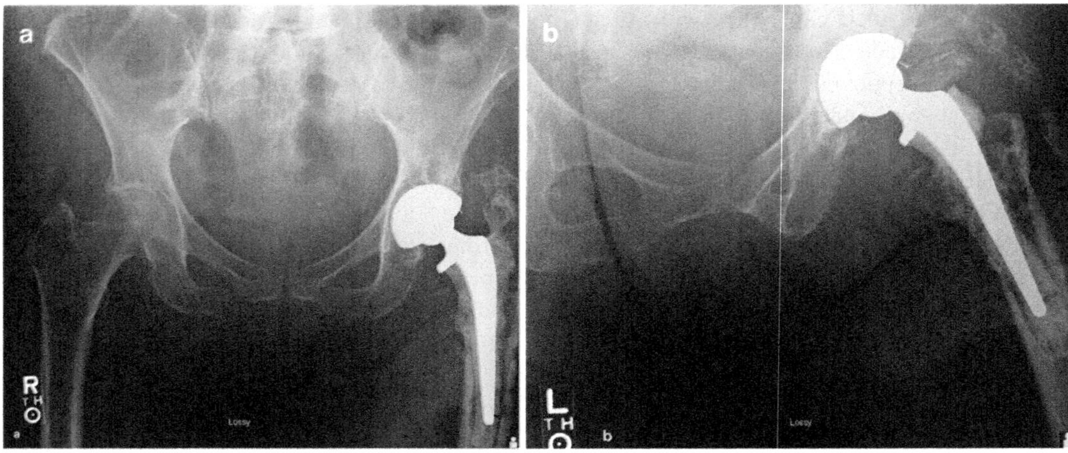

Fig. 17.1 (**a**, **b**) This patient was an 86-year-old female nearly 16 years status post left total hip arthroplasty. She suffered from numerous chronic medical conditions including non-Hodgkin's lymphoma, diabetes mellitus and congestive heart failure. On presentation she reported greater than 18 months of hip pain and had been nonambulatory for 6 months. Twelve months prior to presentation, she was admitted to the hospital following a ground-level fall and was found to be bacteremic. She was treated with a prolonged course of parenteral antibiotics and then transitioned to oral antibiotics. She was still taking oral antibiotics. Other remarkable surgical history included bilateral total knee arthroplasties. She had been wheelchair-dependent for 6 months and reported severe hip pain and fatigue. Her primary care physician was concerned she had a prosthetic joint infection that was failing antibiotic suppression. Her pelvic and left hip radiographs are shown in Fig. 17.1a, b. She had severe osteolysis and a fractured cement mantle. Following a long discussion about treatment options with the patient, her children and her primary care physician, it was felt she was a poor candidate for a complex, two-staged reconstruction of her left hip and she elected to have a resection arthroplasty of her left hip

and preventing potentially fatal complications from systemic sepsis (Figs. 17.1a, b and 17.2a, b). Most studies report >90 % success by this measure. Although removal of all foreign material is expected to improve infection treatment results, several published studies have reported no significant correlation in eradication rates in those patients with retained cement [10]. Kantor did show a significant difference in a 1986 study, with 59 % of hips with persistent infection having retained cement versus 33 % that did not [11]. Most surgeons advocate removal of all foreign material. These results are predictable and have been reported by numerous authors.

If the success of the procedure is measured by pain relief, patient function or ambulation and patient satisfaction, then the results are significantly worse compared to a one- or two-stage reimplantation. Pain relief after resection arthroplasty isn't entirely predictable. The intractable, unrelenting pain of the hip that is not infrequently associated with the prosthetic joint infection should logically be improved when this infection has been eradicated as the result of surgical debridement, removal of the prosthesis and excision of infected and necrotic tissue. Unfortunately, after resection arthroplasty the hip may be painful because of other factors including articulation of two irregular surfaces (the proximal intertrochanteric area and remaining acetabular bone), muscle pain and spasm as the pelvic musculature contracts to maintain hip stability, alignment and function or because of other poorly understood causes of pain. Bourne et al. determined pain relief was common after resection arthroplasty for prosthetic joint infection [2]. Of the 33 patients he and his authors followed for 3–13 years, 30 were free from pain or satisfied with their relief from pain because of the surgical procedure.

Ballard reported on 27 patients with 29 resection arthroplasties for infected THA. Eight (29.6 % of patients) had no pain at all, 14 (51.9 %) had pain only with fatigue, three

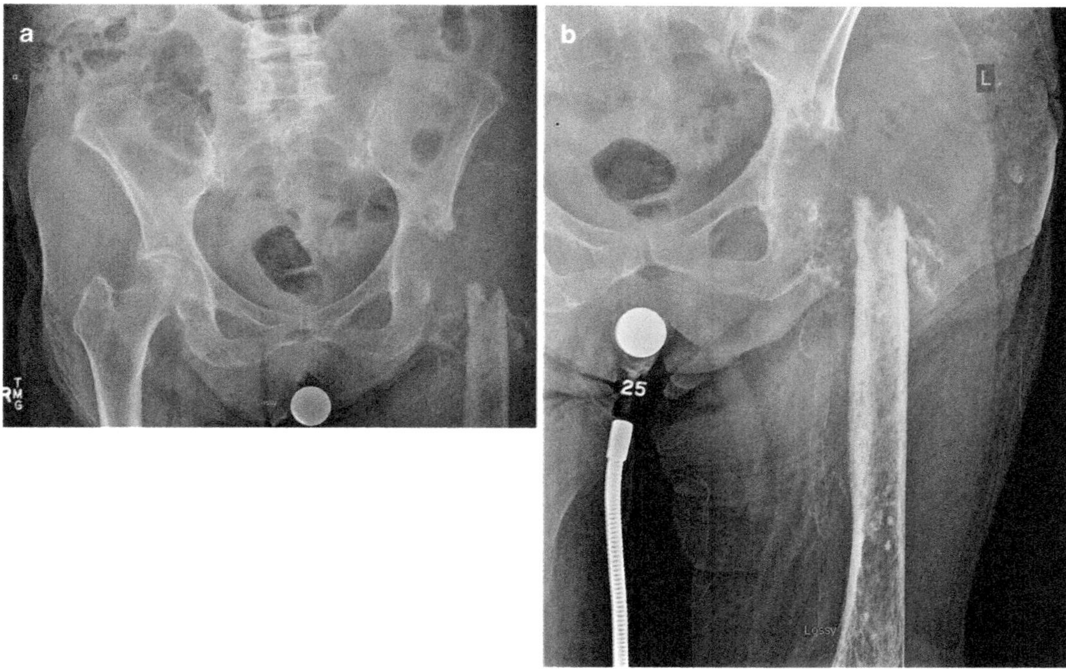

Fig. 17.2 (**a**, **b**) This patient presented with a chronic infection of the left hip, as seen in Fig. 17.1a, b. Following a resection arthroplasty her wound healed, her pain was significantly improved, and although she was wheelchair-dependent, she appeared clinically infection-free. Postoperative radiographs demonstrated a stable resection arthroplasty

(11.1 %) had pain only with weight bearing, and only two patients (7.4 %) had pain with sitting or in bed. Their functional status was also more promising. One patient walked without any assistive device, four patients reported unlimited walking distance ability and the average walking distance limitation was 2.9 blocks. Only one patient was limited to household ambulation and no patients changed occupational status as a result of the surgery. The postoperative average Iowa Hip Rating score was 76; 72 % said they were satisfied with the result; and 59 % actually felt they were better at this point compared to before the index arthroplasty [10].

A recent report by Barbaric et al. who studied 53 resection arthroplasties also performed for prosthetic joint infection had conflicting results [12]. Seven of the patients died and 22 had pain or were dissatisfied. It's not possible to separate the causes of the patients' dissatisfaction based on this report but the 42 % of dissatisfied patients is remarkable. The results of the studies are strikingly dissimilar as other authors report relief of pain for the majority of their patients (70–80 %) (Table 17.2).

Failure to restore function and leg length inequality resulting in instability are the greatest problems of resection arthroplasty. Essentially all patients will require the use of a walking aid such as a crutch or a walker and a lift of their shoe to help equalize the leg length so that this extremity can be used for balance and support.

A more alarming result of resection arthroplasty is the mortality of the patients who are candidates for the procedure. A recent report of frequent repeat surgeries, high complication risk and mortality can be attributed to the patients who are candidates for the procedure. Unlike Bourne's et al. population of patients from the 1970s and 1980s, recent reports find that these patients are older and have more comorbidities. Malcolm's population was 5–10 years older than the typical primary total hip arthroplasty patients with a very high Charlson comorbidity index

Table 17.2 Results of resection arthroplasty for diseases of the hip

Study	Number of patients/hips	Average age of patients (years)	Prosthetic joint infection	Aseptic implant failure	Relief from pain No	Infection eradicated	Function:ambulate without aid	Death <2 years after resection arthroplasty	Other complications
Clegg (1977) [13]	29/30	67 (39–82)	30	0	26	N/S	0	N/S	–
Mallory (1978) [14]	10/10	63	10	0	9	10	0	0	–
Ahlgren et al. (1980) [15]	27/27	64	27	0	24	27	0	0	–
Petty and Goldsmith (1980) [16]	21/21	58 (32–82)	21	0	0	16	0	0	–
Bourne et al. (1984) [2]	33/33	72 (34–89)	33	0	30	32	2	N/S	–
Sharma et al. (2005) [17]	43/43	76 (57–94)	23	20	12	14	0	25	–
Barbaric et al. (2014) [12]	53/53	63 (35–87)	53	0	24	53	0	7	–
Malcolm et al. (2015) [4]	36/38	71	26	12	9	9	N/S	N/S	–

(CCI) of 6.6. One study of primary total hip arthroplasty reported a CCI of 0 and a second study found a CCI of less than 3 in 93 % of the patients. Death of the patient in one series occurred on an average of 26 months after resection and was also associated with male gender and the increase in number of comorbidities (P=0.01 and P=0.04).

Alternatives to Resection Arthroplasty

The role of chronic suppression using antibiotics for patients with a prosthetic joint infection has not been well defined. The countless factors contributing to the decision to use antibiotics to suppress the infection or to perform an operation are related to the health of the patient, the risk of surgery, the antibiotic's effectiveness for a particular bacteria and the complexity of the surgery. The early reports of suppressive antibiotics associated the use of antibiotics with surgical debridement. The combination of surgical debridement and antibiotics was effective in more than half of the patients [18]. Since the report by Goulet et al., most studies anecdotally include a very small number of patients who have been managed with long-term suppressive antibiotics. A 2003 study by Rao evaluated 36 patients with infected arthroplasties that underwent surgical irrigation and debridement and parenteral antibiotics followed by oral antibiotic suppressive therapy. The mean duration of therapy was 52.6 months (range 6–128). Three patients discontinued antibiotics on their own and remained asymptomatic. Five patients discontinued antibiotics due to clinical failure. All five failures had *Staphylococcus* infections. The remaining 31/36 (86 %) were successfully pain free and had well-functioning prostheses at mean follow-up of more than 60 months (range 16–128 months) [19]. Other recent studies have shown more promising results in treatment of bone and joint *Staphylococcus* infections by adding oral rifampin, oral linezolid or with once weekly IV teicoplanin infusions [20–22]. However, in patients that are healthy enough to tolerate a revision surgery, exchange arthroplasty remains the recommended treatment over chronic suppression at this time.

Prostalac Implants and Local Antibiotic Delivery

The first stage of treatment for a prosthetic joint infection is thorough debridement, prosthetic joint removal and excision of the infected and necrotic tissue. The procedure is typically completed by placement of a prosthesis laden with antibiotic-impregnated polymethylmethacrylate. The femoral and acetabular components are laden with high doses of antibiotics (10–12 g of tobramycin and vancomycin) [23]. Occasionally if the patient's symptoms resolve, the implant may be definitive and allow the patient to be free of infection and pain with acceptable ambulation.

Amputation

In rare circumstances a hip disarticulation is required to treat a severe soft-tissue infection. Hip disarticulation is most commonly performed for malignant tumors, limb ischemia, and severe trauma [24]. While several authors have reported successful prosthetic rehabilitation in patients with a hip disarticulation, most studies are small cohorts and mix all indications (malignancy, trauma, and infection) [25, 26]. Hip disarticulation for infection is usually considered only after failure of numerous previous hip operations. The high rate of major complications and death also discourage the use of amputation for chronic prosthetic hip infections.

Conclusion

While it is likely one can achieve a functional result with infection eradication and decent ambulatory ability after resection arthroplasty for failed THA infection, the risk of complications and mortality is high. Indeed, the role and indications for resection arthroplasty are limited and it is typically reserved as a last option. This small subset of patients that currently present as candidates for this treatment are often severely medically compromised and frail.

References

1. Girdlestone GR. Acute pyogenic arthritis of the hip: an operation giving free access and effective drainage. Lancet. 1943;241(6240):419–21.
2. Bourne RB, Hunter GA, Rorabeck CH, Macnab JJ. A six-year follow-up of infected total hip replacements managed by Girdlestone's arthroplasty. J Bone Joint Surg Br. 1984;66(3):340–3.
3. Parvizi J, Mui A, Purtill JJ, Sharkey PF, Hozack WJ, Rothman RH. Total joint arthroplasty: when do fatal or near-fatal complications occur? J Bone Joint Surg Am. 2007;89(1):27–32.
4. Malcolm TL, Gad BV, Elsharkawy KA, Higuera CA. Complication, survival, and reoperation rates following girdlestone resection arthroplasty. J Arthroplasty. 2015;30(7):1183–6.
5. Berend KR, Lombardi Jr AV, Morris MJ, Bergeson AG, Adams JB, Sneller MA. Two-stage treatment of hip periprosthetic joint infection is associated with a high rate of infection control but high mortality. Clin Orthop Relat Res. 2013;471(2):510–8.
6. Toulson C, Walcott-Sapp S, Hur J, Salvati E, Bostrom M, Brause B, et al. Treatment of infected total hip arthroplasty with a 2-stage reimplantation protocol: update on "our institution's" experience from 1989 to 2003. J Arthroplasty. 2009;24(7):1051–60.
7. Lim S, Park J, Moon Y, Park Y. Treatment of periprosthetic hip infection caused by resistant microorganisms using 2-stage reimplantation protocol. J Arthroplasty. 2009;24(8):1264–9.
8. Nelson CL. Femoral head and neck excision arthroplasty. Orthop Clin North Am. 1971;2(1):127–37.
9. Murray WR, Lucas DB, Inman VT. Femoral head and neck resection. J Bone Joint Surg Am. 1964;46:1184–97.
10. Ballard WT, Lowry DA, Brand RA. Resection arthroplasty of the hip. J Arthroplasty. 1995;10(6):772–9.
11. Kantor GS, Osterkamp JA, Dorr LD, Perry J, Conaty JP. Resection arthroplasty following infected total hip replacement arthroplasty. J Arthroplasty. 1986;1(2):83–9.
12. Barbaric K, Aljinovic A, Dubravcic ID, Delimar D, Bicanic G. Patient satisfaction after revision hip arthroplasty or resection hip arthroplasty due to periprosthetic infection. Coll Antropol. 2014;38(2):605–10.
13. Clegg J. The results of the pseudarthrosis after removal of an infected total hip prosthesis. J Bone Joint Surg Br. 1977;59(3):298–301.
14. Mallory TH. Excision arthroplasty with delayed wound closure for the infected total hip replacement. Clin Orthop Relat Res. 1978;137:106–11.
15. Ahlgren SA, Gudmundsson G, Bartholdsson E. Function after removal of a septic total hip prosthesis. A survey of 27 Girdlestone hips. Acta Orthop Scand. 1980;51(3):541–5.
16. Petty W, Goldsmith S. Resection arthroplasty following infected total hip arthroplasty. J Bone Joint Surg Am. 1980;62-A:889–96.
17. Sharma H, Dreghorn CR, Gardner ER. Girdlestone resection arthroplasty of the hip: current perspectives. Curr Orthopaedics. 2005;19(5):385–92.
18. Goulet JA, Pellicci PM, Brause BD, Salvati EM. Prolonged suppression of infection in total hip arthroplasty. J Arthroplasty. 1988;3(2):109–16.
19. Rao N, Crossett LS, Sinha RK, Le Frock JL. Long-term suppression of infection in total joint arthroplasty. Clin Orthop Relat Res. 2003;414:55–60.
20. Allen J, Adams K, Thompson F, Cullen L, Barlow G. Long-term, once-weekly outpatient teicoplanin use for suppression of chronic prosthetic joint infection. Int J Antimicrob Agents. 2013;41(2):200–1.
21. Zimmerli W, Widmer AF, Blatter M, Frei R, Ochsner PE. Role of rifampin for treatment of orthopedic implant-related staphylococcal infections: a randomized controlled trial. Foreign-Body Infection (FBI) Study Group. JAMA. 1998;279(19):1537–41.
22. Bassetti M, Di Biagio A, Cenderello G, Del Bono V, Palermo A, Cruciani M, et al. Linezolid treatment of prosthetic hip infections due to Methicillin-resistant Staphylococcus aureus (MRSA). J Infect. 2001;43(2):148–9.
23. Springer BD, Lee G, Osmon D, Haidukewych GJ, Hanssen AD, Jacofsky DJ. Systemic safety of high-dose antibiotic-loaded cement spacers after resection of an infected total knee arthroplasty. Clin Orthop Relat Res. 2004;427:47–51.
24. Dillingham TR, Pezzin LE, MacKenzie EJ. Limb amputation and limb deficiency: epidemiology and recent trends in the United States. South Med J. 2002;95(8):875–83.
25. Kralovec ME, Houdek MT, Andrews KL, Shives TC, Rose PS, Sim FH. Prosthetic rehabilitation after hip disarticulation or hemipelvectomy. Am J Phys Med Rehabil. 2015;94(12):1035–40.
26. Unruh T, Fisher Jr DF, Unruh TA, Gottschalk F, Fry RE, Clagett GP, et al. Hip disarticulation. An 11-year experience. Arch Surg. 1990;125(6):791–3.

Part VI

The Knee Joint

Acute Periprosthetic Joint Infections: Diagnostic Considerations

18

Valentin Antoci Jr., Hany Bedair, and Craig J. Della Valle

Abstract

Acute post-operative infections occur within first 6 weeks after surgery and are challenging to diagnose due to the heightened inflammatory state of normal healing. Wound erythema, fevers, and swelling may be expected findings in the early postoperative period and can be difficult to differentiate from infection, deep venous thrombosis, or other diagnoses. The first step in determining an accurate diagnosis is avoiding the administration of antibiotics until an appropriate evaluation for periprosthetic joint infection (PJI) has been performed.

Recent work has shown that the serum C-reactive protein (CRP), while normally elevated in the early postoperative period, is an excellent screening test for identifying deep infection. Specifically, a serum CRP of greater than approximately 100 mg/L (normal <10 mg/L) has been shown to be an excellent screening test in the first 6 weeks postoperatively. If there is any question regarding an early infection, a serum CRP is obtained and if above or near this value, an arthrocentesis should be performed. The synovial fluid white blood cell count (WBC) and differential have been shown to be the best tests in the early postoperative period, albeit at threshold levels that are higher than those used for diagnosing chronic PJI. While in the setting of chronic PJI the typical threshold for the synovial fluid WBC

V. Antoci Jr., MD, PhD
Hip and Knee Reconstruction Surgeon University Orthopedics, Providence, RI Alpert Medical School of Brown University, Providence, RI 02903, USA
e-mail: Valentin.Antoci@gmail.com

H. Bedair, MD
Department of Orthopaedic Surgery, Massachusetts General Hospital, Harvard Medical School, Boston, MA, USA

C.J. Della Valle, MD (✉)
Department of Orthopaedic Surgery, Rush University Medical Center, Chicago, IL, USA
e-mail: craigdv@yahoo.com

D. Kendoff et al. (eds.), *Periprosthetic Joint Infections: Changing Paradigms*,
DOI 10.1007/978-3-319-30091-7_18

count and differential is 3000 WBC/uL and 80 %, in the early postoperative period we utilize thresholds of greater than 10,000 WBC/uL and a differential of greater than 90 %. If the diagnosis is still unclear, cultures obtained from the aspirated fluid can be observed to confirm or refute the diagnosis of PJI.

Keywords
Acute infection • Periprosthetic infection • Postoperative • Serology • Biomarkers • Wound • Drainage • Synovial WBC • ESR • CRP

Introduction

Joint replacement is one the most widely-used surgical procedures in medicine and has high success rates and tremendous benefits to the well-being of a large patient population. More than two million cases of hospital-acquired infection are reported annually in the United States, with more than half associated with implants [1]. Periprosthetic joint infection (PJI), one of the most dreaded complications in orthopedics, often results in repeat surgeries, patient distress and disability, increased cost and utilization of medical resources [2, 3]. Half a century ago, Sir John Charnley considered the 7 % rate of infection unacceptable – yet, to date, that incidence has only dropped to 1–2 % [4–6]. As far back as 1989, the annual cost of infection exceeded $200 million dollars [7]. More recent data shows that joint revisions due to infection cost more than $50,000 per case. Financial analysis estimates that as little as 1 % decrease in revision rate for total joint arthroplasty would save as much as $211 million in US health care costs [8]. Considering the costs of revisions, the additional hospital time and disability and the loss of the work force due to sick leave, the costs of periprosthetic infection easily surpasses one billion dollars.

Diagnosis of Acute Infection

Despite extensive progress, the diagnosis of periprosthetic infection remains elusive with no "perfect" test for PJI. Laffer et al. [9] proposed that 45 % of infections present early, 23 % delayed, and 32 % represent late infections [10]. Fulkerson et al. [11] reviewed 146 patients, with 70 % of infection cases being chronic, 17 % acute postoperative, and 13 % acute hematogenous. Infection originates from bacterial contamination of the implant either during surgery, or later through hematogenous transfer or local dissemination [12]. Attention to the timing of initial clinical presentation can divide infections into either acute postoperative, acute hematogenous, or chronic, with each having their own diagnostic challenges [13, 14]. Diagnosis in the early postoperative period is particularly difficult as symptoms are short lived or confused with normal healing.

The American Academy of Orthopaedic Surgeons (AAOS) proposed a set of diagnostic guidelines for the diagnosis of periprosthetic infection in 2011 [15]. The recommendations rely on a consensus workgroup and form a framework for decision making in cases of suspected PJI. The decisions are stratified based on the risk and probability of infection. All patients that are evaluated for possible periprosthetic infection should have a physical exam, appropriate imaging, and inflammatory markers including erythrocyte sedimentation rate (ESR) and C-reactive protein (CRP). Positive values merit an aspiration for further evaluation.

Risk Factors for Acute Infection

Peel et al. [16] looked at the predictive risk factors for prosthetic hip and knee infection according to the arthroplasty site. They identify 63 patients over an 8-year period with 36 infected hips and 27 infected knees. Certain comorbidities increase the risk of infection. Obesity is associated with a three-fold increased risk of infection in total hip patients [17], with every 1 kg/m^2 increase in body mass index resulting in a 10 % increased risk of prosthetic hip joint infection. Rheumatoid arthritis, diabetes mellitus, obesity, sickle cell disease, psoriasis, poor nutrition and a compromised immune system, as well as previous surgeries in the affected limb, are often linked to higher risks of implant associated infection [7, 18–20]. Rheumatoid arthritis is associated with a 2.6-fold increase in infection rates compared to uncomplicated osteoarthritis [21]. Revision surgeries lead to an almost three-fold increase in infection risk [22, 23]. Patients with a postoperative surgical site infection had up to a 36-fold increase in the risk of the subsequent development of PJI [16]. These data allow surgeons to assess the pre-test probabilities of infection and provide the necessary support for a diagnosis.

It is common for patients to have several prosthetic joints, which raises the question of cross-contamination and subsequent infection at different sites, as well as the predictive value of previous PJI. Over 50 % of total knee patients and 40 % of total hip arthroplasty patients have an additional total hip or knee artificial joint [24]. Murray et al. [25], in a retrospective review of 159 joint replacements in 68 patients with PJI, found that patients presenting with PJI have a 15 % risk of infection at a second site. Recent systemic infections increased the risk of infection at the site of other joints. Over 80 % of infections at other sites occurred within the first year after the first infection suggesting a possible common etiology.

Previous PJI also increases the risk of infection in future total joint arthroplasties. Bedair et al. [26], in a retrospective matched cohort study, reviewed 90 patients who had a history of a successfully treated PJI and subsequently underwent another total joint. The relative risk of developing an infection in a subsequent total joint was 21, significantly higher than patients with no such history. These results align with the work of Cierny et al. [27] and McPherson et al. [28], with the host playing an important role in severity and thus classification of infection. The organism is also important, as Bedair et al. [26] identified Staphylococcal species having a 4.26 relative risk of causing a second infection compared to other infecting organisms. Recent intra-articular cortisone injections before arthroplasty surgery may also increase infection rates in total joints. A review of 224 primary total hip patients with a cortisone injection within 1 year of the arthroplasty surgery found a hazard ratio of 3 for PJI, with infected joints having had an injection within 44 days from surgery [29].

Infection associated with surgical contamination manifests within 6–12 weeks from surgery [30, 31]. The importance of surgical contamination is documented by an infection rate of 1–5 % that drops to less than 0.5–1 % using modern prophylactic measures including pre-operative antibiotics and improved attention to sterility [22, 32, 33]. Surgeon experience [34, 35], antibiotic timing and dosing, surgery duration (especially if over 2.5 h), operating-room traffic, and the complexity of reconstruction are all important factors determining the probability of infection [7].

Patient Presentation

Any patient presenting with concerning symptoms including fevers, drainage, or progressive pain associated with a total joint should be ruled out for infection. Establishing the diagnosis of infection in a patient with an exposed implant or a draining sinus is simple and does not require extensive workup. This can occur in acute post-operative infections with complete wound breakdown.

The question of culturing either the wound or draining sinus for a microbiological diagnosis is controversial with the current consensus recommending against it [36]. Surgeons are concerned regarding the reliability of superficial sampling, presence of contaminants, and the diagnostic validity of the test. Mousa et al. [37] in a prospective review of 55 patients with bone infections, found an 88.7 % correlation between the sinus tract and bone cultures, showing 95.7 % specificity and a 90.3 % predictive value. Very few authors have looked at the correlation between sinus or wound culture and the operative results in total joints. Cune et al. [38] examined 56 patients, including 30 hips and 26 knees. Superficial wound cultures were taken at admission and compared to intra-operative cultures during debridement. The cultures showed concordance in 80.3 % of cases, and there was no significant difference between hips and knees. Superficial swabs were 93.7 % sensitive at picking up *Staphylococcus aureus*, 90 % sensitive for gram-negative bacilli, but only 50 % sensitive and non-specific for other gram-positive microorganisms. Tetreault et al. [39] reviewed 55 patients with a draining wound or sinus after total joint arthroplasty with a equal distribution of hips and knees. All patients were off antibiotics at the time of evaluation. Unfortunately, only 47.3 % of superficial cultures correlated with deep cultures. The superficial cultures were typically polymicrobial, which would have resulted in an antibiotic regimen change in 41.8 % of cases. More importantly, superficial cultures yielded microbial growth in 80 % of cases deemed negative for deep infection. The authors thus recommend against wound or sinus swabs for diagnosis due to possible overtreatment.

The patient should be asked about wound healing and any history of drainage or delayed healing, as well as the presence of any other wounds. A general as well as focal exam can help differentiate between mechanical complains and more generalized pain. An infected knee joint may present with swelling, warmth, as well as limited range of motion. Subclinical infections are also possible, with limited clinical manifestations. A cellulitis is difficult to differentiate from a deep joint infection. Nevertheless, a high index of suspicion should be maintained, and additional studies should be entertained to rule out PJI.

Post-operative Complications

Post-operative fevers and swelling are probably the most frequent significant complaints outside of pain. As many as 50 % of patients after total joints may experience a febrile response, which sometimes leads to concerns of infection and prompts extensive workup [40]. Postoperative fever workup often delays discharges and provides an unnecessary burden on the cost of healthcare [41]. Fever can be a normal response to surgical intervention, but fever can also represent a manifestation of infection, pneumonia, or deep venous thrombosis.

The differential is further complicated by the variable serology and exam. Shaw et al. [42] evaluated 100 patients who underwent total hip arthroplasty and 100 patients after total knee arthroplasty, suggesting fevers in the immediate postoperative period as a normal inflammatory response with no significant correlation with late deep infection. As expected, revision surgeries tend to mount a higher fever curve. Athanassious et al. [40] evaluated 341 patients after total joint arthroplasty and found that 36 % of the cohort showed fevers after surgery. Only 16 % of those with fevers had a positive urinalysis but subsequently all patients had negative urine cultures. All patient records were reviewed at 1 year after the index procedure and no deep infections were documented. Nevertheless, others suggested fevers to be a finding of atelectasis, hematoma, wound infection, urinary tract infection, and fat emboli – all complications with significant mortality and morbidity [43].

Blood cultures are often part of the workup. Bindelglass et al. [41] studied 453 patients with blood cultures drawn in the setting of infection and total joint arthroplasty. Blood cultures were obtained for persistent fever, at least 2 readings greater than 101 F. Only two patients had positive blood cultures and an infectious disease consultation deeming them contaminants with no management and no subsequent development of active infection. An appropriate clinical exam and history taking can elucidate an appropriate differential and limit reliance on fever as a single marker of disease. The current clinical thinking suggests that post-operative pyrexia without specific physical examination findings should not trigger further workup and has very poor correlation with infection [44].

Fever and a draining wound are significantly more concerning. The incidence of superficial wound infection progressing to deep periprosthetic infection is difficult to assess. Limited soft tissue coverage makes a wound complication much more concerning in a total knee compared to total hips [45]. Gaine et al. [46] reviewed 530 patients with either total hip or total knee arthroplasty and found an over 15 % rate of wound complications. Six patients had deep wound infections that required operative debridement and two patients required removal of prosthesis. The rate of post-operative infection ranges from 1.3 to 50 % in patients with persistent wound drainage [47, 48]. Post-operative drainage correlates to body mass index and type of anticoagulation used. Each day of prolonged drainage is associated with up to 42 % increased risk of wound infection in total hip patients and 29 % increase in the risk of postoperative infection in total knee patients [49]. Ultimately, deep wound infections have been shown to highly correlate to superficial surgical site infection [50], but they are a poor predictor of ongoing problems or periprosthetic infection at 1 year post-surgery [51]. As such it is very difficult to make a diagnosis of infection during the early post-operative period. Wound complications in themselves do not confirm the presence of deep infection, and additional studies are often required to define a diagnosis.

Serology

Serology can help further stratify patients at risk of periprosthetic joint infection. Inflammatory markers have a well-characterized curve in the post-operative period. Bilgen et al. [52] describe the normal distribution of C-reactive protein (CRP) and erythrocyte sedimentation rate (ESR) in total hip and total knee patients. The highest CRP levels were recorded on day 2 after surgery, with a rapid decrease over the first 3 weeks, and return to normal by the end of the third month. Total knee patients tend to express a higher CRP production compared to total hip arthroplasty patients during the first post-operative week after which the difference is insignificant [53]. Mean ESR levels were the highest on day 5 after surgery and show a rapid decrease over the first month but remain elevated compared to pre-operative levels even at 1 year after surgery. CRP levels thus react more rapidly and are likely more helpful in following the inflammatory response after surgery. More importantly, CRP response is not correlated with type of anesthesia, estimated blood loss, operative time, transfusions, medications, age, or gender [54]. As such, any late reversal of downtrend should raise suspicion and be concerning for infection or other process.

The value of ESR and CRP can be difficult to interpret in the early post-operative period. Bedair et al. [55] reviewed 11,964 primary total knee arthroplasties and identified 146 with an aspiration within 6 weeks from surgery. Infection was diagnosed in 19 of the 146 knees by positive cultures or gross purulence. While the mean CRP was significantly higher among patients with PJI, the ESR values were not different between the infected and non-infected groups. This discrepancy may be related to the fact that the CRP normalizes faster compared to ESR, which would still be elevated early post-operatively. A cutoff value of 95 mg/L (normal <10 mg/L) provides a negative predictive value of 91 %, thus helpful in ruling out infection.

Similarly, Yi et al. [56] reviewed 6033 consecutive primary total hip arthroplasties, identifying 36 patients with a deep infection within 6 weeks from surgery based on the MSIS criteria. In contrast to the work by Bedair et al., significantly higher ESR values were observed in the infected compared to the non-infected cohorts. While an ESR cutoff of 44 mm/h showed 92 % sensitivity, the specificity was only 53 %. The ESR differences were small compared to a dramatic difference in CRP in the infected cohort. Using 93 mg/L as the cutoff for CRP leads to 88 % sensitivity and 100 % specificity for periprosthetic infection. This cutoff has an 83 % negative predictive value. Based on these two works, CRP is the most helpful serological value in diagnosing infection within first 6 weeks after surgery. Values near or above 93–95 mg/L prompt an aspiration of the joint.

Joint Aspiration

Joint aspiration is considered a key test for the diagnosis of PJI in the setting of a chronic infection with the synovial fluid WBC count, differential and cultures all being useful to establish the diagnosis. The MSIS has determined that a cut-off value of 3000 WBC/uL and a differential of greater than 80 % polymorphonuclear cells is suggestive of PJI. In the early postoperative period, however, one would expect these values to be elevated given inflammation and an expected hematoma around the wound.

To determine the value of the synovial fluid WBC count and differential within the first 6 weeks postoperatively, Bedair et al. [55] reviewed 11,964 primary total knee arthroplasties in 9826 patients. As previously described, all knees were aspirated based on physical exam and concerning signs including drainage, fever, erythema, effusion, and the new onset of pain. The synovial fluid WBC count was the best test for the diagnosis of infection in the early post-operative period. Most patients diagnosed with infection had a WBC count of greater than 10,700 cells/uL. Most non-infected patients had a WBC count of less than 27,800 cell/uL. Using 10,700 cell/uL as a threshold for diagnosis of infection yielded a 95 % sensitivity and 91 % specificity. Using 27,800 cell/uL as a threshold for diagnosis yielded a 84 % sensitivity but 99 % specificity. A synovial fluid polymorphonuclear cell percentage higher than 89 % had a 84 % sensitivity and 69 % specificity. The authors did examine if the synovial fluid WBC count needed to be "corrected" for the red blood cells often present in an aspiration in the early postoperative period (secondary to an expected postoperative hematoma) and found that this correction was not necessary.

Similarly, Yi et al. [56] reviewed 6033 primary total hip arthroplasties with 36 hips reoperated for periprosthetic infection. Compared to the non-infected cohort, the mean preoperative serum ESR, CRP, as well as synovial fluid WBC count and %PMNs were all significantly higher in the infected group. ROC analysis supported the synovial WBC count as the best test for the diagnosis of acute infection, with a cutoff value of 12,800 cells/uL. This cutoff was associated with 89 % sensitivity and 100 % specificity with an 88 % negative predictive value for infection. The average value of synovial WBC was 84,954 WBC/uL in the infected group compared to 2391 in the non-infected group. A synovial fluid polymorphonuclear cell percentage higher than 89 % had a 81 % sensitivity and 90 % specificity. Interestingly, if using a traditional cutoff value of 80 % for polymorphonuclear cell percentages, more than one-third of the patient population would be diagnosed with infection. Nevertheless, PMN% can be a good secondary test when the synovial fluid WBC count is close to but not clearly above or below the recommended cut off value.

In cases where the diagnosis is still unclear, the clinician can also observe the results of cultures obtained at the time of aspiration. It is important to keep in mind, however, that the administration of antibiotics is highly discouraged if an acute postoperative infection has been suspected until an appropriate evaluation for PJI has been performed as described above. The indiscriminate use of antibiotics only clouds the diagnosis. Even though there is no clearly defined effect of antibiotic administration on serologic tests and synovial fluid analysis, there is a clear detrimental effect of antibiotics on the results of synovial fluid cultures.

Future Tests

New tests are being explored to improve the diagnosis of infection. Biomarkers provide an easy and rapid test but current methods lack sensitivity and specificity in the stetting of acute infection. In addition to the clinically available alpha defensin, other potential markers include interleukin-6 (IL6), neutrophil elastase 2 (ELA2), bactericidal-permeability increasing protein (BPI), neutrophil gelatinase-associated lipocalin (NGAL), lactoferrin, and leukocyte esterase. Berbari et al. [57], in a metanalysis, reviewed 2909 revision total hip and knee arthroplasties with 32.5 % infection, identifying interleukin-6 as most predictive for infection, followed by CRP and ESR.

Parvizi et al. [58] and Deirmengian et al. [59] have explored simple and rapid diagnostic methods for effectively detecting periprosthetic infection. Using urinary test strips often used for detection of pyuria were used in the setting of joint aspiration with good results. Leukocyte esterase is an enzyme secreted by neutrophils that have been recruited to the site of infection. A colorimetric strip tests for this enzyme with results available within seconds. In a study of 108 total knees undergoing revision arthroplasty, leukocyte esterase test strips were 80.6 % sensitive and 100 % specific in predicting infection when using culture as the gold standard 58. Similarly, Omar et al. [60], in a prospective study of 146 joints, found leukocyte esterase to be 89.5 % sensitive and 99.2 % specific. Nevertheless, the test may be technically difficult as any blood or other contaminant may obscure the colorimetric reading and centrifugation may be required to clarify the result [61]. While these results are exciting as they offer a test that is effective, rapid, and easily available in the office, this test has not been validated in the acute postoperative period.

Attempting to capture a larger group of markers elevated in septic conditions, Deirmengian et al. [59] screened 43 different biomarkers, identifying alpha defensing, ELA-2, BPI, NGAL, and lactoferrin as 100 % sensitive and 100 % specific using the MSIS criteria for infection as the gold standard. Furthermore, they have shown that the results were superior to other available markers, including leukocyte esterase [62]. The effectiveness of these markers in acute post-operative infection has not been established or described [63].

Conclusion

The diagnosis of an acute postoperative infection can be particularly challenging as normal postoperative pain and wound healing can be difficult to differentiate from PJI. Based on the work of Bediar et al. [55] and Yi et al. [56], we recommend a serum CRP in all cases where an acute postoperative infection is suspected. Serum CRP values approaching or above 100 mg/L (normal <10 mg/L) should prompt an aspiration of the joint with the fluid obtained sent for a synovial fluid WBC count, differential and culture. A synovial WBC count >10,000 cells/uL and PMN% >90 % [64] are considered concerning for PJI.

References

1. Darouiche RO. Treatment of infections associated with surgical implants. N Engl J Med. 2004;350(14):1422–9.
2. Barrack RL. Economics of revision total hip arthroplasty. Clin Orthop Relat Res. 1995;319:209.
3. Gómez J, Rodríguez M, Baños V, Martínez L, Claver MA, Ruiz J, et al. Orthopedic implant infection: prognostic factors and influence of long-term antibiotic treatment on evolution. Prospective study, 1992–1999. Enferm Infecc Microbiol Clin. 2003;21(5):232–6.
4. Charnley J, Eftekhar N. Postoperative infection in total prosthetic replacement arthroplasty of the hip-joint. With special reference to the bacterial content of the air of the operating room. Br J Surg. 1969;56(9):641–9.
5. Charnley J. Total hip replacement by low-friction arthroplasty. Clin Orthop Relat Res. 1970;72:7–21.
6. Warth LC, Callaghan JJ, Liu SS, Klaassen AL, Goetz DD, Johnston RC. Thirty-five-year results after Charnley total hip arthroplasty in patients less than fifty years old. A concise follow-up of previous reports. J Bone Joint Surg Am. 2014;96(21):1814–9.
7. Bozic KJ, Ries MD. The impact of infection after total hip arthroplasty on hospital and surgeon resource utilization. J Bone Joint Surg. 2005.
8. Kurtz S, Mowat F, Ong K, Chan N, Lau E, Halpern M. Prevalence of primary and revision total hip and knee arthroplasty in the United States from 1990 through 2002. J Bone Joint Surg Am. 2005;87(7):1487–97.
9. Laffer RR, Graber P, Ochsner PE, Zimmerli W. Outcome of prosthetic knee-associated infection: evaluation of 40 consecutive episodes at a single centre. Clin Microbiol Infect. 2006;12(5):433–9.
10. Tsukayama DT, Estrada R, Gustilo RB. Infection after total hip arthroplasty. A study of the treatment of one hundred and six infections. J Bone Joint Surg. 1996;78(4):512–23.
11. Fulkerson E, Valle CJD, Wise B, Walsh M, Preston C, Di Cesare PE. Antibiotic susceptibility of bacteria infecting total joint arthroplasty sites. J Bone Joint Surg. 2006;88(6):1231–7.
12. Trampuz A, Widmer AF. Infections associated with orthopedic implants. Curr Opin Infect Dis. 2006;19(4):349–56.
13. Fitzgerald RH. Reduction of deep sepsis following total hip arthroplasty. Ann N Y Acad Sci. 1980;353:262–70.

14. Fitzgerald RH, Nolan DR, Ilstrup DM, Van Scoy RE, Washington JA, Coventry MB. Deep wound sepsis following total hip arthroplasty. J Bone Joint Surg. 1977;59(7):847–55.
15. Valle Della C, Parvizi J, Bauer TW, DiCesare PE, Evans RP, Segreti J, et al. Diagnosis of periprosthetic joint infections of the Hip and knee. J Am Acad Orthop Surg. 2010;18(12):760–70.
16. Peel TN, Dowsey MM, Daffy JR, Stanley PA, Choong PF, Buising KL. Risk factors for prosthetic hip and knee infections according to arthroplasty site. J Hosp Infect. 2011;79(2):129–33.
17. Kim YH, Cho SH, Kim RS. Drainage versus nondrainage in simultaneous bilateral total knee arthroplasties. Clin Orthop Relat Res. 1998;347:188–93.
18. Berbari EF, Hanssen AD, Duffy MC, Steckelberg JM, Ilstrup DM, Harmsen WS, et al. Risk factors for prosthetic joint infection: case-control study. Clin Infect Dis. 1998;27(5):1247–54.
19. Garvin KL, Hanssen AD. Infection after total hip arthroplasty. Past, present, and future. J Bone Joint Surg. 1995;77(10):1576–88.
20. Wilson MG, Kelley K, Thornhill TS. Infection as a complication of total knee-replacement arthroplasty. Risk factors and treatment in sixty-seven cases. J Bone Joint Surg. 1990.
21. Poss R, Thornhill TS, Ewald FC, Thomas WH, Batte NJ, Sledge CB. Factors influencing the incidence and outcome of infection following total joint arthroplasty. Clin Orthop Relat Res. 1984;182:117.
22. Peersman G, Laskin R, Davis J, Peterson M. Infection in total knee replacement: a retrospective review of 6489 total knee replacements. Clin Orthop Relat Res. 2001;392:15.
23. Zhan C, Kaczmarek R, Loyo-Berrios N, Sangl J, Bright RA. Incidence and short-term outcomes of primary and revision hip replacement in the United States. J Bone Joint Surg Am. 2007;89(3):526–33.
24. Shao Y, Zhang C, Charron KD, MacDonald SJ, McCalden RW, Bourne RB. The fate of the remaining knee(s) or hip(s) in osteoarthritic patients undergoing a primary TKA or THA. J Arthroplasty. 2013;28(10):1842–5.
25. Murray RP, Bourne MH, Fitzgerald RH. Metachronous infections in patients who have had more than one total joint arthroplasty. J Bone Joint Surg. 1991;73(10):1469–74.
26. Bedair H, Goyal N, Dietz MJ, Urish K, Hansen V, Manrique J, et al. A history of treated periprosthetic joint infection increases the risk of subsequent different site infection. Clin Orthop Relat Res. 2015;473(7):2300–4.
27. Cierny GI, DiPasquale D. Periprosthetic total joint infections: staging, treatment, and outcomes. Clin Orthop Relat Res. 2002;403:23.
28. McPherson EJ, Woodson C, Holtom P, Roidis N, Shufelt C, Patzakis M. Periprosthetic total hip infection: outcomes using a staging system. Clin Orthop Relat Res. 2002;403:8.
29. McIntosh AL, Hanssen AD, Wenger DE, Osmon DR. Recent intraarticular steroid injection may increase infection rates in primary THA. Clin Orthop Relat Res. 2006;451:50–4.
30. Zimmerli W. Prosthetic-joint-associated infections. Best Pract Res Clin Rheumatol. 2006;20(6):1045–63.
31. Fehring TK, Odum SM, Berend KR, Jiranek WA, Parvizi J, Bozic KJ, et al. Failure of irrigation and débridement for early postoperative periprosthetic infection. Clin Orthop Relat Res. 2013;471(1):250–7.
32. Ritter MA. Operating room environment. Clin Orthop Relat Res. 1999;369:103–9.
33. Ritter MA, Eitzen H, French ML, Hart JB. The operating room environment as affected by people and the surgical face mask. Clin Orthop Relat Res. 1975;111:147–50.
34. Dimick JB, Welch HG, Birkmeyer JD. Surgical mortality as an indicator of hospital quality: the problem with small sample size. JAMA. 2004;292(7):847–51.
35. Stewart GD, Stewart PC, Nott ML, Long G. Total joint replacement surgery in a rural centre. Aust J Rural Health. 2006;14(6):253–7.
36. Parvizi J, Gehrke T, Chen AF. Proceedings of the international consensus on periprosthetic joint infection. Bone Joint J. 2013;95-B(11):1450–2.
37. Mousa HA. Evaluation of sinus-track cultures in chronic bone infection. J Bone Joint Surg Br. 1997;79(4):567–9.
38. Cuñé J, Soriano A, Martínez JC, García S, Mensa J. A superficial swab culture is useful for microbiologic diagnosis in acute prosthetic joint infections. Clin Orthop Relat Res. 2009;467(2):531–5.
39. Tetreault MW, Wetters NG, Aggarwal VK, Moric M, Segreti J, Huddleston III JI, et al. Should draining wounds and sinuses associated with hip and knee arthroplasties be cultured? J Arthroplasty. 2013;28(8):133–6.
40. Athanassious C, Samad A, Avery A, Cohen J, Chalnick D. Evaluation of fever in the immediate postoperative period in patients who underwent total joint arthroplasty. J Arthroplasty. 2011;26(8):1404–8.
41. Bindelglass DF, Pellegrino J. The role of blood cultures in the acute evaluation of postoperative fever in arthroplasty patients. J Arthroplasty. 2007;22(5):701–2.
42. Shaw JA, Chung R. Febrile response after knee and hip arthroplasty. Clin Orthop Relat Res. 1999;367:181–9.
43. Summersell PC, Turnbull A, Long G, Diwan A, Macdessi S, Cooke PJ, et al. Temperature trends in total hip arthroplasty: a retrospective study. J Arthroplasty. 2003;18(4):426–9.
44. Kennedy JG, Rodgers WB, Zurakowski D, Sullivan R, Griffin D, Beardsley W, et al. Pyrexia after total knee replacement. A cause for concern? Am J Orthop. 1997;26(8):549–52, 554.
45. Dennis DA. Wound complications in total knee arthroplasty. Orthopedics. 1997;20(9):837–40.
46. Gaine WJ, Ramamohan NA, Hussein NA, Hullin MG, McCreath SW. Wound infection in hip and knee arthroplasty. J Bone Joint Surg Br. 2000;82(4):561–5.

47. Poss R, Maloney JP, Ewald FC, Thomas WH, Batte NJ, Hartness C, et al. Six- to 11-year results of total hip arthroplasty in rheumatoid arthritis. Clin Orthop Relat Res. 1984;182:109–16.
48. Eveillard M, Mertl P, Canarelli B, Lavenne J, Fave MH, Eb F, et al. Risk of deep infection in first-intention total hip replacement. Evaluation concerning a continuous series of 790 cases. Presse Med. 2001;30(38):1868–75.
49. Patel VP, Walsh M, Sehgal B, Preston C, DeWal H, Di Cesare PE. Factors associated with prolonged wound drainage after primary total hip and knee arthroplasty. J Bone Joint Surg. 2007;89(1):33–8.
50. Saleh K, Olson M, Resig S, Bershadsky B, Kuskowski M, Gioe T, et al. Predictors of wound infection in hip and knee joint replacement: results from a 20 year surveillance program. J Orthop Res. 2002;20(3): 506–15.
51. Lidwell OM, Lowbury EJL, Whyte W, Blowers R, Stanley SJ, Lowe D. Infection and sepsis after operations for total hip or knee-joint replacement: influence of ultraclean air, prophylactic antibiotics and other factors. J Hygiene. 1984;93(03):505–29.
52. Bilgen O, Atici T, Durak K, Karaeminoğullari, Bilgen MS. C-reactive protein values and erythrocyte sedimentation rates after total hip and total knee arthroplasty. J Int Med Res. 2001;29(1):7–12.
53. White J, Kelly M, Dunsmuir R. C-reactive protein level after total hip and total knee replacement. J Bone Joint Surg Br. 1998;80(5):909–11.
54. Larsson S, Thelander U, Friberg S. C-reactive protein (CRP) levels after elective orthopedic surgery. Clin Orthop Relat Res. 1992;275:237–42.
55. Bedair H, Ting N, Jacovides C, Saxena A, Moric M, Parvizi J, et al. The Mark Coventry Award: diagnosis of early postoperative tka infection using synovial fluid analysis. Clin Orthop Relat Res. 2011;469(1):34–40.
56. Yi PH, Cross MB, Moric M, Sporer SM, Berger RA, Valle Della CJ. The 2013 Frank Stinchfield award: diagnosis of infection in the early postoperative period after total hip arthroplasty. Clin Orthop Relat Res. 2014;472(2):424–9.
57. Berbari E, Mabry T, Tsaras G, Spangehl M. Inflammatory blood laboratory levels as markers of prosthetic joint infection. J Bone Joint Surg Am. 2010;92(11):2102–9.
58. Parvizi J, Jacovides C, Antoci V, Ghanem E. Diagnosis of periprosthetic joint infection: the utility of a simple yet unappreciated enzyme. J Bone Joint Surg. 2011;93(24):2242–8.
59. Deirmengian C, Kardos K, Kilmartin P, Cameron A, Schiller K, Parvizi J. Diagnosing periprosthetic joint infection: has the era of the biomarker arrived? Clin Orthop Relat Res. 2014;472(11):3254–62.
60. Omar M, Ettinger M, Reichling M, Petri M, Lichtinghagen R, Guenther D, et al. Preliminary results of a new test for rapid diagnosis of septic arthritis with use of leukocyte esterase and glucose reagent strips. J Bone Joint Surg. 2014;96(24):2032–7.
61. Aggarwal VK, Tischler E, Ghanem E, Parvizi J. Leukocyte esterase from synovial fluid aspirate: a technical note. J Arthroplasty. 2013;28(1):193–5.
62. Deirmengian C, Kardos K, Kilmartin P, Cameron A, Schiller K, Booth Jr RE, et al. The alpha-defensin test for periprosthetic joint infection outperforms the leukocyte esterase test strip. Clin Orthop Relat Res. 2015;473(1):198–203.
63. Springer BD. CORR Insights(®): the alpha-defensin test for periprosthetic joint infection responds to a wide spectrum of organisms. Clin Orthop Relat Res. 2015;473(7):2236–7.
64. Zmistowski B, et al. Diagnosis of periprosthetic joint infection. J Orthop Res. 2014;32:S98–107. doi:10.1002/jor.22553.

Irrigation and Debridement with Component Retention

19

Myra Trivellas and Michael B. Cross

Abstract
A periprosthetic joint infection is a devastating complication after total joint arthroplasty. While patients with a chronic infection are treated with one-stage or two-stage revision, some patients with an acute infection may be treated with irrigation and debridement with component retention. The purpose of this chapter is describe the indications, contraindications, surgical technique and published results on irrigation and debridement with polyethylene liner exchange and component retention.

Keywords
Acute • Periprosthetic joint infection • Irrigation and debridement • Component retention • Outcomes

Introduction

Debridement has been a key aspect of the treatment of infection in orthopedics since before World War I. The term initially meant the drainage of a wound to remove foreign material and to release pressure. Originally derived from the French word *débrider,* the unbridling of a horse [1], the association with the French *débriser*, from which the word debris is derived, allowed for the technique's modern connotations to expand. As the theory of infection and contamination of wounds advanced, the word debridement evolved to the now recognized meaning of "the aseptic excision of all devitalized tissue" [2]. A substantial, quality debridement today is acknowledged to be the foundation of a successful treatment of a deep infection after an orthopaedic procedure.

Managing PJI is challenging due to the aggressive nature of bacterial inoculation and spread, as well as the bacterial biofilm. Irrigation Debridement and Component Retention (IDCR) is a *relatively* conservative

M. Trivellas, BS
Department of Biomechanics, Hospital for Special Surgery, New York, NY, USA

M.B. Cross, MD (✉)
Department of Adult Reconstruction Joint Replacement, Hospital for Special Surgery, New York, NY, USA
e-mail: crossm@hss.edu

D. Kendoff et al. (eds.), *Periprosthetic Joint Infections: Changing Paradigms*,
DOI 10.1007/978-3-319-30091-7_19

surgical option that provides the surgeon with access to the joint space to clean out the infected tissues and exchange the modular components, while still allowing the patients to retain the primary implants firmly fixed to their bone. Balancing the desire to clear the infection quickly and completely, while recognizing the additional risks and recovery required from added surgeries, is paramount in the approach to treating PJI. IDCR is a procedure that limits the morbidity associated with explantation, while still allowing for access to the deep joint space to adequately treat and debride an acute infection. The ultimate goal of treatment is still to eradicate the infection and achieve a pain-free, functional joint. Appropriate care involves both surgical and medical therapies and an invested team monitoring progression and improvement. Surgical options beyond IDCR for a PJI include one-stage and two-stage revision. This chapter will review irrigation and debridement with component retention (IDCR) as a treatment for an acute periprosthetic joint infection (PJI), and will discuss the advantages and disadvantages of IDCR, the indications and contraindications, and the success and reported outcomes.

Pros of IDCR

When comparing options for surgical treatment of PJI, IDCR is an attractive choice due to the lower morbidity associated with the procedure. First, the procedure is bone preserving, saving the patient from the bone loss associated with the removal of implants and preparation of the bony surfaces for re-implantation. Successful IDCR also reduces hospitalization time, immobility, and physical/emotional discomfort, the psychological implications of which cannot be underestimated. Further, the technical demands of IDCR are lower than one or two stage revisions that would require removal of implants, and as a result, the healthcare costs are notably decreased. With the changing healthcare climate, these are highly relevant considerations, provided successful eradications results can be obtained.

Cons of IDCR

Most importantly, the success rate with IDCR is less than that of one-stage or two-stage revision surgeries [3]. Due to variations in treatment failure definitions and combining total knee arthroplasty (TKA) and total hip arthroplasty (THA) together, success rates for IDCR are largely reported 15–80 %, whereas success rates for two-stage revisions are generally around 75–90 %. Significant predictors of decreased success include more virulent organisms (e.g., MRSA), symptom duration as it increases beyond 5 days (up to 4 weeks in some studies), and obesity [4]. Furthermore, if the initial IDCR fails to eradicate the infection, the subsequent two-stage operation also has reduced success at successfully treating the infection [5]. Therefore, although its prevalence varies in the literature, failure of IDCR is not uncommon and failure results in increased recovery time and morbidity with greater cost to the patient and the healthcare system.

Indications

The patient characteristics and the presenting bacteria best suited for IDCR has been characterized in the literature and discussed amongst international leaders in orthopedics at the PJI consensus meeting in 2013. Historically, timing has been classified into early-onset and delayed or late-onset. The timeframe is a significant factor, as it can dictate severity of the infection, and therefore categorizing the timing of the infection has previously been considered helpful in determining possible approaches to treatment. Early-onset infections (less than 4 weeks after surgery) are typically acquired during the initial arthroplasty and commonly result from virulent organisms, such as *Staph. aureus*, gram-negative bacilli, anaerobic organisms, or mixed infections. Delayed and late, chronic infections present in an indolent fashion greater than 4 weeks after surgery. They can also be acquired during primary arthroplasty, but are generally caused by less virulent organisms, such as coagulase-negative

Staphylococci or Enterococci. Late haematogenous infections (over 12 months after surgery) are classically due to seeding of the joint, of which S. aureus, beta-hemolytic Streptococci, gram-negative bacilli, and Enterobacteriaceae are the most common culprits [6–9]. Although these categories can be helpful because they suggest the microbiology and pathophysiology of the infection, they should not be used alone to decide the fate of component retention. Generally, IDCR is accepted as a viable option for *acute* symptoms after primary arthroplasty or for late haematogenous spread with a short duration of symptoms [10]. More specifically, patients presenting with an acute infection, defined as either (1) less than 2–4 weeks of acute symptoms in a previously well-functioning total joint arthroplasty (TJA) or (2) presentation within the first 2–6 weeks from the primary TJA would be the ideal candidates for IDCR [4, 11, 12].

Furthermore, to be a candidate for IDCR, the prosthesis must be well-fixed and should be well-positioned. There should be no evidence of a sinus tract, and there should be a good soft-tissue envelope to cover the prosthesis. An additional reason to consider IDCR as the treatment of PJI is for those patients that are at high risk of medical complications if another more aggressive surgery was performed [13]. In a retrospective study of 42 patients treated with IDCR, comorbidities specifically analyzed such as diabetes, malignancy, vascular disease, thyroid disease, connective tissue disease, pulmonary disease, smoking, psychiatric disorders, chronic liver disease, and stage 2 or 3 chronic kidney failure have not been shown to have significant effects on IDCR outcomes [4].

Contraindications

Timing, as previously mentioned, can be helpful with cut offs for indications for IDCR. However, various classification systems that categorize infections based on timeframe of presenting symptoms alone do not have sufficient evidence to support their use as the guide to which infections can be treated conservatively and which require more aggressive management. There is a consensus that an infection with presenting symptoms lasting longer than 4 weeks is a contraindication to IDCR. Co-existing patient risk factors must be considered when evaluating whether or not a patient is a good candidate for IDCR. Not only have obesity [14] and immunosuppression been shown to increase the likelihood of initial infection after total arthroplasty, but they have also been shown to be independent predictors of IDCR failure [4, 6].

The etiologic organism can be a contraindication to IDCR as well. Virulence of the infecting organism (s), which as discussed is tied to presentation timeframe, has a statistically significant effect on successful treatment with IDCR [11]. An infection known to be polymicrobial, suggesting a sinus tract, or due to MRSA is recognized as a contraindication to IDCR due to high failure rates [6, 13, 15]. Other virulent infection etiologies shown to have high failure rates with IDCR are MRSE and VRE, and are best treated with a two-stage revision [16].

Due to high re-infection rates, IDCR is also not recommended for fungal PJI. Fungal PJI is rare and has been reported to make up about 1 % of all PJI, nevertheless treatment requires aggressive management [17]. Risk factors for fungal infection include immunosuppression, neutropenia, and chronic or prolonged antibiotic use. Treatment depends on severity of the infection, patient medical status and existing comorbidities. Generally, resection arthroplasty is the procedure of choice to eliminate the infection, and is either followed by a staged re-implantation or arthrodesis depending on individual patient factors. IDCR has been attempted in fungal PJI; however, in the small populations studied retrospectively, reinfection rates after this procedure have been reported to be from 67 to 75 % [17]. Therefore, two-stage revision is considered the gold standard for treatment, as it has the potential to remove organisms sheltered in a biofilm and subsequently provide function and mobility, once the infection has cleared [18]. The technical challenges of the extensive debridement and dedicated follow-up care required in these cases demands an experienced surgeon and specialized team for proper management.

Additional contraindications for IDCR are as previously mentioned, the presence of a sinus tract, if the prosthesis is loose, and if there is inadequate closure for the wound. The patient's soft tissue quality must be suitable for recovery, so that the local tissues remain viable and capable of fighting off infection. An open wound has the potential for contamination of the joint which will progress to chronic infection; therefore, IDCR should not be performed in these circumstances, as it will fail. With PJI after a revision surgery, IDCR can be considered for patients [19]; however, implants with long stems, or patients that have previously failed two-stage revisions are not good candidates for IDCR.

Pre-OP

Irrespective of the planned procedure in treating an infected joint, the approach requires a systematic and meticulous method to ensure removal of the maximum bacterial bioburden and devitalized tissue. As with all elective surgery, a proper IDCR starts with optimization of the patient before the operation. Time to initiate antibiotic treatment of an infection is crucial. However, IDCR is not considered an emergent procedure if the patient is not septic. The 2013 International Consensus Meeting on PJI advised that optimization should not be short-changed to emergently address the infection with surgery [13]. Attending to any medical comorbidities, that could potentially lead to complications is an important first step, especially when dealing with the likely systemic involvement of a deep PJI. Notably, nutritional status, hyperglycemia, anemia, and any coagulopathies should be controlled before the patient undergoes an operation.

In the OR

As in primary THA and TKA, provided that the bacteria is known, prophylactic antibiotics can be given prior to surgery and should not be withheld due to concern over inconclusive culture results [20]. Studies have shown that perioperative antibiotics do not affect the ability to obtain accurate cultures in an infected TJA [20]. The only exception to this rule is culture negative infections. If the patient has an infection based on international consensus guidelines for diagnosis but negative cultures, then perioperative antibiotics should be held until adequate tissue cultures are obtained in the operating room.

With aseptic technique and using separate, clean instruments for each sample, surgeons should obtain five to six cultures from the involved joint, tissue, and fluid from the superficial and deep periprosthetic regions. In order to obtain a quality sample for anaerobic and aerobic cultures and post-operative directed antibiotic therapy, no less than three cultures from the macroscopically most affected tissues should be sent to pathology lab [13]. In a patient with concern for atypical organisms such as in an immunosuppressed patient, notifying the lab to hold specimens for special culture plating techniques using various enriched media for potential isolation of fungi can be helpful.

Debridement

Good visualization must be obtained, and a thorough debridement of all compartments should be performed. An adequate debridement include excision of the prior skin incision (for early infections), a total synovectomy, extensive removal of all necrotic regions in the joint including the tissue in the posterior capsule, and drainage of any periarticular abscesses. However, one must still protect important structures such as the collateral ligaments of the knee and the periarticular muscles and neurovascular structures around the hip. After debridement, the joint should be irrigated with 9 L of normal saline with additional antibiotics (type of antibiotic depends on the hospitals pharmacy) added to the fluid, using low-pressure pulsatile lavage. In patients that have fascial defects or deep fluid pockets confirmed by aspiration, the fascia should be opened and all fluid, purulent, edematous, or hematoma should be evacuated. The modular components of the prosthesis should be removed to gain access to posterior compartments (e.g., of the knee) and to treat all interfaces. A Cobb elevator or similar instrument should be used to safely scrape the necrotic, infected tissue from the posterior capsule. A laminar spreader with a lap sponge protecting the metal femur and tibia can be used to help improve visualization of the posterior capsule. The remaining components should be examined for gross loosening of the protheses; however, aggressive testing of the fixation of the implants is not usually performed, as it is usually determined preoperatively if the components are well fixed. If any of the components are loose, they should be removed, and the procedure would then be converted to either a one-stage or a two-stage revision/re-implantation depending on the surgeon's assessment of the infection. In addition to the 9 L of fluid, some surgeons have recommend using a diluted betadine solution, Dakin's Solutions, or hydrogen peroxide to further clean the joint and the components. Further, some surgeons have begun using a sterile brush to scrape the metallic surfaces of the components, in an effort to remove the biofilm of the bacteria. While there is much variation in the additional methods employed (on top of the irrigation and debridement) to try to improve the success of the procedure, none of the adjunctive procedures have been proven to be harmful to the patient and. thus, all can be considered.

The extracellular polymeric substance matrix that the bacteria produce is the nemesis of successful management and cure of infection, as it is impenetrable with current antibiotic therapy or with the host immune system alone. Of note, in the lab, biofilm has been found to form within hours, and therefore complete removal cannot be expected with solely irrigation and debridement [21, 22]. The conservative treatment of IDCR works to decrease the bioburden as much as possible, so that in combination with ensuing antibiotic therapy, the host immune system can clear the infection.

Localized Antibiotic Agents

Although one-stage and two-stage surgeries successfully employ antibiotic impregnated bone cement in the component revision, local administration of antibiotics in IDCR is not recommended due to lack of specific evidence showing significance in improvement [13]. Success with intra-articular administration via Hickman catheter of antibiotics after IDCR has been described [23]; however, there is limited evidence to support this as an independent factor leading to a successful outcome. Therefore, the value of this procedure is debatable, as it adds cost, an additional procedure to remove the catheter, and potential drug reactions. Similarly, no randomized control trials have shown that resorbable antibiotic-laden beads or dissolvable gentamicin loaded collagen sponges have an independent significant effect on improving outcomes with IDCR. The value of these products should be judged as they increase costs and harbor additional risks including associated local tissue reactions and wound exudates with calcium sulphate pellets. Developments of materials and delivery systems such as hydroxyapatite nanoparticles require further study and proof of efficacy, but beckon advancements in biotechnology.

Overall, scrupulous debridement is known to be the most significant component of success with IDCR.

Antimicrobial Management Following IDCR

Together surgical and medical treatments are allies in abolishing PJI. Antibiotic therapy is a crucial element in the consistent follow up after IDCR. Although there is no decisive evidence dictating the length of therapy, the recommended duration of pathogen-specific IV antibiotic treatment is 2–6 weeks, with the majority of the literature suggesting 6 weeks. Shortening the treatment decreases cost and, with proper treatment compliance, could decrease the development of resistance. The Infectious Diseases

Society of America released clinical practice guidelines in 2013 suggesting either highly bioavailable oral antibiotics or IV therapy could be used in certain PJI circumstances. Intravenous administration allows for faster and more controlled drug delivery systemically. However, if indicated, oral antibiotics reduce costs, allow patients to manage their treatment at home, and decrease complications associated with vascular access. The main concern for challenges with oral antibiotic therapy is related to patient compliance. Due to the notorious potential of resistant organisms as proven predictors of negative outcomes in PJI, the decision to treat with oral antibiotics must be weighed thoughtfully.

The protocol for antibiotic treatment after IDCR for PJI due to Staphylococcal species has more specific recommendations. The Infectious Diseases Society of America recommends 300–450 mg of oral rifampin be given twice daily along with the initial IV antibiotic treatment. Following the IV treatment, rifampin should be continued in combination with another oral antibiotic for a total of 3 months for a THA infection and 6 months for a TKA infection. Ciprofloxacin or levofloxacin are generally good oral antibiotic choices in conjunction with rifampin, if the sensitivity of the bacteria is appropriate [24]. Rifampin is known to promote resistance development if used as monotherapy and is therefore recommended to be used as an adjunct therapy and should only be started after the patient is first established on a primary antibiotic drug. Furthermore, if bacteremia exists, rifampin should not be initiated until this has cleared to decrease the potential development of resistance. Rifampin has significant side effects such as hepatotoxicity and gastrointestinal intolerance, which should be monitored accordingly with the extended therapy [13].

Chronic Suppression

Although not ideal, depending on the patient, indefinite chronic suppression therapy can be utilized. If patient comorbidities or patient preferences rule out further surgery, yet clinical signs of infection are still present, medical therapy alone is the alternative. This option is generally reserved for patients who are surgically unfit for, or refuse, two-stage revision, excision arthroplasty, or amputation. Concerns surrounding chronic antimicrobial suppression involve patient adherence, selection of resistant organisms, and high cost. The antimicrobial regimen is chosen for the patient based on the isolated organism(s) and sensitivities, and the patient's allergies and intolerances.

With IDCR, it is accepted that not all the bacteria will be removed with the surgical procedure, and thus, many orthopaedic surgeons and infectious disease specialists like the idea of chronic suppression provided the patient can tolerate the antimicrobial therapy. However, there can be detrimental side effects with long-term antibiotic therapy, which should be discussed between the physician and the patient when deciding against more aggressive treatment approaches. The hazards of long-term use of various antibiotics include nephrotoxicity, ototoxicity, and disturbance of normal gastrointestinal microflora, which impairs the natural defense mechanisms of the colonic microbiome. Depending on the antibiotic drug used, specific toxicities have been observed such as neurotoxicity with penicillins and tendinopathy with fluoroquinolones. Other bactericidal agents can cause oxidative damage to DNA, proteins, and membrane lipids due to the formation of reactive oxygen species causing mitochondrial dysfunction [25]. Furthermore, since total joint arthroplasty patients are often older, evaluation of hepatic and renal function is imperative due to the metabolism and elimination of antimicrobial drugs. In addition to toxicity to the liver and kidneys, poor initial function of these organs can lead to impaired clearance, and variations in systemic drug concentrations, which compounds toxicities. As a result, clinical follow-up and patient laboratory values should be monitored regularly. Likewise, because of interactions with other drugs and effect on metabolism via the cytochrome P450 system, patient medication regimens and changes should be reviewed carefully.

Management of chronic infection status and drug therapy requires a multidisciplinary team including orthopedic and plastic surgeons, infectious disease specialists, microbiologists, the patient's primary care physician, and rehabilitation physiotherapists and occupational therapists.

Culture-Negative PJI

Reiterating the importance of adequate intra-op specimen collection, up to 35 % of PJI cases can result in negative culture results [13]. In the diagnostic work-up, beyond histology and gram-staining, advanced testing such as polymerase chain reaction (PCR), reverse transcriptase polymerase chain reaction (RT-PCR), mass spectrometry, microarray identification, and fluorescence in situ hybridization (FISH), may aid in determining the etiologic organism. Preserving the cultures for at least 14 days may also help to identify a low virulence pathogen, such as Propioibacterium Acnes (s) [13].

In the case that the organism remains elusive, broad-spectrum antimicrobial therapy with MRSA coverage is recommended. Treatment should encompass gram-negative, gram-positive, anaerobic organisms, and potentially fungal etiologies. An accepted choice amongst infectious disease specialists is a combination of vancomycin and either ceftriaxone or a fluoroquinolone [13].

Following Recovery

Clinical signs of improvement are not guaranteed predictors of clearance of the infection. Likewise, although normalizing or decreasing ESR and CRP values can be helpful in obtaining a clinical picture of the patient, they cannot be depended on to declare that the patient has eradicated the infection. There is no ideal cut off for these markers, and values have the tendency to vary amongst patients with other medical comorbidities. New inflammatory markers such as pro-calcitonin, leukocyte esterase, and IL-6 have been suggested as potential indicators, however, further study is needed [13].

If IDCR Is Unsuccessful

The biggest concern with IDCR to treat PJI is that it will fail to clear the infection, and the patient will require additional surgery. Risk factors for failure of IDCR have been reported retrospectively to include infection with *Staphylococcus* species, symptoms lasting longer than 5 days, obesity, preoperative ESR above 60, high American Society of Anesthesiologists score, and intra-articular purulence [4, 26, 27]. The only factor consistently significant in all reports is infection due to *Staphylococci.* Following initial failure of IDCR, repeating the same procedure has been shown to have limited success and should be avoided [19]. If IDCR fails, all original implants should be removed. Two-stage revision is more common than one-stage in the United States; however, both are acceptable surgical options. A two-stage revision is generally used for more severe circumstances and progression such as sepsis, development of a sinus tract, no longer viable soft tissue coverage, and either unidentifiable or isolated resistant organisms [13]. If the patient's bone stock is extremely limited, or if their health is poor, and they do not have high expectations of the limb, resection arthroplasty with an arthrodesis can be used.

References

1. Hoover NW, Ivins JC. Wound debridement. A M A Arch Surg. 1959;79(5):701–10. doi:10.1001/archsurg.1959.04320110003001.
2. Huntley JS. Debridement: development of the concept. J Perioper Pract. 2011;21(3):104–5.
3. Shuman EK, Urquhart A, Malani PN. Management and prevention of prosthetic joint infection. Infect Dis Clin North Am. 2012;26(1):29–39.
4. Triantafyllopoulos GK, Poultsides LA, Sakellariou VI, Zhang W, Sculco PK, Ma Y, et al. Irrigation and debridement for periprosthetic infections of the hip and factors determining outcome. Int Orthop. 2015;39(6):1203–9.
5. Sherrell JC, Fehring TK, Odum S, Hansen E, Zmistowski B, Dennos A, Kalore N. The Chitranjan Ranawat Award: fate of two-stage reimplantation after failed irrigation and debridement for periprosthetic knee infection. Clin Orthop Relat Res. 2011;469:18–25.

6. Lora-tamayo J, Murillo O, Iribarren JA, Soriano A, Sánchez-Somolinos M, Baraia-Etxaburu JM, et al. A large multicenter study of methicillin-susceptible and methicillin-resistant Staphylococcus aureus prosthetic joint infections managed with implant retention. Clin Infect Dis. 2013;56(2):182–94.
7. Zimmerli W, Trampuz A, Ochsner PE. Prosthetic-joint infections. N Engl J Med. 2004;351(16):1645–54.
8. Widmer AF. New developments in diagnosis and treatment of infection in orthopedic implants. Clin Infect Dis. 2001;33 Suppl 2:S94–106.
9. Anagnostakos K, Schmid NV, Kelm J, Grün U, Jung J. Classification of hip joint infections. Int J Med Sci. 2009;6(5):227–33.
10. Odum SM, Fehring TK, Lombardi AV, Zmistowski BM, Brown NM, Luna JT, et al. Irrigation and debridement for periprosthetic infections: does the organism matter? J Arthroplasty. 2011; 26(6 Suppl):114–8.
11. Brandt CM, Sistrunk WW, Duffy MC, Hanssen AD, Steckelberg JM, Ilstrup DM, et al. Staphylococcus aureus prosthetic joint infection treated with debridement and prosthesis retention. Clin Infect Dis. 1997;24(5):914–9.
12. Anagnostakos K, Schmitt C. Can periprosthetic hip joint infections be successfully managed by debridement and prosthesis retention? World J Orthop. 2014;5(3):218–24.
13. Parvizi J, Gehrke T, Chen AF. Proceedings of the International Consensus on periprosthetic joint infection. Bone Joint J. 2013;95-B(11):1450–2.
14. Namba RS, Paxton L, Fithian DC, Stone ML. Obesity and perioperative morbidity in total hip and total knee arthroplasty patients. J Arthroplasty. 2005;20: 46–50.
15. Barberán J, Aguilar L, Carroquino G, Giménez MJ, Sánchez B, Martínez D, et al. Conservative treatment of staphylococcal prosthetic joint infections in elderly patients. Am J Med. 2006;119(11):993.e7–10.
16. Buller LT, Sabry FY, Easton RQ, Klika AK, Barsoum WK. The preoperative prediction of success following irrigation and debridement with polyethylene exchange for hip and knee prosthetic joint infections. J Arthroplasty. 2012;27:857-64.el–4.
17. Schoof B, Jakobs O, Schmidl S, Klatte TO, Frommelt L, Gehrke T, et al. Fungal periprosthetic joint infection of the hip: a systematic review. Orthop Rev (Pavia). 2015;7(1):5748.
18. Jakobs O, Schoof B, Klatte TO, Schmidl S, Fensky F, Guenther D, et al. Fungal periprosthetic joint infection in total knee arthroplasty: a systemic review. Orthop Rev (Pavia). 2015;7(1):5623.
19. Triantafyllopoulos G, Poultsides LA, Zhang W, Sculco PK, Ma Y, Sculco TP. Multiple irrigation and debridements for periprosthetic joint infections: facing a necessity or just prolonging the inevitable? J Arthroplasty. 2015. doi:10.1016/j.arth.2015.06.051.
20. Tetreault MW, Wetters NG, Aggarwal V, Mont M, Parvizi J, Della valle CJ. The Chitranjan Ranawat Award: should prophylactic antibiotics be withheld before revision surgery to obtain appropriate cultures? Clin Orthop Relat Res. 2014;472(1):52–6.
21. Archer NK, Mazaitis MJ, Costerton JW, Leid JG, Powers ME, Shirtliff ME. Staphylococcus aureus biofilms: properties, regulation, and roles in human disease. Virulence. 2011;2(5):445–59.
22. Fey PD, Olson ME. Current concepts in biofilm formation of Staphylococcus epidermidis. Future Microbiol. 2010;5(6):917–33.
23. Whiteside LA, Nayfeh TA, LaZear R, Roy ME. Reinfected revised TKA resolves with an aggressive protocol and antibiotic infusion. Clin Orthop Relat Res. 2012;470(1):236–43.
24. Osmon DR, Berbari EF, Berendt AR, Lew D, Zimmerli W, Steckelberg JM, et al. Diagnosis and management of prosthetic joint infection: clinical practice guidelines by the Infectious Diseases Society of America. Clin Infect Dis. 2013;56(1):e1–25.
25. Kalghatgi S, Spina CS, Costello JC, Liesa M, Morones-Ramirez JR, Slomovic S, et al. Bactericidal antibiotics induce mitochondrial dysfunction and oxidative damage in Mammalian cells. Sci Transl Med. 2013;5(192):192ra85.
26. Kim JG, Bae JH, Lee SY, Cho WT, Lim HC. The parameters affecting the success of irrigation and debridement with component retention in the treatment of acutely infected total knee arthroplasty. Clin Orthop Surg. 2015;7(1):69–76.
27. Azzam KA, Seeley M, Ghanem E, Austin MS, Purtill JJ, Parvizi J. Irrigation and debridement in the management of prosthetic joint infection: traditional indications revisited. J Arthroplasty. 2010;25:1022–7.

Late Infections of the Knee Joint: One-Stage Approach with Cement

20

Carl Haasper and Thorsten Gehrke

Abstract

Two major concepts have been established to treat infected knee arthroplasties (TKA) in terms of one- or two-stage exchanges. A single-stage TKA exchange offers some advantages: the need for only one operative procedure without spacers, a general reduced hospitalization time, reduced overall cost (specific reimbursement system) and potential of improved patient. The presence of an organism culture with a sensitivity antibiogram is mandatory for a successful revision. Implant fixation using antibiotic loaded cement is, we believe, the current gold standard for single-stage procedure. A defined period of systemic antibiotic therapy follows and early mobilization should be started as soon as possible.

Keywords

Knee • Bacteria • Sepsis • Total joint • Exchange • Revision • Arthroplasty

Introduction

Total knee arthroplasty (TKA) is considered to be one of the most successful procedures in orthopaedic surgery nowadays. However, complications like infection often result in poor clinical outcome. Periprosthetic infections are reported in the literature with prevalence between 1 and 2 % in primary and between 3 and 5 % in revision total knee arthroplasty [1, 2]. Operative management of periprosthetic infection after TKA remains a very challenging procedure and devastating problem not only for the surgeon but especially for the patient. Thus, prevention of infection in TKA is of paramount importance.

Concepts that have been established to treat delayed and late infections include one- and two-stage exchanges. Two-stage revision technique in late TKA infection has become the gold standard worldwide with described published success rates ranging from 70 to 90 %. There are only very few institutions which focus a one-stage revision approach like ours [2–4].

Although very few studies or clinical reports have been published, the one–staged

C. Haasper, MD, PhD, MSc (✉) • T. Gehrke, MD
Department of Orthopaedic Surgery, Helios ENDO-Klinik, Hamburg, Germany
e-mail: carl.haasper@helios-kliniken.de

D. Kendoff et al. (eds.), *Periprosthetic Joint Infections: Changing Paradigms*,
DOI 10.1007/978-3-319-30091-7_20

revision technique was established at our institution over 35 years ago, for all major septic arthroplasty revisions. Over the last three decades more than 85 % of our infected TKA patients were treated using a one-stage revision technique with a comparable high success rate [3, 4].

Generally all mentioned revision techniques should be adapted to the clinical situation, local clinical set-up, surgeon's preference and previous expertise. In the most frequent two-stage scenarios, TKA implant removal is followed by a 6–8 weeks course of antibiotics and consequent delayed revision arthroplasty. Articulating spacers have shown to improve the functional outcome of the two-stage approach, however with ongoing controversy. There seems to be a marginal improvement of postoperative ROM, but without statistical significance [5]. Identified potential problems associated with articulating spacers include bone loss, cement fracture, wound healing problems and even spacer dislocations [6]. Although antibiotic loaded spacers do show sufficient local release of these antibiotics up to 6 weeks after implantation, there is evidence of material abrasion of these spacers, which can be detected in the synovial membrane [7–9]. Substantial amounts of zirconium oxide can be detected in the synovial membrane, which implies a further radical synovectomy and extensive lavage at the time of re-implantation [7].

Articles describing the two staged technique as the gold standard in infection eradication, comment on remaining controversies, e.g., duration of antibiotic treatment, static vs. mobile spacer, interval of spacer retention, cemented vs. uncemented implant fixation, and are based on level IV to III evidence studies or even expert opinions, rather than on prospective randomized or comparative data [4, 10]. In direct contrast a one-stage TKA exchange offers some advantages: This mainly includes the need for only one operative procedure without spacers, a general reduced hospitalization time, reduced overall cost (specific reimbursement system) and potential of improved patient satisfaction [1, 3].

In this chapter the authors try to establish a practical guide for performing a successful one-stage approach and try to highlight the key differences between one-stage and two-stage revision surgeries in treating periprosthetic knee infections.

Diagnostics

Recent clinical practice guidelines, our own experience and current evidence published by the American Academy of Orthopaedic Surgeons and International Consensus Group recommend the following mandatory preoperative testing in **every single** unclear painful TKA patient [11, 12]:

- Laboratory monitoring of C-reactive protein (CRP)
- Knee joint aspiration with prolonged microbiologic culture time of at least 14 days, while patients being off antibiotics for a minimum of 14 days [13, 14]
- Synovial fluid analyzing of white blood cell count and percentage of neutrophils
- Repeated aspiration in cases of own negative cultural results in combination with either obvious infections signs or pre-existing external positive cultural results
- Biopsy of the knee joint in cases of persistent negative aspiration results, with obvious infections signs

Joint Aspiration

The most relevant preoperative and mandatory diagnostic test needed in any planned one-stage TKA exchange, is based on the knee joint aspiration with an exact identification of the organism. The antibiogram is required for the one-stage procedure. Only then is it possible to define a specific antibiotic-loaded acrylic cement (ALAC) to achieve a high therapeutic level of antibiotic elution at the surgical side [15].

In a previous unpublished study from our institution looking at results of preoperative aspirations before revision knee and hip surgery we were able to show that 4–7 % of patients had positive results even when clinical symptoms or relevant changes in laboratory were missing [16].

Imaging

We consider serial radiographs and CT scans to be the most helpful imaging tools in the diagnosis of infection at our institution. In serial radiographs we look for signs of infection, loosing, implants etc. Nuclear imaging as a routine tool is not included in our setup. Bone scans, e.g., labeled leukocyte imaging, Gallium imaging or PET imaging have shown to be non-specific, although highly sensitive [11]. Those could detect physiological bone remodeling and may be misleading. There is only limited evidence for the use of PET in the literature and we therefore consider this technology to be secondary in the diagnosis of infection and probably more helpful when planning for revision THA due to infection.

Preoperative Preparation and Planning for the TKA Revision

Preoperative preparation and planning for revision knee surgery have been well documented and published elsewhere. In infections, however, several additional points need to be considered. These include evaluation of the patient, anaesthesia and surgery. Again we would like to underline the mandatory presence of a positive bacterial culture and respective antibiogram for the procedure. The proposed cemented fixation using ALAC is considered to be the treatment of choice in order to achieve a high therapeutic level of antibiotic elution from the cement [17].

Patient

Specific sources of patient related infection should be evaluated. Malnutrition and diabetes are endocrinoligical predispositions associated with poor outcome. General signs of infection in terms of SIRS and sepsis should be ruled out prior elective septic exchange.

Anaesthesia

Clinical and anesthesiology assessment of the general operative risk is mandatory. An adequate quantity of additional donor blood should be available. In cases of time extensive operations preoperative administration of fibrinolysis inhibitors (e.g., tranexamic acid) might be helpful [18]. Monitoring body temperature and heating blankets should be recommended.

Surgery

The surgical success of a one staged approach depends on the complete removal of all hardware material, furthermore the aggressive and complete debridement of any infected bone and soft tissues. A full synovectomy, including the most posterior aspects of the knee capsule is also extremely important and needs to be performed routinely. Consequently, resection of the PCL, if still existing, and even in some rare cases of the collateral ligaments needs to be considered, to perform this radical and complete soft tissue resection. Thus, the definitive preoperative planning should consider the use of a condylar constraint or hinged implant, also based on the surgeon's preference and technique. A distinct knowledge of the implant in situ and knowledge how to remove and disassemble it is required (e.g., hinge mechanism). Occasionally the use of implant-specific instrumentation becomes necessary. Principally a variety of implants should be available, from primary total condylar to hinged designs, depending on the requirements for reconstruction. As mentioned above, pre-existing ligament deficiencies require constraint implants; however, ligament deficiency may also result during an aggressive intraoperative debridement. Based on our own aggressive soft tissue debridement, this happens to be the case in over 90 % of our one-stage TKA revisions. Inadequate bone stock, possible intraoperative complications as femoral or tibial shaft fractures, perforations of the cortex and osseous windows must be taken into consideration when choosing an appropriate implant. Distal femoral or proximal tibial replacement implants may have to be chosen in patients with significant bone deficiency. Bone loss is usually significantly more extensive than radio graphically evident. Custom made implants with extra long or narrow stems may have to be ordered prior to surgery. Today we also use tantalum based cones in our one-stage revisions, to achieve an adequate metaphyseal rotational stabilization of the revision implant. Significant damage to the extensor mechanism might necessitate the use of an arthrodesis nail, also in a one staged technique. However, a distinct preoperative patient communication and consent should be assured in those rare cases (less than 0.5 % per year in our clinic). Cement with additional antibiotics in powder form, added intraoperatively, is mandatory in all cases. Mostly two to three mixes of cement (40–80 g) per femur and also per tibia are required per case. Larger mixing systems and appropriate cement guns are required, while a narrow diaphysis might necessitate extra narrow nozzles for an appropriate retrograde cementing technique. Distinct knowledge of type and antibiotic adding of the cement used at the primary implantation should exist, as resistance to the previously used antibiotic must be expected. In consequence, a variation of ALAC should be considered, although in many cases, even an industrially pre-manufactured ALAC might still be appropriate.

Indications One-Stage Approach

Principally we do see only very few arguments against our one-stage revision protocol, consequently we are able to fulfill over 85 % of all infected cases with the one-stage approach. An experienced microbiologist is essential to develop a distinct patient specific plan for the local and systemic antibiotic treatment.

Contraindications One-Stage Approach

We defined to following criteria to deviate from our one-stage approach to a two-stage procedure:

- Failure of ≥2 previous one-stage procedures
- Infection spreading to the posterior nerve-vessel bundle
- Unclear pre-operative bacteria specification
- Non-availability of appropriate antibiotics
- High antibiotic resistance

Surgical Technique

Skin Incision and Debridement

Old scars in the line of the skin incision should be excised (Fig. 20.1). The prior incision from the last operative approach should be used, if possible. In cases of multiple scars, the most lateral one should be considered. If crossing of scars by incision is necessary try to be as rectangular as possible. Existing fistulae should be integrated into the incision and radically excised to the joint capsule. In cases of increased distances of the fistulae to the lateral or posterior aspects, a separate excision should be used. Try to form full-thickness flaps. Consider plastic consultation, expanders and sham incisions in severe cases. It is important

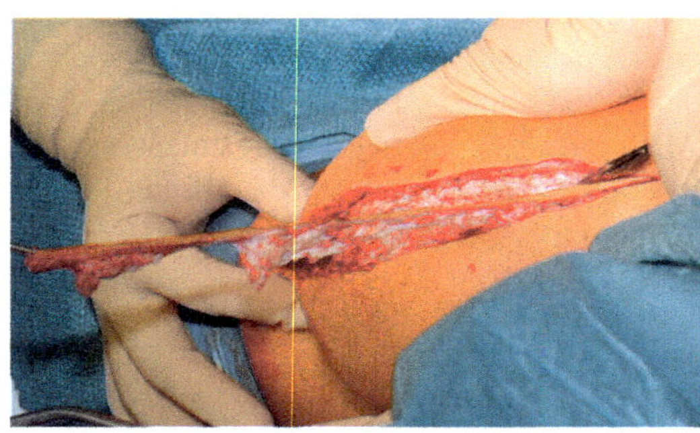

Fig. 20.1 Excision of the scar from the prior incision should be performed. In case of multiple scars, the most lateral one should be considered. Between two incisions, one should maintain sufficient distance between them

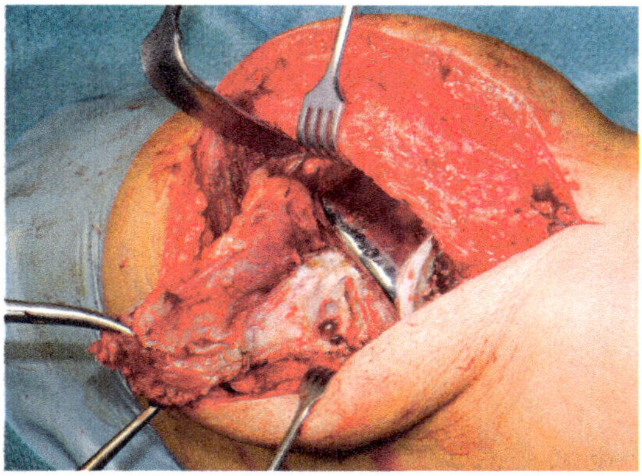

Fig. 20.2 A full synovectomy, including the most posterior aspects of the knee capsule, needs to be performed. All non-bleeding tissues and related bone need to be excised

to be gentle to the skin. The thinner the flap is it is more prone to infection. In difficult cases of exposure consider quad-snip, extensor plasty and/or tibial tubercle osteotomy. For bony exposure banana peel (femoral peel) and medial subperiostal exposure with external rotation of the tibia are helpful.

The procedure should be started without tourniquet; consequently boundaries between infected tissue, scar and surrounding healthy bleeding soft tissue (and bone) can be distinguished easier during the debridement. All non-bleeding tissues and related bone needs to be excised (Fig. 20.2). After completion of debridement and implant removal, the tourniquet can be helpful for the final intramedullary cement removal as well as for the process of re-cementation.

Biopsies

Early in the operation biopsy material, preferably five to six samples, should be taken from all relevant areas for combined microbiological and histological evaluation [19], before the defined intravenous antibiotics are administered. This commonly consists of any wide-spectrum cephalosporin with further specifications, based on the arteriogram.

Implant Removal and Debridement Completion

For implant removal start first with removal of the inlay, then femoral component and afterwards the tibial component. For the femoral component retrograde slap hammers are helpful. In cases of well-fixed uncemented components, rarely cortical windows are required to gain access to the bone-implant interface. High-speed burrs and curved saw blades can simplify the removal; however, even in experienced hands, occasionally significant collateral osseous destruction can occur. Alternatively, a Gigli saw or small bladed electric saw can be useful to cut around the femoral shield and the tibial base plate of the implant. A full range of narrow and wide osteotomes of various thicknesses should be available. Utilizing multiple osteotomes, which are carefully driven between the tibial base plate and cement from medial and lateral, even if stemmed, can be gradually wedged/forced out of its cement mantle. This is usually less destructive than aggressive extraction with the mallet. In cemented cases, narrow straight osteotomes with symmetrically coned blades should remove all accessible bone cement, without causing further loss of bone stock. In order to achieve longer intramedullary cement mantles, special curved chisels, long rongeurs, curetting instruments, extra long drills and cement taps should be used to remove residual cement.

Successful one-stage re-implantation necessitates a radical debridement of bone and posterior soft tissues This must include all areas of osteolysis and non-viable bone, thus finalisation of the aggressive debridement often exceeds the amount of resected materials compared to a two-stage approach (Figs. 20.3 and 20.4). We recommend the general use of pulsatile lavage throughout the procedure. After all implant removal and completed debridement; the intramedullary canals are packed with polymeric biguanid-hydrochlorid (polyhexanid)–soaked swabs. Furthermore, the swabs are placed over the wound area before re-draping the patient.

The complete surgical team should now re-scrub, while new instruments are used for re-implantation. A second dose of recommended antibiotics is administered after 1.5 h operating

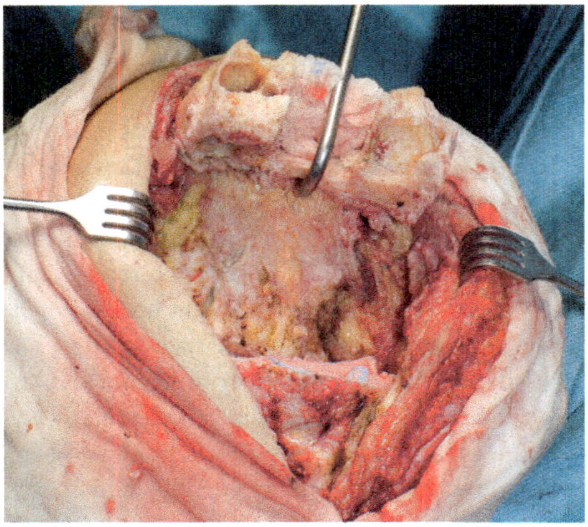

Fig. 20.3 Successful one-stage re-implantation necessitates a radical debridement of bone and posterior soft tissues This must include all areas of osteolysis and non-viable bone; thus, finalisation of the aggressive debridement often exceeds the amount of resected materials compared to a two-stage approach

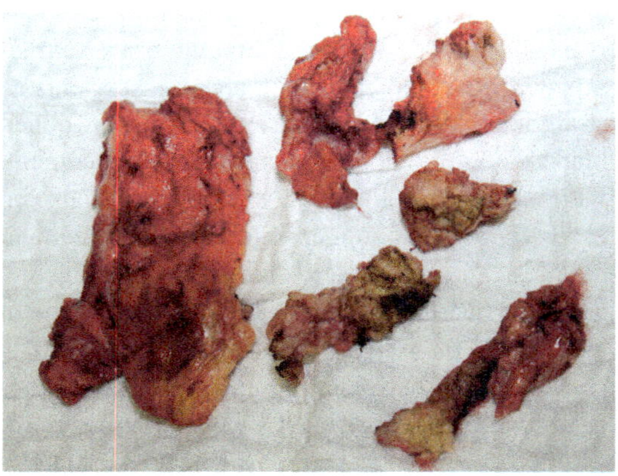

Fig. 20.4 The surgical success of a one-stage approach depends on the distinct and complete removal of all hardware material and the aggressive and complete debridement of any infected bone and soft tissue

time, or if the perioperative blood loss exceeds 1 l. In case of a two-stage approach a cement-loaded spacer should be implanted and the first step of surgical treatment ends.

Reimplantation

For the two-stage procedure an aggressive and radical debridement is absolutely mandatory at the time of re-implantation. The procedure continues as for the one-stage exchange: In cases of inadequate metaphyseal bone stock we preferred to fill large defects with cement in the past, instead of using allograft bone. Although it has been shown, that allografts can effectively be thoroughly lavaged and impregnated with antibiotics and potential of a high local antibiotic carrier, especially in a suggested cementless approach, we personally have only very limited experience with this technique [20].

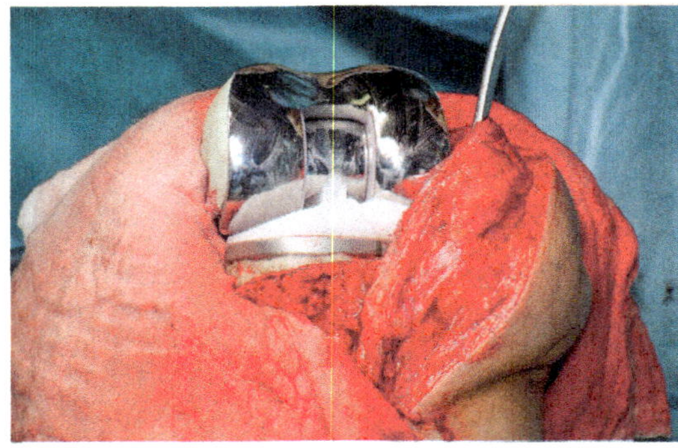

Fig. 20.5 Finally, we use a hinged knee with combined fixation of the cemented prosthesis and, if indicated, tantalum cones

Alternatively the use of tantalum based femoral and tibial cones have been implemented in our regular clinical use and one-stage approaches in recent years. Variations of depth and width of those augments allow for a proper reconstruction of the resulting bone loss, including an excellent biocompatibility and related stiffness and cellular structure comparable to bone [21]. Consequently a combined fixation of the cement with the prosthesis and tantalum cone becomes possible, even in infected cases (Fig. 20.5).

Cement

The antibiotic loaded cement is prepared fulfilling the following criteria:

- Appropriate antibiotics (antibiogram, adequate elusion characteristics)
- Bactericidal (exception clindamycin)

- Powder form (never use liquid antibiotics)
- Maximum addition of 10 % to the PMMA powder

It should always be considered, that antibiotics might change the polymerization behavior of the cement, causing acceleration of the curing process and weaken the mechanical properties. The current principles of modern cementing techniques should be applied under all circumstances. To achieve an improved cement bone interface, the tourniquet should be inflated prior to cementing.

Postoperative Antibiotics

The in-hospital time postoperatively ranges from 12 to 20 days (mean 14), whereas the associated postoperative systemic antibiotic administration is 10–14 days (exception: streptococci). Whereas a prolonged administration of intravenous antibiotics for 6 weeks is common in the two-stage approach, the rational for this prolongation has not been clarified in studies. In contradiction, there is clear evidence about possible relevant systemic and organ specific complications after any prolonged antibiotic administration [18].

Postoperative Rehabilitation

The physiotherapeutic plan in any one staged approach cannot be generalized. Based on the variety of osseous defects, soft tissue compromise, extent of infection and further patient specific circumstances, an individual patient plan is developed. Although compromises between necessary immobilization due to structural damage and general attempts of early mobilization have to be made, we recommend a mobilization within the first 8 days postoperatively. Weight bearing is adapted to the intraoperative findings; thus, a similar mobilization strategy compared to primary TKA is attempted. In defined patients without bone grafting, adequate bone stock and relative low soft tissue involvement, an immediate mobilization under full weight bearing becomes possible.

Postoperative Complications

Persistence or recurrence of infection remains the most relevant complication in the one-stage technique. As failures rates with a two-stage exchange have been described between 9 and 20 % in non-resistant bacteria, our unpublished data shows comparative results after 8 years of follow-up, using the one-stage approach (unpublished data) [2, 6, 22]. Consequently, we discuss at the time of patients consent a possible risk of recurrent or new infection of about 10–20 %. Postoperative stiffness and reduction of knee function remains the other most relevant complication postoperatively. Although we are unable to present comparative data evaluating the functional outcome under a two- vs. one-stage approach, we truly believe that neither any articulating spacer nor partial or complete immobilization of the knee joint will result in better functional outcome.

We consider the risk of direct damage to the peroneal nerve or main vessels as relatively low to an experienced surgeon, even in such an extended aggressive debridement. Further damage to the extensor mechanism is mainly based on the number of previous operations and relative stiffness of the knee. In rare cases if combined infection and distinct stiffness, we perform a tibial tubercle osteotomy.

We have no experience with the use of patellar tendon allografting in the infected scenario of a defective extensor mechanism. The general risk of intra- and postoperative fractures should be comparable to the two- or more stage exchange.

Conclusion

It remains mandatory to obtain a culture, based on a joint aspiration, with a respective antibiogram for a successful one-stage approach and every revision. Cemented implant fixation using local antibiotics is currently the gold standard for single-stage procedure. In addition, the success of the surgical procedure is related to the experience of a designated microbiologist, including development of a patient specific treatment plan with specifications of the systemic and topic antibiotic regime. Explantation of the infected implant is followed by an aggressive local debridement. In general, "a one-stage exchange is a two-stage in one session," as Prof. Michael Freeman likes to state, and the preoperative algorithms are equal. Consequently, implantation of the new cemented implant with patient-specific loaded antibiotics becomes possible in one-stage.

References

1. Buechel FF, Femino FP, D'Alessio J. Primary exchange revision arthroplasty for infected total knee replacement: a long-term study. Am J Orthop (Belle Mead NJ). 2004;33(4):190–8; discussion 8. Epub 2004/05/11. eng.
2. Kilgus DJ, Howe DJ, Strang A. Results of periprosthetic hip and knee infections caused by resistant bacteria. Clin Orthop Relat Res. 2002;404:116–24. Epub 2002/11/20. eng.
3. von Foerster G, Kluber D, Kabler U. Mid- to long-term results after treatment of 118 cases of periprosthetic infections after knee joint replacement using one-stage exchange surgery. Orthopade. 1991;20(3):244–52. Epub 1991/06/01. Mittel- bis langfristige Ergebnisse nach Behandlung von 118 periprothetischen Infektionen nach Kniegelenkersatz durch einzeitige Austauschoperation. ger.
4. Gehrke T, Haasper C. Comment on: Two-stage revision of septic knee prosthesis with articulating knee spacers yields better infection eradication rate than one-stage or two-stage revision with static spacers. Knee Surg Sports Traumatol Arthrosc Off J ESSKA. 2014;22(8):1958–9.
5. Pietsch M, Wenisch C, Traussnig S, Trnoska R, Hofmann S. Temporary articulating spacer with antibiotic-impregnated cement for an infected knee endoprosthesis. Orthopade. 2003;32(6):490–7. Die temporare Antibiotikaspacerprothese bei der infizierten Knieendoprothese. ger.
6. Jacobs C, Christensen CP, Berend ME. Static and mobile antibiotic-impregnated cement spacers for the management of prosthetic joint infection. J Am Acad Orthop Surg. 2009;17(6):356–68. Epub 2009/05/29. eng.
7. Fink B, Rechtenbach A, Buchner H, Vogt S, Hahn M. Articulating spacers used in two-stage revision of infected hip and knee prostheses abrade with time. Clin Orthop Relat Res. 2011;469(4):1095–102. Pubmed Central PMCID: 3048284, Epub 2010/07/29. eng.
8. Citak M, Argenson JN, Masri B, Kendoff D, Springer B, Alt V, et al. Spacers. J Arthroplasty. 2014; 29(2 Suppl):93–9.
9. Citak M, Citak M, Kendoff D. Dynamic versus static cement spacer in periprosthetic knee infection : a meta-analysis. Orthopade. 2015;44(8):599–606. Dynamischer vs. statischer Zementspacer in der Knietotalendoprotheseninfektion : Eine Metaanalyse.
10. Lichstein P, Gehrke T, Lombardi A, Romano C, Stockley I, Babis G, et al. One-stage vs two-stage exchange. J Arthroplasty. 2014;29(2 Suppl):108–11.
11. Della Valle C, Parvizi J, Bauer TW, Dicesare PE, Evans RP, Segreti J, et al. AAOS Clinical Practice Guideline Summary: diagnosis of periprosthetic joint infections of the hip and knee. J Am Acad Orthop Surg. 2010;18(12):760–70. Epub 2010/12/02. eng.
12. Parvizi J, Gehrke T, International Consensus Group on Periprosthetic Joint I. Definition of periprosthetic joint infection. J Arthroplasty. 2014;29(7):1331.
13. Frommelt L, editor. Periprosthetic infection – bacteria and the interface between prosthesis and bone. New York: Springer; 2004.
14. Mont MA, Waldman BJ, Hungerford DS. Evaluation of preoperative cultures before second-stage reimplantation of a total knee prosthesis complicated by infection. A comparison-group study. J Bone Joint Surg Am. 2000;82-A(11):1552–7. Epub 2000/11/30. eng.
15. Hanssen AD, Spangehl MJ. Practical applications of antibiotic-loaded bone cement for treatment of infected joint replacements. Clin Orthop Relat Res. 2004;427:79–85. Epub 2004/11/24. eng.
16. Kordelle J, Klett R, Stahl U, Hossain H, Schleicher I, Haas H. Infection diagnosis after knee-TEP-implantation. Z Orthop Ihre Grenzgeb. 2004;142(3):337–43. Epub 2004/07/14. Infektdiagnostik nach Knie-TEP-Implantation. ger.
17. Gehrke T, Frommelt L, G. vF, editors. Pharmakokinetik study of a gentamycin/clindamycin bone cement used in one stage revision arthroplasty. In: Bone cement and cementing technique. New York: Springer; 1998.
18. MacGillivray RG, Tarabichi SB, Hawari MF, Raoof NT. Tranexamic acid to reduce blood loss after bilateral total knee arthroplasty: a prospective, randomized double blind study. J Arthroplasty. 2011;26(1):24–8. Epub 2010/02/23. eng.
19. Zimmerli W, Trampuz A, Ochsner PE. Prosthetic-joint infections. N Engl J Med. 2004;351(16):1645–54. Epub 2004/10/16. eng.
20. Winkler H, Kaudela K, Stoiber A, Menschik F. Bone grafts impregnated with antibiotics as a tool for treating infected implants in orthopedic surgery – one stage revision results. Cell Tissue Bank. 2006;7(4):319–23. Epub 2006/05/20. eng.
21. Lachiewicz PF, Bolognesi MP, Henderson RA, Soileau ES, Vail TP. Can tantalum cones provide fixation in complex revision knee arthroplasty? Clin Orthop Relat Res. 2012;470(1):199–204. doi: 10.1007/s11999-011-1888-9.
22. Azzam K, McHale K, Austin M, Purtill JJ, Parvizi J. Outcome of a second two-stage reimplantation for periprosthetic knee infection. Clin Orthop Relat Res. 2009;467(7):1706–14. Pubmed Central PMCID: 2690747, Epub 2009/02/19. eng.

Uncemented Revision Total Knee Arthroplasty for Peri-prosthetic Joint Infection

21

Rhidian Morgan-Jones

Abstract

Uncemented fixation in revision total knee arthroplasty for peri-prosthetic infection is discussed by covering several key issues. Firstly, what is and how to undertake a systematic and effective debridement. Secondly, reviewing the concept of zonal reconstruction and fixation, looking at the options for dealing with bone loss. Finally, a discussion of the role of antibiotics and published outcomes.

Keywords

Debridement • Uncemented revision knee arthroplasty • Zonal fixation • Antibiotic delivery

Introduction

De-bride-ment is the surgical removal of foreign matter and dead tissue from a wound. It derives from the original French debridement (1835–1845), equivalent to debride, literally to take away the bridle. In modern management of orthopaedic infection we must understand what debridement involves and have reproducible steps that can be applied to each anatomical region. Here we will discuss debridement as it applies to revision of infected total knee replacement. Its importance cannot be overstated, as the commonest cause of re-revision is infection, between 30 and 50 % in one series [1]. Once debridement has been completed thoroughly, reconstruction and fixation should proceed by the surgeons chosen method, with cemented or uncemented fixation being unimportant provided it is methodically done, using and respecting the remaining bone stock and a multizone strategy [2–5]. In this chapter we will cover debridement, reconstruction and fixation, antibiotic delivery and finally outcome in the infected knee arthroplasty using uncemented techniques.

Debridement

Extensile Approach

Debridement begins with an extensile approach to the infected knee, and must consider the

R. Morgan-Jones, MBBCh, MMedSci, FRCS(Ed/Tr&Orth)
Department of Trauma and Orthopaedics, University Hospital of Wales, Cardiff, Wales, UK
e-mail: rhidianmj@hotmail.com

D. Kendoff et al. (eds.), *Periprosthetic Joint Infections: Changing Paradigms*,
DOI 10.1007/978-3-319-30091-7_21

previous skin incision or incisions. As a general rule, use the previous incision if adequate and extend proximally and distally as needed. Be prepared to excise broad scars in a mobile joint, but proceed with caution in the stiff and tethered knee. Sinuses in the line of incision can be excised, elsewhere isolated sinuses can be curetted and the deep sinus tract excised. All curetted sinuses will heal if the infected source is removed and debrided adequately. Occasionally, the need for plastic surgical coverage must be planned for when potential non-viable or necrotic skin loss is present, a medial Gastocnemius rotational or pedicled flap is generally sufficient. The author favours a tibial crest osteotomy to improve access to both explant and debride all corners, whilst protecting the extensor mechanism.

Methods of Debridement [6–8]

Debridement can be divided into superficial and deep. Superficial wound debridement can be subdivided into *autolytic,* which includes hydrogels and auto-enzymes; *enzymatic,* which includes streptokinase and collagenase; and *biological,* which includes maggot therapy.

Deep wound debridement can similarly be sub-divided into *surgical,* which includes explantation and sharp dissection; *mechanical,* including curettage and reaming, power lavage and H_2O_2 [9]; and *chemical,* which can include acetic acid [10] and honey [11, 12].

It is with deep debridement we should concentrate when discussing the management of the infected knee replacement. However, we should always consider the soft tissue envelope, as failure to do so may lead to poor wound healing and subsequent compromise of deep tissues [13, 14].

Surgical Debridement

Explantation when dealing with infected arthroplasty is akin to sequestrectomy and must include all implants and necrotic bone. Sharp dissection involves a thorough synovectomy and excision of all visible infected membrane/biofilm. Only when explantation and sharp dissection have been completed can the next stage of debridement begin.

Mechanical Debridement

Mechanical debridement has several distinct stages. The femoral and tibial joint surfaces and intra-medullary canals are curetted of any residual membrane, avascular bone and cement residue. Once complete the femoral and tibial intra-medullary canals are reamed under power to remove persistent neo-cortex and membrane in a compartmental debridement as described by Prof. Charles Lautenbach [15–18] from Johannesburg, South Africa. Once complete, all joint surfaces and canals are lavaged under power. Pulse lavage has a tidal effect of washing loose debris away from the operating field but more importantly lavage under power makes any infected, membrane adherent to bone, oedematous. Oedematous membrane is easier to both see and to debride by a further pass of curettage and reaming. Mechanical debridement should be seen as cyclical, with a minimum of two and possibly three cycles required to adequately debride. The volume of power lavage is less important than where and how the operative field is lavaged. Lavage of the soft tissues, joint surfaces and the intra-medullary canals must be performed in sequence. Most surgeons prefer normal saline, but other solutions with added chemicals or antibiotics can be used as the surgeon prefers.

H_2O_2 has been used for the mechanical effect of O_2 release producing effervescent cleaning and theoretically degrading biofilm and penetrating the cell wall. Controversy remains over the risk of air embolus whilst using H_2O_2, although this is mitigated by the use of a tourniquet. If H_2O_2 is used, it would make sense to use it after cyclical mechanical debridement with curettage, reaming and power lavage, to create biofilm and organisms susceptible to chemical debridement.

Chemical Debridement

Chemical debridement is the final part of deep debridement and seeks to create a hostile chemical environment that further degrades residual biofilm, kills bacteria and prevents future bacterial growth. Several options are available, the author prefers 3 % Acetic Acid [19] which lowers the environmental pH and has both Gram −ve and +ve activity. Generally a 10 min acetic acid soak before reimplantion is sufficient. Another option is SurgiHoney™ [11, 12] which works by a local osmolar effect but also produces H_2O_2. SurgiHoney also has the potential to be used as an antibacterial coating after re-implantation. Other potential chemical debriding agents include alcoholic betadine/chlorhexidine and hypochlorite.

Zonal Fixation and Reconstruction [2]

Solid fixation of the implant is important for long-term survival but also early on for immediate rehabilitation and function, and is irrespective of whether uncemented or cemented techniques are used. The larger the bone defect the more difficult the fixation. Three zones of fixation exist: the joint surface or epiphysis (zone 1), the metaphysis (zone 2) and the diaphysis (zone 3). In most revision knee replacements, zone 1 is compromised and therefore the zones 2 and 3 need to be used. The concept of zonal fixation and reconstruction is applicable to both tibia and femur (Figs. 21.1 and 21.2).

Fixation in Zone 1: The Epiphysis (Joint Surface)

In most revisions and all re-revisions, zone 1 is compromised by implant failure and removal. To enhance the use of fixation in zone 1, it is necessary to establish a stable surface, free of cement debris, avascular bone and fibrous membrane. Where possible, flat aligned cuts with augmentation of defects aides implant stability and fixation. Augmentation can be by cement, bone graft or metal block but in zone 1 fixation can only be reliably achieved with PMMA cement. As a rule, where augmentation is needed, fixation in at least

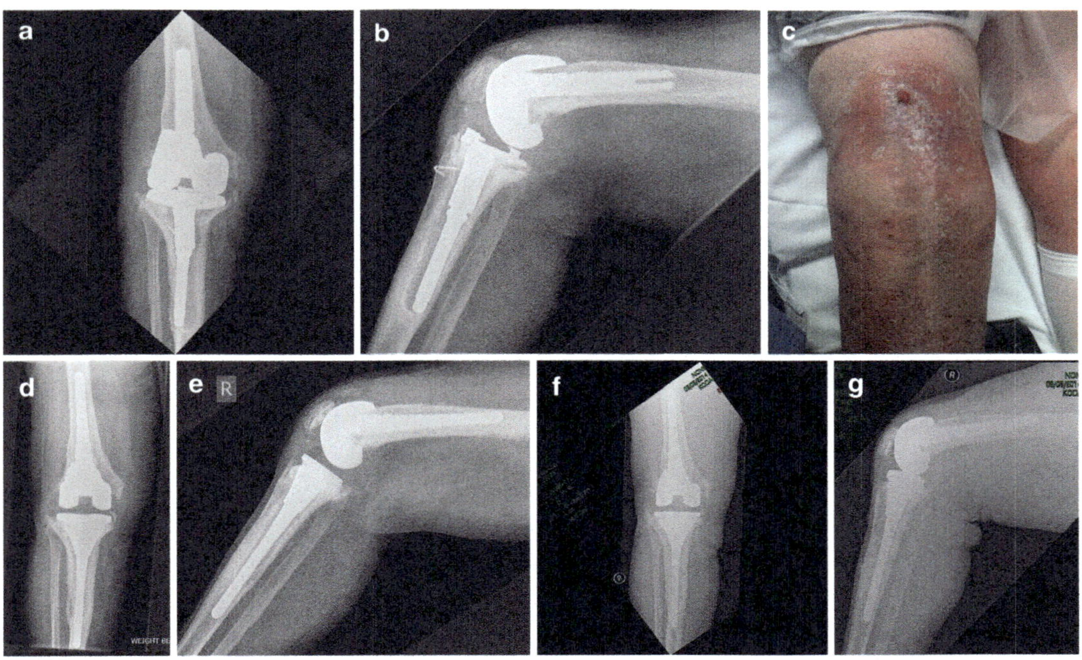

Fig. 21.1 (**a**, **b**) An infected, loose revision TKA 18 months post two-stage revision. (**c**) Clinical photograph of draining sinus and inflamed soft tissue envelope. (**d**, **e**) X-rays post one-stage revision using uncemented fixation with metaphyseal sleeves in zone 2 and diaphyseal stem in zone 3. (**f**, **g**) X-rays at 3 year review showing fixation and physiological loading leading to femoral and tibial bone remodelling

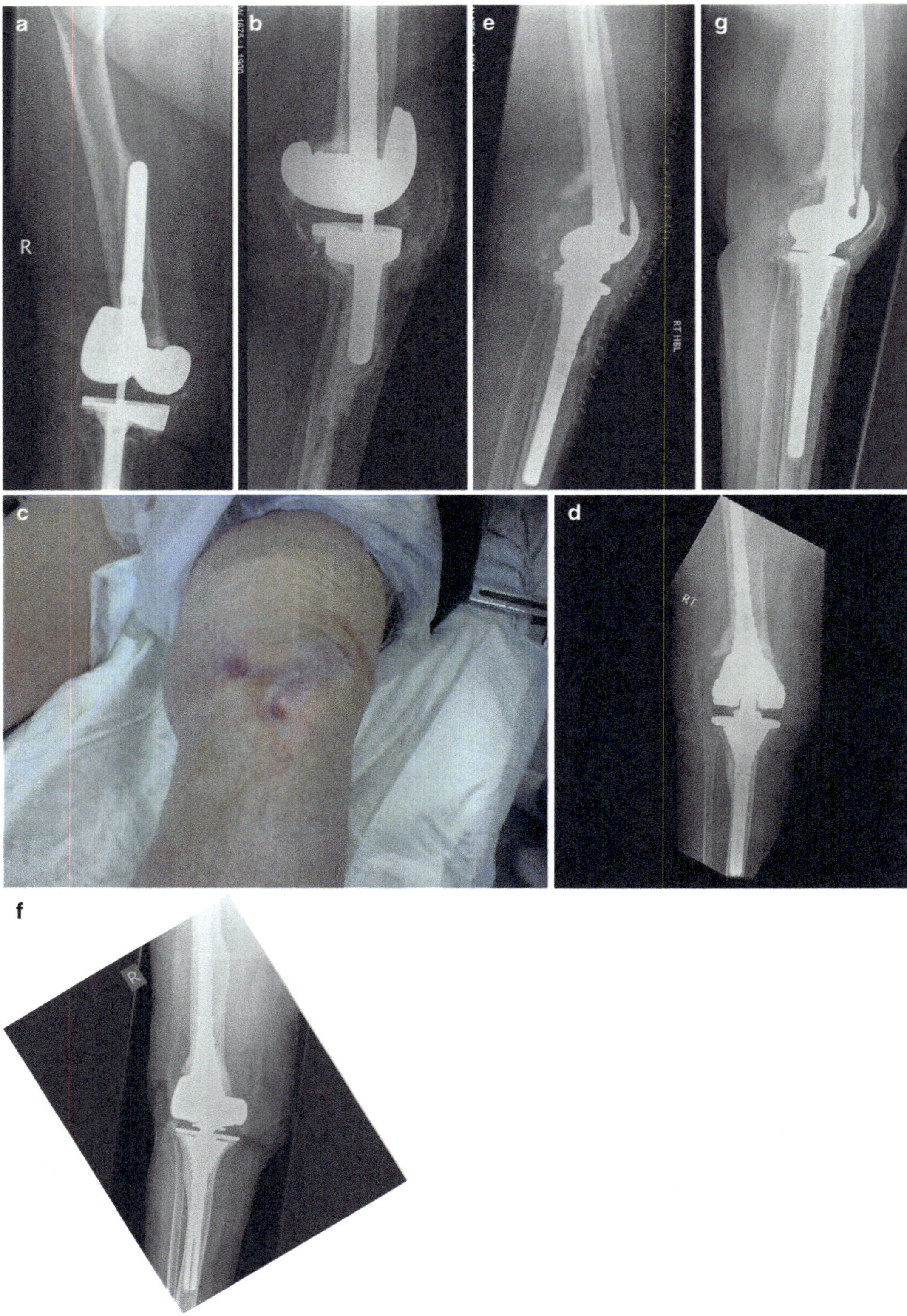
a
b
e
g
R
RT HBL
c
d
RT
f
R

1 other zone is necessary. Offset stems allow zones 1 and 3 to be linked. The geometry of the diaphysis and that of the epiphysis are not congruent, therefore an offset is sometimes needed to optimize zone 1 coverage and avoid medial overhang of the tray.

Fixation in Zone 2: The Metaphysis

Since Julius Wolff described the law which bears his name in 1892 [20, 21], we know that bone reacts to loading with increased bone density and when unloaded, bone will be reabsorbed. Traditional revision knee replacement systems bypass the metaphysis concentrating on diaphyseal and joint surface (zones 3 and 1) fixation. However, fixation in the metaphysis (zone 2) allows fixation closer to the point of articulation and makes restoration of the joint line easier. The geometry of the metaphysis and that of the joint surface are similar therefore obviating the need for an offset on the tibial implant. Similarly, fixation in zone 2 allows posterior translation of the femoral component and the use of shorter stems, to mitigate against femoral bowing which moves implants anteriorly. Failure to utilise zone 2 can lead to uncontrolled biomechanical sheer stress and instability of augment fixation in zone 1 potentially leading to early failure of the revision [22–24].

There are currently only two options for direct fixation in zone 2, cement [25] or metaphyseal sleeves (DePuy-Synthes) [26, 27]. Cement fixation in metaphyseal bone is not costly, readily available and can be used with either cemented or uncemented stems. Metaphyseal sleeves have been available since 1975 but have been most widely used as part of the S-ROM Noiles, rotating hinge system which has shown good mid-term results [26]. Metaphyseal sleeve fixation optimises load transfer to improve bone re-growth ('Wolff's law') and on-growth [27]. Fixation closer to the joint space provides better restoration of joint line and axial/rotational fixation stability even in the presence of cortical or cancellous bone defects and are an alternative to long stems [28, 29]. Metaphyseal sleeves as part of mobile bearing revision systems have been available for over 30 years but have only belatedly gained popularity, showing good early to mid-term results [4, 30, 31]. If zone 1 is sufficiently preserved to accept a worthwhile cement mantle, additional fixation in zone 3 might not be necessary. However, insufficient data on stemless metaphyseal sleeve fixation exist for general use to be recommended.

Metaphyseal sleeves are the only method available that provides both bone reconstruction and direct implant fixation. Indirect metaphyseal fixation in zone 2 is possible when reconstruction has been achieved first. As with zone 1 augmentation, zone 2 reconstruction can be achieved with cement, bone graft (bulk allograft or morsellised impaction graft) [32] or by the use of trabecular metal (TM) cones (Zimmer) which acts as metal bone graft and is used as a reconstruction ring. Trabecular metal has a structure similar to cancellous bone, is highly biocompatible and osteoconductive [33, 34]. Once metaphyseal reconstruction is secure and stable, secondary zone 2 fixation is achieved with bone cement. Trabecular metal cones offer the advantages of availability and intra-operative press-fit stability, allowing immediate weight bearing [35, 36]. Bone ingrowth has been demonstrated even in tibial TM retrieval specimens revised for infection [37]. Zone 2 reconstruction, however achieved, should be supported by secure zone 3 fixation with either cemented or uncemented stems.

Fig. 21.2 (**a**, **b**) Chronically infected revision TKR with massive bone loss. AORI classification grade 3 femur and tibia. (**c**) Clinical image of multiple sinuses draining chronically infected revision knee arthroplasty. (**d**, **e**) Post-operative x-rays after 1-stage revision using uncemented fixation: zone 2 metaphyseal sleeve, zone 3 diaphyseal stem. (**f**, **g**) Four-year review showing fixation and physiological loading leading to femoral and tibial bone regeneration

Fixation in Zone 3: The Diaphysis

Fixation in zone 3 by diaphyseal stems have been shown to offload the metaphysis where augmentation may have been necessary thus protecting the implant/cement interface areas from failure. Stems may be cemented or uncemented, both can offer long-term survival but both have individual limitations. In cemented stem fixation, bone resorption occurs in the metaphysis over time [38]. Using cementless stems seems to be beneficial for the bone of the metaphysis [39].

The geometry of the diaphysis and that of the epiphysis is not congruent, therefore an offset is occasionally needed. With this concept an optimized coverage of the joint surface can be assured. However it is still unclear whether a cemented or an uncemented fixation of the stems is advantageous and optimal length as well as optimal thickness of the stems are also still unclear [40]. Cementless diaphyseal engaging stems have been reported with lower radiographic failure than cemented stems in two-stage re-implantation, with similar re-infection rates despite the absence of antibiotic cement in cementless construct [5].

Treatment Options

Management options are based on the severity of defect and the chosen method of bone reconstruction, which range from bone cement, allograft, metal augmentation, and mega prosthesis. Recently, new alloys with high porosity have been introduced with satisfactory short-term results [41, 42]; however, it should be recognised that all methods of managing bone loss have different pros and cons [43]. Selection of the best treatment method is based on many factors, including defect size and location, the patient's age and health, and ability to participate in the necessary postoperative rehabilitation. Metaphyseal sleeves and porous tantalum cones are a major addition in dealing with large, central, contained and uncontained defects. The use of stem extensions in cases of bone deficits is helpful in enhancing fixation and lessening stresses to weakened condylar bone [44].

Cement Augmentation

This has limited clinical use and is indicated for small defects that are 5–10 mm. The advantages of cement are economical (affordable) and universal availability. The disadvantages include difficulty with uncontained defects, early radiolucent lines due to poor fixation and a failure to reconstitute bone for future surgery. However, in the elderly, low-demand patients and for expediency there remains a role for cement augmentation. Cement augmentation has been combined with metallic screw secured into the bone cortex as a reinforced hybrid construct [45] but this has not found widespread or sustained clinical use.

Bone Graft

When bone grafting, the host bone must be debrided to a viable layer and well cleaned. The graft must be contained and/or compressed, and preferably both. The aim, whenever possible, is to produce graft that has inherent structural stability although it always needs protecting with stems. High complications rates have been reported which include graft-host non-union, aseptic loosening, peri-prosthetic fractures, infections, and implant instability [46]. Allografts have several advantages. They are versatile and can be contoured to fill any shape and size (bulk or morsellised impaction grafts). Bone graft has the potential to restore bone stock provided that incorporation occurs, although this is always unpredictable [47, 48].

Disadvantages, however, are many. Excellent load transfer with bulk graft is seen, although this may lead to collapse unless revascularisation and incorporation occur. Outcome is technique and surgeon dependant and remains biologically unpredictable. In many countries and institutions the supply is limited and expensive. The risk of disease transmission is a real but statistically a minor concern. Failure to re-vascularise and incorporate will give an on-going risk of non-union and collapse. However, acceptable mid-term results have been published by several authors for both massive allografts [49] and impaction bone grafting [50]. Other reports have been less favourable for both [51–54]. The risk of infection is minimised by the use of antibiotic coated cancellous allograft [55–57].

Autograft have some advantage over allograft. It is more biologically active and carries no risk of disease transmission, and contouring is easy with a lower risk of non-union. The disadvantages, however, are a limited supply and provide only small bulk and limited morcellised graft. Autografts are usually only appropriate for complex primary TKR. Bone substitutes are commercially available with both osteoconductive and osteoinductive properties. They are presented in various consistencies such as putties, pastes, injections. There are, however, major disadvantages of significant cost, uncertain integration and a lack of structural options.

In summary, bone grafting has a place in revision TKR in the chronologically and physiologically young patients to increase bone stock. It offers versatility for differing types of bone loss. Allograft offers bulk for large bone loss, whilst allograft, autograft or bone substitutes may be appropriate for smaller defects.

Prosthetic Augmentation

Most modern revision systems include a complete set of metallic augments and stems. These are designed to reconstruct in zone 1 (joint surface) and zone 2 (metaphysis) and support in zone 3 (diaphysis).

Metal augments have the advantages of availability with no risk of disease transmission, shrinkage or collapse. They offer good load transfer and cutting guides increase ease and accuracy of use. The disadvantages include limited sizes and shapes producing further host bone loss. Augmentation usually necessitates the need for diaphyseal stem fixation. Metal augments may be a poor choice in massive defects, modularity may increase debris and reconstruction without use of metaphyseal and diaphyseal bone may lead to early failure [2]. The role of cemented and uncemented stems continues to be debated but the use of both can be supported [58–62].

The new generation of metaphyseal implants have made a dramatic difference to bone reconstruction. The commonest options include metaphyseal sleeves (DePuy-Synthes) [2, 4] or porous reconstruction cones (Zimmer) [63, 64]. Trabecular metal cones have shown good radiographic osteo-integration at 1 year, mitigating against future collapse or implant migration [65]. Metaphyseal sleeves have a pedigree of over 30 years of biological fixation allowing physiological loading to help regenerate bone stock and secure long-term fixation [4, 27–31, 66–69].

In summary, metal augments are versatile and allow intra-operative customisation and are suitable for moderate-sized, non-contained defects. Tantalum cones allow reconstruction of massive zone 2 defects with predictable osseo-integration and secure cement implant fixation. Metaphyseal sleeves offer an excellent option for reconstruction using zone 2 uncemented fixation irrespective of contained or uncontained defects. They offer immediate fixation and reconstruction and obviate the need for bone graft.

Are Antibiotics Important?

Debridement is the key to infection clearance. The more difficult question is what role antibiotics play in the eradication and prevention of recurrence. For eradication, antibiotics can be seen as adjunctive to surgery, treating the soft tissue envelope and attacking residual organisms. For this, antibiotics should be at bactericidal levels throughout the surgical period. For prevention of implant contamination/infection, antibiotics should prevent the establishment of a biofilm and must therefore be used for a sufficient time postoperatively. The time frame for antibiotics post revision can vary from a 2 weeks to 6 months, depending on whether the surgery is a one- or two-stage, a debride and implant retention procedure and whether the organism and host are favourable or not [70–72].

Antibiotic delivery can be systemic or local and each can used for varying lengths of time. All surgeons use intravenous systemic antibiotics to cover the initial operation, but conversion to oral can at

5 days to 6 weeks depending on the host and organism variables. The duration of oral therapy again varies from 6 weeks to 6 months. Local antibiotics can be delivered by a variety of media. Bone cement can be pre-mixed or hand mixed intra-operatively. In the uncemented revision knee replacement, antibiotic cement is often used in zone 1 to provide hybrid fixation and eradicate any dead space between implant and bone. Biodegradable implants such as Calcium Sulphate or Collagen fleece have been used to increase the intra-capsular antibiotic levels. Local antibiotics have the advantage of providing bespoke antibiotic usage at high concentration. Antibiotic impregnated bone graft has been reported successfully in the one-stage management of infected revision total hip replacements [55–57] and revision total knee arthroplasty [73] albeit in two stages.

Published Outcomes on Uncemented Revision TKA for PJI

Once a thorough debridement has been achieved, the remaining issues for the operating surgeon are: one- vs. two-stage, reconstruction of bone loss and long-term fixation. Regrettably there are so many variables that no randomised trials are possible to compare all the options. Common sense and experience tells us, however, that excellent outcomes can be achieved by a variety of means. Hence, provided the surgeon adheres to the good principles of infection clearance, antibiotic usage and delivery, and zonal reconstruction and fixation, an argument can be made for all philosophies. Other chapters will use literature to support their position and similarly we can review the published experience of uncemented revision TKA for infection.

Edwards et al. [5] in a retrospective study, compared cemented and uncemented diaphyseal stems at the second stage of revision for infection. Uncemented diaphyseal-engaging stems had a lower rate of radiographic failure than did cemented stems. This study did not look specifically at infection free survival but stem survival at a minimum 2 year radiographic review. However, reinfection rates were similar despite the absence of antibiotic cement in the cementless constructs. Vince and Long [62], however, reported earlier aseptic loosening in three patients after a two-stage re-implantation, from a small series of 13 patients revised using press-fit medullary stem fixation.

Bourne et al. [74] reported a series of 135 patients revised using uncemented press-fit stems of which 34 (25 %) were revised for infection in two stages. Of the infected revisions two had recurrent infection accompanied by radiolucent lines indicative of loosening. Agarwal et al. [4], looking at uncemented metaphyseal sleeve reconstruction and fixation in a minimum 2 year review, confirmed no recurrent infections in the 31 one-stage infected revisions. Similarly, Hanssen et al. [35] reported bony ingrowth into porous tantalum metaphyseal cones in a small series which included seven second-stage revision TKA. Bone ingrowth was unaffected by previous infection.

Using a two-stage protocol and "antibiotic-soaked" bone graft, Whiteside [59] used uncemented stem and screw fixation. Twenty-nine of 33 revisions were free of infection at mid-term review. Uncemented fixation has also been reported in limb salvage [61]. Using a two-stage protocol, cementless intramedullary nailing, without achieving bone-to-bone fusion, was used for treating chronically infected total knee arthroplasty. At 2 year review 89.5 % showed no recurrence of infection. No aseptic loosening or implant failure was reported.

Conclusion

Debridement is as much a formal part of any revision as is the reconstruction and soft tissue balance. By having defined stages which include surgical, mechanical and chemical debridement, a thorough and reproducible debridement is possible. The concept of repeated cyclical debridement is also vital to understand, as no surgeon can achieve adequate clearance of infection in a single pass. Finally, debridement should be seen as separate from reconstruction, which should not be prejudiced by inadequate debridement.

The concept of zonal reconstruction and fixation allows the surgeon to use their implants of choice in a methodical manner which should give reproducible outcomes. The published literature, although not extensive, confirms that uncemented fixation is at least as effective as cemented fixation in revision TKA for peri-prosthetic infection.

References

1. Aggarwal VK, Goyal N, Deirmengian G, Rangavajulla A, Parvizi J, Austin MS. Revision total knee arthroplasty in the young patient: is there trouble on the horizon? J Bone Joint Surg Am. 2014;96(7):536–42.
2. Morgan-Jones R, Oussedik SIS, Graichen H, Haddad FS. Zonal fixation in revision total knee arthroplasty. Bone Joint J. 2015;97-B(2):147–9.
3. Whiteside LA. Cementless revision total knee arthroplasty. Clin Orthop Relat Res. 1993;286:160–7.
4. Agarwal S, Azam A, Morgan-Jones R. Metal metaphyseal sleeves in revision total knee replacement. Bone Joint J. 2013;95-B(12):1640–4.
5. Edwards PK, Fehring TK, Hamilton WG, Perricelli B, Beaver WB, Odum SM. Are cementless stems more durable than cemented stems in two-stage revisions of infected total knee arthroplasties? Clin Orthop Relat Res. 2014;472(1):206–11.
6. Leaper DJ, Harding KG, editors. Wounds: biology and management. Oxford: Oxford University Press; 1998.
7. Falanga V, Harding KG, editors. The clinical relevance of wound bed preparation. Berlin/Heidelberg/New York: Springer; 2002.
8. Cherry GW, Hughes MA, Ferguson MWJ, Leaper DJ (2000) Wound healing. In: Morris PJ, Wood WC eds. Oxford Textbook of Surgery, 2nd edn.
9. Al-Ali M, Sathorn C, Parashos P. Root canal debridement efficacy of different final irrigation protocols. Int Endod J. 2012;45(10):898–906.
10. Nagoba BS, Selkar SP, Wadher BJ, Gandhi RC. Acetic acid treatment of pseudomonal wound infections–a review. J Infect Public Health. 2013;6(6):410–5.
11. Dryden M, Milward G, Saeed K. Infection prevention in wounds with Surgihoney. J Hosp Infect. 2014;88(2):121–2.
12. Dryden M, Tawse C, Adams J, Howard A, Saeed K, Cooke J. The use of Surgihoney to prevent or eradicate bacterial colonisation in dressing oncology long vascular lines. J Wound Care. 2014;23(6):338–41.
13. Ågren MS. Wound debridement optimisation. J Wound Care. 2014;23(8):381.
14. Eckardt JJ, Wirganowicz PZ, Mar T. An aggressive surgical approach to the management of chronic osteomyelitis. Clin Orthop Relat Res. 1994;298:229–39.
15. Weber FA, Lautenbach EE. Revision of infected total hip arthroplasty. Clin Orthop Relat Res. 1986;211:108–15.
16. Caesar BC, Morgan-Jones RL, Warren RE, Wade RH, Roberts PJ, Richardson JB. Closed double-lumen suction irrigation in the management of chronic diaphyseal osteomyelitis: long-term follow-up. J Bone Joint Surg Br. 2009;91(9):1243–8.
17. Hashmi MA, Norman P, Saleh M. The management of chronic osteomyelitis using the Lautenbach method. J Bone Joint Surg Br. 2004;86(2):269–75.
18. Zalavras CG, Singh A, Patzakis MJ. Novel technique for medullary canal débridement in tibia and femur osteomyelitis. Clin Orthop Relat Res. 2007;461:31–4.
19. Schaefer P, Baugh RF. Acute otitis externa: an update. Am Fam Physician. 2012;86(11):1055–61.
20. Wolff J. The law of bone remodelling. Berlin: Springer; 1986.
21. Richard A. Brand Biographical Sketch: Julius Wolff, 1836–1902. Clin Orthop Relat Res. 2010;468(4):1047–9.
22. Brigstocke G, Agarwal Y, Bradley N, Crocombe A. Finite element study of augmented total knee replacement. Orthop Proc July. 2012;94-B:55.
23. Brigstocke G, Agarwal Y, Bradley N, Frehill B, Crocombe A. Finite element analysis of cement shear stresses in augmented total knee replacement. Orthop Proc July. 2012;94-B:59.
24. Frehill B, Crocombe A, Cirovic S, Agarwal Y, Bradley N. Initial stability of type-2 tibial defect treatments. Proc Inst Mech Eng H. 2010;224(1):77–85.
25. Sah AP, Shukla S, Della Valle CJ, Rosenberg AG, Paprosky WG. Modified hybrid stem fixation in revision TKA is durable at 2 to 10 years. Clin Orthop Relat Res. 2011;469(3):839–46.
26. Jones RE, Skedros JG, Chan AJ, Beauchamp DH, Harkins PC. Total knee arthroplasty using the S-ROM mobile-bearing hinge prosthesis. J Arthroplasty. 2001;16(3):279–87.
27. Meftah M, Ranawat A, Ranawat CS. Osteointegration of non-cemented metaphyseal sleeves in revision total knee arthroplasty. Bone Joint J. 2013;95-B Suppl 34:492.
28. Jones RE, Barrack RL, Skedros J. Modular, mobile-bearing hinge total knee arthroplasty. CORR. 2001;392:306–14.
29. Jones RE. Mobile bearings in revision total knee arthroplasty. Instr Course Lect. 2005;54:225–31.
30. Ahmed I, Maheshwari R, Walmsley P, Brenkel I. Use of porous stepped metaphyseal sleeves during revision total knee arthroplasty. J Bone Joint Surg (Br). 2012;94-B(suppl XXIX):55.
31. Mullen M, Bell SW, Rooney BP, Leach WJ. Femoral and tibial metaphyseal sleeves in revision total knee arthroplasty. Bone Joint J. 2013;95-B(Suppl):30–45.
32. Toms AD, Barker RL, McClelland D, Chua L, Spencer-Jones R, Kuiper J-H. Repair of defects and containment in revision total knee replacement. J Bone Joint Surg Br. 2009;91-B:271–7.

33. Meneghini RM, Lewallen DG, Hanssen AD. Use of porous tantalum metaphyseal cones for severe tibial bone loss during revision total knee replacement. Surgical technique. Joint Surg Am. 2009;91(Suppl 2 Pt 1):131–8.
34. Lachiewicz PF, Bolognesi MP, Henderson RA, Soileau ES, Vail TP. Can tantalum cones provide fixation in complex revision knee arthroplasty? Clin Orthop Relat Res. 2012;470(1):199–204.
35. Meneghini RM, Lewallen DG, Hanssen AD. Use of porous tantalum metaphyseal cones for severe tibial bone loss during revision total knee replacement. J Bone Joint Surg Am. 2008;90(1):78–84.
36. Long WJ, Scuderi GR. The use of porous tantalum for bone loss in revision total knee arthroplasty: a minimum 2 year follow-up. J Bone Joint Surg Br. 2011;93-B(Suppl IV):418–9.
37. Sambaziotis C, Lovy AJ, Koller KE, Bloebaum RD, Hirsh DM. Kim. Histologic retrieval analysis of a porous tantalum metal implant in an infected primary total knee arthroplasty. J Arthroplasty. 2012;27(7):1413.5–9.
38. Lonner JH, Klotz M, Levitz C, Lotke PA. Changes in bone density after cemented total knee arthroplasty: influence of stem design. J Arthroplasty. 2001;16(1):107–11.
39. Completo A, Simões JA, Fonseca F, Oliveira M. The influence of different tibial stem designs in load sharing and stability at the cement-bone interface in revision TKA. Knee. 2008;15(3):227–32.
40. Completo A, Fonseca F, Simões JA. Strain shielding in proximal tibia of stemmed knee prosthesis: experimental study. J Biomech. 2008;41(3):560–6.
41. Beckmann J, Lüring C, Springorum R, Köck FX, Grifka J, Tingart M. Fixation of revision TKA: a review of the literature. Knee Surg Sports Traumatol Arthrosc. 2011;19(6):872–9.
42. Hongvilai S, Tanavalee A. Review article: management of bone loss in revision knee arthroplasty. J Med Assoc Thai. 2012;95 Suppl 10:S230–7.
43. Lombardi AV, Berend KR, Adams JB. Management of bone loss in revision TKA: it's a changing world. Orthopaedics. 2010;33(9):662.
44. Qiu YY, Yan CH, Chiu KY, Ng FY. Review article: treatments for bone loss in revision total knee arthroplasty. J Orthop Surg (Hong Kong). 2012;20(1):78–86.
45. Daines BK, Dennis DA. Management of bone defects in revision total knee arthroplasty. Instr Course Lect. 2013;62:341–8.
46. Scott RD. Revision total knee arthroplasty. Clin Orthop Relat Res. 1988;226:65–77.
47. Backstein D, Safir O, Gross A. Management of bone loss: structural grafts in revision total knee arthroplasty. Clin Orthop Relat Res. 2006;446:104–12.
48. Franke KF, Nusem I, Gamboa G, Morgan DA. Outcome of revision total knee arthroplasty with bone allograft in 30 cases. TKR Acta Orthop Belg. 2013;79(4):427–34.
49. Lyall HS, Sanghrajka A, Scott G. Severe tibial bone loss in revision total knee replacement managed with structural femoral head allograft: a prospective case series from the Royal London Hospital. Knee. 2009;16(5):326–31.
50. Engh GA, Ammeen DJ. Use of structural allograft in revision total knee arthroplasty in knees with severe tibial bone loss. J Bone Joint Surg Am. 2007;89(12):2640–7.
51. Naim S, Toms AD. Impaction bone grafting for tibial defects in knee replacement surgery. Results at two years. Acta Orthop Belg. 2013;79(2):205–10.
52. Ghazavi MT, Stockley I, Gilbert Y, Davis A, Gross A. Reconstruction of massive bone defects with allograft in revision TKA. J Bone Joint Surg Am. 1997;79:17–25.
53. Clatworthy MG, Ballance J, Brick GW, Chandler HP, Gross AE. The use of structural allograft for uncontained defects in revision total knee arthroplasty. A minimum five-year review. J Bone Joint Surg Am. 2001;83-A(3):404–11.
54. Hilgen V, Citak M, Vettorazzi E, Haasper C, Day K, Amling M, Gehrke T, Gebauer M. 10-year results following impaction bone grafting of major bone defects in 29 rotational and hinged knee revision arthroplasties: a follow-up of a previous report. Acta Orthop. 2013;84(4):387–91.
55. Winkler H. Rationale for one stage exchange of infected hip replacement using uncemented implants and antibiotic impregnated bone graft. Int J Med Sci. 2009;6(5):247–52.
56. Winkler H. Bone grafting and one-stage revision of THR–biological reconstruction and effective antimicrobial treatment using antibiotic impregnated allograft bone. Hip Int. 2012;22 Suppl 8:S62–8.
57. Winkler H, Stoiber A, Kaudela K, Winter F, Menschik F. One stage uncemented revision of infected total hip replacement using cancellous allograft bone impregnated with antibiotics. J Bone Joint Surg Br. 2008;90(12):1580–4.
58. Mabry TM, Hanssen AD. The role of stems and augments for bone loss in revision knee arthroplasty. J Arthroplasty. 2007;22(4 Suppl 1):56–60.
59. Whiteside LA. Cementless reconstruction of massive tibial bone loss in revision total knee arthroplasty. Clin Orthop Relat Res. 1989;248:80–6.
60. Jazrawi LM, Bai B, Kummer FJ, Hiebert R, Stuchin SA. The effect of stem modularity and mode of fixation on tibial component stability in revision total knee arthroplasty. J Arthroplasty. 2001;16(6):759–67.
61. Scarponi S, Drago L, Romanò D, Logoluso N, Peccati A, Meani E, Romanò CL. Cementless modular intramedullary nail without bone-on-bone fusion as a salvage procedure in chronically infected total knee prosthesis: long-term results. Int Orthop. 2014;38(2):413–8.
62. Vince KG, Long W. Revision knee arthroplasty. The limits of press fit medullary fixation. Clin Orthop Relat Res. 1995;317:172–7.

63. Jensen CL, Winther N, Schrøder HM, Petersen MM. Outcome of revision total knee arthroplasty with the use of trabecular metal cone for reconstruction of severe bone loss at the proximal tibia. Knee. 2014;21(6):1233–7.
64. Vasso M, Beaufils P, Cerciello S, Schiavone Panni A. Bone loss following knee arthroplasty: potential treatment options. Arch Orthop Trauma Surg. 2014;134(4):543–53.
65. Rao BM, Kamal TT, Vafaye J, Moss M. Tantalum cones for major osteolysis in revision knee replacement. Bone Joint J. 2013;95-B(8):1069–74.
66. Alexander GE, Bernasek TL, Crank RL, Haidukewych GJ. Cementless metaphyseal sleeves used for large tibial defects in revision total knee arthroplasty. J Arthroplasty. 2013;28(4):604–7.
67. Accardo NJ, Noiles DG, Pena R, Accardo NJ. Noiles total knee replacement procedure. Orthopedics. 1979;2(1):37–45.
68. Flynn LM. The Noiles hinge knee prosthesis with axial rotation. Orthopaedics. 1979;2(6):602–5.
69. Barnett SL, Mayer RR, Gondusky JS, Choi L, Patel JJ, Gorab RS. Use of stepped porous titanium metaphyseal sleeves for tibial defects in revision total knee arthroplasty: short term results. J Arthroplasty. 2014;29(6):1219–24.
70. Byren I, Bejon P, Atkins BL, Angus B, Masters S, McLardy-Smith P, Gundle R, Berendt A. One hundred and twelve infected arthroplasties treated with 'DAIR' (debridement, antibiotics and implant retention): antibiotic duration and outcome. J Antimicrob Chemother. 2009;63(6):1264–71.
71. Hoad-Reddick DA, Evans CR, Norman P, Stockley I. Is there a role for extended antibiotic therapy in a two-stage revision of the infected knee arthroplasty? J Bone Joint Surg Br. 2005;87(2):171–4.
72. Sims AL, Baker P, Bellamy R, McMurtry IA. Outpatient parenteral antibiotic therapy in primary hip and knee arthroplasty infection managed with debridement and retention of prosthesis: a retrospective cohort study. Surg Infect (Larchmt). 2013;14(3):293–6.
73. Whiteside LA. Treatment of infected total knee arthroplasty. Clin Orthop Relat Res. 1994;299:169–72.
74. Wood GC, Naudie DDR, MacDonald SJ, McCalden RW, Bourne RB. Results of press-fit stems in revision knee arthroplasties. Clin Orthop Relat Res. 2009;467:810–7.

Late Infections of the Knee Joint: Two-staged Static Solutions

22

Christopher P. Wilding, Michael C. Parry, and Lee Jeys

Abstract

Appropriate management of the unsalvageable infected total knee replacement remains a challenge, and avoidance of above-knee amputation remains the ultimate goal. In this chapter we look to review the techniques available to achieve arthrodesis of the knee as a means to salvage the limb. We will address the current evidence and clinical outcomes related to arthrodesis using intramedullary nailing, external fixation, plating and vascularised fibular grafts. Common complications and their management will be considered. The functional outcomes of arthrodesis patients will be presented, specifically in comparison to patients having undergone above knee amputation. Finally we will discuss some novel therapies emerging, including discussion of the use of silver-coated arthrodesis nails in this complex cohort of patients, and presenting early follow-up data from our experience.

Keywords

Arthrodesis • Above knee amputation • Intramedullary nail • External fixation • Vascularised fibular graft • Plate • Silver coating

C.P. Wilding, MBBS, BSc (Hons)
Department of Orthopaedics, Royal Orthopaedic Hospital, Birmingham, UK
e-mail: christopher.wilding@nhs.net

M.C. Parry, BSC, MBCHB, PGCME, MD, FRCS (✉)
Department of Oncology and Complex Arthroplasty, Royal Orthopaedic Hospital, Birmingham, UK
e-mail: michael.parry3@nhs.net

L. Jeys, MBCHB, MSc (Ortho Eng), FRCS
Department of Orthopaedic Oncology, Royal Orthopaedic Hospital, Birmingham, UK
e-mail: lee.jeys@btclick.com; lee.jeys@nhs.net

Introduction

The treatment of infection in the multiply revised, recurrent or recalcitrant infection subgroup represents a distinct challenge. The situation is often complicated by poor bone stock, poor soft tissue coverage and often a poor patient co-morbid condition. In such patients, who have undergone multiple revisions, or in whom aggressive limb salvage procedures carry a high risk of failure due to patient or microbial factors, the option of knee

D. Kendoff et al. (eds.), *Periprosthetic Joint Infections: Changing Paradigms*,
DOI 10.1007/978-3-319-30091-7_22

arthrodesis becomes a viable option in an attempt to prevent above knee amputation (AKA).

Knee arthrodesis has been performed since the turn of the 19th century as the treatment modality of choice in patients with septic arthritis, poliomyelitis, tuberculosis of the knee joint and debilitating osteoarthritis, and was first used for the treatment of failed TKA in 1971 [1]. Since then, arthrodesis has become a viable option in the armoury of the orthopaedic surgeon for the group of complex patients presenting with an unsalvageable failed TKA.

On this background, the aims of this chapter are to explore the following topics relating to static solutions in the treatment of PJI of the knee:

- Indications and contraindications for arthrodesis
- Techniques to achieve knee arthrodesis
- The pitfalls and complications of knee arthrodesis and their management
- Functional outcomes following arthrodesis
- Novel techniques related to knee arthrodesis

Indications for Arthrodesis

The current role for knee arthrodesis in relation to TKA remains open to debate, but the recognised indication is for the patient with an unsalvageable TKA on the background of recurrent infection often following multiple revisions, in order to prevent progression to AKA. Debate remains as to which TKAs can be salvaged and which require arthrodesis, and this decision must be made on a case-by-case basis, within a multidisciplinary team environment, to determine the route which will lead to the best clinical outcome.

Infection with multiple or resistant bacteria is one such risk factor with re-infection rates as high as 24 % when methicillin-resistant *Staph. aureus* or methicillin-resistant *Staph. epidermidis* were the infecting organism [2, 3]. Other patient-related factors which have a detrimental impact on revision arthroplasty survival include obesity, immune compromise, rheumatic disease, liver cirrhosis and kidney disease [4–6].

Gross soft tissue instability may also be considered in the decision between arthrodesis and re-implantation. In these cases successful arthrodesis can result in a stable leg through which weight can be borne, thus resulting in acceptable functional outcomes and allowing patients a degree of independence [7, 8]. The alternative to arthrodesis in these cases would be a constrained prosthesis; however, revision of a constrained prosthesis often results in a greater degree of bone resection when compared with the removal of less constrained prostheses [9]. This in turn leads to reduced fusion rates following arthrodesis, 56 % compared to 81 %, which should be taken into account during the decision making process [10].

Deficiency of the extensor mechanism following TKA has been reported as a complication in 1–12 % of arthroplasty procedures [11] and can be the result of patellar tendon disruption, quadriceps tendon disruption, patellar crepitus and soft-tissue impingement, periprosthetic patella fracture, patellofemoral instability, and osteonecrosis of the patella. In the case of deficiency of the extensor mechanism following infection, this is most commonly attributable to sinus formation resulting in erosion of the patella tendon or destruction of the patella tendon insertion. Aggressive debridement of the sinus must always be achieved even with sacrifice of the extensor mechanism. Options for treatment of the deficient extensor mechanism include the use of a brace, direct repair, augmentation with native tissue, allograft, autograft or synthetic material. Non-operative treatment is generally not acceptable due to the poor outcomes associated with a deficient extensor mechanism. The use of allorgraft techniques, sacrificing the extensor mechanism at the time of first stage debridement and reconstructing at the second stage reimplantation, have been reported anecdotally with varying success in small numbers. In such cases where the reconstruction of the extensor mechanism will prove challenging with a small chance of successful function, arthrodesis may be considered.

For patients in whom the soft tissue envelope of the knee and proximal tibia has been significantly violated by infection or repeated surgery, and for those in whom residual stiffness in the knee is likely to compromise function following revision, arthrodesis may be considered. In such cases, wound healing and soft tissue coverage is far more likely in the context of a stable knee. Often, patients in this predicament are significantly affected by pain. In such a context, the prospect of a pain free, albeit stiff knee is often more agreeable to the patient, rather than chronic pain and instability.

Contraindications to Arthrodesis

Contraindications to knee arthrodesis can be considered as relative and absolute. To our mind, the only absolute contraindication to arthrodesis would be in the case of life threatening sepsis form PJI of the knee, AKA may be the only option. Social and cultural factors must be considered when counselling patients considering amputation or arthrodesis. The cultural stigma associated with amputation by some may push patients and surgeons alike towards considering arthrodesis. Patient wishes must be taken into consideration when contemplating limb salvage or sacrificing options for definitive treatment of the PJI.

Following successful knee fusion, compensatory mechanisms occur to allow walking, including increased pelvic tilt, hip abduction and ankle dorsiflexion on the ipsilateral side [12]. As such arthrodesis should be avoided if possible in patients with ipsilateral degenerative changes in the hip or ankle, as these will limit the effect of the compensatory mechanisms. Equally, the presence of degenerative changes in the spine may be considered as a relative contraindication to knee arthrodesis, as the increased degree of pelvic tilt will result in increased loads through the lumbar spine accelerating degenerative wear [13].

Patients with a contralateral amputation may be unsuitable for arthrodesis due to the degree of energy expenditure which would be required to ambulate. Knee fusion requires the exertion of 30 % more energy when walking compared to a normal gait, with amputation 25 % higher still than arthrodesis [12]. This increased degree of energy exertion thus makes arthrodesis unsuitable in these patients due to the degree of difficulty as well as the risk to cardio-vascular fragile patients.

Finally, patients who are medically unfit for such drastic surgeries, or who have decided against arthrodesis, should not be considered.

Current Techniques to Achieve Knee Fusion

Intramedullary (IM) Nailing

The use of a long IM nail has become the most commonly utilised method for arthrodesis (Fig. 22.1). IM arthrodesis is associated with prolonged stability of the joint, allows weight bearing more quickly and has a high rate of fusion. IM nailing has the disadvantage of being a technically challenging procedure and often requires a two-stage procedure in the presence of active infection. Historical methods of attempting to achieve bone-to-bone fusion often left an unacceptably large leg length discrepancy. One method utilised to avoid this is the use of an IM nail as an endoprosthesis with antibiotic-laden cement or bone grafting used to fill the gap between tibia and femur [14–16].

Technically, the knee is approached anteriorly with the joint accessed with the patella everted or retracted. Thorough debridement of any infected soft tissues is vital to reduce the risk of recurrent infection following arthrodesis. Any hardware or cement present following the first stage must be removed. For insertion of the IM nail, the smaller diameter bone of the tibia is reamed followed by the femur, with the aim of this to prevent over-reaming of the femoral canal [17]. Over-reaming of either canal leads to the nail lacking a secure fit and consequently reducing the stability of the arthrodesis. A nail 0.5-mm diameter smaller than the diameter of the final reamer is usually suitable for insertion. Cancellous bone fragments, autologous bone grafts or antibiotic laden cement can be packed around the knee to improve bone fusion and bridge any large gaps between the tibia and femur [18]. The IM nail is anchored proximally in the femur with a locking screw, which has been shown to prevent proximal migration which can be a cause of gluteal pain necessitating nail removal [19].

Table 22.2 shows some of the available evidence reporting outcomes following arthrodesis using IM nails following recurrent PJI of the knee. The group sizes are relatively small as expected due to the rarity of cases necessitating

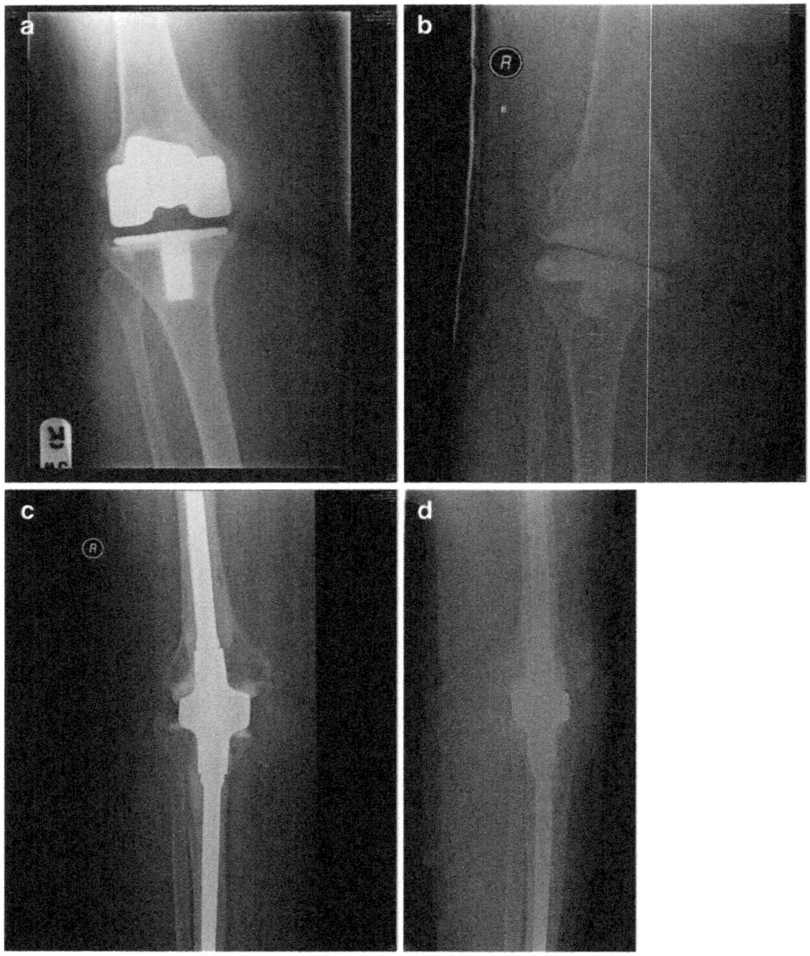

Fig. 22.1 The case of a 78-year-old patient who presented with a late haematogenous periprosthetic joint infection of a primary TKA performed 8 years previously (**a**). The infecting organism was a methicillin resistant *Staphylococcus aureus* and the patient suffered with diabetes mellitus, renal impairment, coronary heart disease and pulmonary disease necessitating regular steroid use. It was, therefore, elected to treat this PJI by staged arthrodesis, the first stage temporised with an articulating antibiotic loaded cement spacer (**b**). The patient underwent second-stage arthrodesis with an intramedullary arthrodesis nail augmented with antibiotic-loaded cement (**c**, **d**)

arthrodesis, which increases the variability when comparing outcomes. Overall the data presented shows that IM nailing is an effective technique to fuse the knee following failed infected TKA, with a solid fusion rate ranging from 68 to 100 % at an average time of 4–11.6 months [17–31, 33]. Length of stay following arthrodesis was on average between 16 and 23 days, and most likely reflects the early mobilisation and weight bearing achieved with this method of arthrodesis [21, 28].

The published complication rates range from 0 to 30 % which represents a low figure when considered in the context that two-stage revision following infected primary TKA carries a failure rate of as high as 36 % [7–12, 24, 26–29, 31, 33–44]. However, it is also worth noting that when recurrent infections occur, the rate of these progressing to AKA is high. As can be seen in Table 22.1, 29 patients developed recurrent infections despite arthrodesis, with ten progressing to AKA, a rate of 34.5 % [15, 16, 22, 23, 26]. This is likely a reflection of the complex patients undergoing arthrodesis, often as a last resort prior to AKA. Nevertheless, eradication of infection remains the greatest challenge when attempting knee arthrodesis using an IM nail.

External Fixation (EF) Devices

First used in knee arthrodesis as a treatment for advanced osteoarthritis and tuberculous arthritis, EF arthrodesis following unsalvageable infected

Table 22.1 Recent published evidence for IM nailing as a modality for arthrodesis following unsalvageable infected TKA

Author	Year	# of patients	# of solid fusions	Time to fusion	Mean LLD	Complication rate	Complications
Miralles-Muñoz [14]	2014	29	–	–	8 mm	13.7 %	2 recurrent infections, 1 periprosthetic fracture, 1 cortical erosion; all successfully revised
Scarponi [15]	2014	38	–	–	13 mm	10.5 %	4 recurrent infections; 2 went on to AKA, 2 went onto revision surgeries
Putman [20]	2013	31	21 (68 %)	–	10 mm	19.4 %	6 recurrent infection (3 removal of metalwork, 3 long-term antibiotics)
Iacono [16]	2013	22	–	–	45 mm	13.6 %	3 recurrent infections all went on to AKA
Lee [18]	2012	9	9 (100 %)	9.9 months	11 mm	0 %	–
Yeoh [21]	2008	11	10 (91 %)	4.4 months	–	9.1 %	1 non-union
De Vil [22]	2008	19	14 (74 %)	–	45 mm	26.3 %	4 recurrent infections; 3 went on to AKA 1 aspetic non-union
Senior [23]	2008	14	13 (93 %)	4 months	>20 mm	14.2 %	1 infected non-union; went on to AKA 1 peroneal nerve palsy; resolved at 5 months
Garcia-Lopez [24]	2008	20	16 (80 %)	9 months	24.5 mm	30 %	4 psuedoarthroses, 1 intra-op fracture, 1 peroneal nerve palsy
Mabry [25]	2007	24	23 (96 %)	–	–	8.3 %	2 recurrent infections
Bargiotas [26]	2006	12	10 (83 %)	5.5 months	55 mm	16.7 %	1 recurrent infection; went on to AKA 1 nail breakage after 3 years
McQueen [27]	2005	7	7 (100 %)	18.7 weeks	–	28.6 %	2 recurrent infections; went on to delayed union
White [28]	2003	5	5 (100 %)	11.6 month	–	0 %	–

(continued)

Table 22.1 (continued)

Author	Year	# of patients	# of solid fusions	Time to fusion	Mean LLD	Complication rate	Complications
Gore [29]	2003	16	12 (75 %)	13.5 weeks	–	25 %	1 aseptic non-union, 1 skin graft 2 recurrent infections; 1 revised and united, 1 removed and now braced
Waldman [17]	1999	21	20 (95 %)	6.3 months	–	9.5 %	1 non-union; treated with bone graft 1 wound dehiscence requiring muscle flap
Lai [30]	1998	33	30 (91 %)	5.2 months	26 mm	9.1 %	2 non unions 1 recurrent infection; debridement + fused
Jørgensen [31]	1995	5	5 (100 %)	4.8 months	–	0 %	–
Knutson [32]	1985	11	10 (91 %)	–	40.1 mm	18.2 %	1 non-union, 1 revision

TKA has been explored, albeit to a lesser extent than IM nails [39]. EF has the advantage that it provides compression across the arthrodesis site when sufficient bone stock is present and also it may be performed as a single stage procedure in the presence of infection (Fig. 22.2). However, EF devices usually require a period of none weight bearing, they are cumbersome for the patient and have a high incidence of complications including pin site infection, pin loosening and fracture.

Technically the application of an EF system is dependent upon the design chosen, with each design having advantages and disadvantages. Single plane EF systems provide minimal stability in the flexion-extension plane and as such biplanar configurations are believed to provide greater stability, and therefore greater rates of fusion, during attempted arthrodesis [40]. Circular EF frame have also been used with the advantage of an all-wire fixation. This offers the greatest stability in cases of poor bone quality as may be expected in the multiply operated and infected knee following failed TKA. Application of a circular frame can, however, be technically challenging and due to its necessary size to accommodate the soft tissues of the thigh, may cause difficulty in walking.

Table 22.2 presents the available evidence for the use of EF devices for arthrodesis of the knee. As a much less widely used technique, there are few case series exclusively assessing the use of EF arthrodesis in unsalvageable TKA. What can be seen, however, is that the incidence of persistent or recurrent infections is low when the EF is used for knee arthrodesis with six papers reporting 100 % success rate of infection eradication [16, 41–44, 49]. Equally, there was only one reported case of AKA following attempted arthrodesis with an EF device [50]. As such in those patients identified as particularly high risk of re-infection, EF may be a more prudent management strategy in preventing progression to AKA when compared to IM nailing, where arthrodesis is considered a viable option.

Pin site infection is a common complication during EF arthrodesis but is often easily treated with local care and oral antibiotics [16, 41, 43, 47, 49, 51, 53, 54]. Other common complications included pin loosening requiring either pin exchange or re-application of the EF device. Although not often mentioned, the use of hydroxyapatite-coated pins is widely accepted to reduce the risk of deep pin site infection and pin loosening necessitating frame revision [55].

Table 22.2 Published evidence for the use of EF systems for knee arthrodesis

Author	Year	Type EF	Patient #	# of fusions	Mean time to fusion	Mean LLD	% pin tract infection	Complication rate	Complications
Iacono [16]	2013	Hoffman II	12	9 (75 %)	5.6 months	45 mm	33.3 %	0 %	–
Raskolnikov [41]	2013	Taylor Spatial Frame	7	5 (71 %)	8.4 months	–	71.4 %	14.3 %	1 wound breakdown requiring gastroc flap cover
Corona [46]	2013	Monolateral EF	21	17 (81 %)	10.3 months	–	–	27.3 %	3 recurrent infection
Reddy [47]	2011	Ilizarov frame	16	15 (94 %)	28.3 weeks	–	31.3 %	12.5 %	1 pseudoarthrosis 1 recurrent infection
Spina [45]	2010	Ilizarov frame	17	13 (76 %)	9.3 months	38 mm	–	23.5 %	2 septic non-unions 2 intolerance of frame
Riouallon [48]	2009	Single frame + Steinmann pins	8	8 (100 %)	3.5 months	–	12.5 %	25 %	1 supracondylar # + pin migration, 1 haematoma
Eralp [49]	2008	Monolateral frame	11	11 (100 %)	8 months	16 mm	45.5 %	9.1 %	1 leg lengthening surgery
Yeoh [21]	2008	Orthofix (4) Hoffman II (3)	7	2 (29 %)	4.3 months	–	–	71.4 %	1 haematoma, 4 recurrent infections; 2 further washouts
Parratte [42]	2007	Double monobar	18	16 (89 %)	5 months	–	–	5.6 %	1 aseptic non-union
Ulstrup [43]	2007	Sheffield ring fixator	10	6 (60 %)	3.6 months	60 mm	70 %	40 %	4 non-unions; 1 fused with an IM nail, 3 permanently braced
Johannsen [50]	2005	Ilizarov frame	8	6 (75 %)	–	–	–	25 %	1 AKA 1 early death
VanRyn [44]	2002	Hybrid frame	2	2 (100 %)	10 weeks	–	–	0 %	–
David [51]	2001	Ilizarov frame	13	13 (100 %)	27.6 weeks	37 mm	38.5 %	7.7 %	1 superficial wound infection
Manzotti [52]	2001	Ilizarov frame	6	6 (100 %)	6.8 months	–	–	0 %	–
Garberina [53]	2001	Circular EF	19	13 (68 %)	4 months	–	52.6 %	31.6 %	6 aseptic non-unions
Oostenbroek [54]	2001	Ilizarov frame	15	14 (93 %)	28 weeks	40 mm	100 %	53.3 %	3 pin track osteomyelitis, 1 non-union, 2 fractures, 2 frame loosening

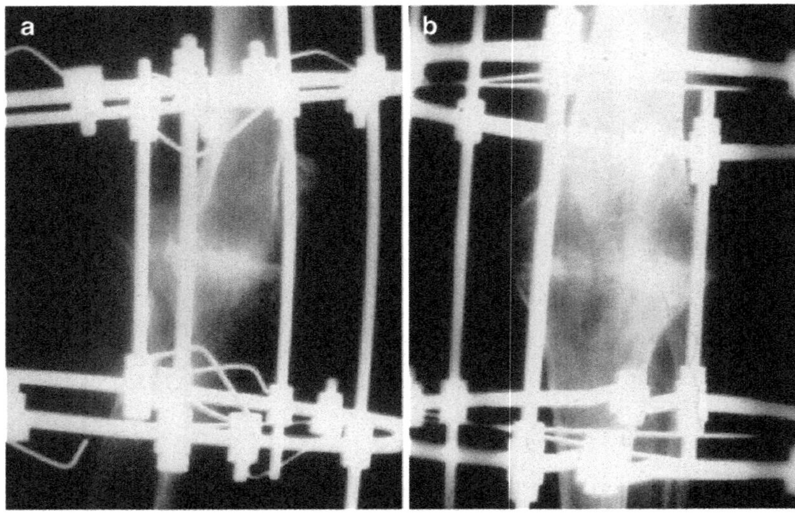

Fig. 22.2 Lateral (**a**) and AP (**b**) plain radiographs of the knee showing successful knee arthrodesis, demonstrated by continuity of the trabecular-medullary pattern, following application of an Ilizarov external fixator in the case series by Spina et al. [45] (With kind permission from Springer Science + Business Media: Spina et al. [45])

Following EF arthrodesis the average length of stay reported by Yeoh et al. was 76 days, greater than that seen following IM nailing [21]. The authors also demonstrated a greater rate of fusion following IM nails compared to EF; however, this paper had a particularly low EF fusion rate of 29 % [21]. Iacono also directly compared IM nailing and EF and found no difference in fusion rate but did demonstrate a significantly greater LLD following EF and also observed a trend towards increased risk of recurrent deep infection following IM nailing [16].

Plates

In theory, arthrodesis using plate osteosynthesis is a useful option for achieving fusion as it is not reliant on the morphology of the tibial or femoral medullary canal, and can provide rigid fixation in the presence of poor bone quality (Fig. 22.3). This said, only a small body of evidence exists for the use of plating techniques for arthrodesis of the knee, but rarely in the exclusive context of infected TKA. In 1961, Lucas and Murray presented 18 cases of knee arthrodesis using two plates on the anterior and medial aspects of the femur and tibia at 90° to each other. With this method they achieved a 94 % fusion rate with the single failure achieving solid fusion after a revision plating procedure [57]. Arthrodesis of the knee has also been demonstrated using a tension band plate system with a single anterior, broad contoured, dynamic-compression plate with screws applied as a tension band. With this arrangement all 26 patients showed osseous union at 2 year follow-up and all could mobilise without aids [58]. The use of a dual-plating technique, with the compression plates on the medial and lateral side of the knee, has also been utilised in two papers of 34 and 11 patients with fusion rates from 80 to 100 %, respectively [59, 60]. The successful use of a locking-compression plate has also been described in three patients with unsalvageable infected TKA, all of whom went on to achieve union [56].

Of these small series, one reported a 28 % incidence of metalwork removal due to pain and metalwork prominence with another reported complications involving 2 of the 11 cases in the form of a femoral stress fracture and persistent infection [56, 60]. Plate arthrodesis is often limited by the protected weight bearing required in the post-operative period, in some cases up to 6 months [56, 57].

Vascularised Fibular Grafts

The use of fibular grafts is more commonly utilised in arthrodesis of the knee following the

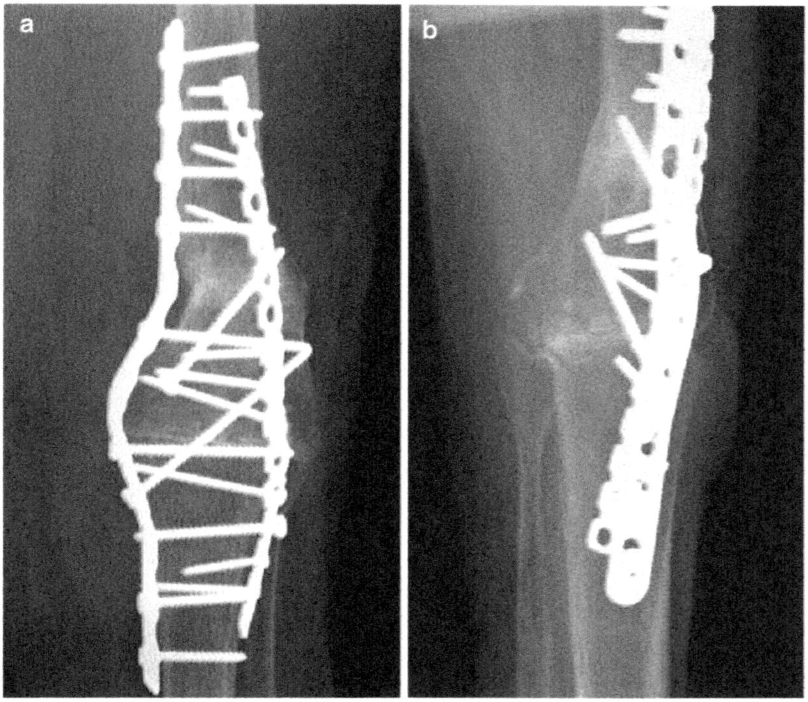

Fig. 22.3 AP (**a**) and lateral (**b**) plain radiographs of a successfully fused knee following dual-plating, with medial and anterolateral plates in situ, in the case series by Kuo et al. [56] (Reprinted from Kuo et al. [56], Copyright 2005)

removal of distal femoral tumours resulting in large bony defects. In the context of the unsalvageable infected TKA, multiple operations and infections may to lead to a significant degree of segmental bone loss in which this technique may be useful in the effort to avoid AKA (Fig. 22.4). Use of the vascularised rotatory fibular transfer provides a biological reconstruction but initially requires mechanical support from an IM nail, external fixator or plate to allow the graft to be adopted and hypertrophy. Reported fusion rates of vascularised fibular grafts range from 75 to 93 %; however, the rate of complications following the procedure is high [61–63]. Following fibular grafts, complications include graft fracture, infection and non-union, however as the literature is mostly related to oncological cases the high rates of infection and poor union may be expected when associated with the adjuvant therapies required to optimally treat the underlying pathology.

Complications Following Arthrodesis and Their Management

As discussed, successful arthrodesis of the knee following failed TKA is an effective treatment option resulting in reasonable function in a complex group of patients. However, complications can occur and the following section aims to highlight the pitfalls associated with arthrodesis and how best to manage them when they occur.

Recurrent Infection

A major risk of arthrodesis in the treatment of infected TKA is that of recurrent infection. Studies have shown that re-infection occurs in as many as 50 % of cases [20, 64, 65]. In these cases it is important to remove the septic metalwork and perform a thorough debridement. Subsequent

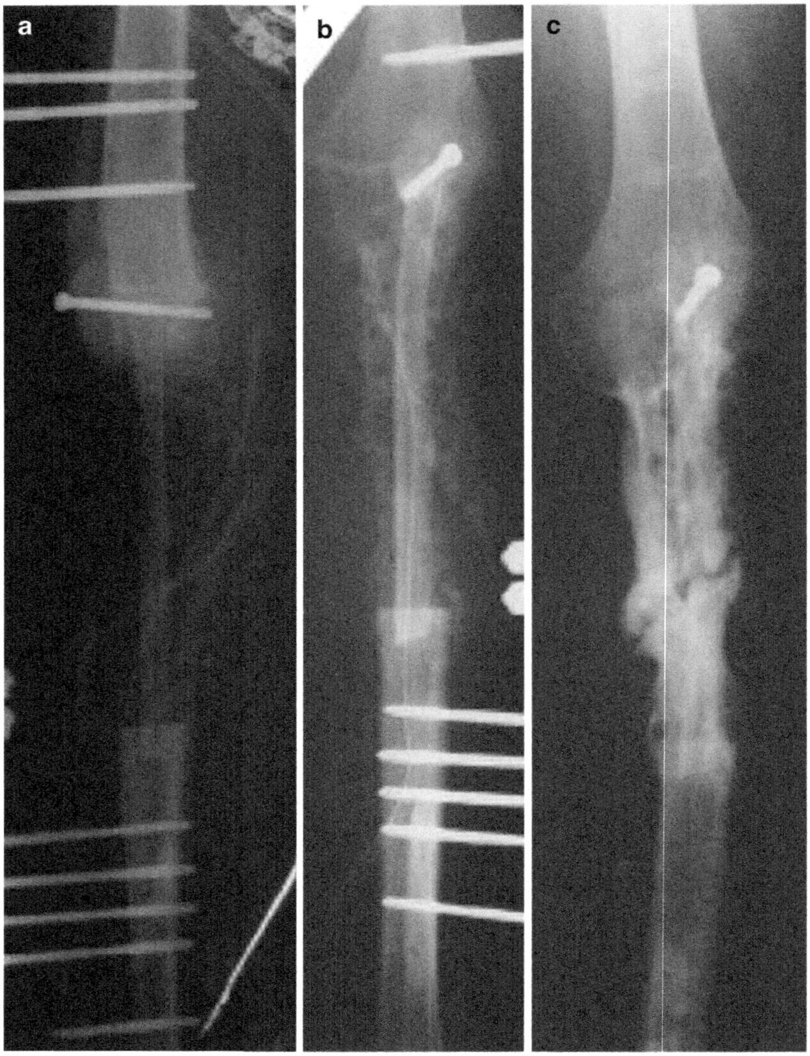

Fig. 22.4 Progressive radiographs following vascularised fibular graft following resection arthroplasty from the case series by Nouri et al. [61]. Initial graft placement stabilised by a monoplanar EF (**a**), subsequent graft consolidation at the extremities with bone graft in situ (**b**), and graft stress fracture following progressive weight bearing after EF removal (**c**)

insertion of an antibiotic coated nail and targeted antibiotic therapy may then be considered. However, recurrent infection following attempted arthrodesis has a high probability of progressing to AKA [15, 16, 22, 26].

One suggested method of treating failed arthrodesis secondary to recurrent infection around an IM nail in situ is the use of a fibular graft [66]. The proposed treatment protocol is a three stage revision with removal of the IM nail, debridement and insertion of a cement spacer ± ipsilateral gastrocnemius flap for soft coverage compromising the first stage. This is then followed by removal of the cement spacer and implementation of a contralateral fibular osteocutaneous flap with EF device for support. The third stage involves exchange of the EF device to internal fixation. A series of five patients who underwent this treatment protocol as a final option prior to AKA showed reasonable results with all five grafts integrating between 6 and 8 months. Complications included one fibular graft stress fracture and two cases of deep infection following the third stage, successfully treated by further debridement and antibiotic therapy, and a cohort mean LLD of 3.8 cm. Importantly, none of the patients required an AKA and all were independently mobile with the aid of one crutch.

Non-union

Following attempted arthrodesis of the knee, the rate of non-union can range from 10 to 80 % and remains a difficult complication to resolve [21, 25, 33]. The treatment of arthrodesis non-union usually involves the use of bone grafting and either fixation with a supplemental plate or exchange intramedullary nailing [67]. Supplemental plate fixation is already commonly used in non-union following long bone fracture augmented with bone graft to the non-union site [68]. This method has the advantages of increasing rotational, bending and torsional stiffness and is effective at achieving solid union in cases where an IM nail may not be placed or where one may not add additional stability [69, 70]. Exchange IM nailing is advantageous in that during the procedure the bony canal is reamed. This allows for a larger diameter IM nail to be inserted increasing rigidity and strength across the non-union site [71]. Additionally, reaming promotes new bone growth adding a biological dimension to the benefits of exchange IM nailing by promoting a more rigid construct and faster union [72, 73].

Leg Length Discrepancies

Although an anticipated effect of arthrodesis and desirable in that it allows easier foot clearance during walking, symptomatic leg length discrepancy usually requires intervention. A shoe lift remains the most common non-surgical intervention; however, patient acceptance of this and issues with balance become problematic as the discrepancy increases with reciprocal increase in orthoses [74]. If surgical intervention is necessitated following arthrodesis, distraction osteogenesis is achievable by lengthening over the nail or exchange nailing with an internal lengthening device [67]. Leg lengthening over a nail has been shown to be an effective method to achieve distraction osteogenesis, with the IM nail offering support to the newly generated bone and as such reducing the time with the external fixator in situ [75, 76]. If this method is chosen to improve leg length discrepancy, great care should be taken to prevent pin site infection which could lead to deep intramedullary sepsis [77]. Exchanging the in situ IM nail for an internal lengthening device can also be considered. These devices alleviate the risk of pin site infections and have been shown to reduce the risk of joint contractures and allow earlier return to normal function [78, 79]. However, there have been reports of a difficulty in controlling the rate of distraction and although debatable, current evidence suggests that lengthening over a nail is a preferable management option [80, 81].

Functional Outcomes Following Knee Arthrodesis

In the unsalvageable failed TKA the management options are arthrodesis or AKA and as such functional comparison between the two must be considered. The decision between limb salvage and amputation is more commonly faced by orthopaedic oncologists and as such the evidence in this field is stronger than in relation to failed TKA, although the question remains the same.

Walking Ability

In terms of ambulatory status, patients undergoing knee arthrodesis have demonstrated good mobility in the literature. Following successful knee fusion, ambulation has been reported in 84 %, 95 % and 100 % of patients [14, 82–84]. Often these patients do require walking aids, however many are able to ambulate independently in the community [24, 49, 51]. In stark contrast, AKA following failed TKA resulted in only 20–50 % of patients mobilising "even to a limited degree" [85, 86]. Obviously, this reduced function following amputation is a function not only of the surgical intervention but also the age and co-morbidities in whom the amputation is often performed.

Pain

Following successful fusion some patients still suffer with pain in and around the fused knee although this is often improved when compared to pre-operative scores [16]. Talmo et al. reported 28 % of patients following successful knee arthrodesis complained of pain in the fused knee, 28 % complained of pain in the ipsilateral hip and 8 % pain in the contralateral hip [82]. Less promising results have been reported, with Röhner et al. observing that 73 % of fused patients complained of permanent pain demonstrated by a visual analogue scale greater than three [64]. This however, still represents a reasonable outcome compared to AKA with Smith et al. reporting that only 9.2 % of patients with an AKA were pain-free in the preceding 4 months, with 36.7 % reporting phantom limb pain and 40.2 % residual limb pain for more than half the time [87].

Physical Health

In terms of the physical health of patients, arthrodesis has been reported to confer a superior level of physical health using the physical component of the validated SF-12 score, with a mean score of 51.4 compared to 26.0 following AKA [85]. Even when compared to patients following revision TKA, arthrodesis performs equally well with a median score of 29.9 on the SF-12 physical outcome measures compared to 28.4 in a patient matched group [8].

Mental Health

The mental wellbeing of patients following knee arthrodesis has also been demonstrated to be better than following AKA with scores of 60.4 and 44.4, respectively, on the mental component of the SF-12 [85]. Again, arthrodesis also performed well when compared with a matched patient cohort following revision TKA, with a median score of 45.1 compared to 36.5 [8].

Patient Satisfaction

Successful arthrodesis of the knee generally leads to a satisfied patient. In a successfully fused knee, up to 82 % claim to be very or somewhat satisfied compared to patients in whom fusion was not achieved with 75 % of these patients being very dissatisfied [46]. Rud et al. also showed a post-arthrodesis satisfaction rate of 80 % and also that 78 % of those whose who were in employment prior to their arthrodesis were able to return to work [88].

Novel Techniques in Implant Arthrodesis

In recent years there has been an expansion of implanted, non-articulating arthrodesis devices. One of the greatest challenges with this technique is the risk of recurrent infection and the subsequent risk of AKA. One method currently under evaluation is the use of a silver coated arthrodesis (SCA) nail in an attempt to reduce infection recurrence.

The presence of silver has been shown to improve resistance to infection and bacterial colonisation as the silver ions are able to attach to bacterial DNA thus preventing protein synthesis [89, 90]. The technique of silver coating orthopaedic prosthesis has been supported in the oncology field with Hardes et al. reporting a reduction in infection rates from 17.6 % in a control group to 5.9 % in the silver coated group [91]. The same study also demonstrated that following infection, an amputation was necessary in 38.5 % of those with an uncoated prosthesis compared to none in the silver coated group.

In our series of eight patients with unsalvageable, multiply revised TKA for

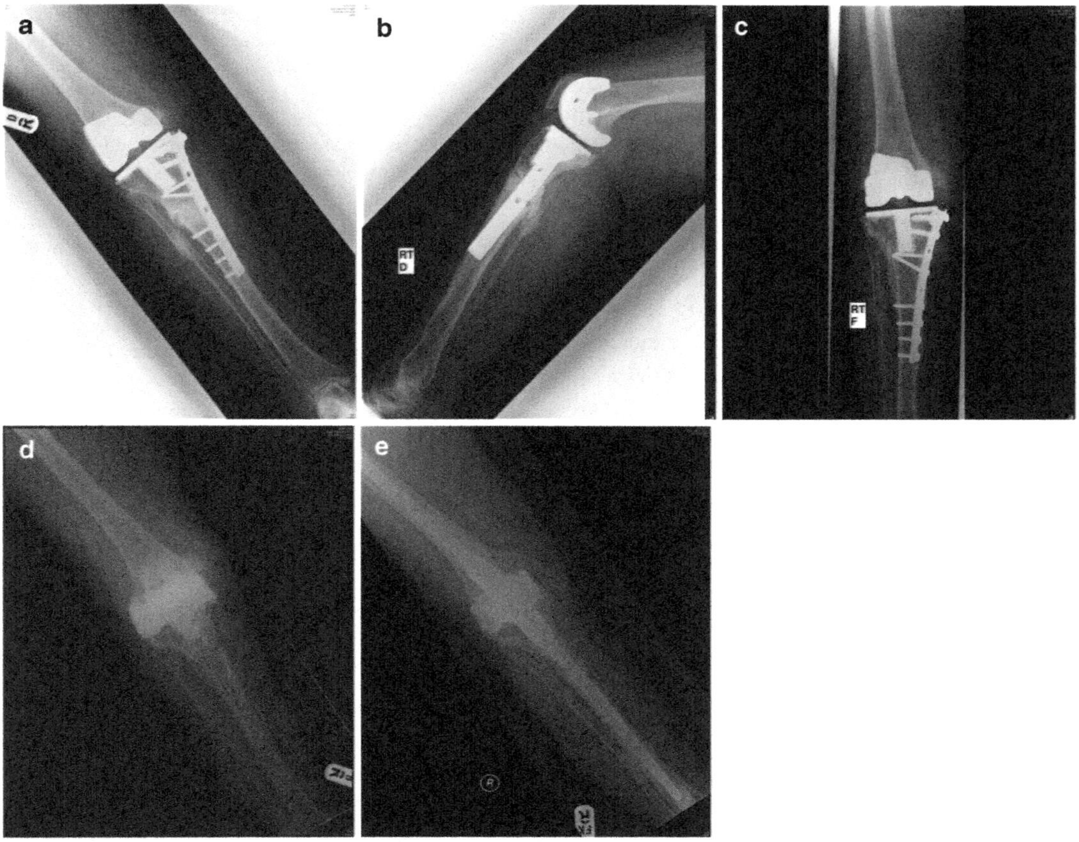

Fig. 22.5 The case of a 65-year-old patient who underwent combined primary TKA and extra-articular osteotomy for correction of a varus malunion following a tibial diaphyseal fracture (**a**, **b**). The patient went on to develop a PJI following union of the osteotomy (**c**) which, due to the poor condition of the soft tissue envelope of the proximal tibia, was treated by two-stage revision with an interval static antibiotic loaded cement spacer (**d**) and subsequent reimplantation with a silver coated arthrodesis nail (**e**). The patient remains free of infection and has returned to a high level of function

infection, with an average five previous procedures, at a mean follow up of 16 months (range 5.2–35.5 months), we have had no patients' progress to amputation (Fig. 22.5). One patient required re-admission, 30 days following SCA nail insertion, due to recurrent deep infection, which was managed successfully with further debridement. One patient developed a superficial wound infection, which was successfully treated with incision, drainage and delayed wound closure. At latest follow-up, the mean Oxford Knee Scores (OKS) was 25.6, a vast improvement on the mean pre-operative OKS of 16.7. Although early in the follow-up period, and only a relatively small group size, the use of an SCA nail for knee arthrodesis may be a promising step forward in reducing the rate of deep infection and subsequent AKA.

Conclusion

Although the multiply infected unsalvageable TKA remains a challenging scenario for the orthopaedic surgeon, knee arthrodesis remains a viable management option over AKA where possible. There are a number of techniques available to achieve arthrodesis, and although IM nailing is currently the most popular, alternative strategies exist if this is not possible. As with any surgical treatment, complications occur, and in the case of arthrodesis, the failure to eradicate infection inevitably results in the need to consider AKA. Functionally, limb salvage with knee fusion has consistently been shown to confer greater functional outcomes when compared with AKA. The use of silver coated prostheses has shown promise in orthopaedic oncology, and the addition of silver to an arthrodesis nail, in our own experience, shows promise in preventing progression to amputation. As the number of TKAs performed worldwide increases, the incidence of unsalvageable multiply revised TKAs is also likely to increase. Therefore, the effective management of the unsalvageable, multiply revised, infected TKA will no doubt become a more pressing issue in the future.

References

1. Nelson CL, Evarts CM. Arthroplasty and arthrodesis of the knee joint. Orthop Clin North Am. 1971;2(1):245–64.
2. Mittal Y, Fehring TK, Hanssen A, Marculescu C, Odum SM, Osmon D. Two-stage reimplantation for periprosthetic knee infection involving resistant organisms. J Bone Joint Surg Am. 2007;89(6):1227–31.
3. Pelt CE, Grijalva R, Anderson L, Anderson MB, Erickson J, Peters CL. Two-Stage Revision TKA Is Associated with High Complication and Failure Rates. Adv Orthop. 2014;2014:659047.
4. Watts CD, Wagner ER, Houdek MT, Osmon DR, Hanssen AD, Lewallen DG, et al. Morbid obesity: a significant risk factor for failure of two-stage revision total knee arthroplasty for infection. J Bone Joint Surg Am. 2014;96(18):e154.
5. Jiang SL, Schairer WW, Bozic KJ. Increased rates of periprosthetic joint infection in patients with cirrhosis undergoing total joint arthroplasty. Clin Orthop Relat Res. 2014;472(8):2483–91.
6. Luque R, Rizo B, Urda A, Garcia-Crespo R, Moro E, Marco F, et al. Predictive factors for failure after total knee replacement revision. Int Orthop. 2014;38(2):429–35.
7. Benson ER, Resine ST, Lewis CG. Functional outcome of arthrodesis for failed total knee arthroplasty. Orthopedics. 1998;21(8):875–9.
8. Barton TM, White SP, Mintowt-Czyz W, Porteous AJ, Newman JH. A comparison of patient based outcome following knee arthrodesis for failed total knee arthroplasty and revision knee arthroplasty. Knee. 2008;15(2):98–100.
9. Behr JT, Chmell SJ, Schwartz CM. Knee arthrodesis for failed total knee arthroplasty. Arch Surg. 1985;120(3):350–4.
10. Brodersen MP, Fitzgerald RH, Peterson LF, Coventry MB, Bryan RS. Arthrodesis of the knee following failed total knee arthroplasty. J Bone Joint Surg Am. 1979;61(2):181–5.
11. Parker DA, Dunbar MJ, Rorabeck CH. Extensor mechanism failure associated with total knee arthroplasty: prevention and management. J Am Acad Orthop Surg. 2003;11(4):238–47.
12. Conway JD, Mont MA, Bezwada HP. Arthrodesis of the knee. J Bone Joint Surg Am. 2004;86-A(4):835–48.
13. Damron TA, McBeath AA. Arthrodesis following failed total knee arthroplasty: comprehensive review and meta-analysis of recent literature. Orthopedics. 1995;18(4):361–8.
14. Miralles-Muñoz FA, Lizaur-Utrilla A, Manrique-Lipa C, López-Prats FA. Arthrodesis without bone fusion with an intramedullary modular nail for revision of infected total knee arthroplasty. Rev Esp Cir Ortop Traumatol. 2014;58(4):217–22.
15. Scarponi S, Drago L, Romanò D, Logoluso N, Peccati A, Meani E, et al. Cementless modular intramedullary nail without bone-on-bone fusion as a salvage procedure in chronically infected total knee prosthesis: long-term results. Int Orthop. 2014;38(2):413–8.
16. Iacono F, Francesco I, Raspugli GF, Francesco RG, Bruni D, Danilo B, et al. Arthrodesis After Infected Revision TKA: Retrospective Comparison of Intramedullary Nailing and External Fixation. HSS J. 2013;9(3):229–35.
17. Waldman BJ, Mont MA, Payman KR, Freiberg AA, Windsor RE, Sculco TP, et al. Infected total knee arthroplasty treated with arthrodesis using a modular nail. Clin Orthop Relat Res. 1999;367:230–7.
18. Lee S, Jang J, Seong SC, Lee MC. Distraction arthrodesis with intramedullary nail and mixed bone grafting after failed infected total knee arthroplasty. Knee Surg Sports Traumatol Arthrosc. 2012;20(2):346–55.
19. Donley BG, Matthews LS, Kaufer H. Arthrodesis of the knee with an intramedullary nail. J Bone Joint Surg Am. 1991;73(6):907–13.
20. Putman S, Kern G, Senneville E, Beltrand E, Migaud H. Knee arthrodesis using a customised modular intramedullary nail in failed infected total knee arthroplasty. Orthop Traumatol Surg Res. 2013;99(4):391–8.
21. Yeoh D, Goddard R, Macnamara P, Bowman N, Miles K, East D, et al. A comparison of two techniques for knee arthrodesis: the custom made intramedullary Mayday nail versus a monoaxial external fixator. Knee. 2008;15(4):263–7.
22. De Vil J, Almqvist KF, Vanheeren P, Boone B, Verdonk R. Knee arthrodesis with an intramedullary nail: a retrospective study. Knee Surg Sports Traumatol Arthrosc. 2008;16(7):645–50.
23. Senior CJ, da Assunção RE, Barlow IW. Knee arthrodesis for limb salvage with an intramedullary coupled nail. Arch Orthop Trauma Surg. 2008;128(7):683–7.
24. Garcia-Lopez I, Aguayo MA, Cuevas A, Navarro P, Prieto C, Carpintero P. Knee arthrodesis with the

Vari-Wall nail for treatment of infected total knee arthroplasty. Acta Orthop Belg. 2008;74(6):809–15.
25. Mabry TM, Jacofsky DJ, Haidukewych GJ, Hanssen AD. Comparison of intramedullary nailing and external fixation knee arthrodesis for the infected knee replacement. Clin Orthop Relat Res. 2007;464: 11–5.
26. Bargiotas K, Wohlrab D, Sewecke JJ, Lavinge G, Demeo PJ, Sotereanos NG. Arthrodesis of the knee with a long intramedullary nail following the failure of a total knee arthroplasty as the result of infection. J Bone Joint Surg Am J Bone Joint Surg Inc. 2006;88(3):103–10.
27. McQueen DA, Cooke FW, Hahn DL. Intramedullary compression arthrodesis of the knee: early experience with a new device and technique. J Arthroplasty. 2005;20(1):72–8.
28. White SP, Porteous AJ, Newman JH, Mintowt-Czyz W, Barr V. Arthrodesis of the knee using a custom-made intramedullary coupled device. J Bone Joint Surg Br. 2003;85(1):57–61.
29. Gore DR, Gassner K. Use of an intramedullary rod in knee arthrodesis following failed total knee arthroplasty. J Knee Surg. 2003;16(3):165–7.
30. Lai KA, Shen WJ, Yang CY. Arthrodesis with a short Huckstep nail as a salvage procedure for failed total knee arthroplasty. J Bone Joint Surg Am J Bone Joint Surg Inc. 1998;80(3):380–8.
31. Jørgensen PS, Tørholm C. Arthrodesis after infected knee arthroplasty using long arthrodesis nail. A report of five cases. Am J Knee Surg. 1995;8(3):110–3.
32. Knutson K, Lindstrand A, Lidgren L. Arthrodesis for failed knee arthroplasty. A report of 20 cases. J Bone Joint Surg Br. 1985;67(1):47–52.
33. Knutson K, Hovelius L, Lindstrand A, Lidgren L. Arthrodesis after failed knee arthroplasty. A nationwide multicenter investigation of 91 cases. Clin Orthop Relat Res. 1984;191:202–11.
34. Barrack RL, Butler RA, Andrews P, Rorabeck CH, Engh G. Managing the infected knee: as good as it gets. Orthopedics. 2000;23(9):991–2.
35. Wasielewski RC, Barden RM, Rosenberg AG. Results of different surgical procedures on total knee arthroplasty infections. J Arthroplasty. 1996;11(8):931–8.
36. Kubista B, Hartzler RU, Wood CM, Osmon DR, Hanssen AD, Lewallen DG. Reinfection after two-stage revision for periprosthetic infection of total knee arthroplasty. Int Orthop. 2012;36(1):65–71.
37. Suarez J, Griffin W, Springer B, Fehring T, Mason JB, Odum S. Why do revision knee arthroplasties fail? J Arthroplasty. 2008;23(6 Suppl 1):99–103.
38. Hossain F, Patel S, Haddad FS. Midterm assessment of causes and results of revision total knee arthroplasty. Clin Orthop Relat Res. 2010;468(5):1221–8.
39. Charnley J, Lowe HG. A study of the end-results of compression arthrodesis of the knee. J Bone Joint Surg Br. 1958;40-B(4):633–5.
40. Brooker AF, Hansen NM. The biplane frame: modified compression arthrodesis of the knee. Clin Orthop Relat Res. 1981;160:163–7.
41. Raskolnikov D, Slover JD, Egol KA. The use of a multiplanar, multi-axis external fixator to achieve knee arthrodesis in a worst case scenario: a case series. Iowa Orthop J. 2013;33:19–24.
42. Parratte S, Madougou S, Villaba M, Stein A, Rochwerger A, Curvale G. Knee arthrodesis with a double mono-bar external fixators to salvage infected knee arthroplasty: retrospective analysis of 18 knees with mean seven-year follow-up. Rev Chir Orthop Reparatrice Appar Mot. 2007;93(4):373–80.
43. Ulstrup AK, Folkmar K, Broeng L. Knee arthrodesis with the Sheffield external ring fixator: fusion in 6 of 10 consecutive patients. Acta Orthop. 2007; 78(3):371–6.
44. VanRyn JS, Verebelyi DM. One-stage débridement and knee fusion for infected total knee arthroplasty using the hybrid frame. J Arthroplasty. 2002;17(1):129–34.
45. Spina M, Gualdrini G, Fosco M, Giunti A. Knee arthrodesis with the Ilizarov external fixator as treatment for septic failure of knee arthroplasty. J Orthop Traumatol. 2010;11(2):81–8.
46. Corona PS, Hernandez A, Reverte-Vinaixa MM, Amat C, Flores X. Outcome after knee arthrodesis for failed septic total knee replacement using a monolateral external fixator. J Orthop Surg (Hong Kong). 2013;21(3):275–80.
47. Reddy VG, Kumar RV, Mootha AK, Thayi C, Kantesaria P, Reddy D. Salvage of infected total knee arthroplasty with Ilizarov external fixator. Indian J Orthop. 2011;45(6):541–7.
48. Riouallon G, Molina V, Mansour C, Court C, Nordin J-Y. An original knee arthrodesis technique combining external fixator with Steinman pins direct fixation. Orthop Traumatol Surg Res. 2009;95(4):272–7.
49. Eralp L, Kocaoğlu M, Tuncay I, Bilen FE, Samir SE. Knee arthrodesis using a unilateral external fixator for the treatment of infectious sequelae. Acta Orthop Traumatol Turc. 2008;42(2):84–9.
50. Johannsen HG, Skov O, Weeth ER. Knee arthrodesis with external ring fixator after infected knee arthroplasty. Ugeskr Laeger. 2005;167(35):3295–6.
51. David R, Shtarker H, Horesh Z, Tsur A, Soudry M. Arthrodesis with the Ilizarov device after failed knee arthroplasty. Orthopedics. 2001;24(1):33–6.
52. Manzotti A, Pullen C, Deromedis B, Catagni MA. Knee arthrodesis after infected total knee arthroplasty using the Ilizarov method. Clin Orthop Relat Res. 2001;(389):143–9.
53. Garberina MJ, Fitch RD, Hoffmann ED, Hardaker WT, Vail TP, Scully SP. Knee arthrodesis with circular external fixation. Clin Orthop Relat Res. 2001;382:168–78.
54. Oostenbroek HJ, van Roermund PM. Arthrodesis of the knee after an infected arthroplasty using the Ilizarov method. J Bone Joint Surg Br. 2001;83(1):50–4.
55. Pommer A, Muhr G, Dávid A. Hydroxyapatite-coated Schanz pins in external fixators used for distraction osteogenesis: a randomized, controlled trial. J Bone Joint Surg Am. 2002;84-A(7):1162–6.

56. Kuo AC, Meehan JP, Lee M. Knee fusion using dual platings with the locking compression plate. J Arthroplasty. 2005;20(6):772–6.
57. Lucas DB, Murray WR. Arthrodesis of the knee by double-plating. J Bone Joint Surg J Bone Joint Surg Inc. 1961;43(6):795–808.
58. Pritchett JW, Mallin BA, Matthews AC. Knee arthrodesis with a tension-band plate. J Bone Joint Surg Am J Bone Joint Surg Inc. 1988;70(2):285–8.
59. Munzinger U, Knessl J, Gschwend N. Arthrodesis following knee arthroplasty. Orthopade. 1987;16(4): 301–9.
60. Nichols SJ, Landon GC, Tullos HS. Arthrodesis with dual plates after failed total knee arthroplasty. J Bone Joint Surg Am J Bone Joint Surg Inc. 1991;73(7):1020–4.
61. Nouri H, Meherzi MH, Jenzeri M, Daghfous M, Hdidane R, Zehi K, et al. Knee arthrodesis using a vascularized fibular rotatory graft after tumor resection. Orthop Traumatol Surg Res. 2010;96(1): 57–63.
62. Wada T, Usui M, Nagoya S, Isu K, Yamawaki S, Ishii S. Resection arthrodesis of the knee with a vascularised fibular graft. Medium- to long-term results. J Bone Joint Surg Br. 2000;82(4):489–93.
63. Rasmussen MR, Bishop AT, Wood MB. Arthrodesis of the knee with a vascularized fibular rotatory graft. J Bone Joint Surg Am. 1995;77(5):751–9.
64. Röhner E, Windisch C, Nuetzmann K, Rau M, Arnhold M, Matziolis G. Unsatisfactory outcome of arthrodesis performed after septic failure of revision total knee arthroplasty. J Bone Joint Surg Am. 2015;97(4):298–301.
65. Schwarzkopf R, Kahn TL, Succar J, Ready JE. Success of different knee arthrodesis techniques after failed total knee arthroplasty: is there a preferred technique? J Arthroplasty. 2014;29(5):982–8.
66. Cavadas PC, Thione A, Perez-Garcia A, Lorca-García C, Aranda-Romero F. Salvage of infected intramedullary knee arthrodesis with vascularized free fibula and staged fixation. Injury. 2014;45(11):1772–5.
67. Wood JH, Conway JD. Advanced concepts in knee arthrodesis. World J Orthop. 2015;6(2):202–10.
68. AO Surgery Reference. https://www2.aofoundation.org/wps/portal/surgery.
69. Choi YS, Kim KS. Plate augmentation leaving the nail in situ and bone grafting for non-union of femoral shaft fractures. Int Orthop. 2005;29(5): 287–90.
70. Birjandinejad A, Ebrahimzadeh MH, Ahmadzadeh-Chabock H. Augmentation plate fixation for the treatment of femoral and tibial nonunion after intramedullary nailing. Orthopedics. 2009;32(6):409.
71. Hak DJ, Lee SS, Goulet JA. Success of exchange reamed intramedullary nailing for femoral shaft nonunion or delayed union. J Orthop Trauma. 2000;14(3):178–82.
72. Pape H-C, Giannoudis P. The biological and physiological effects of intramedullary reaming. J Bone Joint Surg Br. 2007;89(11):1421–6.
73. Chapman MW. The effect of reamed and nonreamed intramedullary nailing on fracture healing. Clin Orthop Relat Res. 1998;355(Suppl):S230–8.
74. Danbert RJ. Clinical assessment and treatment of leg length inequalities. J Manipulative Physiol Ther. 1988;11(4):290–5.
75. Simpson AH, Cole AS, Kenwright J. Leg lengthening over an intramedullary nail. J Bone Joint Surg Br. 1999;81(6):1041–5.
76. Chaudhary M. Limb lengthening over a nail can safely reduce the duration of external fixation. Indian J Orthop. 2008;42(3):323–9.
77. Kim S-J, Cielo Balce G, Huh Y-J, Song S-Y, Song H-R. Deep intramedullary infection in tibial lengthening over an intramedullary nail. Acta Orthop Belg. 2011;77(4):506–15.
78. Rozbruch SR, Birch JG, Dahl MT, Herzenberg JE. Motorized intramedullary nail for management of limb-length discrepancy and deformity. J Am Acad Orthop Surg. 2014;22(7):403–9.
79. Karakoyun O, Küçükkaya M, Sökücü S. Intramedullary skeletal kinetic distractor in lower extremity lengthening. Acta Orthop Traumatol Turc. 2014;48(3):307–12.
80. Lee DH, Ryu KJ, Song HR, Han S-H. Complications of the Intramedullary Skeletal Kinetic Distractor (ISKD) in distraction osteogenesis. Clin Orthop Relat Res. 2014;472(12):3852–9.
81. Mahboubian S, Seah M, Fragomen AT, Rozbruch SR. Femoral lengthening with lengthening over a nail has fewer complications than intramedullary skeletal kinetic distraction. Clin Orthop Relat Res. 2012;470(4):1221–31.
82. Talmo CT, Bono JV, Figgie MP, Sculco TP, Laskin RS, Windsor RE. Intramedullary arthrodesis of the knee in the treatment of sepsis after TKR. HSS J. 2007;3(1):83–8.
83. Watanabe K, Minowa T, Takeda S, Otsubo H, Kobayashi T, Kura H, et al. Outcomes of knee arthrodesis following infected total knee arthroplasty: a retrospective analysis of 8 cases. Mod Rheumatol. 2014; 24(2):243–9.
84. Chen AF, Kinback NC, Heyl AE, McClain EJ, Klatt BA. Better function for fusions versus above-the-knee amputations for recurrent periprosthetic knee infection. Clin Orthop Relat Res. 2012;470(10):2737–45.
85. Fedorka CJ, Chen AF, McGarry WM, Parvizi J, Klatt BA. Functional ability after above-the-knee amputation for infected total knee arthroplasty. Clin Orthop Relat Res. 2011;469(4):1024–32.
86. Sierra RJ, Trousdale RT, Pagnano MW. Above-the-knee amputation after a total knee replacement: prevalence, etiology, and functional outcome. J Bone Joint Surg Am. 2003;85-A(6):1000–4.
87. Smith DG, Ehde DM, Legro MW, Reiber GE, del Aguila M, Boone DA. Phantom limb, residual limb, and back pain after lower extremity amputations. Clin Orthop Relat Res. 1999;361:29–38.
88. Rud B, Jensen UH. Function after arthrodesis of the knee. Informa UK Ltd UK; 2009.

89. Park H-J, Kim JY, Kim J, Lee J-H, Hahn J-S, Gu MB, et al. Silver-ion-mediated reactive oxygen species generation affecting bactericidal activity. Water Res. 2009;43(4):1027–32.
90. Kim JS, Kuk E, Yu KN, Kim J-H, Park SJ, Lee HJ, et al. Antimicrobial effects of silver nanoparticles. Nanomedicine. 2007;3(1):95–101.
91. Hardes J, von Eiff C, Streitbuerger A, Balke M, Budny T, Henrichs MP, et al. Reduction of periprosthetic infection with silver-coated megaprostheses in patients with bone sarcoma. J Surg Oncol. 2010; 101(5):389–95.

Late Infections of the Knee Joint: Two-Stage Articulating Solutions

23

O. Brant Nikolaus and Matthew P. Abdel

Abstract

Two-stage exchange is the gold standard for the treatment of chronic total knee arthroplasty (TKA) infections in North America. Cement spacers impregnated with high- dose antibiotics have successfully been utilized in the interim period of the two-stage exchange. A number of non-articulating and articulating spacers have been described. With an intact extensor mechanism, a reasonable soft-tissue envelope, and adequate bone, articulating antibiotic spacers provide several advantages. These include an infection eradication rate of approximately 90 %, a higher range of motion after reimplantation, and lower complication rates when compared with non-articulating spacers. In the appropriate patient, articulating antibiotic spacers are an effective and a safe treatment choice in the two-stage exchange process for infected TKAs.

Keywords

Total knee arthroplasty (TKA) • Periprosthetic joint infection (PJI) • Two-stage exchange • Articulating antibiotic spacer • Non-articulating antibiotic spacer

Introduction

Total knee arthroplasty (TKA) is one of the most successful procedures, with excellent pain relief and good functional outcomes [1–3]. However, there are still perioperative complications that occur and can be very difficult to manage. Periprosthetic joint infection (PJI) is one of the most devastating and expensive complications, occurring in 1–2 % of TKAs [4–7]. It is one of the top three reasons for TKA failures, accounting for up to 40 % of all revision TKAs [8–12].

Two-stage exchange for infected TKAs was first described in the early 1980s, and is now considered the gold standard for treatment of chronic PJI in North America. In 1983, Insall et al. [13]

O.B. Nikolaus, MD • M.P. Abdel, MD (✉)
Department of Orthopedic Surgery, Mayo Clinic, 200 First Street SW, Rochester, MN 55905, USA
e-mail: nikolaus.oliver@mayo.edu; Abdel.Matthew@mayo.edu

D. Kendoff et al. (eds.), *Periprosthetic Joint Infections: Changing Paradigms*,
DOI 10.1007/978-3-319-30091-7_23

reported on 11 two-stage revisions for infection, with no recurrence of the original organism. However, one patient did have an acute hematogenous infection with a different organism. While the component resection and joint debridement helped eradicate the infection, the knee in the interim was usually painful, with limited weight bearing and motion allowed. Reimplantation was frequently difficult given the poor bone quality and the degree of adhesions that formed in the knee joint between stages. In addition, the delivery of antibiotics to the local tissues was difficult given the debridement of the vascular synovium.

To address these issues, antibiotic-impregnated polymethylmethacrylate (PMMA) cement spacers were introduced into the joint during the exchange interval. The first usage of these were non-articulating spacers, which included antibiotic-impregnated PMMA beads, followed by spacer blocks [14–16]. The main advantage of these spacers was the local delivery of high-dose antibiotics [17]. In addition, non-articulating spacers had the potential benefit of maintaining the joint space by preserving the tension on the collateral ligaments and surrounding soft-tissues, preventing contracture formation for the subsequent reimplantation. Moreover, the non-articulating spacer blocks helped maintain bone stock. However, a number of problems occurred with the block spacers, including quadriceps shortening, arthrofibrosis, extensor mechanism disruptions, spacer block migration, significant bone loss, and difficulty with exposure secondary to joint contractures [18–23]. In addition, patients had functional difficulties with a knee locked in near full extension during the interval period [18, 24].

To overcome these disadvantages, articulating spacers were popularized in the mid-1990s [25]. Since then, there have been a number of different articulating spacers described in the literature, including cement-on-cement, cement-on-polyethylene, and metal-on-polyethylene articulations. The potential advantages of these articulating spacers are (1) a preserved joint space allowing for delivery of high-dose antibiotics to the local tissues, (2) a mobile knee with greater range of motion, (3) partial weight bearing and greater patient comfort during the exchange period, and (4) an easier reimplantation due to the reduced incidence of quadriceps and ligament contractures, reduced arthrofibrosis, and minimal bone loss [18, 24, 26, 27].

Indications and Contraindications

The primary indication for the use of an articulating spacer is the treatment of a chronic periprosthetic knee infection in patients with adequate bone stock (Anderson Orthopaedic Research Institute [AORI] [28] Classification Type 2A or less), an intact extensor mechanism, and an adequate soft-tissue envelope. In addition, an articulating spacer can be utilized as the first stage in a planned two-stage primary TKA to treat patients with recalcitrant native septic arthritis with secondary end-stage joint destruction.

The absolute contraindication for use of an articulating spacer is the lack of an intact extensor mechanism. Relative contraindications include severe bone loss (AORI Type 2B or greater), large soft tissue defects such as those requiring flap coverage, morbid obesity, collateral ligament insufficiency, non-compliant patients, and previous failure of a two-stage revision for chronic PJI [27].

Articulating Antibiotic-Impregnated Spacer Techniques

There are a number of different possible techniques that have been described for articulating spacers. These can be classified largely into three different groups based on the articulating surfaces in each implant: cement-on-cement, cement-on-polyethylene, and metal-on-polyethylene.

Cement-on-cement femoral-tibial articulations have been effective in infection eradication [18, 29, 30]. However, there is not a consensus on the best technique to produce a cement-on-cement spacer, leading to a number of different techniques. The first type can be classified as a customized cement spacer. These spacers are built and fitted to the host bone, and then the components are molded and customized with a high-speed burr to shape the spacer into functional articulating components [29, 31–33]. Another type of cement-on-cement spacer allows for intraoperative molding. Some authors have reported using heavy aluminum foil to make a mold of the bony ends to better match the bony defects [34]. Others have reported on the use of the articulating portions of the resected femoral and tibial components to make custom molds of different materials such as bone cement [35, 36] or a putty matrix composed of polydimethyl siloxane and silica [37]. There are also studies that use metal molds [18, 38], polypropene molds [39], and silicone molds [40]. A third technique involves utilizing commercially available intraoperative molds such as the StageOne Spacer Mold (Biomet Orthopaedics, Inc; Warsaw, IN) [30, 41, 42]. The last type of cement-on-cement articulating spacer involves using femoral and tibial components that are manufactured in the factory, coming pre-formed as an ultracongruent condylar knee prosthesis design made exclusively of acrylic cement impregnated with gentamicin and/or vancomycin antibiotics (InterSpace Knee, Exactech Inc., Gainesville, FL; Spacer-K, TECRES S.P.A, Verona, Italy). These cement spacers have been approved by the United States (US) Food and Drug Administration (FDA) for use in two-stage exchanges for infected TKAs. However, the dosage of gentamicin in these components ranges from 0.8 to 1.7 g per 40 g of cement, which is well below the recommended dose of 3.6 g of gentamicin per 40 g of cement [27, 43]. Regardless, such spacers have been biomechanically tested to verify that they were adequate for clinical use [44–48].

Independent of the type of cement-on-cement spacer utilized, all have the advantage of a large surface area of antibiotic impregnated cement being exposed to the knee tissues. They also have the distinct advantage of allowing for adjustable antibiotic dosing, adding a combination of antibiotics, and the ability to add an anti-fungal agent if desired [21]. However, they also have the potential mechanical problems of increased wear debris and fragmentation from a high coefficient of friction with cement-on-cement articulation. In addition, cement-on-cement articulations in the knee cannot provide the stability of a posterior-stabilized (PS) post [49]. Another disadvantage of customized and intraoperatively molded spacers is that they require additional time in the operating room to construct [21].

The second group of articulating spacers is that with a cement-on-polyethylene articulation. There is only one study that has described this technique [49]. In this study, the authors report use of a handmade cement femoral component or a disposable femoral mold to make a cement femoral component. Then, a stemmed PS all-polyethylene tibial component is covered in cement.

The third, and most popular, group of articulating spacers is that of a metal-on-polyethylene construct. Hofmann et al. [25] introduced this technique in 1995. This technique involved sterilization and reimplantation of the original femoral component. The sterilized femoral component and a new tibial polyethylene insert were then fixed with high-dose antibiotic impregnated cement. However, most institutions in the US now limit the use of a previously sterilized femoral component. As such, the most common technique is opening a new, sterile femoral component that is similar in size to the one removed along with a tibial polyethylene insert without its tibial tray, both being cemented in place with high-dose antibiotic impregnated cement [50, 51]. Another technique involves the prosthesis of antibiotic-loaded acrylic cement (PROSTALAC) knee spacer system (DePuy; Warsaw, IN). This system includes separate femoral and tibial components composed of antibiotic impregnated cement. In addition, it features a bi-compartmental stainless steel femoral component that articulates with a PS polyethylene tibial component [52, 53]. A similar technique was recently reported by Carulli et al. [54] with two Oxford III unicompartmental implants (Biomet) along with the StageOne Spacer Mold system (Biomet). The advantage of using a metal-on-polyethylene articulating spacer is that the articulating surface is much smoother. It also allows for adjustable antibiotic dosing, adding a combination of antibiotics, and the ability to add an antifungal agent if needed [21]. By using a new femoral component and tibial insert, the surgeon can save time in the operating room and can also improve overall stability by being able to use more constraint such as posterior stabilized components. However, this can limit the available antibiotic impregnated cement surface area, which is important for antibiotic elution from the cement. It also places exposed metallic and polyethylene surfaces in a contaminated wound, which can be worrisome for further infection risk [49]. In addition, using all new components is more expensive than some of the other techniques [55].

Authors Preferred Technique and Tips

The senior author's (MPA) preferred technique for an articulating spacer is a metal-on-polyethylene articulation with the use of a new femoral component and a new tibial polyethylene insert, both cemented in place with high-dose antibiotic impregnated cement. This technique is simple and reliable, while allowing for delivery of high-dose local antibiotics, preserving knee motion and patient function during the intervening period, and allowing ease of exposure during reimplantation.

After removing the femoral, tibial, and patellar components, it is essential to complete an aggressive irrigation and debridement, including removal of all foreign bodies and debris. This includes all cement from the prior arthroplasty, as well as any non-viable bone and soft-tissues down to a bleeding surface. All bony surfaces on the femur and tibia are freshened. A trial femoral component is then placed on the femur, and trial inserts are placed in the knee to determine which size is most optimal to allow full extension and flexion to approximately 120°, with varus-valgus stability throughout the arc of motion. After a thorough repeat irrigation and debridement and gentle trialing, the femoral and tibial canals are gently reamed to bleeding bone. Data has shown that in an infected TKA, the infection can exist in the intramedullary canals in up to one-third of the patients [56]. However, excessive reaming to cortical bone is avoided, as this does not allow for appropriate cementation at the reimplantation.

Due to the possible colonization of the intramedullary canals, we prefer to use high-dose antibiotic impregnated cement dowels in both the intramedullary canals. These can be easily fashioned by using the nozzles of two cement guns. Since each cement gun nozzle holds approximately 20 g of cement, one 40 g pack of cement with 3 g of vancomycin and 3.6 g of gentamicin is mixed with methylene blue to create two tapered cement dowels (Fig. 23.1). A nipple is fashioned at the end of each dowel to prevent migration. Intramedullary beads can be extremely difficult to remove at the time of reimplantation. In our opinion, there is no role for such beads in the management of patients with chronic PJI.

After a thorough irrigation and debridement and placement of the intramedullary dowels (Fig. 23.2), the articulating spacer can be formed. It is our preference to cement in two steps. In the first step, one batch of cement with 3 g of vancomycin and 3.6 g of gentamicin, along with methylene blue, is used to coat the tibial surface and condylar surface of the femur where the femoral component will rest. If anti-fungal coverage is required, 150 g of amphotericin b is added to each 40 g batch of cement. It is important to note that it can be quite difficult to mix this amount of antibiotic and cement powder. To facilitate this, it is important to first form the liquid cement by mixing the polymethylmethacrylate monomer and powder together before adding the antibiotic powder. In addition, to help facilitate with antibiotic elution, it is acceptable to leave many of the large antibiotic crystals intact so that the cement is more porous [43].

Small divots are then made in the cement while it is curing (Fig. 23.3). This first round of cement allows for macro-interdigitation, rather than micro-interdigitation, facilitating removal of the cement at the time of reimplantation.

In the meantime, the real femoral component and polyethylene insert are opened based upon previous trialing. The back surface of the polyethylene is then scored with a high-speed burr (Fig. 23.4).

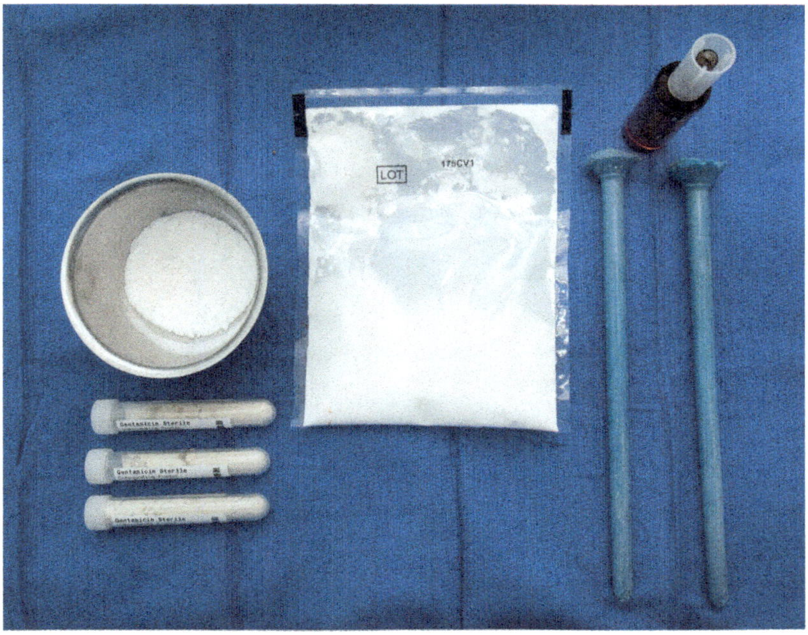

Fig. 23.1 Intramedullary dowels are made utilizing two cement gun nozzles, one 40 g bag of bone cement, 3 g of vancomycin, 3.6 g of gentamicin, and methylene blue

Once the cement is hardened, the second round of cement is mixed with the same proportions of PMMA and antibiotics as described above. The femur should be cemented first, followed by the polyethylene insert (Fig. 23.5). The tibial insert should be inserted in place perpendicular to the long axis of the tibia and in line with the tibial crest for rotation. Additional cement is used to build up to the articular surface of the polyethylene insert (Fig. 23.6a, b).

The knee is then thoroughly irrigated with diluted Betadine [57] and normal saline via the pulsatile lavage. Two intra-articular drains are placed, and usually removed on postoperative day one. The arthrotomy is closed with large absorbable monofilament sutures, and the subdermal layer is closed with smaller absorbable monofilament sutures. The dermal layer is then closed with interrupted vertical mattress sutures with a non-absorbable monofilament suture and Dermabond (Ethicon Inc; Somerville, NJ, USA). It is of the utmost importance to obtain a watertight closure with good apposition of the skin edges to ensure adequate soft tissue and wound healing.

The postoperative regimen allows patients to be out of bed on the day of surgery, and partial weight bearing on postoperative day one. In the vast majority of cases, gentle range of motion is initiated on postoperative day one. Patients are typically treated with 6 weeks of organism-specific IV antibiotics based upon cultures and sensitivities. Throughout this course, inflammatory markers are followed, including the C-reactive protein (CRP) and erythrocyte sedimentation rate (ESR). If improving, antibiotics are discontinued at 6 weeks. Patients are then seen in three additional weeks (i.e., at the 9-week postoperative visit), for a repeat clinical evaluation with CRP and ESR labs. If the patient remains asymptomatic and the exam is benign, combined with improved or normalized inflammatory markers, reimplantation is scheduled in three additional weeks (i.e., at 12 weeks from the resection). Patients are seen the day prior to surgery for a repeat CRP and ESR. Of note, it is important to work closely with an orthopedic infectious disease specialist to ensure appropriate and adequate antibiotic coverage.

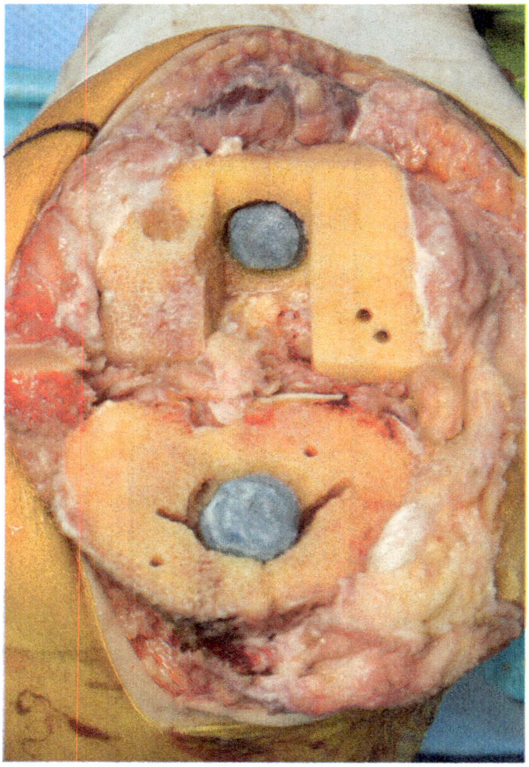

Fig. 23.2 After a thorough irrigation and debridement, including intramedullary reaming, intramedullary dowels with high-dose antibiotics are placed. The nipples on the end of the dowels allow for easier extraction and prevent migration

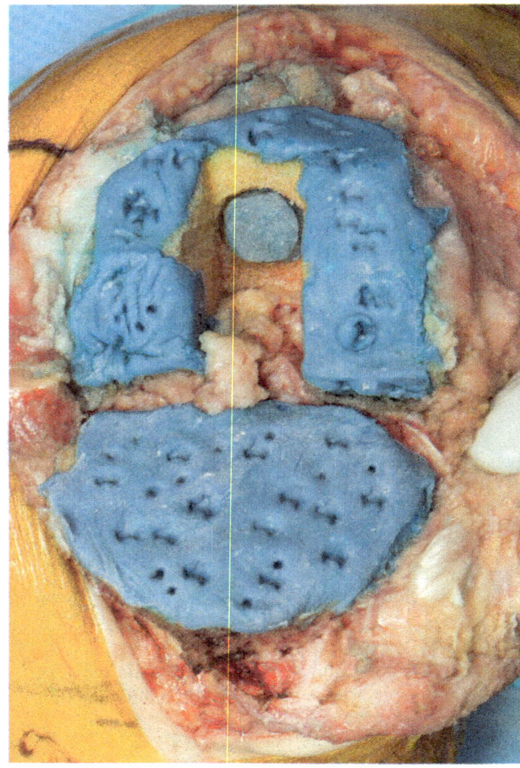

Fig. 23.3 The first stage of the cementation process includes coating the tibial plateau and condylar surfaces of the femur with an additional 40 g batch of cement, 3 g of vancomycin, 3.6 g of gentamicin, and methylene blue

Outcomes

Articulating spacers were originally introduced to overcome the functional difficulties that were seen with non-articulating cement spacers. This led to the development of a number of different types of articulating spacers, which showed infection eradication rates between 88 and 100 % [18, 29, 32–34, 39, 40, 42, 45, 49, 52, 53, 58–62]. While there have not been any published randomized trials comparing non-articulating and articulating spacers, there have been a number of published comparative studies (Table 23.1).

Fehring et al. [18] compared 25 patients with non-articulating static block spacers to 30 patients with articulating all-cement spacers. Static spacers showed an infection eradication rate of 88 % versus 93 % for the articulating spacer group. The difference was not statistically significant. In addition, they did not show any difference in clinical scores, range of motion, or need for extensile exposures between the two groups. However, they did show that 15 (60 %) of the patients who had a non-articulating spacer developed either femoral or tibial bone loss as a result of the block spacer. This is in contrast to the patients with an articulating spacer who did not develop any bone loss. Similarly, Emerson et al. [24] compared 22 patients treated with a non-articulating static spacer with 22 patients treated with an articulating spacer (re-sterilized original femoral component with polyethylene tibial insert). The static spacer group had their surgical procedures performed prior to 1995, while the articulating spacer group had the surgical procedures performed after 1995 due to a change in practice. Due to this timing difference, the non-articulating group has a longer fol-

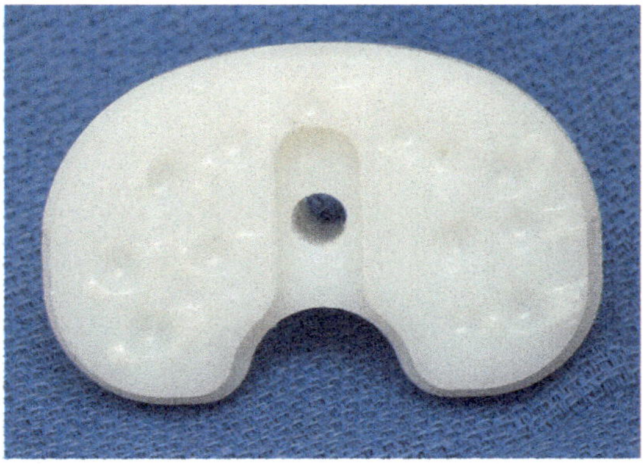

Fig. 23.4 The undersurface of the polyethylene insert should be scored with a high-speed burr to allow for cement interdigitation

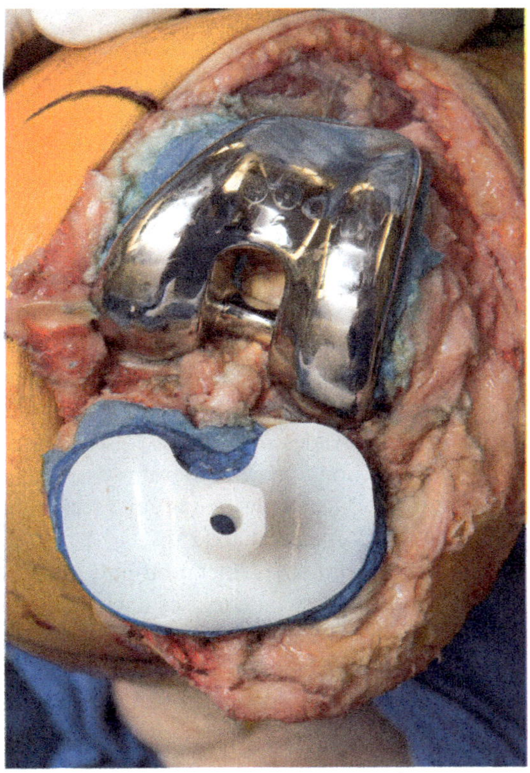

Fig. 23.5 The second stage of the cementation process includes cementing the femoral component and polyethylene insert onto the prior cement mantle. This is completed with a third batch of cement using the previously noted proportions

low-up than the articulating spacers, mandating shorter reported infection eradication rates at 3.6 years. The authors found that static spacers showed an infection eradication rate of 92 % for non-articulating spacers versus 91 % for articulating spacers (not statistically significant). However, the articulating spacer group did have a statistically significant increase in knee flexion (108° vs. 94°, respectively; $p=0.01$).

Chiang et al. [63] also reported on a comparison of articulating and non-articulating spacers in patients with methicillin-resistant *Staphylococcus aureus* (MRSA) and methicillin-resistant coagulase-negative Staphylococcus (MRCNS). Twenty-two patients treated with non-articulating block spacers were compared to 23 patients who were treated with an articulating all cement spacer (intraoperatively molded with specially made molds fabricated from a putty matrix composed of polydimethyl siloxane and silica). There were 19 cases of MRSA and four cases of MRCNS in the articulating spacer group, compared to 20 cases of MRSA and two cases of MRCNS in the non-articulating spacer group. The articulating spacer group only had one reinfection, giving an infection eradication rate of 96 % compared to 91 % in the static group (not significant). They did, however, show that the functional results at a mean of 40 months after surgery were significantly better with the articulating spacer group with better HSS scores and increased postoperative motion (113° vs. 85°, respectively; $p=<0.05$). The non-articulating group also required more extensile approaches upon reimplantation, requiring six quadriceps snips and 1 V-Y turndown, while the articulating group did not require any such extensile approaches. In addition, they also reported that the patient satisfaction rate during the interim stage of the two-stage revision was significantly higher for the articulating group. In summary, this study showed similar infection eradication rates in resistant organisms, but improved functional outcomes with articulating spacers.

In comparing the literature, it is apparent that articulating spacers are at least as effective in infection eradication as non-articulating spacers. However, there is no consensus on how articulating spacers should be made. There are cement-on-cement, cement-on-polyethylene, and metal-on-polyethylene articulating spacers. The largest amount of clinical data available thus far

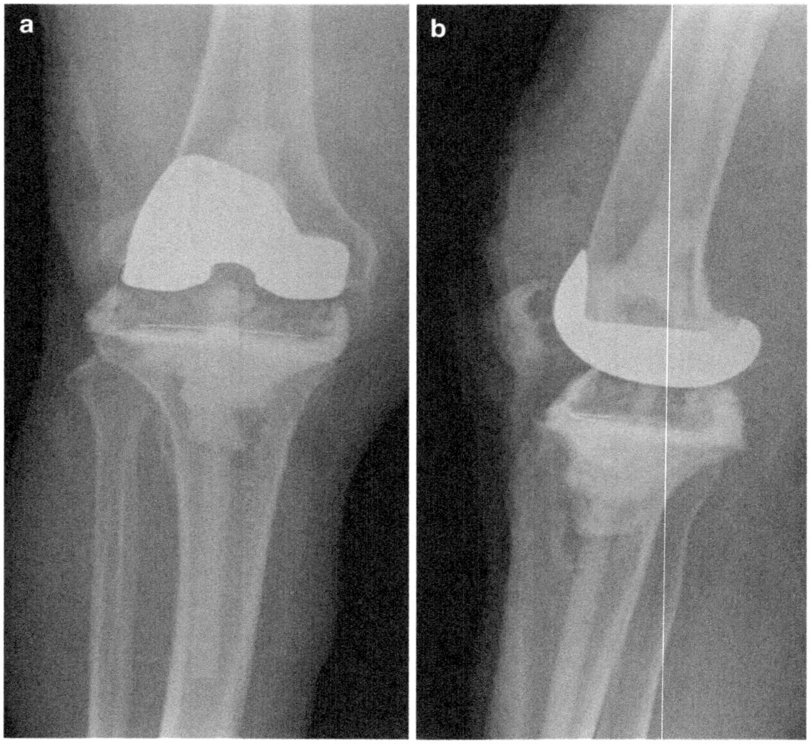

Fig. 23.6 (**a**) Anteroposterior (AP) and (**b**) lateral radiographs of a 56-year-old male with an infected right revision total knee arthroplasty status post resection arthroplasty and placement of an articulating antibiotic spacer

involves the metal-on-polyethylene group. Hofmann et al. [25] first reported a technique in 1995 that involved the sterilization and reimplantation of the removed femoral component along with a new polyethylene tibial insert. The original study reported on 26 patients who underwent two-stage revision for TKA infection with this technique for the interim articulating spacer. There were no reinfections in these original 26 patients at a mean follow-up of 31 months. The authors then reported an update of their results in 2005 [60]. They analyzed a total of 50 patients and reported an infection eradication rate of 88 % with a mean of 74 months of follow-up. These infections occurred at an average of 35 months after reimplantation. There have also been a number of other studies that have reported results with articulating spacers using this particular technique (Table 23.2). Lee and Choi [64] reported a 95 % infection eradication rate at a mean follow-up of 65 months, and they also showed that these patients had significantly improved Knee Society scores after reimplantation. Anderson et al. [58] also reported a 96 % infection eradication rate at a mean follow-up of 54 months using the technique described by Hofmann et al. [25].

Another similar metal-on-polyethylene articulating spacer technique uses a new femoral component rather than sterilizing and reimplanting the removed femoral component. Scott et al. [65] reported the use of a sterile femoral component in conjunction with implanting strings of antibiotic-impregnated cement beads. After insertion of the cement beads into any open medullary canal, tissues, and the knee joint itself, a sterile knee prosthesis was loosely inserted to act as the spacer. There was no reinfection in the group of seven patients in this study. There have since been other studies that have reported their outcomes with the use of a new femoral component in an articulating spacer.

Table 23.1 Literature comparison of articulating and non-articulating spacers

Study	Type of spacer	No. of spacers	Follow-up (months) No. (range)	Infection eradication rate No. (%)	Outcome
Choi et al. [70]	AS	14 (M/PE)	43 (17–102)	10/14 (71 %)	ROM Post-Reimplantation: NAS = 97 vs. AS = 100 Clinical Outcomes: NR Extensile Approaches: NAS = 75 % vs. AS = 29 % Other: 28 % of AS chose to forego second stage reimplantation
	NAS	33	63 (14–118)	22/33 (66 %)	
Fehring et al. [18]	AS	15 (C/C)	27 (24–36)	14/15 (93 %)	ROM Post-Reimplantation: NAS 98 vs. AS 105 Clinical Outcomes: HSS scores NAS 84 vs. AS 83 Extensile Approaches: No difference Other: 60 % w/NAS had significant bone loss[a]
	NAS	25	36 (24–72)	22/25 (88 %)	
Hsu et al. [39]	AS	21 (C/C)	58 (27–96)	19/21 (91 %)	ROM Post-Reimplantation: NAS = 78 vs. AS = 95[a] Clinical Outcomes: KSS for NAS = 81.4 vs. AS = 88.9[a] Extensile Approaches: NAS = 28 % vs. AS = 5 % Other: NAS = 100 % had bone loss vs. AS = 28.7 % had femoral bone loss and 47.6 had tibial bone loss; NAS had larger bony defects than AS[a]
	NAS	7	101 (63–120)	6/7 (86 %)	
Emerson et al. [24]	AS	22 (M/PE)	46 (31–77)	20/22 (91 %)	ROM Post-Reimplantation: NAS = 93.7 vs. AS = 107.8[a] Clinical Outcomes: NR Extensile Approaches: No difference
	NAS	26	90 (34–153)	24/26 (92 %)	
Johnson et al. [68]	AS	34 (C/C and M/PE)	27 (12–72)	28/34 (83 %)	ROM Post-Reimplantation: NAS = 95 vs. AS = 99 Clinical Outcomes: KSS for NAS = 84 vs. 83 Extensile Approaches: NR Other: 12 % of AS had mechanical failure of spacer vs. 0 % for NAS
	NAS	81	66 (12–121)	67/81 (83 %)	
Park et al. [71]	AS	16 (C/C)	29 (24–45)	15/16 (93 %)	ROM Post-Reimplantation: NAS = 92 vs. 108[a] Clinical Outcomes: HSS scores NAS = 80 vs. AS = 87[a]; KSS functional scores NAS = 42 vs. AS = 76[a] Extensile Approaches: NAS = 15 procedures vs. AS = 11 procedures Other: NAS = 75 % had either femoral or tibial bone loss vs. AS = 0 % had bone loss
	NAS	20	36 (24–62)	17/20 (85 %)	
Freeman et al. [59]	AS	48 (C/C)	62 (26–120)	44/48 (92 %)	ROM Post-Reimplantation: NR Clinical Outcomes: KSS function scores NAS = 58 % vs. AS = 36 % good to excellent scores and NAS = 42 % vs. AS = 64 % fair to poor scores[a] Extensile Approaches: NR
	NAS	28	87 (24–196)	25/28 (91 %)	

(continued)

Table 23.1 (continued)

Study	Type of spacer	No. of spacers	Follow-up (months) No. (range)	Infection eradication rate No. (%)	Outcome
Chiang et al. [63]	AS	23 (C/C)	41 (24–61)	22/23 (96 %)	ROM Post-Reimplantation: NAS = 85 vs. AS = 113[a] Clinical Outcomes: HSS scores for NAS = 82 vs. 90[a] Extensile Approaches: NAS = 32 % vs. AS = 0 % Other: NAS = 33 % had patella baja at last f/u vs. AS = 0 %; Satisfaction rate was NAS = 32 % vs. AS = 91 %[a]
	NAS	22	40 (24–59)	21/22 (95 %)	

[a]Statistically significant; *AS* articulating spacer, *NAS* non-articulating spacer, *ROM* range of motion, *HSS* hospital for special surgery, *KSS* knee society score, *NR* not reported, *C/C* cement-on-cement articulating spacer, *M/PE* metal-on-polyethylene articulating spacer

Prasad et al. [51] evaluated 60 patients who underwent a resection arthroplasty with insertion of an articulating spacer, where the spacer consisted of a new femoral component and a new tibial rotating platform polyethylene insert that was used as the tibial component. This specific tibial insert was chosen because the rotating platform portion can serve as the "keel" to add more stability to the tibial component. These components were cemented into place with a double mix of Palacos cement with gentamicin (Palacos R; Zimmer, UK) with the addition of 1 g of vancomycin per mix. Thirty-four of these patients (57 %) actually underwent the full two-stage revision, while the remaining 26 patients (43 %) opted out of the second stage of the procedure. At a mean follow-up of 60 months, there were two reinfections among the 34 patients who underwent reimplantation (94 % infection eradication rate). There were three reinfections among the 26 patients at an average follow-up of 48 months who had elected to not undergo the second stage reimplantation (89 % infection eradication rate). The difference in these eradication rates was not statistically significant. There were also two additional patients in the latter group who underwent subsequent revision surgery due to instability. Trezies et al. [50] reported on 11 patients where they used this technique of a new femoral component and tibial insert for the articulating spacer. Of the 11 patients, there was one reinfection (91 % eradication rate). They also had an even higher rate of patients choosing to forego the second stage of the procedure, with 8 of the 11 (73 %) choosing this option.

Both Prasad et al. and Trezies et al. studies had high rates of patients choosing to forgo the second-stage surgery of reimplantation. These patients opted not to have the second procedure because they were free of infection and they had a functional and pain-free knee with the interim prosthesis. Another study by Choi et al. [66] looked specifically at the fate of the unplanned retention of the articulating spacers for infected total hip and knee arthroplasty. There were 18 hips and knees in this study where the articulating spacers were retained. Sixteen of these patients chose to forgo the second-stage revision surgery because they were happy with the painless and functional spacer, while the other two patients could not undergo the second stage due to poor general health. There were seven retained knee metal-on-polyethylene spacers among this group. There was one knee articulating spacer that developed loosening at 50 months follow-up. The spacer was replaced by a cemented TKA revision. The remaining six knees had an average Knee Society score of 92 for the knee score and 88 for the function score at an average of 43 months. While it is not the standard practice to leave the articulating spacer in place for the long term, this study along with the studies from Prasad et al. and Trezies et al. show that this can be an option for a particular group of patients.

Table 23.2 Literature review of articulating spacers

Type of spacer	Study	No. of knees	Mean follow-up (months) mean (range)	Infection eradication rate no. (%)	Flexion with spacer (°) mean (range)	Flexion at final follow-up (°) mean (range)	Clinical outcomes	Complications
Cement-on-Cement	Castelli et al. [44]	50	84 (24–156)	46/50 (92 %)	77 (10–100)	94 (0–120)	KSS improved from 73 with spacer to 75 at last f/u	1-spacer dislocation, 1-delayed wound healing
	Durbhakula et al. [40]	24	33 (28–51)	22/24 (92 %)	NR	104 (89–122)	KSS of 82 (63–96) at last f/u	None
	Ha et al. [36]	12	>24 (24–42)	12/12 (100 %)	85 (40–130)	102 (75–140)	KSS improved from 30 preop to 87 at last f/u	None
	Pascale et al. [33]	14	12	14/14 (100 %)	NR	120 (97–130)	HSS at last f/u 84	NR
	Pitto et al. [45]	21	24 (12–43)	21/21 (100 %)	77 (10–100)	94 (0–120)	KSS improved from 74 (50–83) with spacer and 81 (30–92) at last f/u Patient reported quality of life during interim phase16% excellent, 68 % good, and 16 % poor	NR
	Shaikh et al. [72]	15	48 (24–84)	15/15 (100 %)	87 (60–135)	115 (75–150)	Improved KSS, WOMAC, and VAS scores from preop to last f/u	NR
	Van Thiel et al. [42]	60	35 (24–51)	53/60 (88 %)	91 (10–125)	101 (0–130)	KSS improved from 53 (10–100) preop to 79 (37–100) at last f/u	2-wound problems, 1-spacer fracture
	Villanueva et al. [32]	30	36 (24–60)	30/30 (100 %)	80 (55–100)	107 (90–120)	KSS were excellent or good (70–100) in 25 patients, fair or poor (<70) in four patients	2-spacer subluxation, 1-spacer fracture
Cement-on-polyethylene	Evans et al. [49]	31	>24 months	29/31 (94 %)	Arc of Motion −10-82	ROM −2-111	NR	1-spacer subluxation, 2-spacer fragmentation

(continued)

Table 23.2 (continued)

Type of spacer	Study	No. of knees	Mean follow-up (months) mean (range)	Infection eradication rate no. (%)	Flexion with spacer (°) mean (range)	Flexion at final follow-up (°) mean (range)	Clinical outcomes	Complications
Metal-on-polyethylene	Anderson et al. [58]	25	54 (24–108)	24/25 (96 %)	Arc of Motion 5–112	ROM 2-115	HSS scores improved from 60 (27–80) preop, to 68 (35–80) with spacer, to 91 (65–100) at last f/u	None
	Lee et al. [64]	20	67 (50–81)	19/20 (95 %)	Arc of Motion 9–73	ROM 3–108	KSS improved from 52 (34–78) with spacer in place to 86 (50–99)	None
	Gooding et al. [53]	115	108 (60–144)	101/115 (88 %)	NR	93.2 (30–140)	Improved mean WOMAC, Oxford, UCLA, and Patient Satisfaction scores at last f/u	3-wound problems, 2-spacer fracture, 1-intraoperative fracture, 1-Knee dislocation, 1-tibial component dislocation
	Haddad et al. [52]	45	48 (20–112)	41/45 (91 %)	76 (20–115)	95 (20–135)	HSS scores improved from 42 preop, to 56 during the interim stage, to 72 at last f/u	1-wound problem, 4-instability, 2-ruptured patellar tendons, 4-knee dislocation, 1-femur fracture
	Hofmann et al. [60]	50	74 (24–150)	44/50 (88 %)	Arc of Motion 6–91	ROM 4–104	HSS scores improved from 64 (30–85) preop to 89 (70–100) at last f/u Patients reported 90 % excellent or good results	1-instability, 1-patellar dislocation
	Prasad et al. [51]	60	#1: 60 (24–96) #2: 48 (24–64)	#1: 32/34 (94 %) #2: 24/26 (88 %)	NR	#1: 98° (70–115) #2: 95° (range 80–115)	Cohort was split into two Groups: #1 underwent second stage reimplantation surgery; #2 opted to not undergo the second stage surgery	NR
	Trezies et al. [50]	11	33.6 (7–116)	10/11 (91 %)	NR	NR	Total KSS 167 (115–193)	1-Quadriceps rupture
	Cuckler et al. [73]	44	65 (24–120)	43/44 (98 %)	110 (45–125)	120 (60–130)	KSS improved from 36 (7–48) preop to 84 (45–98) 1 year after reimplantation	NR

NR not reported, *HSS* hospital for special surgery, *KSS* knee society score, *WOMAC* Western Ontario and McMaster Universities Arthritis Index, *VAS* visual analogue scale

While there are several different options for articulating spacers, there are very few studies that directly compare the different types of articulating spacers [55, 67]. Kalore et al. [55] reported the results for three different articulating spacer techniques in fifty-three knees. Fifteen patients had the re-sterilized femoral component with a new polyethylene insert spacer, 16 patients had a new femoral component with a new polyethylene insert spacer, and 22 patients had a cement-on-cement articulating spacer that was molded intraoperatively with manufactured molds (StageOne Knee Cement Spacer Molds; Biomet). They make note that all of these techniques utilized three to four packs of bone cement with 4 g of tobramycin powder and 6 g of vancomycin powder. In addition, intramedullary cement dowel or beads were used in every patient. The overall reinfection rate was 9.4 % at a mean follow-up time of 39 months when using surgery for infection as the definition for reinfection. They found no difference in infections between the groups, with the re-sterilized component group having an infection eradication rate of 87 % at a mean follow-up of 73 months, while the new component group and the silicone molded cement-on-cement group had infection eradication rate of 91 % at 32 months. There was also no difference in range of motion between the three different techniques either just before reimplantation surgery or at the time of final follow-up. The mean flexion achieved before reimplantation was 77° for the cement-on-cement group, 78° for the new component group, and 79° for the re-sterilized group. The mean flexion seen at the time of final follow-up in patients in whom the infection was controlled 96° for the cement-on-cement group, 98° for the new component group, and 94° for the re-sterilized group. They also performed a cost analysis where they looked at the direct costs of each technique that included the cement, antibiotics, along with the implant cost or the cost of the silicone molds. They reported that the total direct cost was $3945 for the cement-on-cement silicone molded technique, $3589 for the new component technique, and $932 for the re-sterilized technique. Overall, they found that no specific articulating spacer technique was superior to the others.

Complications

There are multiple reported complications of articulating spacers. These include spacer subluxation, spacer dislocation, arthrofibrosis, arthrodesis, extensor lag, extensor mechanism failure, fractured spacer components, amputation, periprosthetic fracture, wound healing complication, flexion contracture, and instability [68]. However, the key is determining if such complications are related to the complex nature of treating deep PJI, and are mitigated by utilizing an articulating spacer. Several recent systematic reviews have compared complications occurring with articulating and non-articulating antibiotic impregnated spacers [26, 69]. When considering complications of any type, Guild et al. [26] reported that the articulating spacer group had statistically fewer adverse events than the non-articulating spacer group (16 % vs. 20 %; $p = <0.04$). However, when further analysis was performed specifically to assess the mechanical complications that could potentially be attributed to the spacer, there was no significant difference between the two groups. Pivec et al. [69] broke the articulating spacers into complex and simple. They found that the non-articulating spacers did have a higher percentage of overall complications compared to the complex and simple articulating spacers, but this was not statistically significant. It is also thought that many of the complications that are seen with articulating spacers, specifically the subluxations and dislocations, could be improved with better cementation technique when placing the articulating spacer [68].

Conclusion

Articulating spacers have been used in two-stage exchange arthroplasties for the treatment of infected TKAs for more than 20 years. While there have not been any published randomized controlled trials comparing non-articulating and articulating spacers, there have been several comparative studies. In addition, there have been numerous studies during this time period that have reported on the efficacy of the different techniques of articulating spacers. Based on the available literature, articulating spacers have been shown to have equal infection eradication rates when compared to non-articulating spacers. During the interim stage of the two-stage exchange, patients with articulating spacers have better function and higher satisfaction rates. They have also been shown to have improved range of motion at last follow-up after reimplantation. So while there is not a consensus in the literature that they are superior, they have at least been shown to be effective and safe to use in the two-stage exchange process when treating an infected TKA.

References

1. Lavernia CJ, Guzman JF, Gachupin-Garcia A. Cost effectiveness and quality of life in knee arthroplasty. Clin Orthop Relat Res. 1997;345:134–9.
2. Jenkins PJ, Clement ND, Hamilton DF, Gaston P, Patton JT, Howie CR. Predicting the cost-effectiveness of total hip and knee replacement: a health economic analysis. Bone Joint J. 2013;95-B(1):115–21.
3. Jones CA, Beaupre LA, Johnston DW, Suarez-Almazor ME. Total joint arthroplasties: current concepts of patient outcomes after surgery. Rheum Dis Clin North Am. 2007;33(1):71–86.
4. Pulido L, Ghanem E, Joshi A, Purtill JJ, Parvizi J. Periprosthetic joint infection: the incidence, timing, and predisposing factors. Clin Orthop Relat Res. 2008;466(7):1710–5.
5. Kurtz SM, Lau E, Schmier J, Ong KL, Zhao K, Parvizi J. Infection burden for hip and knee arthroplasty in the United States. J Arthroplasty. 2008;23(7):984–91.
6. Kurtz SM, Ong KL, Lau E, Bozic KJ, Berry DJ, Parvizi J. Prosthetic joint infection risk after TKA in the medicare population. Clin Orthop Relat Res. 2009;468(1):52–6.
7. Jämsen E. Risk factors for infection after knee arthroplasty. A register-based analysis of 43,149 cases. J Bone Joint Surg Am. 2009;91(1):38.
8. Mortazavi SM, Molligan J, Austin MS, Purtill JJ, Hozack WJ, Parvizi J. Failure following revision total knee arthroplasty: infection is the major cause. Int Orthop. 2011;35(8):1157–64.
9. Sierra RJ, Cooney WP, Pagnano MW, Trousdale RT, Rand JA. Reoperations after 3200 revision TKAs. Clin Orthop Relat Res. 2004;425:200–6.
10. Hossain F, Patel S, Haddad FS. Midterm assessment of causes and results of revision total knee arthroplasty. Clin Orthop Relat Res. 2010;468(5):1221–8.
11. Bozic KJ. The epidemiology of revision total hip arthroplasty in the United States. J Bone Joint Surg Am. 2009;91(1):128.
12. Sharkey PF, Hozack WJ, Rothman RH, Shastri S, Jacoby SM. Insall award paper. Why are total knee arthroplasties failing today? Clin Orthop Relat Res. 2002;(404):7–13.
13. Insall JN, Thompson FM, Brause BD. Two-stage reimplantation for the salvage of infected total knee arthroplasty. J Bone Joint Surg Am. 1983;65(8):1087–98.
14. Booth RE, Lotke PA. The results of spacer block technique in revision of infected total knee arthroplasty. Clin Orthop Relat Res. 1989;248:57–60.
15. Borden LS, Gearen PF. Infected total knee arthroplasty. A protocol for management. J Arthroplasty. 1987;2(1):27–36.
16. Cohen JC, Hozack WJ, Cuckler JM, Booth RE. Two-stage reimplantation of septic total knee arthroplasty. Report of three cases using an antibiotic-PMMA spacer block. J Arthroplasty. 1988;3(4):369–77.
17. Salvati EA, Callaghan JJ, Brause BD, Klein RF, Small RD. Reimplantation in infection. Elution of gentamicin from cement and beads. Clin Orthop Relat Res. 1986;207:83–93.
18. Fehring TK, Odum S, Calton TF, Mason JB. Articulating versus static spacers in revision total knee arthroplasty for sepsis. The Ranawat Award. Clin Orthop Relat Res. 2000;380:9–16.
19. Hanssen AD, Rand JA, Osmon DR. Treatment of the infected total knee arthroplasty with insertion of another prosthesis. The effect of antibiotic-impregnated bone cement. Clin Orthop Relat Res. 1994;309:44–55.
20. Pietsch M, Hofmann S, Wenisch C. Treatment of deep infection of total knee arthroplasty using a two-stage procedure. Oper Orthop Traumatol. 2006;18(1):66–87.
21. Burnett RS, Kelly MA, Hanssen AD, Barrack RL. Technique and timing of two-stage exchange for infection in TKA. Clin Orthop Relat Res. 2007;464:164–78.
22. Struelens B, Claes S, Bellemans J. Spacer-related problems in two-stage revision knee arthroplasty. Acta Orthop Belg. 2013;79(4):422–6.
23. Calton TF, Fehring TK, Griffin WL. Bone loss associated with the use of spacer blocks in infected total knee arthroplasty. Clin Orthop Relat Res. 1997;345:148–54.
24. Emerson RH, Muncie M, Tarbox TR, Higgins LL. Comparison of a static with a mobile spacer in total knee infection. Clin Orthop Relat Res. 2002;404:132–8.
25. Hofmann AA, Kane KR, Tkach TK, Plaster RL, Camargo MP. Treatment of infected total knee arthroplasty using an articulating spacer. Clin Orthop Relat Res. 1995;321:45–54.
26. Guild 3rd GN, Wu B, Scuderi GR. Articulating vs. static antibiotic impregnated spacers in revision total knee arthroplasty for sepsis. A systematic review. J Arthroplasty. 2014;29(3):558–63.
27. Jacobs C, Christensen CP, Berend ME. Static and mobile antibiotic-impregnated cement spacers for the

management of prosthetic joint infection. J Am Acad Orthop Surg. 2009;17(6):356–68.
28. Engh GA, Parks NL. The management of bone defects in revision total knee arthroplasty. Instr Course Lect. 1997;46:227–36.
29. McPherson EJ, Lewonowski K, Dorr LD. Techniques in arthroplasty. Use of an articulated PMMA spacer in the infected total knee arthroplasty. J Arthroplasty. 1995;10(1):87–9.
30. Lombardi AV, Karnes JM, Berend KR. A motion maintaining antibiotic delivery system. J Arthroplasty. 2007;22(4 Suppl 1):50–5.
31. Villanueva M, Ríos A, Pereiro J, Chana F, Fahandez-Saddi H. Hand-made articulating spacers for infected total knee arthroplasty: a technical note. Acta Orthop. 2006;77(2):329–32.
32. Villanueva-Martínez M, Ríos-Luna A, Pereiro J, Fahandez-Saddi H, Villamor Á. Hand-made articulating spacers in two-stage revision for infected total knee arthroplasty: good outcome in 30 patients. Acta Orthop. 2008;79(5):674–82.
33. Pascale V, Pascale W. Custom-made articulating spacer in two-stage revision total knee arthroplasty. An early follow-up of 14 cases of at least 1 year after surgery. HSS J. 2007;3(2):159–63.
34. Goldstein WM, Kopplin M, Wall R, Berland K. Temporary articulating methylmethacrylate antibiotic spacer (TAMMAS). A new method of intraoperative manufacturing of a custom articulating spacer. J Bone Joint Surg Am. 2001;83-A(Suppl 2 Pt 2):92–7.
35. Shen H, Zhang X, Jiang Y, Wang Q, Chen Y, Wang Q, et al. Intraoperatively-made cement-on-cement antibiotic-loaded articulating spacer for infected total knee arthroplasty. Knee. 2010;17(6):407–11.
36. Ha C-W. A technique for intraoperative construction of antibiotic spacers. Clin Orthop Relat Res. 2006;445:204–9.
37. Su Y-P, Lee OK, Chen W-M, Chen T-H. A facile technique to make articulating spacers for infected total knee arthroplasty. J Chin Med Assoc. 2009;72(3):138–45.
38. Kohl S, Evangelopoulos DS, Kohlhof H, Krueger A, Hartel M, Roeder C, et al. An intraoperatively moulded PMMA prostheses like spacer for two-stage revision of infected total knee arthroplasty. Knee. 2011;18(6):464–9.
39. Hsu YC, Cheng HC, Ng TP, Chiu KY. Antibiotic-loaded cement articulating spacer for 2-stage reimplantation in infected total knee arthroplasty: a simple and economic method. J Arthroplasty. 2007;22(7):1060–6.
40. Durbhakula SM, Czajka J, Fuchs MD, Uhl RL. Antibiotic-loaded articulating cement spacer in the 2-stage exchange of infected total knee arthroplasty. J Arthroplasty. 2004;19(6):768–74.
41. Jaekel DJ, Day JS, Klein GR, Levine H, Parvizi J, Kurtz SM. Do dynamic cement-on-cement knee spacers provide better function and activity during two-stage exchange? Clin Orthop Relat Res. 2012;470(9):2599–604.
42. Van Thiel GS, Berend KR, Klein GR, Gordon AC, Lombardi AV, Valle Della CJ. Intraoperative molds to create an articulating spacer for the infected knee arthroplasty. Clin Orthop Relat Res. 2010;469(4):994–1001.
43. Hanssen AD, Spangehl MJ. Practical applications of antibiotic-loaded bone cement for treatment of infected joint replacements. Clin Orthop Relat Res. 2004;427:79–85.
44. Castelli CC, Gotti V, Ferrari R. Two-stage treatment of infected total knee arthroplasty: two to thirteen year experience using an articulating preformed spacer. Int Orthop. 2014;38(2):405–12.
45. Pitto RP, Castelli CC, Ferrari R, Munro J. Pre-formed articulating knee spacer in two-stage revision for the infected total knee arthroplasty. Int Orthop. 2005;29(5):305–8.
46. Villa T, Carnelli D. Experimental evaluation of the biomechanical performances of a PMMA-based knee spacer. Knee. 2007;14(2):145–53.
47. Mutimer J, Gillespie G, Lovering AM, Porteous AJ. Measurements of in vivo intra-articular gentamicin levels from antibiotic loaded articulating spacers in revision total knee replacement. Knee. 2009;16(1):39–41.
48. Wan Z, Karim A, Momaya A, Incavo SJ, Mathis KB. Preformed articulating knee spacers in 2-stage total knee revision arthroplasty. J Arthroplasty. 2012;27(8):1469–73.
49. Evans RP. Successful treatment of total hip and knee infection with articulating antibiotic components: a modified treatment method. Clin Orthop Relat Res. 2004;427:37–46.
50. Trezies A, Parish E, Dixon P, Cross M. The use of an articulating spacer in the management of infected total knee arthroplasties. J Arthroplasty. 2006;21(5):702–4.
51. Prasad N, Paringe V, Kotwal R, Ghandour A, Morgan Jones R. Two-stage revision for infected total knee arthroplasty: our experience with interval prosthesis. Eur J Orthop Surg Traumatol. 2014;24(7):1279–83.
52. Haddad FS, Masri BA, Campbell D, McGraw RW, Beauchamp CP, Duncan CP. The PROSTALAC functional spacer in two-stage revision for infected knee replacements. Prosthesis of antibiotic-loaded acrylic cement. J Bone Joint Surg Br. 2000;82(6):807–12.
53. Gooding CR, Masri BA, Duncan CP, Greidanus NV, Garbuz DS. Durable infection control and function with the PROSTALAC spacer in two-stage revision for infected knee arthroplasty. Clin Orthop Relat Res. 2011;469(4):985–93.
54. Carulli C, Villano M, Civinini R, Matassi F, Nistri L, Innocenti M. A novel technique to preserve range of motion in two-stage revision of infected total knee arthroplasty. Int Orthop. 2013;37(6):1069–74.
55. Kalore NV, Maheshwari A, Sharma A, Cheng E, Gioe TJ. Is there a preferred articulating spacer technique

for infected knee arthroplasty? A preliminary study. Clin Orthop Relat Res. 2011;470(1):228–35.
56. Mont MA, Waldman BJ, Hungerford DS. Evaluation of preoperative cultures before second-stage reimplantation of a total knee prosthesis complicated by infection. A comparison-group study. J Bone Joint Surg Am. 2000;82-A(11):1552–7.
57. Brown NM, Cipriano CA, Moric M, Sporer SM, Valle Della CJ. Dilute betadine lavage before closure for the prevention of acute postoperative deep periprosthetic joint infection. J Arthroplasty. 2012;27(1):27–30.
58. Anderson JA, Sculco PK, Heitkemper S, Mayman DJ, Bostrom MP, Sculco TP. An articulating spacer to treat and mobilize patients with infected total knee arthroplasty. J Arthroplasty. 2009;24(4):631–5.
59. Freeman MG, Fehring TK, Odum SM, Fehring K, Griffin WL, Mason JB. Functional advantage of articulating versus static spacers in 2-stage revision for total knee arthroplasty infection. J Arthroplasty. 2007;22(8):1116–21.
60. Hofmann AA, Goldberg T, Tanner AM, Kurtin SM. Treatment of infected total knee arthroplasty using an articulating spacer. Clin Orthop Relat Res. 2005;(430):125–31.
61. Jämsen E, Stogiannidis I, Malmivaara A, Pajamäki J, Puolakka T, Konttinen YT. Outcome of prosthesis exchange for infected knee arthroplasty: the effect of treatment approach. Acta Orthop. 2009;80(1):67–77.
62. Ocguder A, Firat A, Tecimel O, Solak S, Bozkurt M. Two-stage total infected knee arthroplasty treatment with articulating cement spacer. Arch Orthop Trauma Surg. 2010;130(6):719–25.
63. Chiang E-R, Su Y-P, Chen T-H, Chiu F-Y, Chen W-M. Comparison of articulating and static spacers regarding infection with resistant organisms in total knee arthroplasty. Acta Orthop. 2011;82(4):460–4.
64. Lee JK, Choi CH. Two-stage reimplantation in infected total knee arthroplasty using a re-sterilized tibial polyethylene insert and femoral component. J Arthroplasty. 2012;27(9):1701–1706.e1.
65. Scott IR, Stockley I, Getty CJ. Exchange arthroplasty for infected knee replacements. A new two-stage method. J Bone Joint Surg Br. 1993;75(1):28–31.
66. Choi HR, Freiberg AA, Malchau H, Rubash HE, Kwon YM. The fate of unplanned retention of prosthetic articulating spacers for infected total hip and total knee arthroplasty. J Arthroplasty. 2014;29(4):690–3.
67. Jämsen E, Sheng P, Halonen P, Lehto MU, Moilanen T, Pajamäki J, et al. Spacer prostheses in two-stage revision of infected knee arthroplasty. Int Orthop. 2006;30(4):257–61.
68. Johnson AJ, Sayeed SA, Naziri Q, Khanuja HS, Mont MA. Minimizing dynamic knee spacer complications in infected revision arthroplasty. Clin Orthop Relat Res. 2011;470(1):220–7.
69. Pivec R, Naziri Q, Issa K, Banerjee S, Mont MA. Systematic review comparing static and articulating spacers used for revision of infected total knee arthroplasty. J Arthroplasty. 2014;29(3):553–557.e1.
70. Choi HR, Malchau H, Bedair H. Are prosthetic spacers safe to use in 2-stage treatment for infected total knee arthroplasty? J Arthroplasty. 2012;27(8):1474–1479.e1.
71. Park S-J, Song E-K, Seon J-K, Yoon T-R, Park G-H. Comparison of static and mobile antibiotic-impregnated cement spacers for the treatment of infected total knee arthroplasty. Int Orthop. 2009;34(8):1181–6.
72. Shaikh AA, Ha C-W, Park Y-G, Park Y-B. Two-stage approach to primary TKA in infected arthritic knees using intraoperatively molded articulating cement spacers. Clin Orthop Relat Res. 2014;472(7):2201–7.
73. Cuckler JM. The infected total knee: management options. J Arthroplasty. 2005;20(4 Suppl 2):33–6.

Late Infections of the Knee Joint: Arthrodesis or Other Solutions

24

Eduardo García-Rey, Enrique Gómez-Barrena, and Eduardo García-Cimbrelo

Abstract

One- or two-stage revision procedures are currently the best options to eradicate peri-prosthetic joint infection of the knee while maintaining the best functional outcome. Alternatives are required when infection control or joint reconstruction fail. In this chapter, the current status of alternative solutions to revision surgery is discussed, from the prolonged, suppressive antibiotic therapy after debridement for medically impaired patients, to the salvage alternative surgical procedures. Among these, resection arthroplasty or amputation have limited indications and may not be well tolerated by most patients, which enhances the role of knee arthrodesis. Today, knee arthrodesis is confined to an alternative salvage procedure after previous attempts of one- or two-stage revision total knee replacement (TKR), in the presence of severe soft-tissue and bone defects, in patients who request functional limb salvage, will not accept amputation, and demand independent function. Surgeons must be aware of different external fixator and intramedullary nail (IMN) devices, their published results, and the potentially high number of complications that may occur after these procedures. As definite bone healing is difficult to achieve due to poor status of the bone and soft tissues in the knee joint line, recent IMNs without the need for bone union at the fusion site may have to be considered, while research and innovation in these complex reconstructions may provide alternative future solutions.

Keywords

Chronic knee infections • Salvage procedures • Antibiotic suppression Knee resection arthroplasty • Above-knee amputation • Knee arthrodesis External fixation • Uncemented intramedullary nailing • Cemented intramedullary nailing • Fusion after knee arthrodesis • Re-infection

E. García-Rey, MD, PhD, EBOT (✉)
E. Gómez-Barrena, MD, PhD • E. García-Cimbrelo, MD, PhD
Department of Orthopaedic Surgery, Hospital La Paz-Idi Paz, Pº Castellana 261, Madrid 28046, Spain
e-mail: edugrey@yahoo.es; egomezbarrena@gmail.com; gcimbrelo@yahoo.es

D. Kendoff et al. (eds.), *Periprosthetic Joint Infections: Changing Paradigms*, DOI 10.1007/978-3-319-30091-7_24

Introduction

Total knee replacement (TKR) is one of the most cost-effective procedures in terms of quality of life [1], including decreased post-operative mortality rates in the last years [2]. However, infection remains the most devastating complication [3]. To eradicate the infection, most patients require revision and removal of the prosthesis, affecting clinical outcome. To date, the rates of infection after revision TKR, a procedure that is also increasing nowadays, are higher than after primary TKR and results are usually poor. Despite improvements in surgical environment, technique and antibiotic prophylaxis, data from Registries show that during the last years, the rate of revision due to infection is not decreasing [4, 5]. As mentioned above, the increased incidence of primary and revision TKR in many countries also leads to a higher number of infection cases, particularly in immuno-compromised patients who are prone to infection [6]. Although mechanical reasons are the first cause for revision surgery, in many tertiary centres infection is the most common etiology for revision TKR before or after 2 years from the primary procedure [7].

Consequently, treatment is also different depending on the type and definition of the infection, physical activity and/or age of the patient, medical conditions (immune system, concomitant drugs, the existence of diabetes, obsesity) and osteo-articular status (osteopenic bone, soft tissue status, instability).

Alternative Methods for Management in Chronically Infected Total Knee Replacement

Since the diagnosis of peri-prosthetic joint infection (PJI) may be difficult, the clinician must be alert in order to suspect the possible existence of infection. During the last years, different reported criteria help to identify PJI [8–12]. Once the infection is diagnosed, the removal of the prosthesis is the most preferred option of treatment due to the formation of biofilm on the implant [13–18]. However, alternative treatments need to be considered in some patients. Prolonged suppressive therapy with retention of the implant may be acceptable for some frail patients who cannot receive standard treatment because of concomitant medical co-morbidity. A prolonged suppressive antibiotherapy, combined with prompt surgical debridement, may be indicated in selected patients, although complications related to antibiotic suppression are not low [19, 20]. Retention of the implant is controversial since the success rate for infection eradication can be very low and delay may affect a standard two-stage procedure [21, 22]. Geurts et al. reported data on prosthesis retention if it was stable after deep post-operative or haematogenous PJIs, regardless of the interval from implantation or the duration of the symptoms [23]. They found good results with debridement and retention of the prosthesis in combination with local and systemic antibiotics, and emphasized the importance of starting treatment within 4 weeks of symptom onset. They noted that symptom onset could be difficult to identify. They attributed their good results to the use of gentamicin-loaded beads (which were removed in a second operation after 2 weeks) or collagen, which are particularly useful as antibiotic carriers in TKR infections, even if they did not replace the polyethylene during debridement. Most authors, however, do not recommend this procedure given the high rates of failure to eradicate infection [24].

The incidence of an above-the-knee amputation (AKA) is low. Sierra et al. reported that the majority of AKAs were performed for reasons other than TKR complications. This means a rate of 0.14 % when AKA was done for causes related to TKR. However, 19 of the 25 were done due to an uncontrollable infection [25]. Although patients with a late infected TKR are relatively satisfied after AKA, functional outcome is poor. When an AKA is indicated, the presence of resistant or gram-negative microorganisms is frequent, and several failed surgical procedures, many medial co-morbidities, and wound healing problems are usually associated [26]. Other problems are in the relatively high mortality rates, and in the difficulties some patients experience in fitting AKA prosthesis. Although custom-made devices are offering more options during the last years, the functional results fol-

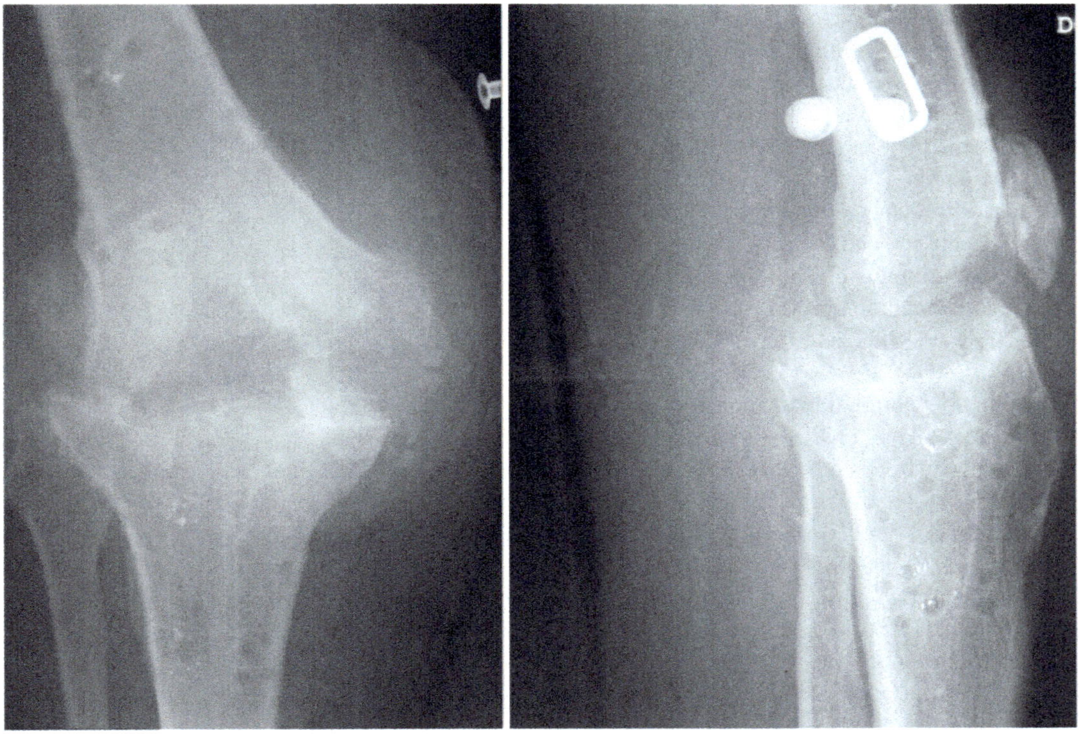

Fig. 24.1 Knee resection arthroplasty after recurrent infection. Note the need for knee orthoses

lowing an AKA after an infected TKR are poor, including a low percentage of the patients been able to walk.

Patients with severe polyarticular disability and a late infected TKR may be treated with a resection arthroplasty of the knee (Fig. 24.1). This first-stage procedure can eradicate infection, and although functional outcome is poor, some of them can walk [27]. If the patient does not tolerate the disability for daily activities, a secondary procedure like an arthrodesis can be performed. However, the functional outcome of resection arthroplasty is very poor, and energy consumption is greater than in patients with an AKA [28]. Resection arthroplasty of the knee with a bolus of bone cement moulded to fill the remaining cavity, the so-called "beefburger" procedure, has also been described as an alternative to arthrodesis or AKA [29]. In a series of 13 patients followed for 5 years, eight did not need any further surgery, three underwent a bone fusion and two an AKA. Although the results were not satisfactory, the procedure can solve infection in medically compromised patients [30].

Arthrodesis of the Knee

Sir John Charnley's first description of the compression arthrodesis of the knee showed good results in terms of bone union using two Steinmann nails connected by special screw-clamps tightened under the compression force; this construct was placed within a Thomas' splint as an external fixation in order to prevent extension and flexion forces [31]. He reported "compression is the simple impaction of cancellous surfaces until trabeculae almost interdigitate" and hypothesized two possible mechanisms for this high compression force: a local transference of bone substance by cellular activity rather than chemical ossification mechanisms, and the response of osteoblasts to the dynamic process of union secondary to compression [32]. This compression method for arthrodesis of the knee confirmed good results in terms of bone consolidation reported by others [33]. The best results in terms of consolidation and functional results were associated with the Charnley method, particularly for the time needed for bone union. The functional results of a fused knee are important to remember. Although better physical activity and stability can be observed when comparing fusion with other salvage procedures like amputation or a resection arthroplasty, sitting is more affected after a knee arthrodesis [34].

When conventional management, the one- or two-stage revision TKR, for a chronic TKR has failed, knee fusion is probably the most accepted method for medically fit patients. The functional results of the rarely indicated knee resection arthroplasty are poor as previously mentioned. The comparative results of above-the-knee-amputation and fusion for recurrent PJI after TKR are similar and the literature reports worse results for the latter in other pathologies like trauma and tumours. However, particularly for infection, a better function and satisfaction can be expected from a successful knee arthrodesis [35]. So, with the wide use of TKR, the most frequent indication for a knee arthrodesis may be as a salvage procedure after recurrent septic failure. Some conditions like severe bone loss, disorders of the extensor mechanism of the knee, repeated previous surgeries, multi-resistant microorganisms and a stiff joint can be considered the current indications in many cases (Table 24.1). Most patients who may be suitable for a knee fusion have undergone several surgeries and usually require multiple medical treatments since infection rates are higher in the presence of significant co-morbidities. Poor skin and other local and general conditions may be apparent and compromise surgical outcome, thus a complete evaluation of the patient is compulsory. Some systems like the Cierny classification may be helpful at the beginning of the management and the local bone defect must also be evaluated [36]. For the latter, it is very important to be sure that previous material has been removed, particularly TKR rather than a cement spacer, most of which are revised long implants and cemented devices and may significantly increase the pre-operatively planned bone defect.

Table 24.1 Current indications for arthrodesis after infected total knee replacement

Salvage procedure	Medically fit patients
	Patient's refusal to other procedures
Microorganism	Multi-resistant gram positive bacteria
	Gram negative
	Polimicrobial
Osteoarticular status	Good hip status
	Moderate-severe bone loss
	Disruption extensor mechanism

Although many authors recommend performing arthrodesis in a two-stage procedure, first extracting the material, debriding and placing a cement spacer during 4–6 weeks before the definite fusion surgery [37–39], others recommended this management depending on the bone defect [40], while, finally, other authors recommend arthrodesis in a one-stage procedure regardless of bone loss [41–43].

Two different fixation techniques are currently used: external fixation (EF) and intramedullary nailing (IMN), internal fixation with plates has been abandoned when infection is present. Mabry et al. reported a high number of complications for both EF and IMN procedures, but better union rates with the use of IMN, although with higher re-infection rates than external fixation [44]. In their comparative study, 41 of 61 knees achieved fusion with external fixation and a 4.9 % infection rate and 23 of 24 knees consolidate with IMN but with an infection rate of 8.3 %; nevertheless, the authors emphasized that although a knee arthrodesis is suitable as a salvage procedure for an infected TKR, the number of complications is high. Alternatively, Vlasak et al. recommended IMN due to better union rates, and six of their patients with non-union after external fixation achieved consolidation with INM [45] (Table 24.2).

Some of the early reports for knee arthrodesis following failed TKR included the use of external

Table 24.2 Different series for knee arthrodesis after failed total knee replacement

Authors	Number of cases	Fixation	Union rates	Remarks
Mabry et al. [44]	61	EF	67 %	Better re-infection rates
	24	IMN	95.8 %	Better union rates
Vlasak et al. [45]	13	EF	38 %	Two-stages procedure
	12	IMN	100 %	
Brodersen et al. [46]	40	EF	81 %	Recommend EF for infection
Knutson et al. [48]	7	EF	71.4 %	Two-stages procedure
	10	IMN	90 %	
Oostenbroeck and Van Roermund [43]	15	EF	93 %	Ilizarov one-stage procedure
Salem et al. [50]	21	EF	95.2 %	Ilizarov, no bone grafting
Puranen et al. [41]	33 (15 after failed TKR)	IMN	87.8 %	No infections
Ellingsen and Rand [51]	18	IMN	88.9 %	Frequent complications
Bargiotas et al. [38]	12	IMN	83.3 %	Two-stages, convex-to-concave preparation of bone ends
McQueen et al. [52]	44	IMN-C	100 %	3 infection, 20 % complication rate
Scarponi et al. [39]	38	IMN-M	–	89 % no –re-infected, no pain, no mechanical complications
Putman et al. [55]	31	IMN-M	–	19 % re-infected, no mechanical failures

fixation as the most common method, particularly for infection revisions [46]. The use of an external fixator is based on the compression mechanism developed by Charnley regardless of the type of device used, although better fusion rates can be expected after an external double frame [47–49] (Fig. 24.2). The use of the Ilizarov frame has also shown high union rates, without a need for bone grafting and success has been reported even in cases of an active chronic infection [40, 43, 50]. Although some of the disadvantages of this frame include the long treatment time, the need for patient cooperation, the complications related to pins, and the learning curve, circular external fixation can correct misalignment of the leg and even allow lengthening during fusion to avoid leg-length discrepancies.

IMN has the advantages of shorter treatment duration than external fixation, and less leg length discrepancy. However, the infection must be eradicated to obtain the femoro-tibial fusion. Good union rates with the use of long intramedullary nails have been reported if good contact is established between bones [38]. Although the number of cases evaluated is not high in the different

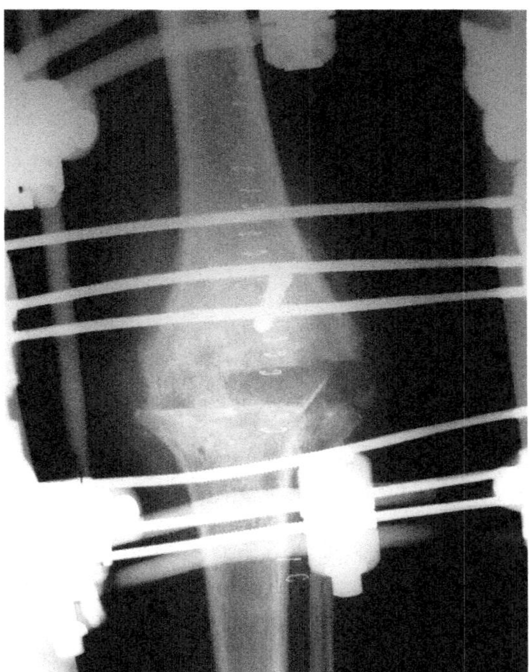

Fig. 24.2 External fixator (double frame) in an arthrodesis procedure (under compression)

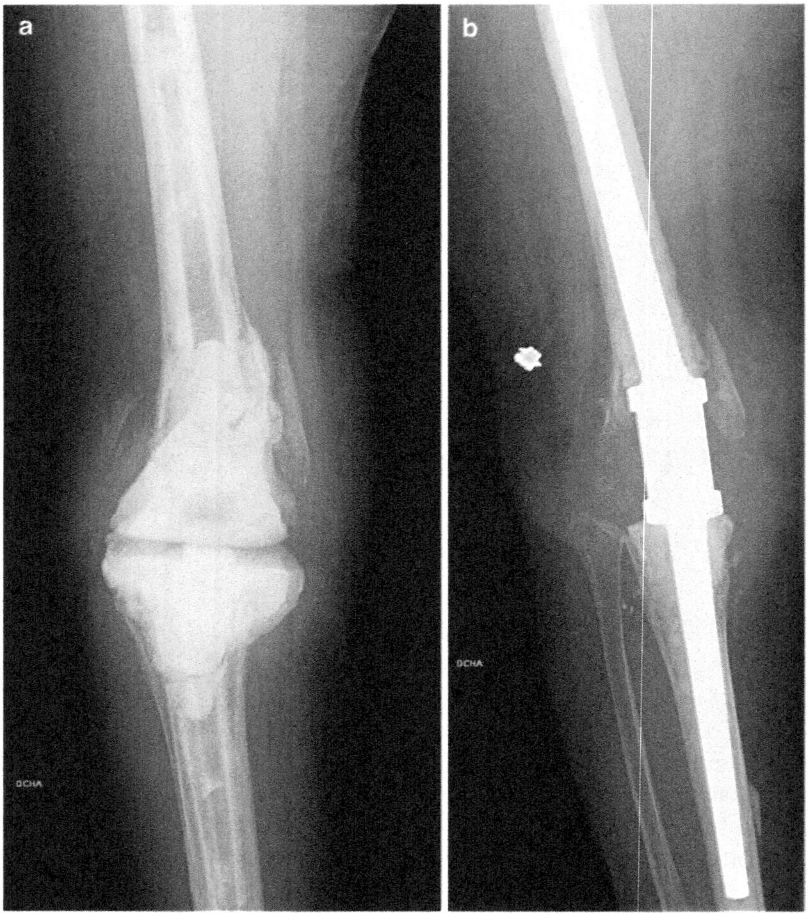

Fig. 24.3 Significant bone loss after recurrent knee infection (revision of cemented stems in a constrained knee replacement), requiring a cemented intramedullary nail after the infection healed. (**a**) During spacer treatment after implant revision. (**b**) Three-year follow-up after implantation of cemented intramedullary device

series, most arthrodesis consolidated despite a relatively high number of re-interventions and a large amount of blood loss [38, 41, 51]. New intramedullary compression nails provided high union rates and were reported as reliable procedures with limited learning curves. However, the re-infection rate remains as major disadvantage for IMN [52].

Cemented intramedullary modular nails have also been considered to salvage the limb in severe cases and can give acceptable functional results regardless of radiographic union [53]. The possible advantages are that bone union is not needed for a good result and there is less leg length discrepancy. In a two-stage procedure, a cementless modular nail can be inserted after reaming in a press-fit manner in both the femur and tibia, and linked at the knee joint line. Instead of bone grafting, antibiotic-loaded cement is inserted and a conventional partial weight-bearing regime can be started [39]. Although insufficient literature is available, a recent series of 22 cases proved its feasibility and efficacy to maintain the limb when severe bone loss and soft tissue damage may preclude bone fusion at the knee [54]. Our own experience confirms the capacity of this technique to solve extremely complex cases (Fig. 24.3), particularly when the reconstruction occurs after cemented intramedullary fixation of the revised prosthesis. Caution should be recommended in that the risk of re-infection is always

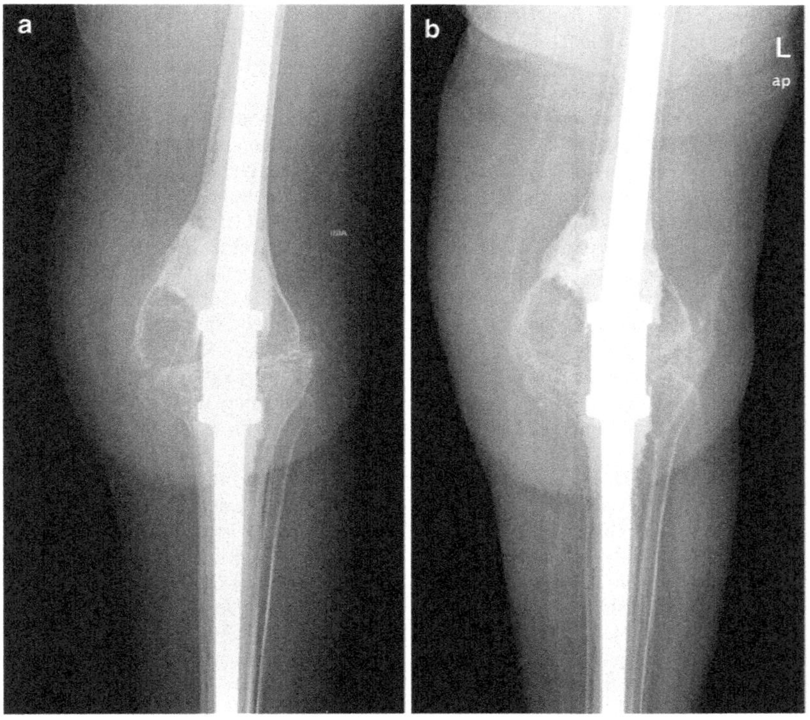

Fig. 24.4 Arthrodesis intended after knee infection through cemented intramedullary nail. (**a**) Six weeks after implantation, note satisfactory femoro-tibial bone contact. (**b**) Four years after implantation, note maintained stability with significant femoral and tibial bone resorption

present (3 cases out of 22 in the Neuerburg et al. series) and that stress shielding may impact in unloaded epiphyso-metaphyseal bone around the knee (Fig. 24.4), with unknown future consequences. However, the eradication of infection is again the most important limitation [55] to date.

Recently, very poor results using IMN for a knee arthrodesis after revision TKR were reported, half of the knees showed a persistent infection, and the incidence of pain and functional impairment was high [56].

Final Remarks

Chronic, late infections of the knee may lead to treatment failures, particularly if a severe local compromise remains due to resistant microorganisms and deteriorated tissues, and more often in frail patients with comorbidities further compromised by infection. In these cases, alternative and salvage treatments will also be needed. Current experience on arthrodesis and salvage procedures, reviewed in this chapter, will need reinforcement as the patients and the infections under treatment become more complex. Although bone fusion is not always possible, more proposals are required to combine limb salvage with durable solutions, while maintaining sufficient function to allow independent stance and gait. More research and innovation will hopefully reinforce this area of difficult lower limb reconstruction techniques.

References

1. Lavernia CJ, Guzman JF, Gachupin-Garcia A. Cost effectiveness and quality of life in knee arthroplasty. Clin Orthop Relat Res. 1997;345:134–9.
2. Hunt LP, Ben-Shlomo Y, Clark EM, Dieppe P, Judge A, MacGregor AJ, Tobias JH, Vernon K, Blom AW, National Joint Registry for England and Wales. 45-day mortality after 467,779 knee replacements for

osteoarthritis from the National Joint Registry for England and Wales: an observational study. Lancet. 2014;384(9952):1429–36.
3. Blom AW, Brown J, Taylor AH, Pattison G, Whitehouse S, Bannister GC. Infection after total knee arthroplasty. J Bone Joint Surg Br. 2004;86(5):688–91.
4. Jämsen E, Huotari K, Huhtala H, Nevalainen J, Konttinen YT. Low rate of infected knee replacements in a nationwide series—is it an underestimate? Review of the Finnish Arthroplasty Register on 38,676 operations performed in 1997 through 2003. Acta Orthop. 2009;80(2):205–12.
5. Sundberg M, Lidgren L, Dahl A, Robertsson O. The Swedish Arthroplasty Register—Annual Report 2013. Lund: Elvins Grafiska AB, Helsingborg; 2013.
6. Leta TH, Lygre SH, Skredderstuen A, Hallan G, Furnes O. Failure of aseptic revision total knee arthroplasties. Acta Orthop. 2015;86(1):48–57.
7. Hossain F, Patel S, Haddad FS. Midterm assessment of causes and results of revision total knee arthroplasty. Clin Orthop Relat Res. 2010;468(5):1221–8.
8. Berbari EF, Hanssen AD, Duffy MC, Seckelberg JM, Ilsturp DM, Harmsen WS, et al. Risk factors for prosthetic joint infection: case–control study. Clin Infect Dis. 1998;27(5):1247–54.
9. Ghanem E, Parvizi J, Burnett RS, Sharkey PF, Keshavarzi N, Aggarwal A, et al. Cell count and differential or aspirated fluid in the diagnosis of infection at the site of total knee arthroplasty. J Bone Joint Surg Am. 2008;90:1637–43.
10. Parvizi J, Zmistowski B, Berbari EF, Bauer TW, Springer BD, Della Vale CJ, et al. New definition for periprosthetic joint infection: from the Workgroup of the Musculoeskeletal Infection Society. Clin Orthop Relat Res. 2011;469:2992–4.
11. Fink B, Makowiak C, Fuerst M, Berger I, Schäfer P, Frommelt L. The value of synovial biopsy, joint aspiration and C-reactive protein in the diagnosis of late peri-prosthetic infection of total knee replacements. J Bone Joint Surg Br. 2008;90:874–8.
12. Parvizi J, Gehrke T, Chen AF. Proceedings of the international consensus on periprosthetic joint infection. Bone Joint J. 2013;95-B(11):1450–2.
13. Gristina AG, Costerton JW. Bacterial adherence and the glycocalix and their role in musculoeskeletal infection. Orthop Clin North Am. 1984;15:517–35.
14. Trampuz A, Osmon DR, Hanssen AD, Steckelberg JM, Patel R. Molecular and antibiofilm approaches to prosthetic joint infection. Clin Orthop Relat Res. 2003;414:69–88.
15. Gómez-Barrena E, Esteban J, Medel F, Molina-Manso D, Ortiz-Pérez A, Cordero-Ampuero J, et al. Bacterial adherence to separated modular components in joint prostheses: a clinical study. J Orthop Res. 2012;30:1634–9.
16. Tsukayama DT, Goldberg VM, Kyle R. Diagnosis and management of infection after total knee arthroplasty. J Bone Joint Surg Am. 2003;85-B:75–80.
17. Cordero-Ampuero J, Esteban J, García-Rey E. Results after late polymicrobial, gram-negative, and methicilin-resistant infections in knee arthroplasy. Clin Orthop Relat Res. 2010;468:1229–36.
18. Haddad FS, Sukeik M, Alazzwai S. Is single-stage revision according to a strict protocol effective in treatment of chronic knee arthroplasty infections? Clin Orthop Relat Res. 2015;473:8–14.
19. Segreti J, Nelson JA, Trenholme GM. Prolonged suppressive antibiotic therapy for infected orthopaedic prostheses. Clin Infect Dis. 1998;27:711–3.
20. Rao N, Crossett LS, Sinha RK, Le Frock JL. Long-term suppression of infection in total joint arthroplasty. Clin Orthop Relat Res. 2003;414:55–60.
21. Marculescu CE, Berbari EF, Hanssen AD, Steckelberg JM, Harmsen SW, Mandrekar JN, et al. Outcome or prosthetic joint infection treated with débridement and retention of the components. Clin Infect Dis. 2006;42:471–8.
22. Sherrell JC, Fehring TK, Odum S, Hansen E, Zmistowski B, Dennos A, et al. The Chitranjan Ranawar Award: fate of two-stage reimplantation after failed irrigation and debridement for periprosthetic knee infection. Clin Orthop Relat Res. 2011;469:18–25.
23. Geurts JA, Janssen DM, Kessels AG, Walenkamp GH. Good results in postoperative and hematogenous deep infections of 89 stable total hip and knee replacements with retention of prosthesis and local antibiotics. Acta Orthop. 2013;84:509–16.
24. Vanhegan IS, Morgan-Jones R, Barrett DS, Haddad FS. Developing a strategy to treat stablished infection in total knee replacement. J Bone Joint Surg Br. 2012;94-B:875–81.
25. Sierra RJ, Trousdale RT. Above-the-knee amputation after total knee replacement. J Bone Joint Surg Am. 2003;85-A:1000–4.
26. Fedorka CJ, Chen AF, McGarry WM, Parvizi J, Klatt BA. Functional ability after above-the-knee amputation for infected total knee arthroplasty. Clin Orthop Relat Res. 2011;469:1024–32.
27. Falahee MH, Matthews LS, Kaufer H. Resection arthroplasty as a salvage procedure for a knee with infection after total arthroplasty. J Bone Joint Surg Am. 1987;69:1013–21.
28. Kantor GS, Osterkamp JA, Dorr LD, Fischer D, Perry J, Conaty JP. Resection arthroplasty following infected total hip replacement arthroplasty. J Arthroplasty. 1986;1:83–9.
29. Jones WA, Wroblewski BM. Salvage of failed total knee arhtroplasty: the "beefburger" procedure. J Bone Joint Surg Br. 1989;71-B:856–7.
30. Scott SJ, Hennessey MS, Parkinson RW, Molloy AP. Long-term outcome of the "Beefburger" procedure in patients unsuitable for two-stage revision following infected total knee arthroplasty. Knee. 2001;8:281–6.
31. Charnley J. Possitive pressure in arthrodesis of the knee joint. J Bone Joint Surg Br. 1948;30-B:478–86.
32. Charnley J, Baker SL. Compression arthrodesis of the knee. A clinical and histologic study. J Bone Joint Surg Br. 1952;34-B:187–99.

33. Salenius P, Kivilaakso R. Follow-up examination of a series of arthrodesis of the knee-joint. Acta Orthop Scand. 1968;39:91–100.
34. Harris IE, Left AR, Gitelis S, Simon MA. Function after amputation, arthrodesis, or arthroplasty for tumours about the knee. J Bone Joint Surg Am. 1990;72-A:1477–85.
35. Chen AF, Kinback NC, Heyl AE, McClain EJ, Klatt BA. Better function for fusions versus above-the-knee-amputations for recurrent periprosthetic knee infection. Clin Orthop Relat Res. 2012;470:2737–45.
36. Cierny G, DiPasquale D. Periprosthetic total joint infections: staging, treatment, and outcomes. Clin Orthop Relat Res. 2002;403:23–8.
37. Waldman BJ, Mont MA, Payman KR, Freiberg AA, Windsor RE, Sculco TP, Hungerford DS. Infected total knee arthroplasty treated with arthrodesis using a modular nail. Clin Orthop Relat Res. 1999;367:230–7.
38. Bargiotas K, Wohlrab D, Sewecke JJ, Lavinge G, Demeo PJ, Sotereanos NG. Arthrodesis of the knee with a long intramedullary nail following the failure of a total knee arthroplasty as the result of infection. J Bone Joint Surg Am. 2006;88-A:553–8.
39. Scarponi S, Drago L, Romanò D, Logoluso N, Peccati A, Meani E, Romanò CL. Cementless modular intramedullary nail without bone-on-bone fusion as a salvage procedure in chronically infected total knee prosthesis: long-term results. Int Orthop. 2014;38:413–8.
40. Spina M, Gualdrini G, Fosco M, Giunti A. Knee arthrodesis with the Ilizarov external fixator as treatment for septic failure of knee arthroplasty. J Orthop Traumatol. 2010;11:81–8.
41. Puranen J, Kortelainen P, Jalovaara P. Arthrodesis of the knee with intramedullary nail fixation. J Bone Joint Surg Am. 1990;72-A:433.
42. Conway JD, Mont MA, Bezwada HP. Arthrodesis of the knee. J Bone Joint Surg Am. 2004;86-A:835–48.
43. Oostenbroeck HJ, Van Roermund PM. Arthrodesis of the knee after an infected arthroplasty using the Ilizarov method. J Bone Joint Surg Br. 2001;83-B:50–4.
44. Mabry TM, Jacofsky DJ, Haidukewych GJ, Hanssen AD. Comparison of intramedullary nailing and external fixation knee arthrodesis for the infected knee replacement. Clin Orthop Relat Res. 2007;464:11–5.
45. Vlasak R, Gearen PF, Petty W. Knee arthrodesis in the treatment of failed total knee replacement. Clin Orthop Relat Res. 1995;321:138–44.
46. Brodersen MP, Fitzgerald Jr RH, Peterson LF, Coventry MB, Bryan RS. Arthrodesis of the knee following failed total knee arthroplasty. J Bone Joint Surg Am. 1979;61-A:181–5.
47. Fidler MW. Knee arthrodesis following prosthesis removal. Use of the Wagner apparatus. J Bone Joint Surg Br. 1983;65-B:29–31.
48. Knutson K, Hovelius L, Lindstrand A, Lidgren L. Arthrodesis after failed knee arthroplasty. A nationwide multicenter investigation of 91 cases. Clin Orthop Relat Res. 1984;191:201–11.
49. Knutson K, Lindstrand A, Lidgren L. Arthrodesis of the knee arthroplasty. A report of 20 cases. J Bone Joint Surg Br. 1985;67:47–52.
50. Salem KH, Keppler P, Kinzl L, Schmelz A. Hybrid external fixation for arthrodesis in knee sepsis. Clin Orthop Relat Res. 2006;451:113–20.
51. Ellingsen DE, Rand JA. Intramedullary arthrodesis of the knee after failed total knee arthroplasty. J Bone Joint Surg Am. 1994;76-A:870–7.
52. McQueen DA, Cooke FW, Hahn DL. Knee arthrodesis with the Wichita Fusion Nail: an outcome comparison. Clin Orthop Relat Res. 2006;446:132–9.
53. Sundgren K. Cemented modular intramedullary nail in failed knee arthroplasty–a report of 2 cases. Acta Orthop Scand. 1999;70:305–7.
54. Neuerburg C, Bieger R, Jung S, Kappe T, Reichel H, Decking R. Bridging knee arthrodesis for limb salvage using an intramedullary cemented nail: a retrospective outcome analysis of a case series. Arch Orthop Trauma Surg. 2012;132:1183–9.
55. Putman S, Kern G, Senneville E, Beltrand E, Migaud H. Knee arthrodesis using a customised modular intramedullary nail in failed infected total knee arthroplasty. Orthop Traumatol Surg Res. 2013;99(4):391–8.
56. Röhner E, Windisch C, Nuetzmann K, Rau M, Arnhold M, Matziolis G. Unsatisfactory outcome of arthrodesis performed after septic failure of revision total knee arthroplasty. J Bone Joint Surg Am. 2015;18:298–301.

25 Late Infections of the Knee Joint: Local Antibiotic Treatment

Leo A. Whiteside

Abstract

Prolonged bactericidal levels of antibiotics are difficult to achieve in infected total joint arthroplasty when intravenous antibiotics or antibiotic-loaded cement spacers are used, but intra-articular delivery of antibiotics by means of an intra-articular cannula has been effective in several studies. This chapter describes a protocol for intra-articular delivery of antibiotics in infected knee arthroplasty, and summarizes the results of a pharmacokinetic study and two clinical follow-up studies of especially difficult groups (total knees infected with methicillin resistant *Staphylococcus aureus* or with failed two-stage revision). In the pharmacokinetic study, the mean synovial fluid vancomycin peak concentration was 9242 ± 7608 μg/mL (range of 3956–32,150 μg/mL) among the 11 patients studied. Significant serum concentration was achieved as well (4.2–25.2 μg/mL [mean, 12.3 μg/mL]), which exceeded minimal inhibitory concentration. Success rate exceeded 95 % in the two challenging clinical groups. Intra-articular delivery of antibiotics is shown to be safe and effective, and should be considered as a first option for treatment of infected total joint arthroplasty.

Keywords

Total knee arthroplasty • Infection • Intra-articular • Antibiotic delivery • Vancomycin • Periprosthetic infection

Introduction

Revision for infected total knee arthroplasty (TKA) generally is performed in two stages, first removing the infected implants and treating with antibiotics (usually through an antibiotic-loaded spacer), and then implanting the final components

L.A. Whiteside, MD
Department of Surgery, Des Peres Hospital, St. Louis, MO, USA

Missouri Bone and Joint Center, Missouri Bone and Joint Research Foundation, St. Louis, MO, USA
e-mail: whiteside@whitesidebio.com

D. Kendoff et al. (eds.), *Periprosthetic Joint Infections: Changing Paradigms*,
DOI 10.1007/978-3-319-30091-7_25

6–12 weeks later [1–5]. High intra-articular (IA) concentration of antibiotics is well accepted as essential for effective treatment of bacterial infections of joints. Antibiotics in polymethylmethacrylate cement spacers can produce fairly high concentrations of antibiotics in the knee joint, but the levels rapidly decrease during the first 3 days as the antibiotics leach from the surface layer of the cement spacer [4, 6, 7]. Intravenous (IV) administration of antibiotics also allows concentrations of antibiotics in joint fluid that exceed minimal inhibitory concentration (MIC) for susceptible organisms, but the levels achieved are modest and the time duration above MIC is short [8, 9], which may explain why IV antibiotics do not appear to interfere with the isolation of organisms from intraoperative tissue biopsies in patients with infected TKA [10]. The effectiveness of glycopeptide antibiotics is proportional to both the concentration and the length of time the concentration is maintained at a lethal level [11]. This issue is important for management of total joint replacements whether the antibiotic is used as a prophylactic agent in clean cases, or to eradicate bacteria in infected cases.

Reinfection is common, ranging from 24 % to 82 % in cases involving resistant bacteria [12–15]. Treatment of reinfection after two-stage revision for infection is especially daunting with reports of high complication rates including repeated reinfection [16–18], repeat re-revision for loosening, pain, and infection (52 % of one series [17]), and chronic pain in 50 % of revisions for reinfection in the knees that did achieve infection control [18].

In an effort to achieve sustained high concentrations of antibiotics in the synovial fluid of an infected joint, a method to inject antibiotics directly into the joint was developed using Hickman catheters implanted into the joint cavity at the time of surgical treatment for infection, leaving an external portal for injection [19, 20]. Direct intra-articular (IA) injection of antibiotics has been used effectively for treatment of pyarthrosis in veterinary medicine for decades [8, 21–23], and the reported IA concentration is higher by a factor of many hundreds than that achieved by IV administration [9]. Direct injection of antibiotics also has been used successfully in humans to salvage acutely and chronically infected TKA [19, 20, 24–27]. Infection in the knee joint may not be restricted to the local area, but also may involve the adjacent tissues or distant sites such as the regional lymph nodes. Therefore, the concentration of antibiotics in the serum that can be achieved by direct IA injection also is important. Previous studies have reported mean serum peak (4.1–6.1 μg/mL) and trough (3.2–3.3 μg/mL) values [19, 20].

This chapter describes a technique developed to treat infected TKA by immediate exchange arthroplasty using uncemented implants and IA infusion of antibiotics into the knee, and summarizes clinical findings in three cohorts. (1) the technique was evaluated in an IRB-approved study of basic pharmacokinetics in a group of patients to determine antibiotic concentration in the joint and serum. The protocol also was applied to (2) a group of patients with methicillin-resistant *Staphylococcus aureus* (MRSA) and (3) a group of patients with reinfection after failed two-stage revision for infected TKA.

Summary of Three Study Groups

Pharmacokinetic Study [11]

We enrolled 11 patients (11 knees) referred for treatment of infected TKA in a study to evaluate IA and serum concentration of vancomycin in response to IA injection. Two Hickman catheters (Bard Access Systems, Inc., Salt Lake City, UT) (Fig. 25.1) were inserted into the IA space intraoperatively to allow for direct vancomycin injection. These catheters are silicon tubes with a fibrous cuff that allows fibrous tissue ingrowth to seal the entry point and prevent ingress and egress of fluid around the catheter; they have a Luer-lock module and cap (ALARIS Medical Systems, Inc., San Diego, CA) to allow injection with a syringe. Two catheters were used to ensure that one would remain viable for the 6-week term. Both catheters were used for injection only; the only egress of the antibiotics from the joint was through the local venous and lymphatic system.

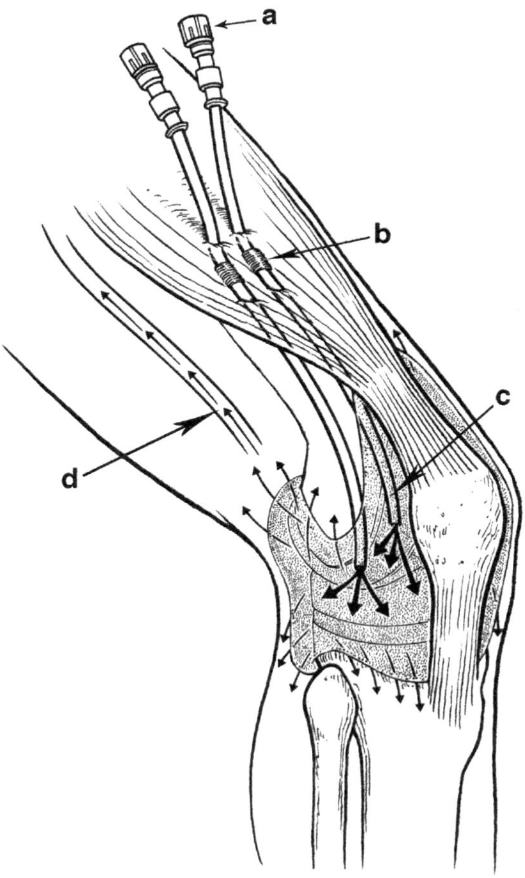

Fig. 25.1 This drawing illustrates the injection portals (*a*) that are outside the skin, the fibrous cuffs that are approximately 5-mm deep to the dermis (*b*), the catheters outside the synovial cavity of the knee (*c*), and outflow of the antibiotic through the synovial membrane and into the regional veins (*d*). The fibrous cuffs seal the catheters so that contaminants do not enter the knee and joint fluid does not leak out. (With kind permission from Springer Science+Business Media: Clinical Orthopaedics and Related Research, Whiteside et al. [19])

IA antibiotics were begun the evening of the first day after surgery if the incision was dry. The beginning dose was small (100 mg vancomycin in 3 cc sterile water) and gradually increased over 3–5 days to 250–500 mg of vancomycin in 3–5 cc sterile water every 12 or 24 h. IV antibiotics were discontinued when the IA route was established (3–5 days). Peak and trough serum vancomycin levels were measured using fluorescent polarization immunoarray (FPIA) [28, 29], after the third dose and twice weekly during treatment. The dosages were decreased if concern arose that serum levels were excessive. In three patients receiving 500 mg of vancomycin every 12 h, serum trough level was reported in excess of 20 μg/mL. Their dosages were decreased to 250 mg, and their trough levels decreased to less than 10 μg/mL. At the conclusion of the treatment (6 weeks), the Hickman catheters were removed in the operating room with local anesthesia as an outpatient hospital procedure. An elliptical incision was made around the catheters, the fibrous cuffs were sharply dissected from the surrounding subcutaneous tissue, and the catheters were extracted gently from the knee. The catheters, made of soft silicon, were handled with care to avoid cutting them and allowing the tip to escape into the knee.

At the time of the Hickman catheters removal, synovial fluid samples were taken by arthrocentesis immediately before the catheters were removed to determine the trough concentration, and immediately after the injection of the final IA antibiotic dose to determine the peak antibiotic concentration. For one patient, synovial fluid samples also were obtained at the 1-month follow-up visit by arthrocentesis. These samples were diluted by a factor of 10, 100, 1000, and 5000 to achieve a concentration that could be measured by the FPIA method. Elimination half-life ($t_{1/2}$) for IA-administered vancomycin was measured by employing a biphasic two-compartment model and biexponential equations, with a distribution stage and an elimination stage [30–32]. The elimination constant β (which is proportional to the clearance rate) and elimination half-life ($t_{1/2}$, in hours) of vancomycin in synovial fluid can be calculated for each pair of IA peak (C_{max}) and trough (C_{min}) measurements:

$$\beta = \{\ln(C_{max}) - \ln(C_{min})\} / ti \qquad (25.1)$$

$$t_{1/2} = \ln(2) / \beta \qquad (25.2)$$

The elimination constant β also can be measured as the slope of an exponential curve fit when the ratio C_{min}/C_{max} from different patients is plotted as a function of time since each patient's last dose, which in turn allows the average elimination half-life ($t_{1/2}$) to be calculated from Eq. 25.2 [30].

Patients who received IA vancomycin to treat infected TKA exhibited very high joint vancomycin levels. Following injection, the mean synovial vancomycin peak level was 9242 ± 7608 μg/mL (range of 3956–32,150 μg/mL) among the 11 patients studied. Synovial trough level (mean of 377 μg/mL, range of 8.4–1610 μg/mL) varied with time but exceeded MIC in all samples. Serum trough level ranged from 4.2 to 25.2 μg/mL (mean, 12.3 μg/mL; average of 9.6 % of the joint trough value), which exceeded MIC. Among individual patients, the elimination half-life ($t_{1/2}$) of IA vancomycin ranged from 1.61 to 4.70 h (mean 3.22 h). Among all patients, using β as the slope of the exponential regression curve, $t_{1/2}$ was 3.06 h ($r^2 = 0.52$, $p < 0.001$) (Fig. 25.2). No adverse events were reported; however, 3 of 11 patients had high vancomycin trough serum levels and their dosage was reduced. No patient had elevated BUN or creatinine concentrations in the serum.

Resistant Organism Study [19]

A prospective study evaluated direct IA injection of vancomycin as treatment for MRSA in 18 patients (18 TKAs) referred to the author January 2001–January 2007. All patients had established chronic infections of greater than 3 months' duration. Eleven patients were women and seven were men. Mean age was 69 ± 6 years (range, 58–84 years). All patients had important comorbidities: nine patients had Type II diabetes, 12 had chronic dependency edema and stasis dermatitis, 9 had morbid obesity, and 15 had malnutrition and hypoalbuminemia. Seventeen of the 18 patients had two or more comorbidities. Four of these patients had previous two-stage revisions for infection with antibiotic cement spacers and antibiotic cement with revision implants. Seven patients had primary total knee components and a previous infection treated by incision and drainage followed by 2–6 weeks IV antibiotics. Four patients had previous surgery after primary TKA for patellar tendon avulsion or patellar subluxation.

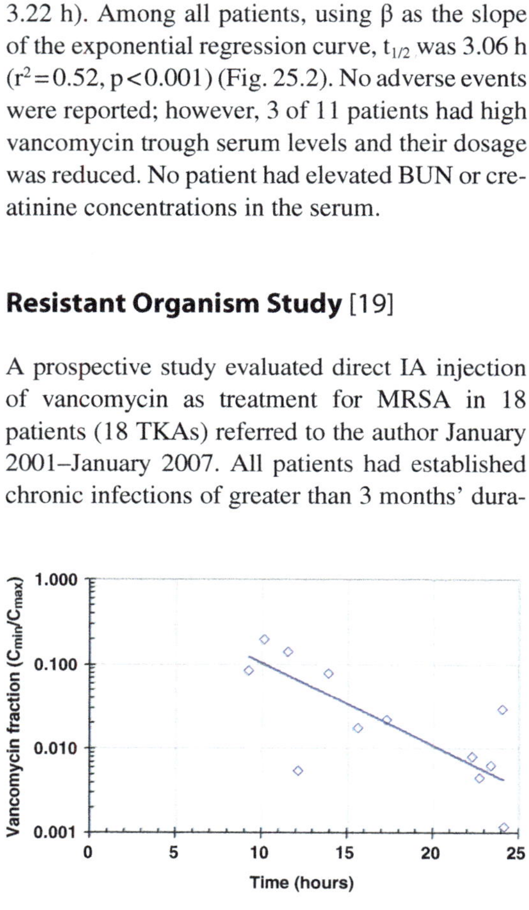

Fig. 25.2 Vancomycin concentration, expressed as a fraction of the peak concentration, plotted on a log scale as function of time since the previous IA dose was administered. The dotted line is an exponential regression curve ($r^2 = 0.52$) whose slope is the elimination constant β $= 0.2265\ h^{-1}$, from which the elimination half-life $t_{1/2}$ can be calculated as 3.06 h (Reprinted from Roy et al. [11], Copyright 2014, with permission from Elsevier)

All patients were treated with a protocol that included debridement, revision TKA with uncemented components, and IA antibiotics. Eleven patients had cemented components removed that included cemented diaphyseal engaging stems in the femur and tibia. The minimum follow-up was 27 months (mean, 62 months; range, 27–96 months). No patients were lost to follow-up.

Surgical treatment included thorough removal of non-absorbable sutures; complete synovectomy; vascularized osteoperiosteal flap osteotomy to expose diaphyseal cement mantles if necessary; and meticulous cement removal using a three-phase debridement starting with rongeurs, followed by curettes, and finishing with high torque reamer to burr away all bone surfaces that had been exposed to cement. During debridement, hand-pump irrigation with saline solution of vancomycin (1 g/L), polymyxin B (250,000 units/L), and bacitracin (50,000 units/L) was performed repeatedly. After debridement, the surgical area was cleaned and re-draped, surgical gowns and gloves were changed, and new sterile instruments were brought into the sterile field. Revision total knee implants had porous-coated surfaces applied directly to available bone and used a diaphyseal-engaging titanium alloy stem. No cement was used for fixation and no bone graft was used to fill defects. Intraoperatively the patients received 1 g vancomycin intravenously and the same dose was given twice postoperatively at 12-h intervals. Vancomycin (100 mg vancomycin in 100 mL sterile water) was started into the knee through the Hickman catheters the first day after surgery if the incision was dry and sealed, then increased in 100 mg/L increments to as much as 500 mg in 5 mL sterile water. IV vancomycin was discontinued once the maintenance dose was established into the knee.

Seven of the 18 knees lost one of the Hickman catheters inserted for IA administration during the 6-week infusion interval, but none lost both catheters. Peak and trough serum vancomycin levels were measured using FPIA [28, 29] after the third dose and twice weekly until the catheters were removed. After 6 weeks, the Hickman catheters were removed surgically and the joint fluid was cultured. The patients were seen at 2 weeks for suture removal, and evaluated at 3 months for tenderness, erythema, and induration, and at yearly intervals. Serum C-reactive protein concentration and sedimentation rate were evaluated at 3 months. C-reactive protein level less than 25 % above normal and sedimentation rate less than 50 % elevated were considered signs of resolved infection.

Seventeen of 18 patients had no clinical sign of infection at last follow-up. All patients except one had laboratory evidence of resolved infection by 3 months postoperative. None of the synovial fluid cultures taken at the time of catheter removal was positive for bacteria. One patient had elevated sedimentation rate and C-reactive protein concentration at 3 months postoperatively and redeveloped clinically apparent infection with MRSA 5 months after initial revision and debridement. The knee was re-operated and a fragment of necrotic bone measuring 2–3 cm on the anterior surface of the femur was found. Complete re-debridement was done, the polyethylene component was exchanged, and the metal components were retained. Hickman catheters were inserted, and the knee was treated for 6 weeks with IA vancomycin. At 42 months postoperatively, this knee had no clinical signs of infection. None of the implants has been revised for loosening.

Mean serum vancomycin peak concentration was 6.1 ± 4.1 μg/mL and mean serum vancomycin trough concentration level was 3.2 ± 1.0 μg/mL at 2 weeks postoperatively. Because of elevated serum vancomycin concentration, five patients required decreasing the dosage to 500 mg given once daily, and one required stopping the antibiotics for 4 days. Three required discontinuation of the antibiotic infusion for 2–3 days because of local inflammatory response to precipitated vancomycin. Six patients (six knees) (33 %) had elevated blood urea nitrogen and creatinine levels during the 6 weeks of antibiotic infusion and required temporary discontinuation of IA vancomycin for 2 days. IA infusion then was resumed at a lower dose. None required complete discontinuation of vancomycin infusion for more than 4 days.

Revision for Reinfection Study [20]

A retrospective study was done to evaluate the success rate of an aggressive protocol to treat infection in 18 patients (18 knees; 12 women, 6 men) that had failed previous two-stage revision for infected TKA January 1999 through January 2008. A surgical protocol was used that included tibial tubercle osteotomy for exposure when necessary in stiff knees to avoid extensive soft-tissue stripping, bivalve osteotomy of the femur and tibia to extirpate extensive cement mantles, cementless fixation, closure with muscle flaps and subfascial skin flaps in cases with deficient capsule and skin, and IA antibiotics with Hickman catheters.

Mean time to initial revision was 7 months (range, 1.5–13 months) and to re-revision was 5 months (range, 1–18 months). All knees were re-infected with the original organism(s): methicillin-resistant *Staphylococcus aureus* (11 patients/11 knees), methicillin-resistant *Staphylococcus epidermidis* (two patients/two knees), methicillin-sensitive *Staphylococcus aureus* (two patients/two knees), and mixed *Proteus mirabilis* and *Escherichia coli* (three patients/three knees). All Staphylococcus organisms were sensitive to vancomycin in concentrations of 2–5 μg/mL, and the three *E. coli* and *P. mirabilis* organisms were sensitive to gentamycin in concentrations of 2 μg/mL. The minimum follow-up was 2.3 years (mean, 6.1 years; range, 2.3–12.0 years). No patient was lost to follow-up.

Ten knees (56 %) had one-stage revision (Fig. 25.3). Five knees (28 %) had debridement, cement spacer, and definitive revision arthroplasty 3–4 months later; and three knees (16 %) had multiple extensive soft tissue reconstruction including tissue expanders to produce enough skin for closure and external fixators to achieve adequate limb length before their definitive revision arthroplasty. Two patients (two knees) required debridement of the edge of a muscle flap and repeat closure within the first week postoperatively. Three patients (three knees) had open drainage of hematoma and re-closure during the first 2 weeks postoperatively. If the bone and soft tissue quality had adequate circulation to sustain healing, and adequate soft tissue was available for closure, then we performed revision TKA using nonporous, fluted, diaphyseal-engaging titanium stems and porous-coated implants applied directly to available bone. No cement was used to fix the implants to bone, and no bone graft was used to fill bone defects. In cases in which bone stock and soft tissue were not deemed adequate for stable fixation of the implants and secure closure of the joint, implants were not inserted, Hickman catheters were inserted for delivery of antibiotics, and closure completed using available skin and muscle flaps, allowing the extremity to shorten if necessary. These patients were managed postoperatively to achieve bone healing of the osteotomies, restore leg length, and gain skin for closure. Three patients (three knees) underwent external fixation for gradual lengthening to regain limb length, and three patients (three knees) had sub-fascial soft tissue expanders to provide skin for closure.

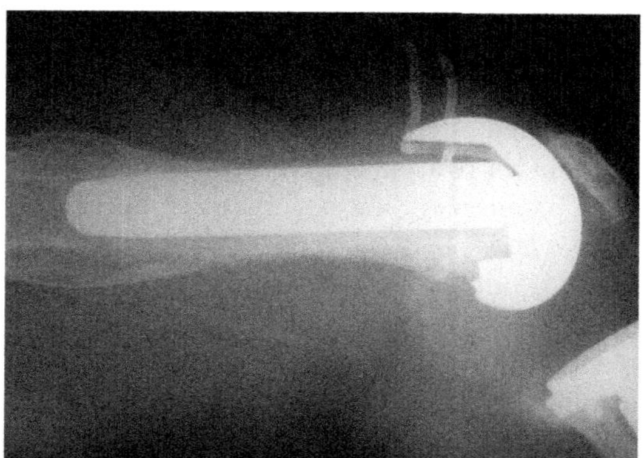

Fig. 25.3 Lateral radiograph performed at 6 weeks after revision with uncemented implants and Hickman catheters for antibiotic infusion. The infection resolved, and the patient progressed to full weightbearing (With kind permission from Springer Science+Business Media: Clinical Orthopaedics and Related Research, Whiteside et al. [20])

Two Hickman catheters were inserted in all knees for IA antibiotic delivery. Postoperatively the patients received 1 g vancomycin or 80 mg gentamicin intravenously every 12 h for at least 48 h postoperatively. IA infusion of antibiotics began the evening of the first day after surgery and the IV antibiotics were discontinued after IA administration was established. 100 mg vancomycin in 3 mL sterile water or 20 mg gentamicin in 3 mL saline was given as a test dose, and the concentration and volume were increased daily if the wound remained sealed and quiescent.

Infection was controlled in 17 of 18 knees. One patient had recurrent infection 13 months after one-stage debridement, revision, and primary closure of the knee. This knee was debrided again, infused with vancomycin for 6 weeks with no implant in place, and re-implanted with cementless implants 6 weeks after catheter removal. The CRP and sedimentation rate were normal at re-implantation with no sign of infection at 28 months follow-up. One knee failed to obtain soft tissue closure, drained continuously, and finally had above-knee amputation 2 months after beginning treatment. CRP and sedimentation rate were within normal limits at 2-year follow-up in 16 of the 17 patients. One patient, who has chronic gingivitis, stasis dermatitis, and arteriosclerotic coronary artery disease, had 24 % elevation of CRP and a high normal sedimentation rate at 1-year follow-up. His knee was asymptomatic and benign to examination. Aspiration revealed no WBCs in the synovial fluid. No patient required chronic suppressive antibiotics.

Serum vancomycin levels within appropriate ranges indicated the safety and efficacy of IA antibiotic delivery. Mean serum vancomycin peak level at 1 month postoperatively was 4.1 ± 1.2 μg/mL, and mean trough level was 3.3 ± 1 μg/mL. Mean serum peak gentamicin level was 1.1 ± 1 μg/mL and trough level was 0.2 ± 0.1 μg/mL. Three patients with vancomycin and one with gentamicin infusion required temporary cessation of antibiotic infusion and resumption at a lower dosage because of excessively high serum antibiotic levels or rising blood urea nitrogen and creatinine levels.

Discussion

Infection control with the described protocol was attained in a high percentage of patients in each cohort. Intra-articular delivery of antibiotics produced peak levels of concentration many orders of magnitude higher than those achieved after IV administration, and the trough levels remained therapeutic for 24 h. Therapeutic levels also were achieved in the serum. The 11 patients in the pharmacokinetic study had vancomycin concentration in the synovial space ranging from 3956 to 32,150 μg/mL. These values are comparable to the high IA levels of amikacin reported by Perry et al. [25]. In contrast to the synovial fluid levels achieved from IV dosing, which likely would become sub-therapeutic in the knee after 6 h, IA administration was shown to maintain concentration of vancomycin within the knee joint above MIC for at least 24 h following the previous dose. IV administration of vancomycin produced joint levels that were 35 % of serum levels on average, while IA administration of vancomycin produced a peak joint concentration that on average was 750 times higher than serum concentration. In addition, serum trough levels following IA administration of vancomycin likewise remained therapeutic, with the mean value greater than the 10 μg/mL recommended to avoid resistance [33].

Extremely high antibiotic concentration in the synovial fluid has a distinct advantage in treating IA infections involving a metal implant. The killing power of antibiotics such as vancomycin that inhibit cell wall and RNA synthesis is proportional to the area under the concentration vs. time curve [33–36], and this factor is especially important for eradication of existing organisms that form a glycocalyx on implant surfaces [37]. Since formation of small colony variants with long reproductive intervals contributes to antibiotic resistance in treatment [38, 39], it seems likely that the sustained high concentrations of antibiotics that are achieved with daily IA injection is important for managing IA infections that involve metallic implants.

Direct IA antibiotic infusion with single-stage revision and porous-surface implants safely and effectively eradicated MRSA and provided a well-fixed implant without the morbidity and inconvenience of an antibiotic spacer and second surgical procedure. Infection was controlled in 17 of 18 patients with the first procedure, and in the failed procedure after debridement and repeat revision. Two-stage revision, using IV antibiotics and antibiotic-loaded PMMA spacer to deliver antibiotics into the joint is considered the conservative surgical approach to this condition [3, 4, 16, 40], but its clinical results are disappointing. Reinfection rates varying from 11 % to 24 % have been reported in centers experienced in care of these difficult cases using two-stage debridement and re-implantation [12, 13, 15, 41].

Cemented fixation of implants consistently is less successful in revision than in primary cases [16, 42–46], and likely is more difficult with persistent infection from indolent bacteria. Cementless fixation with porous devices in revision arthroplasty has had a high rate of successful fixation in the hip and knee and has become the dominant mode of fixation in revision THA [47–49]. Results using cementless fixation for revision of infected TKA resemble those of cementless revision THA [50] and appear to offer an advantage over cemented fixation.

The reinfection cohort involving treatment of failed two-stage revision for infected TKA demonstrates the magnitude of deficiency and the scope of surgical effort required to manage reinfection, and illustrates that treatment has a high success rate when proven surgical procedures are combined with IA antibiotic infusion. Infection was controlled in 17 of 18 knees. The types of cases in this cohort involve problems that cannot be solved only with high levels of antibiotics, but also require aggressive exposure and limb salvage techniques and often multiple procedures to prepare the extremity for re-implantation of the arthroplasty components.

Daily IA injection into the knee achieves and maintains vastly superior antibiotic levels in the synovial fluid throughout the interval between doses as compared with IV infusion. Currently the single-stage procedure—including debridement and use of Hickman catheters for 6 weeks of IA antibiotic administration—is our standard protocol, and it is effective even in difficult cases and with highly resistant organisms.

Acknowledgments The author thanks M.E. Roy, PhD, Michael Peppers, PhD, Renee LaZear, RN, and Tariq Nayfeh, MD, PhD, for their work and collaboration on the studies; William C. Andrea, CMI, for preparation of the illustration; and Diane J. Morton, MS, for assistance with preparation of the manuscript.

References

1. Buchholz HW, Elson RA, Engelbrecht E, Lodenkamper H, Rottger J, Siegel A. Management of deep infection of total hip replacement. J Bone Joint Surg Br. 1981;63:342–53.
2. Buchholz HW, Elson RA, Heinert K. Antibiotic-loaded acrylic cement: current concepts. Clin Orthop Relat Res. 1984;190:96–108.
3. Insall JN, Thompson FM, Brause BD. Two-stage reimplantation for the salvage of infected total knee arthroplasty. J Bone Joint Surg Am. 1983;65:1087–98.
4. Salvati EA, Callaghan JJ, Brause BD, Klein RF, Small RD. Reimplantation in infection: elution of gentamicin from cement and beads. Clin Orthop Relat Res. 1986;207:83–93.
5. Windsor RE, Insall JN, Urs WK, Miller DV, Brause BD. Two-stage reimplantation for the salvage of total knee arthroplasty complicated by infection: further follow-up and refinement of indications. J Bone Joint Surg Am. 1990;72:272–8.
6. van de Belt H, Neut D, Uges DR, Schenk W, van Horn JR, van der Mel HC, et al. Surface roughness, porosity, wettability of gentamicin-loaded bone cements and their antibiotic release. Biomaterials. 2000;21:1981–7.
7. Anguita-Alonso P, Rouse MS, Piper KE, Jacofsky DJ, Osmon DR, Patel R. Comparative study of antimicrobial release kinetics from polymethylmethacrylate. Clin Orthop Relat Res. 2006;445:239–44.
8. Lloyd KC, Stover SM, Pascoe JR, Baggot JD, Kurpershoek C, Hietala S. Plasma and synovial fluid concentrations of gentamicin in horses after intra-articular administration of buffered and unbuffered gentamicin. Am J Vet Res. 1988;49:644–9.
9. McLaren A. Alternative materials to acrylic bone cement for delivery of depot antibiotics in orthopaedic infections. Clin Orthop Relat Res. 2004;427: 101–6.
10. Ghanem E, Parvizi J, Clohisy J, Burnett S, Sharkey PF, Barrack R. Perioperative antibiotics should not be withheld in proven cases of periprosthetic infection. Clin Orthop Relat Res. 2007;461:44–7.
11. Roy ME, Peppers MP, Whiteside LA, LaZear RM. Vancomycin concentration in synovial fluid: direct injection into the knee vs. intravenous infusion. J Arthroplasty. 2014;29:564–8.
12. Kilgus DJ, Howe DJ, Strang A. Results of periprosthetic hip and knee infections caused by resistant bacteria. Clin Orthop Relat Res. 2002;404:116–24.
13. Mittal Y, Fehring TK, Hanssen A, Marculescu C, Odum S, Osmon D. Two-stage reimplantation for periprosthetic knee infection involving resistant organisms. J Bone Joint Surg Am. 2007;89:1227–31.
14. Salgado CD, Dash S, Cantey JR, Marculescu CE. Higher risk of failure of methicillin-resistant Staphylococcus aureus prosthetic joint infections. Clin Orthop Relat Res. 2007;461:48–53.
15. Volin SJ, Hinrichs SH, Garvin KL. Two-stage reimplantation of total joint infections: a comparison of resistant and non-resistant organisms. Clin Orthop Relat Res. 2004;427:94–100.
16. Hanssen AD, Trousdale RT, Osmon DR. Patient outcome with reinfection following reimplantation for the infected total knee arthroplasty. Clin Orthop Relat Res. 1995;321:55–67.
17. Stuart MJ, Larson JE, Morrey BF. Reoperation after condylar revision total knee arthroplasty. Clin Orthop Relat Res. 1993;286:168–73.
18. Wang CJ, Huang TW, Wang JW, Chen HS. The often poor clinical outcome of infected total knee arthroplasty. J Arthroplasty. 2002;17:608–14.
19. Whiteside LA, Peppers MP, Nayfeh T, Roy ME. Methicillin-resistant Staphylococcus aureas in TKA treated with revision and direct intraarticular antibiotic infusion. Clin Orthop Relat Res. 2011;469:26–33.
20. Whiteside LA, Nayfeh TA, LaZear R, Roy ME. Reinfected revised TKA resolves with an aggressive protocol and antibiotic infusion. Clin Orthop Relat Res. 2012;470:236–43.
21. Schneider RK. Treatment of posttraumatic septic arthritis. AAEP Proc. 1988;44:167.
22. Adams SB, Lescun TB. How to treat septic joints with constant intra-articular infusion of gentamicin or amikacin. AAEP Proc. 2000;46:188.
23. Werner L, Hardy J, Bertone A. Bone gentamicin concentration after intra-articular injection or regional intravenous perfusion in the horse. Vet Surg. 2003;32:559–65.
24. Davenport K, Traina S, Perry C. Treatment of acutely infected arthroplasty with local antibiotics. J Arthroplasty. 1991;6:179–83.
25. Perry C, Hulsey R, Mann F, Miller GA, Pearson RL. Treatment of acutely infected arthroplasties with incision drainage, and local antibiotics delivered via an implantable pump. Clin Orthop Relat Res. 1992;281:216–23.

26. Shaw JA. The use of long-term indwelling catheters for local antibiotic administration into infected joints: a concept report. J Orthop Tech. 1995;3:181–4.
27. Fukagawa S, Matsuda S, Miura H, Okazaki K, Tashiro Y, Iwamoto Y. High-dose antibiotic infusion for infected knee prosthesis without implant removal. J Orthop Sci. 2010;15:470–6.
28. Dandliker WB, Feigen GA. Quantification of the antigen-antibody reaction by the polarization of fluorescence. Biochem Biophys Res Commun. 1961;5:299–304.
29. National Committee for Clinical Laboratory Standards. Interference testing in clinical xhemistry; Tentative guideline. NCCLS Publication EP7-T. Villanova: National Committee for Clinical Laboratory Standards; 1986.
30. Greenblatt DJ, Koch-Weser J. Clinical pharmacokinetics. N Engl J Med. 1975;293:964–70.
31. Rotschafer JC, Crossley K, Zaske DE, Mead K, Sawchuk RJ, Solem LD. Pharmacokinetics of vancomycin: observations in 28 patients and dosage recommendations. Antimicrob Agents Chemother. 1982;22:391–4.
32. Marsot A, Boulamery A, Bruguerolle B. Vancomycin: a review of population and morphologic effects of intraarticular ceftiofur sodium in horses. Vet Surg. 2000;29:398–406.
33. Schilling A, Neuner E, Rehm SJ. Vancomycin: a 50-something-year-old antibiotic we still don't understand. Cleve Clin J Med. 2011;78:465–71.
34. Cheung RP, DiPiro JT. Vancomycin: an update. Pharmacotherapy. 1986;6:153–69.
35. Hermans PE, Wilhelm MP. Vancomycin. Mayo Clin Proc. 1987;62:901–5.
36. Rybak MJ. The pharmacokinetic and pharmacodynamic properties of vancomycin. Clin Infect Dis. 2006;42(Suppl1):S35–9.
37. Wymenga AB, Van Dijke BJ, Van Horn JR, Slooff TJ. Prosthesis-related infection. Etiology, prophylaxis and diagnosis (a review). Acta Orthop Belg. 1990;56:463–75.
38. Rusthoven JJ, Davies TA, Lerner SA. Clinical isolation and characterization of aminoglycoside-resistant small colony variants of Enterobacter aerogenes. Am J Med. 1979;67:702–6.
39. Neut D, Hendriks JG, van Horn JR, van der Mei HC, Busscher HJ. Pseudomonas aeruginosa biofilm formation and slime excretion on antibiotic-loaded bone cement. Acta Orthop. 2005;76:109–14.
40. Haleem AA, Berry DJ, Hanssen AD. Mid-term to long-term followup of two-stage reimplantation for infected total knee arthroplasty. Clin Orthop Relat Res. 2004;428:35–9.
41. Hirakawa K, Stulberg BN, Wilde AH, Bauer TW, Secic M. Results of two-stage reimplantation for infected total knee arthroplasty. J Arthroplasty. 1998;13:22–8.
42. Shannon BD, Klassen JF, Rand JA, Berry DJ, Trousdale RT. Revision total knee arthroplasty with cemented components and uncemented intramedullary stems. J Arthroplasty. 2003;18 Suppl 1:27–32.
43. Whiteside LA. Treatment of infected total knee arthroplasty. Clin Orthop Relat Res. 1994;299:169–72.
44. Whiteside LA. Cementless fixation issues in revision total knee arthroplasty. Instr Course Lect. 1999;48:177–82.
45. Whiteside LA. Two-stage exchange for infected TKA—opposes. Semin Arthroplasty. 2008;19:121–5.
46. Whiteside LA, Bicalho PS. Radiologic and histologic analysis of morselized allograft in revision total knee replacement. Clin Orthop Relat Res. 1998;357:149–56.
47. Garazzino S, Aprato A, Baietto L, D'Avolio A, Maiello A, DeRosa FG, et al. Glycopeptide bone penetration in patients with septic pseudoarthrosis of the tibia. Clin Pharmacokinet. 2008;47:793–805.
48. Hamilton WG, Cashen DV, Ho H, Hopper Jr HR, Engh CA. Extensively porous-coated stems for femoral revision: a choice for all seasons. J Arthroplasty. 2007;22(4 suppl1):106–10.
49. Parvizi J, Azzam K, Ghanem E, Austin MS, Rothman RH. Periprosthetic infection due to resistant staphylococci: serious problems on the horizon. Clin Orthop Relat Res. 2009;467:1732–9.
50. Whiteside LA. Major femoral bone loss in revision total hip arthroplasty treated with tapered, porous-coated stems. Clin Orthop Relat Res. 2004;429: 222–6.

Part VII

Perioperative Optimization

Perioperative Optimization

26

Aaron Tande and Elie Berbari

Abstract

Prosthetic joint infection (PJI) is a devastating complication following joint replacement. The risk of PJI may be lowered through careful patient optimization pre and peri-operatively. Proper management of nutritional status, obesity, and diabetes mellitus may yield overall health and perioperative benefits. Preoperative smoking cessation, when achieved, may reduce the rate of postoperative wound complications. Immunosuppressive medications should be modified to provide effective control of underlying inflammatory processes, while minimizing the risk of infection. Elective surgery should be delayed until active clinically diagnosed infections are treated. Selected screening for and decolonization of *Staphylococcus aureus* carriers reduces the rate of surgical site infection, while minimizing the impact on the frequency of community-wide mupirocin resistance. Appropriate perioperative antimicrobial prophylaxis and anticoagulation management are critical. Among patients with significant soft tissue deficits, preoperative plastic surgery consultation should be obtained and a coordinated surgical plan should be developed. A thorough multidisciplinary approach to preoperative evaluation of patients undergoing joint arthroplasty may yield benefits for patient outcomes.

Keywords

Surgical site infection • Prosthetic joint infection • Osteomyelitis • Antimicrobial prophylaxis • Prevention • Risk factors • Diabetes mellitus • Staphylococcal infection • Malnutrition • Obesity • Rheumatoid arthritis

A. Tande, MD (✉) • E. Berbari, MD, FIDSA
Division of Infectious Diseases, Mayo Clinic, Rochester, MN, USA
e-mail: Tande.Aaron@mayo.edu; Berbari.Elie@mayo.edu

D. Kendoff et al. (eds.), *Periprosthetic Joint Infections: Changing Paradigms*, DOI 10.1007/978-3-319-30091-7_26

Introduction

Joint replacement, provides pain relief, restoration of function, and improvement in patient quality of life. In 2010, there were over one million knee and hip arthroplasties performed in the United States alone [1]. Typically, joint replacement is an elective procedure. Accordingly, every effort should be made to optimize a surgical candidate's general health in order to prevent potential complications. A significant proportion of risk factors associated with PJI may be modifiable. Superficial surgical site infection (SSI) as well as deep organ space infection, otherwise known as prosthetic or periprosthetic joint infection (PJI), are associated with significant morbidity and cost [2]. Wound healing abnormalities after surgery are well-established risk factors for both superficial SSI and PJI. A number of different modifiable and non-modifiable risk factors for wound healing problems, superficial SSI, and PJI have been identified. Knowledge and optimization of these will reduce the frequency of these devastating complications.

Nutrition

In the developed world with ample resources in which joint replacement is performed, it seems anathema that malnutrition should be a prevalent finding among patients undergoing joint replacement. However, more than one-quarter of patients undergoing primary joint replacement [3] and more than a third of patients undergoing revision for non-infectious reasons [4] have biochemical evidence of malnutrition. Due to the associated chronic inflammatory state, patients with established PJI may have an even higher prevalence of malnutrition. Numerous prior studies have demonstrated that malnutrition, as defined by either hypoalbuminemia [4–6], low transferrin [7], lymphopenia [4, 6, 8, 9], or low BMI [10] are associated with increased risk of wound healing complications including PJI. Other ways of identifying patients with malnutrition include the use of more complicated anthropomorphic measurements, which may be too cumbersome for clinical practice. Therefore, clinicians have typically relied upon the use of blood tests above. The pathophysiology associating malnutrition to impaired wound healing complications is complex. It likely involves both alterations in the structural building blocks necessary for wound healing, as well as impairment in the inflammatory process, a necessary component of wound healing.

Although somewhat counterintuitive, malnutrition may be coexistent with obesity due to intake of high caloric nutritionally deficient diet. The frequency of malnutrition appears to be similar in both the obese population and the overall population undergoing joint replacement [4, 7]. In addition to the impact of malnutrition on wound healing, the presence of obesity provides an additional set of unique problems which can lead to wound healing difficulties. The increased mechanical tension of the incision can lead to wound dehiscence and create a subsequent portal for initiation of infection. Obesity may result in a blood flow to tissue mismatch, leading to relative tissue hypo-perfusion. Finally, there may be an increase in dead space, creating a potential space for a deep surgical site infection. While preoperative weight loss can be attempted in order to try to minimize these mechanical complications, it must be carefully pursued in order to avoid achieving weight loss at the expense of adequate nutritional intake.

The practical approach to malnutrition and obesity prior to performing joint replacement is not well-defined, but a logical step wise approach could be considered. First, complete blood count with differential (absolute lymphocyte count <1500 cells per microliter), albumin (<3.5 mg/dL) and/or transferrin (<200 mg/dL) are reasonable screening tests to evaluate patients in whom malnutrition is suspected, including patients with obesity. If any of these tests are abnormal, evaluation for uncontrolled chronic infection or a sub-optimally controlled chronic inflammatory state (such as rheumatoid arthritis) should be considered. Among patients with malnutrition, providers should have an in-depth discussion with the patient regarding their current diet. Dietary supplements and a referral to a nutritionist for counseling may be considered. Among patients with obesity in conjunction with malnutrition, referral to a bariatric specialist with expertise in the care of patients with coexistent obesity and malnutrition is appropriate. The role of gastric bypass or gastric banding procedures prior to surgery should be discussed in conjunction with a bariatric medicine specialist.

Diabetes Mellitus

Large studies have suggested that diabetes mellitus is present in up to a quarter of patients undergoing primary total knee or hip replacement [11, 12]. Patients with diabetes mellitus and hyperglycemia may have impaired leukocyte function as well as microvascular dysfunction. Both factors may lead to the development of postoperative infection. Diabetes mellitus is a well-established risk factor for PJI [12–16]. Additionally, perioperative hyperglycemia in patients without diabetes mellitus has been suggested as a risk factor as well [17]. This observation may be related to the experimentally observed increase in biofilm formation in the presence of higher glucose concentrations [18]. It is not clear if the degree of preoperative glycemic control correlates with likelihood of SSI. Hemoglobin A1c is one of the commonly used markers for glycemic control, reflecting the average blood glucose levels over the preceding 3 months. The literature is mixed with regard to whether hemoglobin A1c is predictive of wound complications and infection [15, 19–21]. However, the degree of postoperative hyperglycemia is clearly predictive of wound complications or infection [19]. Studies performed to date (including non-orthopedic surgeries) identified a dose response relationship between the degree of postoperative hyperglycemia and the likelihood of infection [21]. Regardless of the utility of preoperative hemoglobin A1c for predicting subsequent infection, a patient with well-controlled diabetes mellitus prior to surgery will likely have more easily managed blood glucose levels in the immediate postoperative period. Thus, it is our practice to optimize diabetes mellitus control in the preoperative setting.

Optimization of glucose control in the perioperative setting requires close collaboration with the patient's primary care physician and diabetes specialist. At the preoperative visit, the patient should be questioned with regards to their average and range of blood glucose readings at home, diabetes medication regimen, and their most recent hemoglobin A1c levels. If poor glucose control is suspected, it is reasonable to delay surgery and have the patient visit with their provider. Once a surgical date is known, a plan for postoperative diabetes therapy should be put in place. The optimal postoperative glucose targets are not known, as intensive glucose control (random glucose <120–150 mg/dL) has not been shown to be better than the standard control (140–200 mg/dL). Intensive glucose control carries an increased risk of hypoglycemic episodes [22]. Accordingly, a goal of <200 mg/dL is reasonable. Finally, patients receiving corticosteroids who require corticosteroid dose adjustment in the perioperative time period may also require adjustments to their insulin protocol.

Tobacco Use

In addition to the pleotropic adverse effects on human health, tobacco use is associated with impairment in wound healing and subsequent increased risk of SSI [14, 16, 23]. These adverse effects are a function not only of the decreased oxygenation seen with tobacco smoking, but also likely due to the decrease in blood flow directly related to nicotine [24, 25]. A number of different techniques for smoking cessation are available, including counseling techniques, nicotine replacement therapy, varenicline, and bupropion. High-quality randomized control trial data demonstrated an 83 % reduction in wound complications among patients randomized to counseling and nicotine replacement therapy beginning 6–8 weeks prior to elective hip or knee replacements, as compared to placebo [23]. These findings, as well as results of a meta-analysis across a variety of surgeries [26], suggest that arthroplasty surgery should be delayed while smoking cessation is attempted. The use of weekly counseling with a trained smoking cessation counselor in combination with nicotine replacement therapy seems to be a logical approach.

Immunosuppressive Medication Management

Joint replacement in patients with rheumatoid arthritis can provide a significant functional improvement, especially when medical management is no longer effective. Unfortunately, selected immune-modulating therapy used to control rheumatoid arthritis are also associated with an increased risk of SSI [8, 16, 27]. Among the medications used to control rheumatoid arthritis, biologic disease modifying anti-rheumatic drugs (DMARDs) that inhibit tumor necrosis factor alpha (TNF-α) or interleukin-6 (IL-6) appear to significantly increase the risk of SSI compared to other DMARDs [28–30]. Accordingly, the American College of Rheumatology and the British Society for Rheumatology recommend withholding TNF-α inhibitors around the time of arthroplasty surgery or revision [31, 32], with a typical approach of withholding biologic DMARDs for one cycle before surgery. These medications can then be resumed 1 or 2 weeks after joint arthroplasty surgery, provided that wound healing is progressing as expected.

There is mixed data regarding the safety of continuing non-biologic DMARDs through the time of joint arthroplasty surgery [33–35]. Leflunomide and methotrexate are among the most frequently used DMARDS for patients with moderate-severe rheumatoid arthritis and have been evaluated for their impact on postoperative infection. Among 201 patients with rheumatoid arthritis or psoriatic arthritis undergoing elective orthopedic surgery, a significantly higher frequency of wound healing complications was observed among patients receiving leflunomide peri-operatively, as compared to those receiving methotrexate [36]. In contrast, a study of 82 patients undergoing joint replacement observed no difference in infection between patients in whom leflunomide was held 2 weeks before and after surgery and those who continued it through the time of surgery [37]. However, given the half-life of over 14 days of the active metabolite of leflunomide [38], this study design was likely inadequate to observe any true difference between these two strategies. The shorter half-life of methotrexate makes withholding this medication more feasible around the time of surgery. The best data for methotrexate included 160 patients with rheumatoid arthritis undergoing elective orthopedic surgery who were prospectively randomized to hold methotrexate for 2 weeks before and after surgery or continue through surgery [34]. These patients were also compared to a contemporary cohort of patients with rheumatoid arthritis receiving a variety of other non-biologic DMARDS. Somewhat surprisingly, a significantly lower frequency of infection or wound healing complications was observed in those continuing methotrexate, compared with either of the other groups. Additionally, there were significantly fewer disease flares among those continuing methotrexate, a factor that may increase corticosteroid use and inadvertently increase risk of infection. Several smaller, retrospective studies have also found no association with methotrexate and SSI [39–42], while other studies suggested a decrease in SSI when methotrexate was held [43, 44].

The choice to continue DMARDs must be individualized and balanced against the substantial risk of the potential need to increase corticosteroid use. Sometimes used as “bridging agents” during DMARD holidays if flares are expected or occur, corticosteroids have been observed in one large study to be of higher risk for hospitalization for infection than the biologic DMARDs [45]. If corticosteroids are necessary, every effort should be made to maintain a prednisone dose of ≤10 mg daily [46]. A collaborative relationship with a patient’s rheumatologist is critical for developing a strategy to minimize unnecessary immunosuppression, while providing effective control of the underlying disease.

Decolonization and Bacterial Burden Reduction

Staphylococcus aureus is responsible for nearly 40 % of early PJI [2]. The majority of SSIs and early and delayed PJIs result from contamination of the prosthetic joint with the patients' flora at the time of surgery. Accordingly, identifying patients who are carriers of *S. aureus* and attempting decolonization prior to surgery is a reasonable strategy. These strategies typically include the use of mupirocin nasal ointment and chlorhexidine bathing, either alone or in combination. A large, high-quality, randomized double-blind placebo controlled trial demonstrated that a standard protocol of screening for *S. aureus* nasal colonization using PCR, followed by a 5 day protocol of twice daily nasal mupirocin and daily chlorhexidine bathing resulted in a nearly 80 % reduction in deep SSI across a number of different types of surgery [47]. Whether or not these overall results translate to a reduction in surgical site infection or PJI following joint replacement is not clear, given the low baseline rate of infection. A similar protocol of preoperative nasal mupirocin and chlorhexidine bathing reduces nasal *S. aureus* colonization on the day of primary joint arthroplasty [48]. A systematic review including 19 studies using a variety of decolonization protocols in orthopedic surgeries found a decrease in SSI ranging from 13 to 200 % [49]. However, this was a very heterogeneous group of studies, including studies that used selective and universal decolonization. Recent SSI prevention guidelines recommend mupirocin nasal ointment for patients with *S. aureus* nasal colonization [50]. Given the concern about increasing mupirocin resistance among *S. aureus* isolates, the use of povidone iodine nasal decolonization was recently investigated and found to be equally effective to mupirocin nasal decolonization [51].

A universal decolonization strategy avoids the logistical challenges of preoperative screening for *S. aureus* carriers, but increases the medication cost, the number of patients treated, and may lead to an increase in mupirocin resistance. The use of universal mupirocin and chlorhexidine appears to be successful in other settings, such as prevention of infections in patients hospitalized in the intensive care unit [52]. Among patients undergoing a variety of different surgeries, the universal use of mupirocin did not significantly reduce the overall rate of SSI, compared with placebo [53]. However, it did decrease the rate of nosocomial *S. aureus* infections.

Based on the low overall rate of infection, the lack of clear data to support a universal decolonization strategy, and the availability of laboratory services to support *S. aureus* screening, selective screening for and decolonization of *S. aureus* carriers is the authors'preferred strategy. Nasal screening can be performed at the preoperative visit, along with automated prescription delivery and standardized teaching delivered by support staff.

Screening for and Treatment of Active Infection Prior to Surgery

At the preoperative visit, a careful history and physical examination should be performed in order to uncover any signs or symptoms suggestive of an active infection at a site remote from the joint arthroplasty. If infection is suspected, it should be evaluated and managed appropriately, with joint replacement surgery delayed until this has been successfully achieved. Dental health is an important part of prevention of prosthetic joint infection throughout the life of the arthroplasty. A debate remains regarding the use of antimicrobial prophylaxis around the time of dental procedures for patients with arthroplasties. A recent study performed at our institution did not find an association between dental procedures and the risk of PJI [54]. However, both for the benefit of overall patient health and prevention of overt dental infection, routine, proactive dental care should be recommended for all patients undergoing joint replacement.

In the absence of signs or symptoms to suggest remote active infection, there is ongoing debate about the role for laboratory screening for infection, particularly with urinalysis to evaluate for asymptomatic bacteriuria or pyuria. There is conflicting evidence on the association of asymptomatic bacteriuria and the risk of PJI [55–59]. It is important to note that the finding of asymptomatic bacteriuria may simply be a surrogate for other comorbidities that are clearly associated with PJI, such as obesity or diabetes mellitus. Treatment of asymptomatic bacteriuria does not appear to decrease PJI risk [58]. One of the goals of the preoperative visit is to identify patients with symptomatic urinary tract infection (fever, abdominal pain, dysuria, or urinary frequency)., Routine screening of all asymptomatic patients with a urinalysis may not be warranted.

Perioperative Antimicrobial Prophylaxis

The decision to use perioperative antimicrobial prophylaxis depends both on the likelihood of SSI and the consequences if such an infection occurs. While joint arthroplasty procedures are typically associated with a low overall risk of infection, resulting SSI may be associated with significant morbidity and cost, shifting the risk-benefit balance toward providing universal antimicrobial prophylaxis. There is good data to support the efficacy of perioperative antimicrobial prophylaxis for primary joint replacement [60]. The choice of antimicrobial depends on the spectrum of activity, ease of administration, pharmacodynamics, pharmacokinetics, safety and cost of the antimicrobial. Accordingly, first generation cephalosporins, such as cefazolin, are ideal choices. Cefazolin has a short intravenous infusion duration, achieves a peak serum concentration rapidly [61, 62], has excellent anti-staphylococcal activity, is widely available, safe and inexpensive. These factors have led to the recommendation for use of cefazolin by several specialty organizations [50]. While second and third generation cephalosporins have not been shown to be inferior, they tend to be more expensive and may be associated with an increased incidence of *Clostridium difficile* infection [63].

Patients who self-report allergy to β-lactam antimicrobials at the preoperative visits present an opportunity for optimization. Patients with a history of prior positive penicillin skin test or symptoms suggesting a type I hypersensitivity reaction (anaphylaxis, angioedema, bronchospasm, or hives) or exfoliative rash following a β-lactam antimicrobial should not receive cefazolin or other β-lactam antimicrobials. However, the majority of patients with a stated history of self-limited rash or non-allergic adverse effects to β-lactam antimicrobials can safely receive cefazolin. This was illustrated by large study of patients with self-reported penicillin allergy at the preoperative surgical visit, where 85 % were felt to be safe for cefazolin prophylaxis after allergy consultation [64]. The same study demonstrated that same-day allergy consultation can decrease inappropriate vancomycin administration.

When β-lactam antimicrobials cannot be used for prophylaxis, other agents commonly used include vancomycin or clindamycin, although these agents lack the activity of cefazolin against gram-negative bacteria. Vancomycin is reasonable for patients with known methicillin-resistant *Staphylococcus aureus* (MRSA) colonization. However, one study found an increase in the total number of surgical site infections in patients without MRSA nasal colonization when vancomycin was used, as compared to β-lactam antimicrobial prophylaxis [65]. This and other data [66] suggests that vancomycin may be less effective for preventing methicillin-susceptible *Staphylococcus aureus* (MSSA) infections and should be used selectively in patients who can otherwise receive a β-lactam antimicrobial for prophylaxis. Among patients with MRSA nasal colonization, dual prophylaxis with cefazolin and vancomycin may be appropriate. However, the data to guide this practice is lacking [67] and limited retrospective data suggests an increase in acute kidney injury in patients receiving both vancomycin and cefazolin, as compared to cefazolin alone [68]. Vancomycin requires a longer duration of infusion and timing of administration must be adjusted in order to achieve adequate blood and tissue concentrations at the time of incision.

Antimicrobial dosing is of critical importance, particularly in the obese population. Administration of a single 1 g dose of cefazolin results in suboptimal tissue and serum concentrations among morbidly obese patients undergoing gastroplasty, with a marked decline in SSI when a 2 g dose of cefazolin is used [69]. However, among patients with a body mass index above 50, 2 g of cefazolin may not be adequate to maintain sufficient tissue and serum concentrations throughout surgery [70]. Given the favorable therapeutic window, it is reasonable to administer 2 g of IV cefazolin in patients weighing greater than 80 and 3 g of IV cefazolin in patients weighing greater than 120 kg [50]. Vancomycin should be dosed based on actual body weight.

Effective prophylaxis requires effective blood and tissue concentrations of the prophylactic antimicrobial from the time of skin incision to closure. Serum concentrations of cefazolin are well above the minimum inhibitory concentration (MIC) for methicillin-susceptible staphylococci within 15 min after receiving a single 1 g dose of cefazolin [61], also resulting in sufficient levels in bone [71]. However, there are not convincing data to suggest that administration within 30 min prior to incision is superior to administration of 30–60 min prior to incision [72, 73]. Accordingly, cefazolin should be given within 1 h prior to the incision. Vancomycin, which requires a longer infusion time, should be started 60–120 min prior to the incision [50]. With regard to tourniquet inflation, cefazolin is typically administered at least 10 min before the tourniquet is inflated in order to allow adequate penetration of the antibiotic into the operative tissue before ischemia is induced. Mathematical modeling suggests that the optimal time for cefazolin dosing is 10–30 min prior to tourniquet inflation [74]. However, some have questioned whether giving the prophylactic antimicrobial prior to tourniquet inflation may lead to a sub-therapeutic serum level of antimicrobial if a hematoma forms just after tourniquet release, creating a vulnerable window for initiation of infection. An alternate proposed strategy is antimicrobial administration at the end of the procedure but just prior to tourniquet release. This approach was found to be non-inferior to antimicrobial administration prior to tourniquet inflation in a large, randomized trial of knee arthroplasty [75]. However, until further data is available to support this approach, antimicrobial administration 10–60 min prior to tourniquet inflation is recommended.

Repeat administration of antimicrobials during surgery primarily depends upon the clearance of the antimicrobial given prior to surgery. Drug clearance can be affected by the actual half-life of the drug or by significant blood loss leading to increased drug clearance. Given the correlation between blood loss and serum and tissue concentrations of cefazolin [76], an additional dose of antimicrobial should be given if there is blood loss greater than 1500 mL [50]. During prolonged procedures, a repeat dose of antimicrobial should be given if the procedure duration exceeds two times the half-life of the drug. Cefazolin should be re administered approximately 4 h after the initial administration, given the approximately 2 h half-life, a practice that appears to decrease SSI rate in surgeries lasting longer than 4 h [72]. Patients with abnormal renal function and decreased clearance of the antimicrobial may not require repeat antimicrobial administration at the same frequency.

Antimicrobial prophylaxis should be given postoperatively for only the minimal amount of time to prevent infection, in order to minimize costs and adverse effects, such as *C. difficile* infection [77]. There is a growing body of evidence to suggest that no additional dosing is needed after surgery [73, 78, 79]. Current recommendations that perioperative prophylaxis only be given for 24 h or less, regardless of whether a surgical drain remains in place [50].

Anticoagulation Management

Patients undergoing hip or knee replacement are at significant risk for venous thromboembolism (VTE) and accordingly, pharmacologic VTE prophylaxis is typically administered. In addition, patients experiencing postoperative atrial fibrillation or myocardial infarction are sometimes treated with therapeutic anticoagulation. Careful management of anticoagulation is necessary in order to avoid postoperative hematomas, which have been associated with an increased risk of PJI [8, 54, 80]. Additionally, a postoperative International Normalized Ratio (INR) above target at hospital discharge was associated with an increase in risk of PJI in a case–control study [80]. Options for pharmacologic anticoagulation include unfractionated or low molecular weight heparin, fondaparinux or warfarin. Among patients receiving warfarin, several important considerations need to be observed in order to avoid inadvertent increases in the INR which could lead to hematoma development. First, there are numerous drug- drug interactions between warfarin and other medications that are often used in the postoperative setting. Second, many antimicrobials will increase the INR indirectly through alteration in the gastrointestinal microbial flora and a resultant change in vitamin K metabolism. Third, patients with postoperative ileus or poor postoperative nutritional status may have a less predictable response to warfarin and should be accordingly monitored closely. Finally, patients who have never received warfarin may have previously unrecognized genetic polymorphisms that alter its metabolism. Warfarin management should be managed in conjunction with an experienced provider in order to avoid nontherapeutic dosing, a recommendation endorsed by national guidelines [81].

Plastic Surgery and Soft Tissue Coverage

Patients with chronic PJI, particularly those who have undergone multiple revisions, may have extensive soft tissue deficits associated with the arthroplasty. Adequate coverage of the arthroplasty using reconstructive techniques is critical for successful management of the PJI, adequate joint function, and avoidance of amputation. Reconstructive techniques may also be helpful with the management of dead space, particularly with chronic hip PJI [82]. A close collaborative relationship with a plastic or reconstructive surgeon should be developed and the need for reconstructive surgery should be anticipated preoperatively.

Several techniques for soft tissue coverage have been described for use with arthroplasty infection. Free flap or microvascular tissue transfer involves complete detachment of the entire tissue along with its blood supply from the original location of the body and replacement at the location needing coverage. Circulation to the transferred tissue is reestablished at the recipient site using microsurgical techniques. In contrast, a pedicled or local flap leaves a pedicle of tissue with the blood supply intact at the donor site, with a transfer of the tissue to the recipient site. The choice of technique is complex and decided by the plastic surgeon based on the available tissues, blood supply, and coverage needed. Additional skin grafting techniques may be needed. Both free flap and pedicled techniques have been used with success with both knee PJI [83, 84] and hip PJI [82].

Conclusion

While there have been many improvements in the prevention of SSI after joint replacement, significant challenges remain. This chapter has outlined a number of practical strategies for optimization prior to and after joint replacement which may yield further reduction in SSI risk. There is excellent evidence to support smoking cessation, bacterial decolonization and perioperative antimicrobial prophylaxis. Further studies are warranted to delineate the impact in managing the nutritional status, obesity, and glucose control on SSI risk. As the prevalence of these modifiable risk factors rises, it will become increasingly important to develop coordinated, evidence based strategies to improve the delivery of these interventions in order to decrease the risk of SSI in patients undergoing joint arthroplasties.

References

1. CDC. National hospital discharge survey: 2010 table, procedures by selected patient characteristics. Available at: http://www.cdc.gov/nchs/data/nhds/4procedures/2010pro4_numberprocedureage.pdf. Accessed 18 Jan 2014.
2. Tande AJ, Patel R. Prosthetic joint infection. Clin Microbiol Rev. 2014;27(2):302–45.

3. Pruzansky JS, Bronson MJ, Grelsamer RP, Strauss E, Moucha CS. Prevalence of modifiable surgical site infection risk factors in hip and knee joint arthroplasty patients at an urban academic hospital. J Arthroplasty. 2014;29(2):272–6.
4. Yi PH, Frank RM, Vann E, Sonn KA, Moric M, Della Valle CJ. Is potential malnutrition associated with septic failure and acute infection after revision total joint arthroplasty? Clin Orthop Relat Res. 2015;473(1):175–82.
5. Zhu Y, Zhang F, Chen W, Liu S, Zhang Q, Zhang Y. Risk factors for periprosthetic joint infection after total joint arthroplasty: a systematic review and meta-analysis. J Hosp Infect. 2014;89:82–9 [Epub ahead of print].
6. Lavernia CJ, Sierra RJ, Baerga L. Nutritional parameters and short term outcome in arthroplasty. J Am Coll Nutr. 1999;18(3):274–8.
7. Huang R, Greenky M, Kerr GJ, Austin MS, Parvizi J. The effect of malnutrition on patients undergoing elective joint arthroplasty. J Arthroplasty. 2013;28(8 Suppl):21–4.
8. Berbari EF, Hanssen AD, Duffy MC, Steckelberg JM, Ilstrup DM, Harmsen WS, et al. Risk factors for prosthetic joint infection: case–control study. Clin Infect Dis. 1998;27(5):1247–54.
9. Marin LA, Salido JA, Lopez A, Silva A. Preoperative nutritional evaluation as a prognostic tool for wound healing. Acta Orthop Scand. 2002;73(1):2–5.
10. Berbari EF, Osmon DR, Lahr B, Eckel-Passow JE, Tsaras G, Hanssen AD, et al. The Mayo prosthetic joint infection risk score: implication for surgical site infection reporting and risk stratification. Infect Control Hosp Epidemiol. 2012;33(8):774–81.
11. Namba RS, Inacio MC, Paxton EW. Risk factors associated with surgical site infection in 30,491 primary total hip replacements. J Bone Joint Surg Br. 2012;94(10):1330–8.
12. Namba RS, Inacio MC, Paxton EW. Risk factors associated with deep surgical site infections after primary total knee arthroplasty: an analysis of 56,216 knees. J Bone Joint Surg Am. 2013;95(9):775–82.
13. Malinzak RA, Ritter MA, Berend ME, Meding JB, Olberding EM, Davis KE. Morbidly obese, diabetic, younger, and unilateral joint arthroplasty patients have elevated total joint arthroplasty infection rates. J Arthroplasty. 2009;24(6 Suppl):84–8.
14. Everhart JS, Altneu E, Calhoun JH. Medical comorbidities are independent preoperative risk factors for surgical infection after total joint arthroplasty. Clin Orthop Relat Res. 2013;471(10):3112–9.
15. Iorio R, Williams KM, Marcantonio AJ, Specht LM, Tilzey JF, Healy WL. Diabetes mellitus, hemoglobin A1C, and the incidence of total joint arthroplasty infection. J Arthroplasty. 2012;27(5):726–9 e1.
16. Peersman G, Laskin R, Davis J, Peterson M. Infection in total knee replacement: a retrospective review of 6489 total knee replacements. Clin Orthop. 2001;392:15–23.
17. Mraovic B, Suh D, Jacovides C, Parvizi J. Perioperative hyperglycemia and postoperative infection after lower limb arthroplasty. J Diabetes Sci Technol. 2011;5(2):412–8.
18. Seneviratne CJ, Yip JW, Chang JW, Zhang CF, Samaranayake LP. Effect of culture media and nutrients on biofilm growth kinetics of laboratory and clinical strains of Enterococcus faecalis. Arch Oral Biol. 2013;58:1327–34.
19. Stryker LS, Abdel MP, Morrey ME, Morrow MM, Kor DJ, Morrey BF. Elevated postoperative blood glucose and preoperative hemoglobin A1C are associated with increased wound complications following total joint arthroplasty. J Bone Joint Surg Am. 2013;95(9):808–14 S1-2.
20. Jamsen E, Nevalainen P, Kalliovalkama J, Moilanen T. Preoperative hyperglycemia predicts infected total knee replacement. Eur J Intern Med. 2010;21(3):196–201.
21. King Jr JT, Goulet JL, Perkal MF, Rosenthal RA. Glycemic control and infections in patients with diabetes undergoing noncardiac surgery. Ann Surg. 2011;253(1):158–65.
22. Buchleitner AM, Martinez-Alonso M, Hernandez M, Sola I, Mauricio D. Perioperative glycaemic control for diabetic patients undergoing surgery. Cochrane Database Syst Rev. 2012;9:CD007315.
23. Moller AM, Villebro N, Pedersen T, Tonnesen H. Effect of preoperative smoking intervention on postoperative complications: a randomised clinical trial. Lancet. 2002;359(9301):114–7.
24. Sorensen LT, Jorgensen S, Petersen LJ, Hemmingsen U, Bülow J, Loft S, et al. Acute effects of nicotine and smoking on blood flow, tissue oxygen, and aerobe metabolism of the skin and subcutis. J Surg Res. 2009;152(2):224–30.
25. Hopf HW, Hunt TK, West JM, Blomquist P, Goodson 3rd WH, Jensen JA, et al. Wound tissue oxygen tension predicts the risk of wound infection in surgical patients. Arch Surg. 1997;132(9):997–1004; discussion 5.
26. Thomsen T, Villebro N, Moller AM. Interventions for preoperative smoking cessation. Cochrane Database Syst Rev. 2014;3:CD002294.
27. Peel TN, Dowsey MM, Daffy JR, Stanley PA, Choong PF, Buising KL. Risk factors for prosthetic hip and knee infections according to arthroplasty site. J Hosp Infect. 2011;79(2):129–33.
28. Giles JT, Bartlett SJ, Gelber AC, Nanda S, Fontaine K, Ruffing V, et al. Tumor necrosis factor inhibitor therapy and risk of serious postoperative orthopedic infection in rheumatoid arthritis. Arthritis Rheum. 2006;55(2):333–7.
29. Momohara S, Kawakami K, Iwamoto T, Yano K, Sakuma Y, Hiroshima R, et al. Prosthetic joint infection after total hip or knee arthroplasty in rheumatoid arthritis patients treated with nonbiologic and biologic disease-modifying antirheumatic drugs. Mod Rheumatol. 2011;21(5):469–75.

30. Kawakami K, Ikari K, Kawamura K, Tsukahara S, Iwamoto T, Yano K, et al. Complications and features after joint surgery in rheumatoid arthritis patients treated with tumour necrosis factor-alpha blockers: perioperative interruption of tumour necrosis factor-alpha blockers decreases complications? Rheumatology (Oxford). 2010;49(2):341–7.
31. Ding T, Ledingham J, Luqmani R, Westlake S, Hyrich K, Lunt M, et al. BSR and BHPR rheumatoid arthritis guidelines on safety of anti-TNF therapies. Rheumatology (Oxford). 2010;49(11):2217–9.
32. Saag KG, Teng GG, Patkar NM, Anuntiyo J, Finney C, Curtis JR, et al. American College of Rheumatology 2008 recommendations for the use of nonbiologic and biologic disease-modifying antirheumatic drugs in rheumatoid arthritis. Arthritis Rheum. 2008;59(6):762–84.
33. Pieringer H, Stuby U, Biesenbach G. Patients with rheumatoid arthritis undergoing surgery: how should we deal with antirheumatic treatment? Semin Arthritis Rheum. 2007;36(5):278–86.
34. Grennan DM, Gray J, Loudon J, Fear S. Methotrexate and early postoperative complications in patients with rheumatoid arthritis undergoing elective orthopaedic surgery. Ann Rheum Dis. 2001;60(3):214–7.
35. Akkara Veetil BM, Bongartz T. Perioperative care for patients with rheumatic diseases. Nat Rev Rheumatol. 2012;8(1):32–41.
36. Fuerst M, Mohl H, Baumgartel K, Ruther W. Leflunomide increases the risk of early healing complications in patients with rheumatoid arthritis undergoing elective orthopedic surgery. Rheumatol Int. 2006;26(12):1138–42.
37. Tanaka N, Sakahashi H, Sato E, Hirose K, Ishima T, Ishii S. Examination of the risk of continuous leflunomide treatment on the incidence of infectious complications after joint arthroplasty in patients with rheumatoid arthritis. J Clin Rheumatol. 2003;9(2):115–8.
38. Rozman B. Clinical pharmacokinetics of leflunomide. Clin Pharmacokinet. 2002;41(6):421–30.
39. Perhala RS, Wilke WS, Clough JD, Segal AM. Local infectious complications following large joint replacement in rheumatoid arthritis patients treated with methotrexate versus those not treated with methotrexate. Arthritis Rheum. 1991;34(2):146–52.
40. Kasdan ML, June L. Postoperative results of rheumatoid arthritis patients on methotrexate at the time of reconstructive surgery of the hand. Orthopedics. 1993;16(11):1233–5.
41. Jain A, Witbreuk M, Ball C, Nanchahal J. Influence of steroids and methotrexate on wound complications after elective rheumatoid hand and wrist surgery. J Hand Surg Am. 2002;27(3):449–55.
42. Sany J, Anaya JM, Canovas F, Combe B, Jorgensen C, Saker S, et al. Influence of methotrexate on the frequency of postoperative infectious complications in patients with rheumatoid arthritis. J Rheumatol. 1993;20(7):1129–32.
43. Carpenter MT, West SG, Vogelgesang SA, Casey Jones DE. Postoperative joint infections in rheumatoid arthritis patients on methotrexate therapy. Orthopedics. 1996;19(3):207–10.
44. Bridges Jr SL, Lopez-Mendez A, Han KH, Tracy IC, Alarcon GS. Should methotrexate be discontinued before elective orthopedic surgery in patients with rheumatoid arthritis? J Rheumatol. 1991;18(7):984–8.
45. Smitten AL, Choi HK, Hochberg MC, Suissa S, Simon TA, Testa MA, et al. The risk of hospitalized infection in patients with rheumatoid arthritis. J Rheumatol. 2008;35(3):387–93.
46. Stuck AE, Minder CE, Frey FJ. Risk of infectious complications in patients taking glucocorticosteroids. Rev Infect Dis. 1989;11(6):954–63.
47. Bode LG, Kluytmans JA, Wertheim HF, Bogaers D, Vandenbroucke-Grauls CM, Roosendaal R, et al. Preventing surgical-site infections in nasal carriers of Staphylococcus aureus. N Engl J Med. 2010;362(1): 9–17.
48. Chen AF, Heyl AE, Xu PZ, Rao N, Klatt BA. Preoperative decolonization effective at reducing staphylococcal colonization in total joint arthroplasty patients. J Arthroplasty. 2013;28(8 Suppl):18–20.
49. Chen AF, Wessel CB, Rao N. Staphylococcus aureus screening and decolonization in orthopaedic surgery and reduction of surgical site infections. Clin Orthop. 2013;471(7):2383–99.
50. Bratzler DW, Dellinger EP, Olsen KM, Perl TM, Auwaerter PG, Bolon MK, et al. Clinical practice guidelines for antimicrobial prophylaxis in surgery. Am J Health Syst Pharm. 2013;70(3):195–283.
51. Phillips M, Rosenberg A, Shopsin B, Cuff G, Skeete F, Foti A, et al. Preventing surgical site infections: a randomized, open-label trial of nasal mupirocin ointment and nasal povidone-iodine solution. Infect Control Hosp Epidemiol. 2014;35(7):826–32.
52. Huang SS, Septimus E, Kleinman K, Moody J, Hickok J, Avery TR, et al. Targeted versus universal decolonization to prevent ICU infection. N Engl J Med. 2013;368(24):2255–65.
53. Perl TM, Cullen JJ, Wenzel RP, Zimmerman MB, Pfaller MA, Sheppard D, et al. Intranasal mupirocin to prevent postoperative Staphylococcus aureus infections. N Engl J Med The. 2002;346(24):1871–7.
54. Berbari EF, Osmon DR, Carr A, Hanssen AD, Baddour LM, Greene D, et al. Dental procedures as risk factors for prosthetic hip or knee infection: a hospital-based prospective case–control study. Clin Infect Dis. 2010;50(1):8–16.
55. Bouvet C, Lubbeke A, Bandi C, Pagani L, Stern R, Hoffmeyer P, et al. Is there any benefit in pre-operative urinary analysis before elective total joint replacement? Bone Joint J. 2014;96-B(3):390–4.
56. Cordero-Ampuero J, Gonzalez-Fernandez E, Martinez-Velez D, Esteban J. Are antibiotics necessary in hip arthroplasty with asymptomatic bacteriuria? Seeding risk with/without treatment. Clin Orthop. 2013;471:3822–9.
57. Glynn MK, Sheehan JM. The significance of asymptomatic bacteriuria in patients undergoing hip/knee arthroplasty. Clin Orthop. 1984;185:151–4.

58. Sousa R, Munoz-Mahamud E, Quayle J, Dias da Costa L, Casals C, Scott P, et al. Is asymptomatic bacteriuria a risk factor for prosthetic joint infection? Clin Infect Dis. 2014;59(1):41–7.
59. Gou W, Chen J, Jia Y, Wang Y. Preoperative asymptomatic leucocyturia and early prosthetic joint infections in patients undergoing joint arthroplasty. J Arthroplasty. 2014;29(3):473–6.
60. AlBuhairan B, Hind D, Hutchinson A. Antibiotic prophylaxis for wound infections in total joint arthroplasty: a systematic review. J Bone Joint Surg Br. 2008;90(7):915–9.
61. Meter JJ, Polly Jr DW, Brueckner RP, Tenuta JJ, Asplund L, Hopkinson WJ. Effect of intraoperative blood loss on the serum level of cefazolin in patients managed with total hip arthroplasty. A prospective, controlled study. J Bone Joint Surg Am. 1996;78(8):1201–5.
62. Yamada K, Matsumoto K, Tokimura F, Okazaki H, Tanaka S. Are bone and serum cefazolin concentrations adequate for antimicrobial prophylaxis? Clin Orthop Relat Res. 2011;469(12):3486–94.
63. Gulihar A, Nixon M, Jenkins D, Taylor GJ. Clostridium difficile in hip fracture patients: prevention, treatment and associated mortality. Injury. 2009;40(7):746–51.
64. Park M, Markus P, Matesic D, Li JT. Safety and effectiveness of a preoperative allergy clinic in decreasing vancomycin use in patients with a history of penicillin allergy. Ann Allergy Asthma Immunol. 2006;97(5):681–7.
65. Gupta K, Strymish J, Abi-Haidar Y, Williams SA, Itani KM. Preoperative nasal methicillin-resistant Staphylococcus aureus status, surgical prophylaxis, and risk-adjusted postoperative outcomes in veterans. Infect Control Hosp Epidemiol. 2011;32(8):791–6.
66. Bull AL, Worth LJ, Richards MJ. Impact of vancomycin surgical antibiotic prophylaxis on the development of methicillin-sensitive staphylococcus aureus surgical site infections: report from Australian Surveillance Data (VICNISS). Ann Surg. 2012;256(6):1089–92.
67. Sewick A, Makani A, Wu C, O'Donnell J, Baldwin KD, Lee GC. Does dual antibiotic prophylaxis better prevent surgical site infections in total joint arthroplasty? Clin Orthop. 2012;470(10):2702–7.
68. Courtney PM, Melnic CM, Zimmer Z, Anari J, Lee G. Addition of vancomycin to cefazolin prophylaxis is associated with acute kidney injury after primary joint arthroplasty. Clin Orthop. 2014;473:2197–203.
69. Forse RA, Karam B, MacLean LD, Christou NV. Antibiotic prophylaxis for surgery in morbidly obese patients. Surgery. 1989;106(4):750–6; discussion 6–7.
70. Edmiston CE, Krepel C, Kelly H, Larson J, Andris D, Hennen C, et al. Perioperative antibiotic prophylaxis in the gastric bypass patient: do we achieve therapeutic levels? Surgery. 2004;136(4):738–47.
71. Cunha BA, Gossling HR, Pasternak HS, Nightingale CH, Quintiliani R. The penetration characteristics of cefazolin, cephalothin, and cephradine into bone in patients undergoing total hip replacement. J Bone Joint Surg Am. 1977;59(7):856–9.
72. Steinberg JP, Braun BI, Hellinger WC, Kusek L, Bozikis MR, Bush AJ, et al. Timing of antimicrobial prophylaxis and the risk of surgical site infections: results from the Trial to Reduce Antimicrobial Prophylaxis Errors. Ann Surg. 2009;250(1):10–6.
73. van Kasteren ME, Mannien J, Ott A, Kullberg BJ, de Boer AS, Gyssens IC. Antibiotic prophylaxis and the risk of surgical site infections following total hip arthroplasty: timely administration is the most important factor. Clin Infect Dis. 2007;44(7):921–7.
74. Bicanic G, Crnogaca K, Barbaric K, Delimar D. Cefazolin should be administered maximum 30 min before incision in total knee arthroplasty when tourniquet is used. Med Hypotheses. 2014;82(6):766–8.
75. Soriano A, Bori G, Garcia-Ramiro S, Martinez-Pastor JC, Miana T, Codina C, et al. Timing of antibiotic prophylaxis for primary total knee arthroplasty performed during ischemia. Clin Infect Dis. 2008;46(7):1009–14.
76. Swoboda SM, Merz C, Kostuik J, Trentler B, Lipsett PA. Does intraoperative blood loss affect antibiotic serum and tissue concentrations? Arch Surg. 1996;131(11):1165–71; discussion 71–2.
77. Starks I, Ayub G, Walley G, Orendi J, Roberts P, Maffulli N. Single-dose cefuroxime with gentamicin reduces Clostridium difficile-associated disease in hip-fracture patients. J Hosp Infect. 2008;70(1):21–6.
78. Gillespie WJ, Walenkamp GH. Antibiotic prophylaxis for surgery for proximal femoral and other closed long bone fractures. Cochrane Database Syst Rev. 2010;(3):CD000244.
79. Southwell-Keely JP, Russo RR, March L, Cumming R, Cameron I, Brnabic AJ. Antibiotic prophylaxis in hip fracture surgery: a metaanalysis. Clin Orthop Relat Res. 2004;419:179–84.
80. Parvizi J, Ghanem E, Joshi A, Sharkey PF, Hozack WJ, Rothman RH. Does "excessive" anticoagulation predispose to periprosthetic infection? J Arthroplasty. 2007;22(6 Suppl 2):24–8.
81. Holbrook A, Schulman S, Witt DM, Vandvik PO, Fish J, Kovacs MJ, et al. Evidence-based management of anticoagulant therapy: Antithrombotic Therapy and Prevention of Thrombosis, 9th ed: American College of Chest Physicians Evidence-Based Clinical Practice Guidelines. Chest. 2012;141(2 Suppl):e152S–84.
82. Jones NF, Eadie P, Johnson PC, Mears DC. Treatment of chronic infected hip arthroplasty wounds by radical debridement and obliteration with pedicled and free muscle flaps. Plast Reconstr Surg. 1991;88(1):95–101.
83. Manoso MW, Boland PJ, Healey JH, Cordeiro PG. Limb salvage of infected knee reconstructions for cancer with staged revision and free tissue transfer. Ann Plast Surg. 2006;56(5):532–5; discussion 5.
84. Suda AJ, Cieslik A, Grutzner PA, Munzberg M, Heppert V. Flaps for closure of soft tissue defects in infected revision knee arthroplasty. Int Orthop. 2014;38(7):1387–92.

Part VIII

Long-Term Perspectives

Changing Paradigms: Long-Term Perspectives

27

Michael Parry and Clive P. Duncan

Abstract

Whilst lower limb arthroplasty has proven to be a highly efficacious intervention in the treatment of end-stage arthritis of both hip and knee, periprosthetic joint infection can be a devastating complication for the patient and a challenge for those charged with its treatment. Much attention has focused on the surgical and medical management of this complication with outcomes measured in the short term and defined by the recurrence of infection. However, there has been little focus on the long-term effects on the patient both in terms of morbidity and mortality, as well as the long-term function of the revised prosthesis. This chapter aims to review the available evidence in each of these areas identifying, where possible, the long-term effects of periprosthetic joint infection. We have aimed to focus on the morbidity and function of patients treated for periprosthetic joint infections of the hip and knee, as well as the mortality associated with periprosthetic joint infection, concentrating on the outcomes measured in the long term rather than the efficacy of different methods of treatment.

Keywords

Periprosthetic joint infection • Morbidity • Mortality • Functional outcome • Long-term survival • Patient-reported outcome measures

M. Parry, BSC, MBCHB, PGCME, MD, FRCS (✉)
Department of Oncology and Complex Arthroplasty, Royal Orthopaedic Hospital, Birmingham, UK
e-mail: michael.parry3@nhs.net

C.P. Duncan, MB, MSc, FRCSC
Department of Orthopaedics, Vancouver General and University Hospitals, University of British Columbia, Vancouver, BC, Canada
e-mail: cpduncan@gmail.com

Introduction

Total joint arthroplasty of both the hip and knee has evolved to become not only one of the most frequently performed, but also one of the most successful in terms of improving function [1, 2] with high levels of patient satisfaction and cost effectiveness [3, 4]. However, whilst uncommon, periprosthetic joint infection (PJI) remains a

D. Kendoff et al. (eds.), *Periprosthetic Joint Infections: Changing Paradigms*,
DOI 10.1007/978-3-319-30091-7_27

devastating complication for the patient [5] and continues to challenge those involved with their treatment [1] (Fig. 27.1).

PJI places a significant economic and logistic burden on those institutions responsible for their care [6, 7], and with the demand for total hip arthroplasty (THA) and total knee arthroplasty (TKA) projected to increase significantly in the coming years [8], it is expected that the demand on units treating those with PJI will also increase.

Whilst much focus has been directed at the management of PJI, particularly with respects to the surgical approach and the use of single stage or two stage revisions [9, 10], there remains a relative paucity of information on the long term outcomes for patients treated for PJI of the hip or knee. Whilst the focus on outcomes has largely revolved around reinfection, the effect on function, morbidity and mortality has been somewhat overlooked with very little evidence available in the literature measuring these outcomes. Indeed, what limited evidence that does exist suggests that even when infection is eradicated, function is often compromised when compared to non-infected primary arthroplasties.

The aim of this chapter, therefore, is to explore the long-term perspectives and outcomes following PJI of the hip and knee to investigate what effect this potentially devastating complication has on patient and implant survival and function whilst also identifying long term outcomes in terms of reinfection and antibiotic use.

Mortality Following Periprosthetic Joint Infection

The impact of PJI on patient mortality is, of course, multi-factorial and takes into consideration patient co-morbidity and the impact of repetitive surgery and anaesthesia. The effect of PJI on mortality in both the short-term and long-term has been dem-

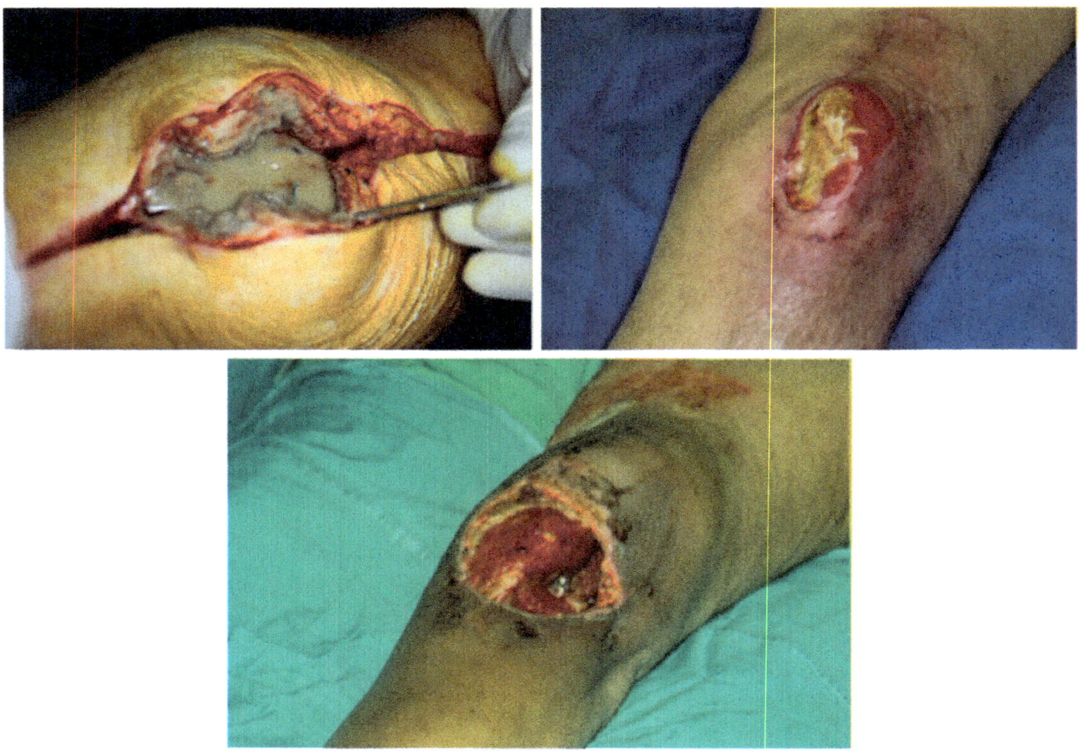

Fig. 27.1 Whilst it thankfully remains a rare complication, infection following lower limb arthroplasty can have devastating effect on the patient and presents a distinct challenge to those responsible for its management

onstrated [11]. It should come as little surprise to find that PJI results in a significant increase in mortality at 90-days, 1-year, 2-years and 5-years, when compared to patients undergoing revision for aseptic causes. When controlling for confounding variables such as patient age, gender, comorbidities, the number of surgical procedures [including single versus two-stage revision], or joint involved, PJI is associated with a five-fold increased risk of death in comparison to revision for non-infective causes [11]. Mortality rates during or following treatment for PJI are often buried within outcomes that report principally, the rates of reinfection or eradication of infection with a treatment algorithm. Berend et al. [12] reported the mortality in association with a two-stage approach for PJI of the hip. A 7 % 90-day mortality was noted after the first-stage procedure with 4 % dying prior to reimplantation. 45 % of patients had died at an average of 4.7 years after treatment, which increased to 50 % in cases of recurrent infection, which is consistent with the 25.8 % rate of mortality within 2 years demonstrated by Toulson et al. [13]. This is higher than reported by others and most likely reflects the longer duration of follow up [14–18].

When comparing one-stage with two-stage revision approaches, there is little evidence to support one over the other in terms of mortality [19, 20]. However, there are obviously a number of confounding variables in each of these approaches. The chosen surgical approach will depend on not only the patient but also the condition of the soft tissue envelope, the degree of bone stock loss, the infecting organism and the facilities available to manage the administration of antibiotics over a prolonged period. In a meta-analysis of the literature examining the reported results of the two-stage exchange compared with a single-stage exchange, Wolf et al. [21] using a Markov decision analysis model, concluded that although a two-stage approach resulted in a greater likelihood of eradication of infection, it also yielded a greater chance of death compared with a single-stage exchange.

The effect of the infecting organism on mortality is demonstrated by the higher rate of death in those treated for resistant organisms when compared to sensitive organisms. Nixon et al. [22] demonstrated that in patients treated for fractures of the femoral shaft, infection with methicillin resistant Staphylococcus aureus (MRSA) was associated with a doubling in the risk of mortality at 1-year. Leung et al. [23] reported a mortality rate of 24 % in patients treated by two-stage revision for PJI due to MRSA at a mean follow-up of 5-years. A significant increase in mortality at 1-year is seen in patients with PJI due to MRSA when compared to those infected by methicillin sensitive Staphylococcus aureus [MSSA] [11], once again highlighting the dismal outcome associated with MRSA PJI [24].

The effect of polymicrobial infection and infection with gram negative organisms also places a higher risk of death on patients [11], which may be a function of increasing age [25, 26] and poor overall health. Indeed, infection by gram-negative organisms is associated with a low success of eradication by two-stage revision due to a high rate of death (26 %) prior to reimplantation [27].

The question remains: is the increased incidence of death in association with PJI a function of poor health status? The risk factors for PJI have been extensively investigated and include male gender, advancing age, obesity, increased number of comorbidities and knee arthroplasty [7, 28–30]. Many of these risk factors may at least in part explain the increased mortality seen following PJI, though this notion was not supported by Zmistowski et al. [11] who identified PJI as a significant predictor of mortality, having controlled for these risk factors. The authors did, however, highlight independent predictors of mortality as advanced age, multiple comorbidities, cardiac disease, and cerebrovascular disease though multiple surgical procedures were not associated with an increased mortality, presumably because patients undergoing multiple procedures were of a higher level of general health. Whilst it would be easy to attribute patient factors to the incidence of PJI, and secondarily relate the increased mortality seen in such patients to their underlying state of health, this does appear to only partly explain the picture. Conventional teaching tells us that there are multiple patient, surgical and extraneous factors that can increase the risk of developing a PJI. However, to attribute these same factors to the detrimental effect on survival appears to only partly explain these findings.

There is no doubt that undergoing treatment for PJI increases the risk of mortality. This increased mortality is not only a reflection of a decreased health status amongst patients, but appears also to be a direct effect of PJI itself. Whilst much effort has been directed towards improving the diagnosis of PJI, as well as controlling infections, reducing their incidence and honing strategies in their management, this should not come at the expense of a tight control on chronic disease. There appears little doubt that perioperative optimization of nutrition, smoking and general health status will result in a reduction in PJI and a concurrent fall in mortality associated with its incidence and treatment.

Function Following Periprosthetic Joint Infection

As with mortality, function following treatment for PJI tends to take a backseat to other outcome measures such as reinfection, when looking at the outcomes of treatment. However, whilst achieving a functional, painless joint is the aim of any revision procedure, the measurement of patient reported or functional outcomes when applied to PJI seems secondary to eradication of infection, despite the importance placed on these measures when applied to other revisions [31].

When assessing functional outcomes following PJI, a number of factors must be taken into consideration. These include the joint, the management strategy and whether this includes an articulating or non-articulating spacer in the case of a two-stage revision, success in eradication of infection, and patient functional requirements, a composite function of age, gender, demand and expectation (Fig. 27.2). Needless to say, the evidence relating to these outcomes are disparate and difficult to compare.

In an attempt to assess the function following revision for infection following single or two-stage revision at both the hip and knee, there have been a number of reports using as breadth of differing functional and patient reported outcome measures. Jamsen et al. [32] in an attempt to identify superiority of either a single-stage or two-stage approach to revision, reported on 25 series looking at outcomes following each approach. Postoperative function was reported in 20 of the included studies, whilst postoperative range of motion was reported in 23. The range of follow-up for included studies, however, ranged from an average of 12–90 months. Comparison of outcomes was complicated by the disparity in outcome measures utilized, though most commonly, Knee Society or Hospital for Special Surgery Score was used. Functional outcomes were no different between approaches but the highest range of motion was seen with two-stage revision with an articulating spacer. Castelli et al. [33] reported function using the Knee Society Score (KSS) at a median follow up of 7 years following two-stage revision for PJI of the knee. The KSS improved from 35.4 (clinical) and 37.96 (functional) at presentation, to 75.38 (clinical) and 80.58 (functional) post reimplantation. Freeman et al. [34] assessing static versus articulating spacers for two-stage revision of PJI of the knee demonstrated no difference between the two implants at final reimplantation, in terms of pain scores, though the articulating spacer group demonstrated better function in the long term. High levels of function, as measured by the Oxford Knee Score and WOMAC, and patient satisfaction have been reported with two-stage revision using an articulating spacer [35–37]. These findings are supported by others who demonstrate an improvement in validated knee outcome scores between pre-revision and definitive reimplantation following two-stage revision [38–45], or a single stage strategy [46]. It should be noted, however, that a consistent feature is that function is reliant on eradication of infection. Whichever measure is used, a consistent feature is for lower scores in the small subsets of patients in whom reinfection occurs, or infection is not eradicated by two-stage revision.

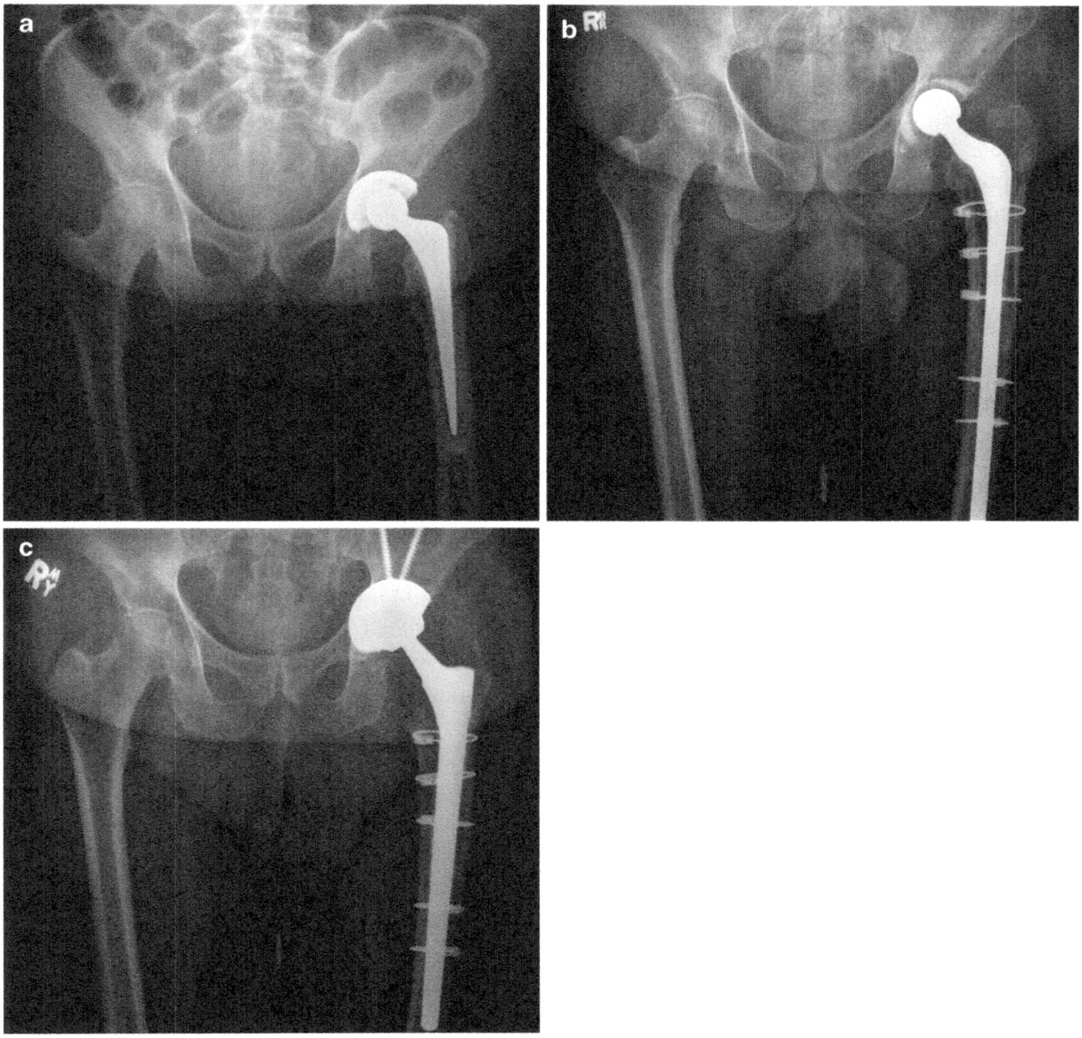

Fig. 27.2 The case of a 76-year-old patient presenting with a late haematogenous periprosthetic joint infection of the left hip (**a**), following successful THA 9 years previously. The patient was treated by two-stage revision with removal of the implant assisted by an extended trochanteric osteotomy and insertion of a temporary antibiotic loaded articulating spacer (**b**). The second stage was completed following a 3-month course of intravenous antibiotics and confirmation of infection by haematogenous markers and aspirate from the hip prior to reinsertion of an uncemented revision hip replacement (**c**). The patient remained free of infection for the remainder of their life but their function was inferior to their initial THA. The patient ambulated with a single stick, a deterioration from their initial post arthroplasty function

Does infection affect the range of motion at a total knee arthroplasty? It would seem logical to suggest that range of motion would be reduced by the presence of infection and should improve following eradication of infection. Gooding et al. [35] demonstrated an improvement in mean knee flexion following two-stage revision from 86.2° to 93.2 post reimplantation, a finding supported by others [36, 43, 45]. However, this is not always the case. Hirakawa et al. [39] in fact demonstrated a reduction in final range of movement after final reimplantation, presumably a product of repeated surgical intervention. With the limited evidence available, the final range of motion does not appear to be improved by a single stage strategy, with flexion comparable between these two approaches [46, 47].

Functional outcome following revision for PJI of the hip follows a similar trend. Whilst there is a great wealth of evidence advocating strategies and defining success in terms of reinfection, measurable functional outcomes are often missing. In their meta analysis of patient reported outcomes following revision hip surgery, Saleh et al. [48] reported improvements in Harris Hip Score [HHS] in 28 studies including both pre and post operative scores, and 18 studies measuring outcome by Global Hip Score, though it should be noted that the indication for revision was not described. Oussedik et al. [49] reported an improvement in HHS between pre operation and 5-years post operation for both single and two-stage revision of the hip, with significant with patients treated by one-stage revision faring better than the two-stage group. The authors also demonstrated an improvement over 5-years in visual analogue scale with improvements significantly higher in the one-stage group. De Man et al. [50] demonstrated improvements in HHS for both one-stage and two-stage revision THA, with one-stage demonstrating only a 4 point better improvement than the two-stage approach. This compares favorably to the reports of others who have demonstrated a mean post operative HHS ranging from 72 to 91 [51, 52]. A consistent feature of these reports is that those who suffer incomplete eradication of infection or in whom reinfection occurs demonstrate poor outcome in terms of function when compared to those in whom infection is successfully treated.

Treatment options for those who have failed multiple previous attempts at infection control are limited to antibiotic suppression, fusion, amputation or resection arthroplasty. Whilst surgical intervention in the management of PJI is often considered the gold standard for management in amenable situations, does conservative treatment confer an improved functional outcome? One would expect that not operating would result in an improved outcome, as patients are not subjected to further surgery. However, medical treatment of PJI, most often on the background of poor host conditioning preventing surgery without significant risk to life, often subjects patients to pain and disability in due to the presence of chronic infection [53]. Often this approach can be combined with initial limited surgical intervention and whilst success in terms of control of infection defined by the relief of pain and continued function can often be achieved [54], patients often find long term antibiotic therapy unsatisfactory. No real evidence exists on the functional outcome following this approach as often these patients number only a few amongst larger series making comparison difficult, and this conservative approach is often only favored in those who would not tolerate more aggressive, definitive surgical treatment.

For patients in whom long-term suppression is not appropriate as a result of risk to life from uncontrolled infection, but in whom aggressive reconstruction is not deemed appropriate, resection arthroplasty with removal of the prosthesis and all foreign material may be considered. Whilst this approach has demonstrated good results in terms of eradication of infection, it is associated with very poor function, to unacceptable levels in some instances [55–57].

When all else has failed, options for control of infection are reliant on either arthrodesis or amputation, in the form of above knee amputation (AKA) in the case of PJI of the knee, or hip disarticulation in the case of the hip, though this is often only reserved for life threatening infection or periprosthetic infection on the background of massive bone loss or megaprosthesis reconstruction. Arthrodesis of the knee remains a reasonable option as it retains the leg as a stable platform for ambulation (Fig. 27.3). If successful in eradicating infection, patients with knee arthrodesis are often able to perform strenuous physical tasks, though the loss of motion at the knee makes sitting difficult [58].

When comparing arthrodesis of the knee with AKA as salvage for failed revision on the background of PJI of the knee, AKA demonstrates a higher energy consumption for ambulation than arthrodesis [59, 60] and also have a reduced capacity for ambulation [59, 60]. Chen et al. [61] compared the ambulatory status as well as physical and mental function in patients undergoing AKA or arthrodesis following failure of treatment for PJI of the knee. Arthrodesis was associated with a higher degree of community ambulation, a feature demonstrated by others [62–64]. Patients undergoing arthrodesis also demonstrate higher mental and physical function when compared to those undergoing AKA [65, 66].

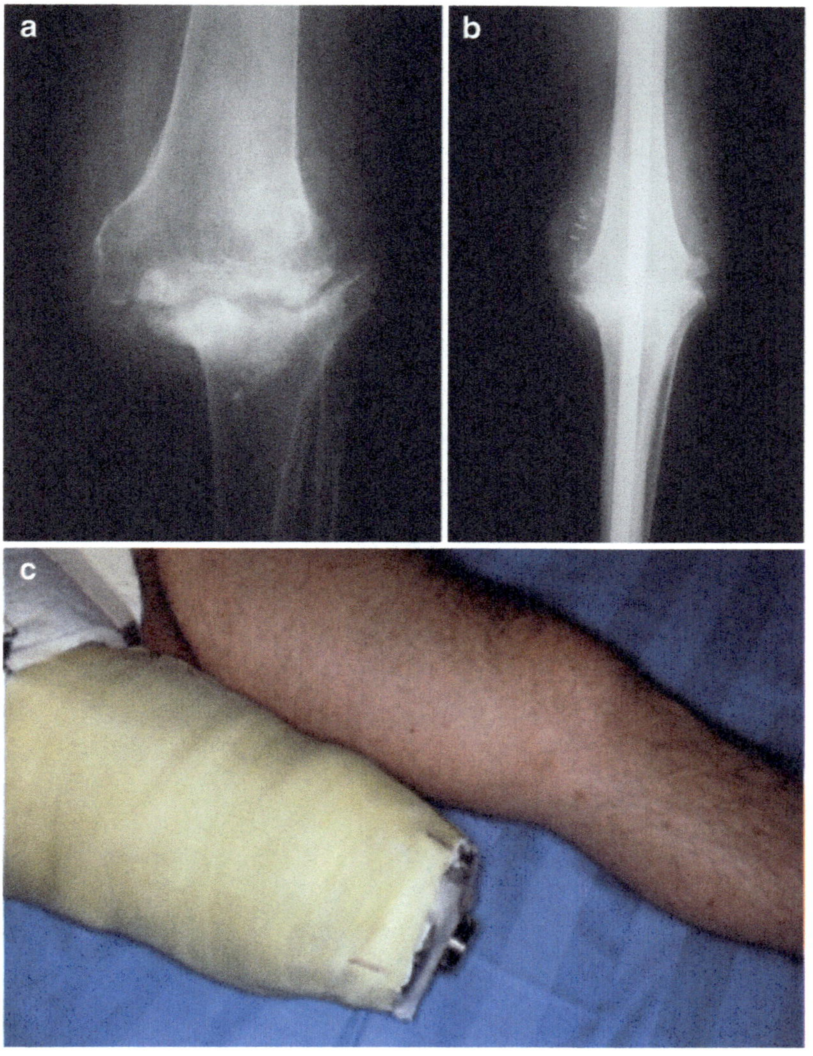

Fig. 27.3 What to do when repeated revision has failed to eradicate infection? Resection arthroplasty and pseudarthrosis (**a**) appears to be associated with a poor function and low levels of patient satisfaction, whilst arthrodesis (**b**) allows the patient to retain the limb and in many cases, return to a good level of function. However, these outcomes are reliant on the eradication of infection, and if this fails the patient is left with the only option, an amputation (**c**), which is associated with a low level of function

When considering salvage options for failed eradication of infection at the knee, the improved mental and physical function, as well as the likelihood of improvements in ambulation following arthrodesis should translate into consideration of this technique in appropriately selected patients. However, this should be tempered by social and cultural considerations where such procedures are not acceptable and chronic suppression may be considered a more appropriate strategy.

Long-Term Outcomes

As previously mentioned, extensive research has gone into trying to define the best surgical treatment option for the management of PJI of the hip or knee (Fig. 27.4), with efforts concentrated on which surgical strategy affords a better rate of eradication of infection. With respects to the knee, rates of reinfection, or treatment failure with a two-stage approach range from 3 to 28 %

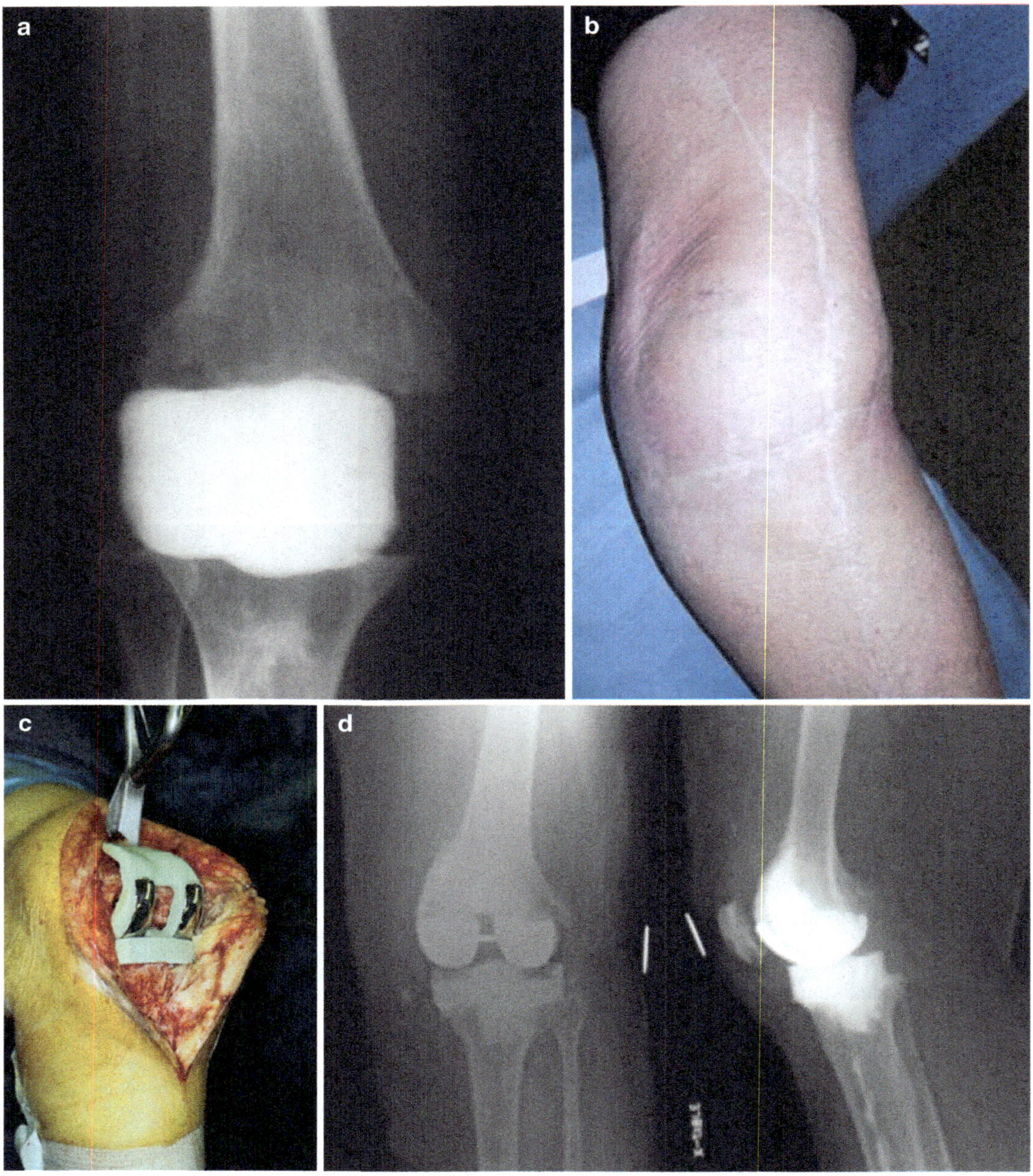

Fig. 27.4 Options for spacers in two-stage revision rely on either a static antibiotic-loaded cement spacer (**a**), which often results in joint stiffness and instability (**b**), or an articulating antibiotic spacer (**c**), which is associated with greater stability and flexibility in the joint (**d**) when it comes to the second-stage reimplantation

across a range of follow up from 24 months to 17 years [19]. Reinfection rates following a single stage approach vary between 0 and 11 % for a follow up period of 12 months to 10 years [46, 47, 67, 68]. With respects to the hip, pooled data suggest a reinfection rate of 8.6 % at a minimum of 2 years for a one-stage approach, and 10.2 % for a two-stage strategy [20, 69]. Significant selection bias exists in the studies included in these meta-analyses making direct comparison difficult. Poor host condition, infection by resistant strains, or unknown pathogens, and significant bone loss or poor soft tissues often pushes surgeons towards the more tried and tested two-stage approach, skewing the final outcome of reinfection in favour of the one-stage approach.

When looking towards the long term, outcomes can be defined in terms of re-infection or failure of the reconstruction. In their long term follow up study of 253 patients with PJI of the knee, Mahmud et al. [41] aimed to identify the fate of patients who failed two-stage revision. The authors demonstrated a rate of infection control of 78 % at 10 years, comparable to others [38, 70]. Over this duration of follow up, patients demonstrated an improvement in functional and patient reported outcome measures, reliant on an eradication of infection. For those that failed the two-stage approach, including those who underwent repeated two-stage revision; treatment comprised either chronic antibiotic suppression or arthrodesis. Patients treated by chronic antibiotic suppression fared poorly in the long term necessitating arthrodesis in 25 %, a feature demonstrated by others [71–73]. This strategy serves only to suppress the infection rather than eradicate it and therefore, should be reserved only for those in whom further surgical intervention is either not desirable or carries significant risk of peri-operative mortality.

Surgical options for treatment of failed revision arthroplasty at the knee for infection are therefore limited to either arthrodesis or amputation. Mahmud et al. [41] reported in their 16 failed two-stage revisions at 10 years, 1 arthrodesis requiring additional antibiotic suppression, 1 successful arthrodesis and 3 AKA. Hanssen et al. [74] described their management of 24 patients treated for failed control of PJI of the knee. 10 were treated successfully with arthrodesis, 5 with chronic antibiotic suppression, 4 above knee amputations, 4 persistent pseudarthroses, 1 resection arthroplasty, and one uninfected prosthesis after reimplantation.

For those implants where infection is successfully eradicated by revision surgery, what is the effect on implant survival in the long term? Haleem et al. [38] identified a comparable implant survival due to aseptic failure as was seen for septic failure following revision for PJI of the knee. Survivorship of TKA implants, free of infection was 93.5 % at 5 years and 85 % at 10 years, whilst survival free of revision for mechanical failure was 96.2 % at 5 years and 91 % at 10 years. This rate of failure at mid to long term follow up is often attributable to failure of fixation, particularly when using uncemented stems, and emphasizes the importance of sound fixation of implants at the second-stage, or at the time of exchange arthroplasty. Whilst the numbers are too small to assess the effect of implant fixation, failure rates for cemented revision prostheses may differ to those for uncemented prostheses whilst conferring the advantage of antibiotic loaded cement. Hybrid fixation of implants at reimplantation may, of course, confer the best of both worlds.

When assessing long-term outcomes following revision for PJI at the hip, the story is similar. Sanchez-Sotelo et al. [75] assessed mid to long-term survival following revision for infection of hip arthroplasty by staged revision with a number of different prostheses. At a mean follow up of 7 years, the rate of reinfection was 7.1 %, which compared to a rate of revision for mechanical failure of 14.2 %. However, at 10 years, the rate of survival free of infection was 87.5 %, and revision free survival for mechanical failure was 75.2 %. As with all studies looking at long-term survivorship, the numbers are often small making meaningful conclusion difficult. A breadth of strategies and implants are included reflecting the change in implant design over time. For example, historically, reimplantation following treatment of infection has relied on cemented fixation, at least for the femoral component, as the use of antibiotic loaded cement was thought to reduce the risk of subsequent reinfection [76], which, by extrapolation, was thought to account for the relatively high rates of reinfection seen following reimplantation using early designs of uncemented femoral components [77]. More recently, however, the use of contemporary designs of uncemented femoral components at reimplantation have been associated with acceptable rates of reinfection, at least in the mid term [78]. Masri et al. [79] reported a reinfection rate of 10.3 % following staged reimplantation with an interval articulating spacer in 29 patients, and an uncemented femoral component. No patients required revision for mechanical failure of the prosthesis at a mean of 4 years, which reflects the improvements made in implant design, particularly around fixation of uncemented femoral prostheses.

The trend for mechanical failure to mirror rates of failure due to reinfection following revision for PJI of the hip reinforces the need for surgeons to achieve sound fixation at the reimplantation stage, whether that be with a single or two-stage approach.

Conclusion

Infection following prosthetic joint replacement remains a devastating complication. Whilst the arthroplasty burden will continue to increase as the population expands and ages, so the infection burden will continue to increase. This coupled with the continued march of multi-drug resistant pathogens will inevitably result in a new set of challenges placed on those charged with the treatment of PJI. Whilst much emphasis has been placed on the outcomes of various treatment strategies, there has been little focus on the impact of PJI and its treatment on patient function, implant survival and ultimately, patient survival. Revision for septic failure presents a raft of challenges to the operating surgeon, not only reliant on eradication of infection, but also on the effective fixation of revision components to often compromised and deficient bone and soft tissue. This translates to inferior implant survival at mid to long term for revision components implanted for the treatment of PJI. There is convincing evidence that, whilst PJI presents challenges to the surgeon, it places an excess mortality on those suffering the infection, above and beyond that expected for patients undergoing prostheses revision for aseptic failure. The reasons for this are, of course, multiple and demonstrate the complex interaction between patient, surgical and pathogenic factors. As time moves on and the projected incidence of PJI continues to rise, it is expected that there will be a resurgence of interventions, often considered historical. In particular, it is expected that the need for more aggressive solutions to recalcitrant infections, including arthrodesis at the knee, and amputation either above knee or through hip disarticulation, will increase. With respects to arthrodesis, if infection can be eradicated and union achieved, this certainly offers a functional advantage over amputation. However, it should be noted that whether prosthesis retention, limb salvage, limb sacrifice or chronic suppression is chosen as the definitive solution, functional benefits are only conferred through infection control and avoidance of repeated surgical intervention.

References

1. Ethgen O, Bruyère O, Richy F, Dardennes C, Reginster J-Y. Health-related quality of life in total hip and total knee arthroplasty: a qualitative and systematic review of the literature. J Bone Joint Surg Am. 2004;86(5):963–74.
2. Learmonth ID, Young C, Rorabeck C. The operation of the century: total hip replacement. Lancet. 2007;370(9597):1508–19.
3. Daigle ME, Weinstein AM, Katz JN, Losina E. The cost-effectiveness of total joint arthroplasty: a systematic review of published literature. Best Pract Res Clin Rheumatol. 2012;26(5):649–58.
4. Chang RW. A cost-effectiveness analysis of total hip arthroplasty for osteoarthritis of the hip. JAMA. 1996;275(11):858.
5. Andersson AE, Bergh I, Karlsson J, Nilsson K. Patients' experiences of acquiring a deep surgical site infection: an interview study. Am J Infect Control. 2010;38(9):711–7.
6. Kurtz SM, Lau E, Watson H, Schmier JK, Parvizi J. Economic burden of periprosthetic joint infection in the United States. J Arthroplasty. 2012;27(S):61–1.
7. Kurtz SM, Lau E, Schmier J, Ong KL, Zhao K, Parvizi J. Infection burden for hip and knee arthroplasty in the United States. J Arthroplasty. 2008;23(7):984–91.
8. Kurtz S, Ong K, Lau E, Mowat F, Halpern M. Projections of primary and revision hip and knee arthroplasty in the United States from 2005 to 2030. J Bone Joint Surg Am. 2007;89(4):780–5.
9. Hanssen AD, Spangehl MJ. Treatment of the infected hip replacement. Clin Orthop Relat Res LWW. 2004;420:63–71.
10. Zimmerli W, Trampuz A, Ochsner PE. Prosthetic-joint infections. N Engl J Med Mass Medical Soc. 2004;351(16):1645–54.

11. Zmistowski B, Karam JA, Durinka JB, Casper DS, Parvizi J. Periprosthetic joint infection increases the risk of one-year mortality. J Bone Joint Surg Am. 2013;95(24):2177.
12. Berend KR, Lombardi AV, Morris MJ, Bergeson AG, Adams JB, Sneller MA. Two-stage treatment of hip periprosthetic joint infection is associated with a high rate of infection control but high mortality. Clin Orthop Relat Res. 2012;471(2):510–8.
13. Toulson C, Walcott-Sapp S, Hur J, Salvati E, Bostrom M, Brause B, et al. Treatment of infected total hip arthroplasty with a 2-stage reimplantation protocol. J Arthroplasty. 2009;24(7):1051–60.
14. McDonald DJ, Fitzgerald RH, Ilstrup DM. Two-stage reconstruction of a total hip arthroplasty because of infection. J Bone Joint Surg Am. 1989;71(6):828–34.
15. Tsukayama DT, Estrada R, Gustilo RB. Infection after total hip arthroplasty. A study of the treatment of one hundred and six infections. J Bone Joint Surg Am. 1996;78(4):512–23.
16. Younger AS, Duncan CP, Masri BA, McGraw RW. The outcome of two-stage arthroplasty using a custom-made interval spacer to treat the infected hip. J Arthroplasty. 1997;12(6):615–23.
17. Nusem I, Morgan DA. Structural allografts for bone stock reconstruction in two-stage revision for infected total hip arthroplasty: good outcome in 16 of 18 patients followed for 5–14 years. Acta Orthop. 2006;77(1):92–7.
18. Stockley I, Mockford BJ, Hoad-Reddick A, Norman P. The use of two-stage exchange arthroplasty with depot antibiotics in the absence of long-term antibiotic therapy in infected total hip replacement. J Bone Joint Surg Br. 2008;90-B(2):145–8.
19. Masters JP, Smith NA, Foguet P, Reed M, Parsons H, Sprowson AP. A systematic review of the evidence for single stage and two stage revision of infected knee replacement. BMC Musculoskelet Disord. 2013;14(1):1–1.
20. Beswick AD, Elvers KT, Smith AJ, Gooberman-Hill R, Lovering A, Blom AW. What is the evidence base to guide surgical treatment of infected hip prostheses? Systematic review of longitudinal studies in unselected patients. BMC Medicine BioMed Central Ltd. 2012;10(1):18–28.
21. Wolf CF, Gu NY, Doctor JN, Manner PA, Leopold SS. Comparison of one and two-stage revision of total hip arthroplasty complicated by infection. J Bone Joint Surg Am. 2011;93(7):631–9.
22. Nixon M, Jackson B, Varghese P, Jenkins D, Taylor G. Methicillin-resistant Staphylococcus aureus on orthopaedic wards: incidence, spread, mortality, cost and control. J Bone Joint Surg Br. 2006;88(6):812–7.
23. Leung F, Richards CJ, Garbuz DS, Masri BA, Duncan CP. Two-stage total hip arthroplasty: how often does It control methicillin-resistant infection? Clin Orthop Relat Res. 2010;469(4):1009–15.
24. Parry MC, Duncan CP. The challenge of methicillin resistant staphylococcal infection after total hip replacement: overlooked or overstated? Bone Joint J. 2014;96-B(11 Supple A):60–5.
25. McGarry SA, Engemann JJ, Schmader K, Sexton DJ, Kaye KS. Surgical-site infection due to Staphylococcus aureus among elderly patients: mortality, duration of hospitalization, and cost. Infect Control Hosp Epid. 2004;25(6):461–7.
26. Marculescu CE, Cantey JR. Polymicrobial prosthetic joint infections: risk factors and outcome. Clin Orthop Relat Res. 2008;466(6):1397–404.
27. Zmistowski B, Fedorka CJ, Sheehan E, Deirmengian G, Austin MS, Parvizi J. Prosthetic joint infection caused by gram-negative organisms. J Arthroplasty. 2011;26(6 Suppl):104–8.
28. Pulido L, Ghanem E, Joshi A, Purtill JJ, Parvizi J. Periprosthetic joint infection: the incidence, timing, and predisposing factors. Clin Orthop Relat Res [Internet]. 2008;466(7):1710–5. Available from: http://link.springer.com/article/10.1007/s11999-008-0209-4.
29. Berbari EF, Hanssen AD, Duffy MC, Steckelberg JM, Ilstrup DM, Harmsen WS, et al. Risk factors for prosthetic joint infection: case-control study. CLIN INFECT DIS. 1998;27(5):1247–54.
30. Bozic KJ. The impact of infection after total hip arthroplasty on hospital and surgeon resource utilization. J Bone Joint Surg Am. 2005;87(8):1746–51.
31. Wylde V, Blom AW. The failure of survivorship. J Bone Joint Surg Br. 2011;93(5):569–70.
32. Jämsen E, Stogiannidis I, Malmivaara A, Pajamäki J, Puolakka T, Konttinen YT. Outcome of prosthesis exchange for infected knee arthroplasty: the effect of treatment approach. Acta Orthop. 2009;80(1):67–77.
33. Castelli CC, Gotti V, Ferrari R. Two-stage treatment of infected total knee arthroplasty: two to thirteen year experience using an articulating preformed spacer. Int Orthop. 2014;38(2):405–12.
34. Freeman MG, Fehring TK, Odum SM, Fehring K, Griffin WL, Mason JB. Functional advantage of articulating versus static spacers in 2-stage revision for total knee arthroplasty infection. J Arthroplasty. 2007;22(8):1116–21.
35. Gooding CR, Masri BA, Duncan CP, Greidanus NV, Garbuz DS. Durable infection control and function with the PROSTALAC spacer in two-stage revision for infected knee arthroplasty. Clin Orthop Relat Res. 2010;469(4):985–93.
36. Meek RD, Masri BA, Dunlop D, Garbuz DS, Greidanus NV, McGraw R, et al. Patient satisfaction and functional status after treatment of infection at the site of a total knee arthroplasty with use of the PROSTALAC articulating spacer. J Bone Joint Surg Am. 2003;85(10):1888–92.
37. Haddad FS, Masri BA, Campbell D, McGraw RW, Beauchamp CP, Duncan CP. The PROSTALAC functional spacer in two-stage revision for infected knee replacements. Prosthesis of antibiotic-loaded acrylic cement. J Bone Joint Surg Br. 2000;82(6):807–12.

38. Haleem AA, Berry DJ, Hanssen AD. Mid-term to long-term followup of two-stage reimplantation for infected total knee arthroplasty. Clin Orthop Relat Res. 2004;428:35–9.
39. Hirakawa K, Stulberg BN, Wilde AH, Bauer TW, Secic M. Results of 2-stage reimplantation for infected total knee arthroplasty. J Arthroplasty. 1998;13(1):22–8.
40. Johnson AJ, Sayeed SA, Naziri Q, Khanuja HS, Mont MA. Minimizing dynamic knee spacer complications in infected revision arthroplasty. Clin Orthop Relat Res. 2011;470(1):220–7.
41. Mahmud T, Lyons MC, Naudie DD, MacDonald SJ, McCalden RW. Assessing the gold standard: a review of 253 two-stage revisions for infected TKA. Clin Orthop Relat Res. 2012;470(10):2730–6.
42. Mont MA, Waldman BJ, Hungerford DS. Evaluation of preoperative cultures before second-stage reimplantation of a total knee prosthesis complicated by infection. A comparison-group study. J Bone Joint Surg Am. 2000;82-A(11):1552–7.
43. Van Thiel GS, Berend KR, Klein GR, Gordon AC, Lombardi AV, Valle Della CJ. Intraoperative molds to create an articulating spacer for the infected knee arthroplasty. Clin Orthop Relat Res. 2010;469(4):994–1001.
44. Westrich GH, Bornstein L, Brause BD. Historical perspective on two-stage reimplantation for infection after total hip arthroplasty at hospital for special surgery, New York City. Am J Orthop (Belle Mead NJ). 2011;40(11):E236–40.
45. Hofmann AA, Goldberg T, Tanner AM, Kurtin SM. Treatment of infected total knee arthroplasty using an articulating spacer. Clin Orthop Relat Res. 2005;430:125–31.
46. Singer J, Merz A, Frommelt L, Fink B. High rate of infection control with one-stage revision of septic knee prostheses excluding mrsa and mrse. Clin Orthop Relat Res. 2011;470(5):1461–71.
47. Goksan SB, Freeman MA. One-stage reimplantation for infected total knee arthroplasty. J Bone Joint Surg Br. 1992;74(1):78–82.
48. Saleh KJ, Celebrezze M, Kassim R, Dykes DC, Gioe TJ, Callaghan JJ, et al. Functional outcome after revision hip arthroplasty. Clin Orthop Relat Res. 2003;416:254–64.
49. Oussedik SIS, Dodd MB, Haddad FS. Outcomes of revision total hip replacement for infection after grading according to a standard protocol. J Bone Joint Surg Br. 2010;92(9):1222–6.
50. De Man FHR, Sendi P, Zimmerli W, Maurer TB, Ochsner PE, Ilchmann T. Infectiological, functional, and radiographic outcome after revision for prosthetic hip infection according to a strict algorithm. Acta Orthop. 2011;82(1):27–34.
51. Lai K-A, Shen W-J, Yang C-Y, Lin R-M, Lin C-J, Jou I-M. Two-stage cementless revision THR after infection: 5 recurrences in 40 cases followed 2.5-7 years. Acta Orthop. 1996;67(4):325–8.
52. Haddad FS, Muirhead-Allwood SK, Manktelow AR, Bacarese-Hamilton I. Two-stage uncemented revision hip arthroplasty for infection. J Bone Joint Surg Br. 2000;82(5):689–94.
53. Toms AD, Davidson D, Masri BA, Duncan CP. The management of peri-prosthetic infection in total joint arthroplasty. J Bone Joint Surg Br. 2006;88(2):149–55.
54. Rao N, Crossett LS, Sinha RK, Le Frock JL. Long-term suppression of infection in total joint arthroplasty. Clin Orthop Relat Res. 2003;414:55–60.
55. Bourne RB, Hunter GA, Rorabeck CH, Macnab JJ. A six-year follow-up of infected total hip replacements managed by Girdlestone's arthroplasty. J Bone Joint Surg Br. 1984;66(3):340–3.
56. Castellanos J, Flores X, Llusà M, Chiriboga C, Navarro A. The Girdlestone pseudarthrosis in the treatment of infected hip replacements. Int Orthop. 1998;22(3):178–81.
57. Scott SJ, Hennessey MS, Parkinson RW, Molloy AP. Long-term outcome of the "Beefburger" procedure in patients unsuitable for two-stage revision following infected total knee replacement. Knee. 2001;8(4):281–6.
58. Harris IE, Leff AR, Gitelis S, Simon MA. Function after amputation, arthrodesis, or arthroplasty for tumors about the knee. J Bone Joint Surg Am. 1990;72(10):1477–85.
59. Conway JD, Mont MA, Bezwada HP. Arthrodesis of the knee. J Bone Joint Surg Am. 2004;86(4):835–48.
60. Waters RL, Perry J, Antonelli D, Hislop H. Energy cost of walking of amputees: the influence of level of amputation. J Bone Joint Surg Am. 1976;58(1):42–6.
61. Chen AF, Kinback NC, Heyl AE, McClain EJ, Klatt BA. Better function for fusions versus above-the-knee amputations for recurrent periprosthetic knee infection. Clin Orthop Relat Res. 2012;470(10):2737–45.
62. Pring DJ, Marks L, Angel JC. Mobility after amputation for failed knee replacement. J Bone Joint Surg Br. 1988;70(5):770–1.
63. Isiklar ZU, Landon GC, Tullos HS. Amputation after failed total knee arthroplasty. Clin Orthop Relat Res LWW. 1994;299:173–8.
64. Fedorka CJ, Chen AF, McGarry WM, Parvizi J, Klatt BA. Functional ability after above-the-knee amputation for infected total knee arthroplasty. Clin Orthop Relat Res. 2010;469(4):1024–32.
65. Klinger H-M, Spahn G, Schultz W, Baums MH. Arthrodesis of the knee after failed infected total knee arthroplasty. Knee Surg Sports Traumatol Arthrosc. 2005;14(5):447–53.
66. Benson ER, Resine ST, Lewis CG. Functional outcome of arthrodesis for failed total knee arthroplasty. Orthopedics. 1998;21(8):875–9.
67. Freeman MA, Sudlow RA, Casewell MW, Radcliff SS. The management of infected total knee replacements. J Bone Joint Surg Br. 1985;67(5):764–8.
68. Buechel FF, Femino FP, D'Alessio J. Primary exchange revision arthroplasty for infected total knee

replacement: a long-term study. Am J Orthop (Belle Mead NJ). 2004;4:190–8; discussion 198.
69. Leonard HAC, Liddle AD, Burke Ó, Murray DW, Pandit H. Single- or two-stage revision for infected total hip arthroplasty? A systematic review of the literature. Clin Orthop Relat Res. 2013;472(3):1036–42.
70. Goldman RT, Scuderi GR, Insall JN. 2-stage reimplantation for infected total knee replacement. Clin Orthop Relat Res. 1996;331:118–24.
71. Johnson DP, Bannister GC. The outcome of infected arthroplasty of the knee. J Bone Joint Surg [Br]. 1986;68(2):289–91.
72. Woods GW, Lionberger DR, Tullos HS. Failed total knee arthroplasty: revision and arthrodesis for infection and noninfectious complications. Clin Orthop Relat Res. 1983;173:184.
73. Grogan TJ, Dorey F, Rollins J, Amstutz HC. Deep sepsis following total knee arthroplasty. Ten-year experience at the University of California at Los Angeles Medical Center. J Bone Joint Surg Am. 1986;68(2):226–34.
74. Hanssen AD, Trousdale RT, Osmon DR. Patient outcome with reinfection following reimplantation for the infected total knee arthroplasty. Clin Orthop Relat Res. 1995;321:55–67.
75. Sanchez-Sotelo J, Berry DJ, Hanssen AD, Cabanela ME. Midterm to long-term followup of staged reimplantation for infected hip arthroplasty. Clin Orthop Relat Res. 2009;467(1):219–24.
76. Duncan CP, Masri BA. The role of antibiotic-loaded cement in the treatment of an infection after a hip replacement. Instr Course Lect. 1995;44:305–13.
77. Nestor BJ, Hanssen AD, Ferrer-Gonzalez R, Fitzgerald RH. The use of porous prostheses in delayed reconstruction of total hip replacements that have failed because of infection. J Bone Joint Surg Am. 1994;76(3):349–59.
78. Kraay MJ, Goldberg VM, Fitzgerald SJ, Salata MJ. Cementless two-staged total hip arthroplasty for deep periprosthetic infection. Clin Orthop Relat Res. 2005;441:243–9.
79. Masri BA, Panagiotopoulos KP, Greidanus NV, Garbuz DS, Duncan CP. Cementless two-stage exchange arthroplasty for infection after total hip arthroplasty. J Arthroplasty. 2007;22(1):72–8.

Paradigm Change in Antibacterial Coatings: Efficacy of Short-Term Local Prophylaxis

28

Carlo Luca Romanò, Delia Romanò, Sara Scarponi, and Lorenzo Drago

Abstract

According to current knowledge, the most critical pathogenic event in the development of implant-related infection is probably biofilm formation, which starts immediately after bacterial adhesion on implanted devices, leading to their irreversible colonization.

A rationale prevention of biomaterial-associated infections should then specifically focus on inhibition of both bacterial adhesion and biofilm formation. Nonetheless, currently available prophylactic measures, although partially effective in reducing surgical site infections, are not based on the pathogenesis of biofilm-related infections and unacceptable high rates of septic complications, especially in high risk patients and procedures are reported.

Traditionally, once demonstrated their biocompatibility, orthopedic implants have been designed as inert mechanical devices, their biological aspects being considered as a byproduct of a stable fixation to the surrounding bone or soft tissues. However, in the last decade, several studies have investigated the ability of implant surface modifications to mitigate possible adverse events, including implant-related infections. Several surface treatment modalities are under development in order to minimize bacterial adhesion, inhibit biofilm formation and provide

Electronic supplementary material The online version of this chapter (doi:10.1007/978-3-319-30091-7_28) contains supplementary material, which is available to authorized users.

C.L. Romanò, MD (✉) • D. Romanò, MD
S. Scarponi, MD
Department of Reconstructive Surgery of Bone and Joint Infections, Galeazzi Orthopedic Institute IRCCS, Milan, Italy
e-mail: carlo.romano@grupposandonato.it

L. Drago, PhD
Department of Biomedical Sciences for Health, IRCCS Galeazzi Hospital, University of Milan, Milan, Italy

D. Kendoff et al. (eds.), *Periprosthetic Joint Infections: Changing Paradigms*,
DOI 10.1007/978-3-319-30091-7_28

effective bacterial killing to protect implanted biomaterials, even if there still is a great discrepancy between proposed and clinically implemented strategies.

Here we provide a brief overview and an original classification of the various technologies under study or already in the market, with particular reference to a novel approach, based on a fast-resorbable hydrogel coating, that may change the paradigm of long-lasting antibacterial implant protection towards a more feasible short-term one, that may minimize the risk of long-term interference with the function of implanted biomaterials and of bacterial resistance induction, while effective protection at an acceptable cost/benefit ratio.

Keywords
Orthopaedic • Implant • Biomaterial • Prosthesis • Joint • Surface • Biofilm • Infection • Coating • Anti-adhesive • Antibacterial • Prophylaxis • Treatment • Silver • Hydrogel • Classification

Introduction

Even if the introduction of various perioperative infection prevention methods, such as antibiotic prophylaxis, have been shown to be effective in reducing surgical site infections (SSI), up to 2.5 % of primary hip and knee arthroplasties and 20 % of revision arthroplasties might be complicated by periprosthetic joint infection (PJI) [1]. Moreover, according to some authors these numbers could be even underestimated and are on the rise [2], while multi-resistant pathogens are often retrieved [3]. Peri-prosthetic infection generally requires implant removal, with increased morbidity and even mortality [4] and high associated costs [5].

The occurrence of an implant-related infection is the results of a variable interaction of different factors, including bacterial load or contamination at the surgical site, host's type, surgical procedure and technique, type of implant and of systemic and local antibacterial prophylaxis.

In fact, even elective surgery may not be performed in a completely bacterial-free environment, since operating rooms have been shown to become contaminated within the first few hours of service [6, 7]. Although the rather low bacterial load eventually present at surgery may still be generally overcome by the combined action of the host's immunological defense and the systemic antibiotic prophylaxis [8], in some patients a surgical site infection may eventually take place, especially in those at higher risk, such as those affected by diabetes, chronic renal insufficiency and other relevant medical conditions, that may increase the relative risk of a SSI by more than ten folds [9–11]. Similarly, the most complex surgical procedures and techniques are more prone to septic complications [12]. In this context, the characteristics of the implanted device, including size, shape, material, topography and intended use also play an important role [13], while local prophylaxis using antibiotic-loaded bone cement or bone grafts has been shown to reduce the incidence of implant related infections [8, 14]. In a recent international Consensus meeting on peri-prosthetic infection, a strong recommendation was delivered concerning the need for developing effective antibacterial surfaces that prevent bacterial adhesion and colonization of implants and proliferation into the surrounding tissues [15].

The aim of this chapter is to provide a brief overview of the technologies under investigation to protect orthopaedic implants in order to mitigate infection, with an original classification and a particular focus on the most recently developed fast-resorbable hydrogel coating, that may offer a novel perspective for short-term local antibacterial prophylaxis, which was first introduced by the authors in 2013.

Antibacterial Coatings

Rationale

Prophylactic systemic antibiotics are administered routinely to patients who receive an orthopaedic device to prevent peri-operative infection [8]. However, systemic administration of antibiotics has many potential disadvantages including the need for a correct timing of administration, the relatively low drug concentration at the target site and the limited ability to kill bacteria eventually present on the implant surface or embedded in biofilms.

When Anthony Gristina first proposed the concept of a "race for the surface", more than three decades ago, he described a simplified model of implant-related infection, whereby host and bacterial cells compete in determining the ultimate fate of the implant [16]. According to this model, when the host cells colonize the implant surface first, the probability of attachment of bacterial cells is very low and vice versa. While this concept has stimulated technological progress and the idea of surface modifications of implants in order to favor host cells and preventing bacterial adhesion, it only provides a static picture of a much more complex process, many variables of which are still poorly understood or completely unknown. In particular, it fails to describe in detail the dynamic process of bacterial versus host's cell implant colonization and is not able to predict the relative host cell *versus* bacterial cell coverage of any implant surface.

The most problematic factor is probably the highly successful and diversified strategy of bacteria to adhere and survive on virtually all natural and synthetic surfaces [17, 18]. Bacterial cell membranes contain various types of adhesins for a wide range of biomaterial surface receptor sites. Environmental and surface characteristics of a biomaterial such as surface roughness, hydrophobicity and electrostatic charge play only conditional roles [19], while a reservoir of several receptors for bacterial adhesive ligands, mediating adhesion of free-floating bacteria to the surface of the biomaterial, offers a conditional protein film covering an implant immediately after its placement into the host body [20–22]. Complement, albumin and several other host proteins and lipids are the main components of this conditional protein film [23–25]. The process of bacterial adhesion can be divided into two basic phases: reversible and irreversible. The former is mechanically and biologically less stable than the latter and lies on nonspecific interactions between implant surface and bacterial adhesins. The second phase is mediated by molecular and cellular interactions closely associated with expression of biofilm specific gene clusters in reversibly attached bacteria [26–29].

On the host site, the details of implant osteo- and tissue-integration are also rather poorly understood [30, 31]. According to the model proposed by Gristina, it is believed that host cells, once attached to fixation implant surfaces, lead to periprosthetic bone regeneration and remodeling, protecting against bacterial colonization [32]. However, neither osteointegration nor fibrous tissue encapsulation of large non-fixation parts of an implant can eliminate long-term survivorship of bacterial micro-colonies. Moreover, peri-implant fibrous barriers can prevent contact between host immunity sentinel cells and bacterial molecules, while is has been demonstrated that implantation of a medical device impairs innate local host response and may facilitate implant-related infections and hence PJI [33–35].

As a result, there is a strong need for intrinsic implant surface antibacterial functionality to overcome the implant-induced defects in the local immune response and to prevent the striking ability of bacteria to quickly adhere on a substrate and immediately produce a protective biofilm barrier, providing a competitive advantage to the host's cells over the contaminating microorganisms. This is of utmost importance especially in patients with underlying compromised immunity [36] and in

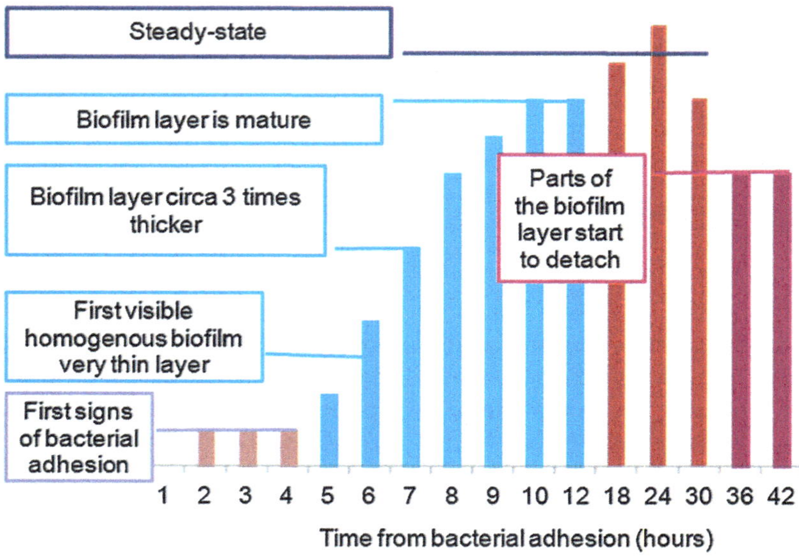

Fig. 28.1 Kinetic of *Staph. epidermidis* biofilm formation (Re-written from Hola et al. [38]). According to current data, the timeframe window to prevent bacterial adhesion and biofilm formation lays within 2–6 h after implant

those undergoing revision surgery [37] in which the relative risk of infection is multiplied. At the same time any coating technology should prove to be safe in the short and long term, should not interfere with osteointegration or induce bacterial resistance in the long run. Moreover, all the bacterial colonization process, from microbial adhesion on an implant surface to the production of an established mature biofilm layer, may only take few hours (Fig. 28.1) [38], so any implant antibacterial functionality should act at the exact time of surgery, that is from the moment the implant is extracted from the sterile package to at least until the very next hours after it is inserted into the body and the skin closed, or, in other words, just before bacteria may adhere on the implant and start producing biofilms.

These observations point out the need for a coating that is able to provide an immediate and complete protection of the implant surface at the time of surgery, but that at the same time is eventually able to completely disappear after few hours or days, to prevent long-term unwanted interference with bone and soft tissue integration of the implanted biomaterial.

This new approach, based on a short-term local implant anti-bacterial protection, compares to traditionally studied permanent or long-lasting surface antibacterial coatings, whose unpredictable long-term effects both on host's cell and bacteria are one of the main limiting factor to their introduction in the clinical use and in the market.

Preclinical and clinical demonstration of the safety and efficacy of the short-term local antibacterial protection of the implants may change the paradigm of antibacterial coating, opening the way to large scale combined local and systemic short-term prophylaxis to further reduce the impact of biofilm-related post-surgical and post-traumatic infections.

Classification

Local antibacterial implant protection can be obtained in many different ways. Currently there is not a single, universally accepted classification of coating technologies and even the validation of these technologies has not been standardized to date, while regulatory aspects appear somewhat inadequate in view of the clinical needs and expectations.

Table 28.1 summarizes the basic requirements that an "ideal" coating technology should fulfill to meet the needs of a widespread clinical use.

Table 28.1 Requirements to be fulfilled by the "ideal" antibacterial implant coating strategy

Requirements	Fulfillments			
Safety	No short-term local toxicity	No short-term systemic toxicity	No detrimental effects on bone healing	No unwanted long-term side effects
In vitro activity	No cytotoxicity or genotoxicity	Bactericidal and antibiofilm activity against various pathogens and on different surfaces	Large spectrum	No resistance induction
Efficacy	Proven *in vivo*	Case series	Multicenter trials	Randomized trials
Ease-of-use	Easy handling	Versatility	Resistance to press-fit insertion	Storage
Market	Acceptable cost	Large availability	Easy to manufacture	Overcomes regulatory issues

Our proposed classification is based on the general strategy of action of different coatings (Table 28.2); while necessarily schematic, this classification may be helpful to compare different technologies and may also be useful both in the clinical practice and concerning regulatory aspects, that may differ substantially for different coating classes.

According to the proposed classification, local antibacterial implant protection can theoretically be achieved in at least three ways:

1. Passive surface finishing/modification. Passive coatings do not release bactericidal agents to the surrounding tissues, but are aimed at preventing or reducing bacterial adhesion through surface chemistry and/or structure modifications. Examples of this approach include modified titanium dioxide surface or polymer coatings.
2. Active surface finishing/modification. Active coatings feature pharmacologically active pre-incorporated bactericidal agents such as antibiotics, antiseptics, metal ions or other organic and inorganic compounds to downregulate implant-related infection. Current clinical successful applications of "contact killing" active surface are silver- or iodine-coated joint implants.
3. Peri-operative antibacterial local carriers or coatings. The local antibacterial carrier or coating, biodegradable or not, is applied during surgery immediately prior or at the same time of the implant and around it; it may have direct or synergistic antibacterial activity or simply deliver high local concentrations of one or more loaded antibacterials. Antibiotic-loaded polymethylmethacrylate is the first example of a successful non-degradable, drug eluting, local carrier and coating for joint prosthesis

Passive Surface Finishing/Modification

A change in the surface chemistry and/or structure of the bulk implant can be achieved either by chemically or physically altering the surface layer in the existing biomaterial (e.g., oxidation or mechanical modifications like roughening/polishing/texturing).

The surface characteristics of implants such as surface roughness and chemistry, hydrophilicity, surface energy, surface potential and conductivity play in fact crucial roles in initial bacterial adhesion to implants and subsequent biofilm formation. Modification of the physiochemical surface properties of the implant is a relatively simple and economic way to counteract bacterial colonization.

For example, ultraviolet light irradiation can lead to an increase in "spontaneous" wettability on titanium dioxide, which can inhibit bacterial adhesion without compromising osteogenesis on titanium alloy implants [39, 40]. A bacterial anti-adhesive surface can also be achieved by modifying the crystalline structure of the surface oxide layer [41].

In addition to physiochemical modifications on the biomaterial surface, certain polymer

Table 28.2 Classification of antibacterial implant protection strategies

Strategy	Features	Examples	Development stage	Limits
Passive surface finishing/ modifications	Prevention in adhesion and adsorption	Hydrophylic surface	Preclinical	Limited antibacterial and antibiofilm activity. Possible interference with osteointegration. Unknown long-term effects Regulatory issues.
		Super-hydrophobic surface		
		Anti-adhesive polymers		
		Nano-patterned surface		
		Albumin		
		Hydrogels		
		Biosurfactants		
Active surface finishing/ modifications	Inorganic	Metal ions and nanoparticles: Silver	Market	Incomplete implant coating Questionable long-term toxicity Limited versatility and applicability Limited large scale applications Possible bacterial resistance. induction Costs
		Other metals (copper, zinc, titanium dioxide etc.)	Preclinical	Questionable long-term toxicity Regulatory issues.
		Non-metals: Iodine	Clinical	Incomplete implant coating Questionable long-term toxicity Challenging large scale application Regulatory issues
		Other non-metal ions (selenium, grapheme, etc.)	Preclinical	Poorly studied compounds. Coating resistance to press-fit insertion. Questionable long-term toxicity Challenging large scale application. Regulatory issues.
	Organic	Coated linked antibiotics	Market	Unique application to nail coating Long-term effects on osteointegration Single antibiotic (gentamicin)
		Covalently linked antibiotics	Preclinical	Incomplete implant coating. Questionable long-term toxicity Challenging large scale application. Regulatory issues.
		Antimicrobial peptides		No data on *in vivo* or clinical effects Coating resistance to press-fit insertion Questionable long-term toxicity Challenging large scale application. Regulatory issues.
		Cytokines		
		Enzymes and biofilm disrupting agents		
		Chitosan derivatives		
	Synthetic	Non-antibiotic antimicrobial compounds		
		"Smart" coatings		
	Combined	Multilayer coating		

Table 28.2 (continued)

Strategy	Features	Examples	Development stage	Limits
Peri-operative antibacterial local carriers or coatings	Not-biodegradable	Antibiotic-loaded polymethylmetacrylate	Market	Resistance and small-colony variants induction No antibiofilm effect Incomplete implant coating May not be used for cementless implants
	Biodegradable	Antibiotic-loaded bone grafts and substitutes	Market	Limited availability Not proven efficacy as implant coating Cost
		Fast-resorbable hydrogel	Market	Early clinical use

coatings such as the hydrophilic polymethacrylic acid, polyethylene oxide or protein resistant polyethylene glycol can be applied to the surface of titanium implants and result in significant inhibition of bacterial adhesion [42–44]. Although some of these coatings may impair local osteoblast function on the surface of implant, the use of additional bioactive molecules such as sericin and RGD motif with the immobilization technique could restore and even improve the impaired cell function [43]. On the other hand, hydrophobic and superhydrophobic surface treatment technologies have shown a great repellent antibacterial effect in preclinical studies [45, 46].

Other research pathways have shown how the biological response to biomaterials can be controlled via alterations in surface structure and design [47, 48]. In this regard, many studies are currently focused on the effect of changing the implant surface at a nanometric scale, at which bacterial adhesion does not simply follow the roughness of the surface but also is dependent on other variables like the quantity of adsorbed proteins. At nanomeric level, when roughness increases, the formation of a thick protein layer on such implant surface could in fact suppress bacteria adhesion [49].

Treating protein-surfaces and/or protein-bacteria interactions may also be a successful strategy of inhibiting bacterial adhesion to a specific biomaterial [50]. Proteins such as albumin, fibronectin, fibrinogen, laminin, denatured collagens, and some plasma/tissue lipids are the first host substances that interact with the surface structure of the biomaterial. Reduction of conditional lipid-protein layer formation can be achieved by changing surface physico-chemical characteristics, and/or surface micro-morphology [51]. Friedman *et al.* using a rabbit model, demonstrated reduced bacterial adherence on pure titanium samples and decreased infection rates of implants coated with cross-linked albumin [52].

More recently, novel strategies include production of self-assembled mono- or multilayers, surface grafting or hydrogels, or the use of biosurfactants and microbial amphiphilic compounds with excellent anti-adhesive properties [53, 54].

In summary, to date a number of anti-adhesive tactics have been proposed for different purposes. Only a few, however, have met the elementary features required for bone implant usage. Specifically, a strong anti-adhesive layer cannot be used for coating of fixation surfaces of total joint arthroplasty because it could also prevent host bone osseointegration and lead to early mechanical failure [46, 47]. Another challenge of designing antiadhesive technologies relates to the current inability to design a universal surface treatment that can be applied to all surfaces, all bacterial species, and under all (ingrowth and noningrowth) implants. Moreover, passive coating methods should be preferred as long as their antibacterial ability is strong enough to prevent biofilm formation. However, the effectiveness of passive coatings for decreasing bacterial adhesion is limited and varies greatly depending on the bacterial species [55].

Moreover, long-term effects of these new technologies both on host's cells and on bacterial resistance are poorly understood and need to be further investigated before clinical applications and market introduction.

Active Surface Finishing/Modification

Surface finishing/modification may include pharmacologically active pre-incorporated antibacterial agents or compounds, like antibiotics, antiseptics, metal ions and organic molecules. Such pharmacologically activated coatings may change the implant from a passive, inert biomaterial, to a new drug formulation, with difficult to predict long-term effects and challenging regulatory issues that prevented until now clinical application of many otherwise promising technologies.

Historically, two main strategies have been proposed for effective antibacterial surface treatment either "contact killing" or drug eluting, while in terms of durability, we can distinguish between degradable and non-degradable coatings. In killing bacteria they rely on diverse mechanisms of action, which may interfere with a cell respiration or division, cell wall formation or bacterial signalling network (e.g., quorum sensing) as well as inhibition of the transition of planktonic phenotype of bacteria into a sessile type [56]. This tactic is aimed at prolonging the window of opportunity for both prophylactic antibiotic activity and the host immune response.

Antibacterial surface technologies can employ metals (silver, zinc, copper, *etc*.), non-metal elements (e.g., iodine, selenium), organic substances (antibiotics, anti-infective peptides, chitosan, other substances), and their combinations.

Antibacterial activity of the majority of metal coatings is closely linked to the ionic or nano form rather than to the bulk material [57]. Silver is the most prevalent metal used in biomedical applications. Dissolved silver cations are biochemically active agents that interfere with bacterial cell membrane permeability and cellular metabolism. Silver also contributes to formation of reactive oxygen species and other mechanisms that potentially influence prokaryotic cells [58]. There has been concern, however, about the toxicity of silver ions. Even in minute levels silver can adversely affect surrounding cells and lead to potentially harmful accumulation in distant locations [59]. Research efforts have focused on the development of silver coating technologies that reduce or even eliminate toxicity while maintaining constructive antibacterial effects [60, 61]. Despite demonstrated clinical efficacy and safety in recent comparative studies [62, 63], routine using of silver coated implants remains rather limited. The main obstacles preventing broader usage of such technology are cytotoxicity on bone cells, that prevented until now coating of the intra-medullary part of the prosthesis. In addition, cost issues and the inability to apply the technology to a variety of prosthetic implants and devices further prevent its application outside oncological or highly selected cases.

Copper and zinc also have potent antibacterial effects on a wide spectrum of bacterial species [64, 65], however, potential toxic side effects of these metals remain a strong concern [66]. Proposed solutions include copper- and zinc-based nanomaterials or, alternatively, controlled release [67]. The risk of bacterial resistance to metallic coatings remains a potential limitation for their widespread use [68]. Concern also exists about the mechanical properties of implant nanocoatings since damage may occur during surgical implantation especially in cementless implants inserted via press-fit methods [69].

Another interesting technology related to modification of commonly used alloys, like titanium. The anti-infective potential of titanium dioxide layers has been widely investigated and proven effective *in vitro* both alone [70] or in combination with other substances [71].

Non-metal elements like hydrogen, chlorine, iodine, or oxygen are commonly used in biomedicine for their anti-infective properties. Selenium bound covalently onto the surface of titanium or titanium alloy implant discs have been shown to prevent *Staphylococcus aureus* and *Staphylococcus epidermidis* attachment without affecting osteoblast viability [72]. Selenium catalyzes the formation of superoxide radicals and subsequently inhibits bacterial adhesion and viability. In addition, selenium nanoparticles can inhibit bacterial growth and biofilm formation [73].

Ongoing research is also directed to determine the clinical applicability of carbon substances like graphene or carbon nanotubes, that can be synthesized in multifunctional layers [74]; however, the most interesting technology today under study, related to non-metal elements, is probably iodine coating of titanium alloys, that has recently demonstrated clinical efficacy in a continuous series of 222 patients with excellent results [75].

Several organic compounds with antibacterial properties have the potential to be linked to the surface of implants conferring them anti-infective properties. A large number of studies have investigated the efficacy of surfaces coated with covalently linked antibiotics [76–80]. Clinical effectiveness of such implants is most likely limited to infections caused by bacteria that are sensitive to the specific antibiotic that has been coupled. In addition, strong forces such as covalent binding are insufficiently sensitive to react to weak external stimuli [81]. In fact, despite the theoretical advantages for non-eluting systems, this concept is limited by the fragility of the coatings and killing activity potential of bacteria which might not be directly adjacent to the implant. To overcome these issues, combinations of antibiotics with other compounds have been proposed either alone or in association with a particular mechanism of controlled release [82]. Antibiotics such as gentamicin, vancomycin and others have been loaded into porous hydroxyapatite (HA) coatings on titanium implants. The antibiotic-HA coatings exhibit significant improvement in preventing infection compared with standard HA coatings in vivo, but there are still many unresolved issues regarding the methodology of antibiotic incorporation into the HA coating and the optimal release kinetics and possible detachment of the coating at the time of press-fit insertion.

Biodegradable polymers and sol–gel coatings are also utilized to form controlled release antibiotic-laden coatings on titanium implants [83, 84]. Clinical applications of antibiotic-loaded D-poly-lactate acid/gentamycin intramedullary coated nail have been recently reported with early positive results [85].

Some antiseptic agent such as chlorhexidine, chloroxylenol or poly-hexamethylenebiguanide have demonstrated efficacy and might be an alternative to avoid the risk of drug resistance. Chlorhexidine can be adsorbed to the TiO2 layer on titanium surfaces and is released gradually over several days [86]. Its release pattern is similar to that of antibiotic-laden coatings with an initial rapid release rate followed by slower but sustained release [87].

Another promising approach involves coating implants with antimicrobial peptides, cytokines or other molecules critical for host response to bacteria invasion. This heterogeneous group of substances has proven experimentally their efficacy against a wide range of pathogens [88]. Antimicrobial peptides, like antibiotics, function via damage of the cell wall and inhibition of key bacterial protein synthesis. In addition, they exert influence upon inflammation, tissue healing, and apoptotic events [89]; resistance to antimicrobial peptides has been reported less frequently than to antibiotics [90]. Initial experiments demonstrated that a thin layer of antimicrobial peptides affixed onto the surfaces of metal alloys exhibit excellent antibacterial effects against typical pathogens related to PJI [91].

Chitosan (CS) is a polycationic polymer derived from chitin that exhibits antibacterial and antifungal activity. The exact mechanism of action remains poorly understood. There is some evidence that CS derivatives can be firmly anchored to titanium alloys and that they have a protective effect against some bacterial species either alone or in combination with other antimicrobial substances like antibiotics or antimicrobial peptides [92, 93]. CS derivatives secured to external fixator pins have been studied as a method of preventing pin tract infections [94]. However, we are not aware a study to date reporting data from clinical setting.

Long-term impact of permanently coated implants with antibiotics and other organic compounds, never used before either for local or general administration, does raise concerns regarding possible induction of bacterial resistance, local and general toxicity and possible detrimental effects on implant osteointegration, ultimately preventing clinical applications until now.

Still more complex approaches involve the development of multifunctional surface layers, like functional polymer brush coating, that combine anti-adhesive and antimicrobial substances and other compounds able to enhance tissue integration [95], while "smart coatings", sensitive and responsive to a variety of stimuli, including the presence of bacteria [96], are another fascinating but futuristic research pathway, that poses a number of open questions, like feasible coating manufacturing process, non-adverse reactions *in vivo*, mechanical resistance and preservation of intended functionalities throughout the life of the device, etc.

Peri-operative Antibacterial Carriers or Coatings

Instead of pre-manufactured surface modifications, either with or without pharmacologically active agents, a different approach to implant protection from bacterial colonization may be to provide a traditional implant with an antibacterial carrier or coating at the time of surgery. The separation of the protective solution from the implant until surgery may reduce the regulatory requirements and increase the applicability of a universal antibacterial coating to many different already existing implants and biomaterials.

Local administration of antibiotics historically attracted much attention in orthopaedics. Buchholz et al. first popularized the incorporation of antibiotics into polymethylmethacrylate (PMMA) bone cement for local antibiotic prophylaxis in cemented total joint arthroplasty [97]. Clinical studies have shown that antibiotic loaded bone cement can decrease deep infection rates of cemented total hip arthroplasties and revision rates due to supposed "aseptic" loosening when combined with systemic antibiotic administration [98] and this solution has been found both effective and economically sound, especially in high risk patients [99, 100],. However, PMMA was not designed as a local delivery carrier of antibiotics and may have some limits. Antibiotic-loaded PMMA may not overcome biofilm formation and may be associated with the development of antibiotic-resistant "small-colony variants" [101, 102], while the increasing use of cementless implants worldwide, especially at the hip site, make this a possible option only for a restricted number of patients.

Other porous materials for local antibiotic delivery like collagen sponges [103], cancellous bone [104] and calcium phosphate cements [105, 106] were not specifically designed to protect implanted biomaterials and their use for routine infection prevention in joint prosthesis is limited by their insufficient *in vitro*, *in vivo* and clinical evidence of efficacy in this specific application, their inability to be applied as a coating to all implants' surfaces, their relatively high costs and possible interference with primary implant fixation and long-term osteointegration.

Based on these examples and in an effort to overcome their limits, a challenging option is to design specific, effective and easy-to-use antibacterial coatings, that can be applied at the time of surgery directly on the implant by the surgeon, either pre-loaded or intra-operatively with antibacterials. In this regard, biocompatible hydrogels do represent a possible attractive solution as they have demonstrated capabilities to deliver local pharmacological agents and may be designed to meet the desired elution pattern [107]. Recently, a fast-resorbable hydrogel coating, that can be loaded intra-operatively with various antibacterials, has been introduced in the European market [108] and may open a novel perspective in the field of antibacterial coatings.

Fast-Resorbable Antibiotic-Loaded Hydrogel Coating: A Paradigm Shift?

Passive and active surface modifications of implants have been traditionally studied in order to provide long-term or permanent antibacterial protection of coated devices. However, the pathogenesis of biofilm-related infections points out how the destiny of an implant, as to regard bacterial colonization, is decided within the very first hours after insertion into the human body and this also explains the equal efficacy of shot- and long-term systemic prophylaxis to prevent PJIs [109]. On the other hand, long-term or permanent antibacterial coating also increases possible unwanted long-term side effects, including local and systemic toxicity or bacterial resistance induction, that may be difficult to predict and control; this has obvious impact on regulatory aspects, preventing widespread acceptance of this strategy and imposing expensive validation studies, that are currently extremely difficult to perform.

A short-term local delivery system, on the contrary, may meet the requirements needed to win the "run to the surface," while limiting possible unwanted side effects. In principle, in fact, the ideal antibiotic delivery coating should release antibiotics at optimal bactericidal levels for a sufficiently long period of time to prevent potential infection, i.e. few hours after surgery as far as post-surgical infections are concerned, and then subsequently antibiotic release should cease quickly to eliminate the risk of developing antibiotic resistance. In addition, any untoward effects of antibiotics on tissue integration of the implant should be minimized [110].

This has been recently put into practice realizing a novel fast-resorbable hydrogel coating, composed of covalently linked hyaluronan and poly-D,L-lactide, "Defensive Antibacterial Coating", DAC® (Novagenit Srl, Mezzolombardo, Italy) (Fig. 28.2), which undergoes complete hydrolytic degradation in vivo and that is able to completely release a variety of different antibacterials at concentrations ranging from 2 to 10 %, including glycopeptides, amynoglycosides, fluoquinolones, etc. within 48–72 h (Table 28.3) (Video 28.1). The hydrogel showed a synergistic antibacterial activity with various antibiotics and antibiofilm effect could be demonstrated in vitro on different substrates and against different common pathogens involved in orthopedic implant-related infections. Moreover, once applied on titanium standard joint prosthesis, the hydrogel coating did show to resist press-fit insertion both in the animal model and in human femurs. Also, histocompatibility studies did show the absence of inflammatory or degenerative signs and physiological bone growth in animal models [111].

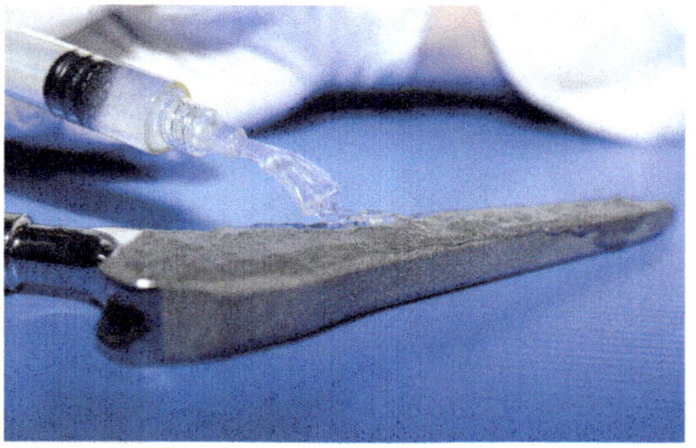

Fig. 28.2 Defensive Antibacterial Coating, DAC® (Novagenit Srl, Mezzolombardo, Italy): a novel fast-resorbable hydrogel coating, composed of covalently linked hyaluronan and poly-D,L-lactide, is spread onto a cementless hip prosthesis. The hydrogel is loaded intra-operatively with one or more antibiotics, that are released within 48–72 h after, thus providing antibacterial and antibiofilm protection to the implant

Table 28.3 Tested antibacterial to be leaded with DAC hydrogel coating at concentrations ranging from 2 to 10 %

Antibacterial family	Tested antibiotics
Aminoglycosides	Gentamicin
	Tobramycin
	Amikacin
Carbapenems	Meropenem
Glicopeptides	Vancomycin
	Teicoplanin
Quinolones	Ciprofloxacin
Glicopeptites	Daptomycin
Rifamycins	Rifampicin
Tetracuclines	Tigecyclin
Oxazolidinones	Linezolid
Antifungals	Amphotericin B
	Fluconazole
	Ketoconazole

113 and Novagenit Srl data on file

Finally, *in vivo* studies have recently demonstrated, for the first time, the efficacy of the short-term local prophylaxis offered by vancomycin-loaded DAC hydrogel in an animal models of highly contaminated implant both with [112] and without systemic prophylaxis [113].

These findings have brought to the introduction of the coating in the market at the end of 2013 and more than 800 implants have been performed until now in different countries in Europe

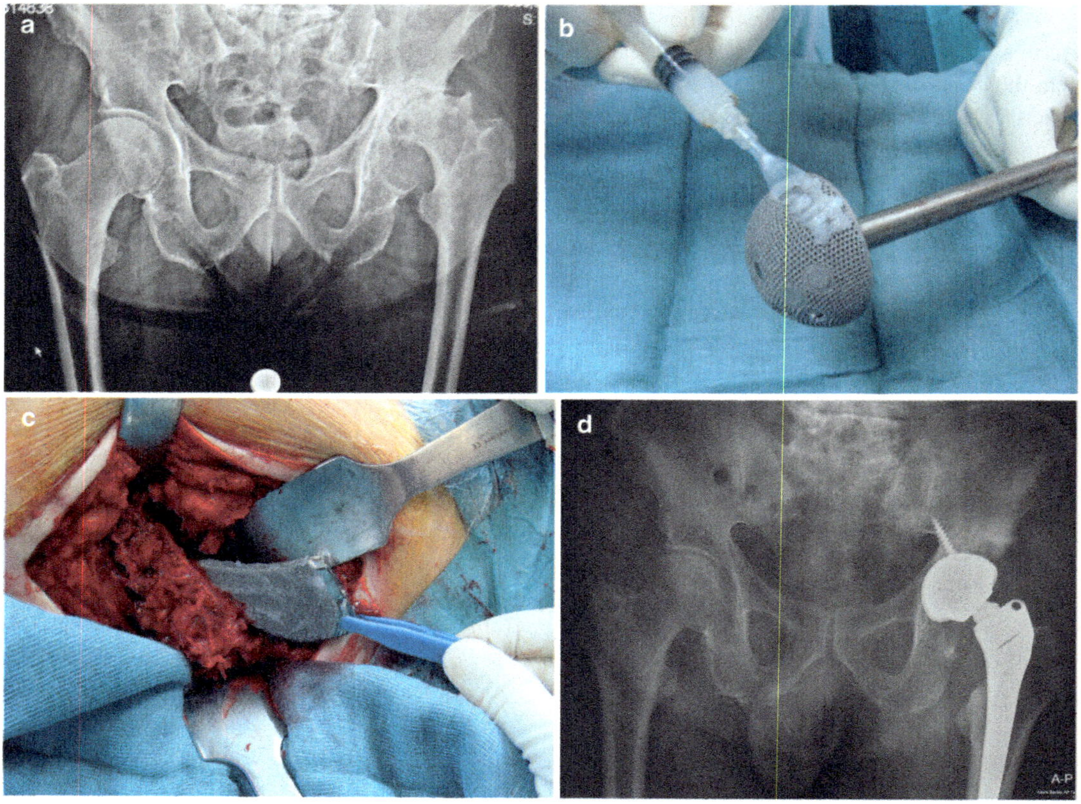

Fig. 28.3 (**a**) Sequelae of septic hip arthritis (*Strept. mutans*) in a young male patient. (**b**) Vancomycin 5 % loaded DAC® hydrogel is applied on the sanded titanium surface of a standard cementless hip prosthesis, both on the acetabular and (**c**) in the femoral component, that is press-fit inserted in the diaphysis according to the normal procedure. (**d**) Control after 12 months shows bone osteo-integration. The patient is pain-free

(Fig. 28.3). Clinical results allow at the moment to confirm the safety of the device, without any reported side effect [114], while the efficacy is still under evaluation in one multicenter trial, partially funded by the European Commission under the Seventh Framework Programme on Research Technological Development and Demonstration (Grant 277988).

If proven effective, this technology may change current perspective in local antibacterial protection of implanted biomaterials in orthopedics and eventually in other disciplines, offering

1. Efficacy toward early bacterial colonization, providing complete protection of the implant for the time needed to win the "race to the surface," i.e, in the first hours after surgery;
2. Safety, as high local concentration and fast and complete release of the antibacterial may avoid induction of antibiotic resistance and possible risks of long-term effects on bone healing;
3. Versatility, through intraoperative mixing with a choice of different antibacterial agents and possible application to virtually all currently used implants and biomaterials (Video 28.2);
4. Ease of handling;
5. Reduced costs for large-scale application.

Conclusion

Examination of published studies on antibacterial coating technologies suggests a striking discrepancy between proposed strategies of antibacterial surface treatment and ultimate completion of *in vitro* and *in vivo* experimentation. In fact, it appears that little progress is being made in the translation of the aforementioned modalities into clinically useful technologies. Barriers to translational medicine in this field are most likely related to economic, medico-legal, regulatory and biotechnological issues.

Most of the studied coatings in fact are not suitable for surface treatment of orthopedic implants due to problems with cytotoxicity, immunoreactivity and genotoxicity [115], while clinical application of those successfully tested *in vitro* and *in vivo* may be limited by a number of various concerns,. Improving collaborative efforts amongst governments, regulatory agencies, industry leaders and health care payers will probably allow more patients to benefit from these technologies.

Another important consideration in designing implants with antibacterial coating relates to the characterization of reasonable and justifiable cost. Theoretically all patients undergoing total joint arthroplasty are at risk for PJI. On the other hand, the risk for PJI is not homogenously distributed among patients and is stratified into the specific groups of "high risk" patients. Therefore, it might be convincing to implant "biofilm resistant" prostheses only in patients at increased risk of PJI. However, a validated tool for screening patients for increased risk of PJI does not currently exist and we have no data to confirm the validity of patient selection with regard to one antibacterial prophylaxis or another. In this panorama, a preventative strategy involving all patients undergoing primary and revision total joint arthroplasty would probably be more justifiable than a more restrictive approach targeting high risk patients, but only as far as the relative cost of any coating technology remains affordable on a large scale.

To this aim, well designed prospective studies on relatively inexpensive and easy-to-use technologies are first necessary, in order to demonstrate the significant reduction of implant-related infections, while cost to benefit analysis may then drive the most correct implementation in the clinical setting.

References

1. Lentino JR. Prosthetic joint infections: bane of orthopedists, challenge for infectious disease specialists. Clin Infect Dis. 2003;36:1157–61.
2. Dale H, Hallan G, Hallan G, Espehaug B, Havelin LI, Engesaeter LB. Increasing risk of revision due to deep infection after hip arthroplasty. Acta Orthop. 2009;80:639–45.
3. Aggarwal VK, Bakhshi H, Ecker NU, Parvizi J, Gehrke T, Kendoff D. Organism profile in periprosthetic joint infection: pathogens differ at two arthroplasty infection referral centers in Europe and in the United States. J Knee Surg. 2014;10:399–406. doi:10.1055/s-0033-1364102.
4. Zmistowski B, Karam JA, Durinka JB, Casper DS, Parvizi J. Periprosthetic joint infection increases the risk of one-year mortality. J Bone Joint Surg Am. 2013;95:2177–84.
5. Kurtz SM, Lau E, Watson H, Schmier JK, Parvizi J. Economic burden of periprosthetic joint infection in the United States. J Arthroplasty. 2012;27:61–5.
6. An YH, Friedman RJ. Prevention of sepsis in total joint arthroplasty. J Hosp Infect. 1996;33:93–108.
7. Humphreys H. Surgical site infection, ultraclean ventilated operating theatres and prosthetic joint surgery: where now? J Hosp Infect. 2012;81:71–2.
8. Jamsen E, Furnes O, Engesaeter LB, Konttinen YT, Odgaard A, Stefansdottir A, et al. Prevention of deep infection in joint replacement surgery. Acta Orthop. 2010;81:660e6.
9. Illingworth KD, Mihalko WM, Parvizi J, Sculco T, McArthur B, el Bitar Y, et al. How to minimize infection and thereby maximize patient outcomes in total joint arthroplasty: a multicenter approach: AAOS exhibit selection. J Bone Joint Surg Am. 2013;95:e50.
10. Pruzansky JS, Bronson MJ, Grelsamer RP, Strauss E, Moucha CS. Prevalence of modifiable surgical site infection risk factors in hip and knee joint arthroplasty patients at an urban academic hospital. J Arthroplasty. 2014;29:272–6.
11. Aggarwal VK, Tischler EH, Lautenbach C, Williams Jr GR, Abboud JA, Altena M, et al. Mitigation and education. J Arthroplasty. 2014;29:19–25.
12. Namba RS, Inacio MC, Paxton EW. Risk factors associated with surgical site infection in 30,491 primary total hip replacements. J Bone Joint Surg Br. 2012;94:1330e8.
13. Moriarty TF, Schlegel U, Perren S, Richards RG. Infection in fracture fixation: can we influence infection rates through implant design? J Mater Sci Mater Med. 2010;21:1031e5.
14. van de Belt H, Neut D, Schenk W, van Horn JR, van der Mei HC, Busscher HJ. Infection of orthopedic implants and the use of antibiotic-loaded bone cements. A review. Acta Orthop Scand. 2001;72:557e71.
15. Cats-Baril W, Gehrke T, Huff K, Kendoff D, Maltenfort M, Parvizi J. International consensus on

periprosthetic joint infection: description of the consensus process. Clin Orthop Relat Res. 2013;471:4065–75.
16. Gristina AG, Naylor P, Myrvik Q. Infections from biomaterials and implants: a race for the surface. Med Prog Technol. 1988;14:205–24.
17. Costerton W, Veeh R, Shirtliff M, Pasmore M, Post C, Ehrlich G. The application of biofilm science to the study and control of chronic bacterial infections. J Clin Invest. 2003;112:1466–77.
18. Busscher HJ, van der Mei HC. How do bacteria know they are on a surface and regulate their response to an adhering state? PLoS Pathog. 2012;8:e1002440.
19. Chen Y, Busscher HJ, van der Mei HC, Norde W. Statistical analysis of long- and short-range forces involved in bacterial adhesion to substratum surfaces as measured using atomic force microscopy. Appl Environ Microbiol. 2011;77:5065–70.
20. Wagner C, Aytac S, Hansch GM. Biofilm growth on implants: bacteria prefer plasma coats. Int J Artif Organs. 2011;34:811–7.
21. Wang Y, Subbiahdoss G, de Vries J, Libera M, van der Mei HC, Busscher HJ. Effect of adsorbed fibronectin on the differential adhesion of osteoblast-like cells and staphylococcus aureus with and without fibronectin-binding proteins. Biofouling. 2012;28:1011–21.
22. Ribeiro M, Monteiro FJ, Ferraz MP. Infection of orthopedic implants with emphasis on bacterial adhesion process and techniques used in studying bacterial-material interactions. Biomatter. 2012;2:176–94.
23. Jenney CR, Anderson JM. Adsorbed serum proteins responsible for surface dependent human macrophage behavior. J Biomed Mater Res. 2000;49:435–47.
24. Thevenot P, Hu W, Tang L. Surface chemistry influences implant biocompatibility. Curr Top Med Chem. 2008;8:270–80.
25. Roach P, Eglin D, Rohde K, Perry CC. Modern biomaterials: a review—bulk properties and implications of surface modifications. J Mater Sci Mater Med. 2007;18:263–1277.
26. Costerton JW, Stewart PS, Greenberg EP. Bacterial biofilms: a common cause of persistent infections. Science. 1999;284:1318–22.
27. Stoodley P, Ehrlich GD, Sedghizadeh PP, Hall-Stoodley L, Baratz ME, Altman DT, Sotereanos NG. Orthopaedic biofilm infections. Curr Orthop Pract. 2011;22:558–63.
28. Laverty G, Gorman SP, Gilmore BF. Biomolecular mechanisms of staphylococcal biofilm formation. Future Microbiol. 2013;8:509–24.
29. Foster TJ, Geoghegan JA, Ganesh VK, Hook M. Adhesion, invasion and evasion: the many functions of the surface proteins of staphylococcus aureus. Nat Rev Microbiol. 2014;12:49–62.
30. Anderson JM, Rodriguez A, Chang DT. Foreign body reaction to biomaterials. Semin Immunol. 2008;20:86–100.
31. Gardner AB, Lee SK, Woods EC, Acharya AP. Biomaterials-based modulation of the immune system. Biomed Res Int. 2013;2013:732182. doi:10.1155/2013/732182.
32. Busscher HJ, van der Mei HC, Subbiahdoss G, Jutte PC, van den Dungen JJ, Zaat SA, Schultz MJ, Grainger DW. Biomaterial-associated infection: locating the finish line in the race for the surface. Sci Transl Med. 2012;4:153rv10.
33. Zimmerli W, Lew PD, Waldvogel FA. Pathogenesis of foreign body infection. Evidence for a local granulocyte defect. J Clin Invest. 1984;73:1191–200.
34. Higgins DM, Basaraba RJ, Hohnbaum AC, Lee EJ, Grainger DW, Gonzalez-Juarrero M. Localized immunosuppressive environment in the foreign body response to implanted biomaterials. Am J Pathol. 2009;175:161–70.
35. Zimmerli W, Sendi P. Pathogenesis of implant-associated infection: the role of the host. Semin Immunopathol. 2011;33:295–306.
36. Berbari EF, Osmon DR, Lahr B, Eckel-Passow JE, Tsaras G, Hanssen AD, Mabry T, Steckelberg J, Thompson R. The Mayo prosthetic joint infection risk score: implication for surgical site infection reporting and risk stratification. Infect Control Hosp Epidemiol. 2012;33:774–81.
37. Engelsman AF, Saldarriaga-Fernandez IC, Nejadnik MR, van Dam GM, Francis KP, Ploeg RJ, et al. The risk of biomaterial-associated infection after revision surgery due to an experimental primary implant infection. Biofouling. 2010;26:761–7.
38. Holá V, Růžička F, Votava M. The dynamics of staphylococcus epidermis biofilm formation in relation to nutrition, temperature, and time. Scr Med. 2006;79:169–74.
39. Gallardo-Moreno AM, Pacha-Olivenza MA, Saldana L, Perez-Giraldo C, Bruque JM, Vilaboa N, et al. In vitro biocompatibility and bacterial adhesion of physico-chemically modified Ti6Al4V surface by means of UV irradiation. Acta Biomater. 2009;5:181e92.
40. Yu JC, Ho W, Lin J, Yip H, Wong PK. Photocatalytic activity, antibacterial effect, and photoinduced hydrophilicity of TiO2 films coated on a stainless steel substrate. Environ Sci Technol. 2003;37:2296e301.
41. Del Curto B, Brunella MF, Giordano C, Pedeferri MP, Valtulina V, Visai L, et al. Decreased bacterial adhesion to surface-treated titanium. Int J Artif Organs. 2005;28:718e30.
42. Zhang F, Zhang Z, Zhu X, Kang ET, Neoh KG. Silk-functionalized titanium surfaces for enhancing osteoblast functions and reducing bacterial adhesion. Biomaterials. 2008;29:4751–9.
43. Harris LG, Tosatti S, Wieland M, Textor M, Richards RG. Staphylococcus aureus adhesion to titanium oxide surfaces coated with non-functionalized and peptide-functionalized poly(L-lysine)-grafted-poly(ethylene glycol) copolymers. Biomaterials. 2004;25:4135–48.

44. Kaper HJ, Busscher HJ, Norde W. Characterization of poly(ethylene oxide) brushes on glass surfaces and adhesion of Staphylococcus epidermidis. J Biomater Sci Polym Ed. 2003;14:313–24.
45. Zhu H, Guo Z, Liu W. Adhesion behaviors on superhydrophobic surfaces. Chem Commun (Camb). 2014;18:3900–13.
46. Braem A, van Mellaert L, Mattheys T, Hofmans D, de Waelheyns E, Geris L, et al. Staphylococcal biofilm growth on smooth and porous titanium coatings for biomedical applications. J Biomed Mater Res A. 2013;102:215–24. doi:10.1002/jbm.a.34688.
47. Bacakova L, Filova E, Parizek M, Ruml T, Svorcik V. Modulation of cell adhesion, proliferation and differentiation on materials designed for body implants. Biotechnol Adv. 2011;29:739–67.
48. Lu T, Qiao Y, Liu X. Surface modification of biomaterials using plasma immersion ion implantation and deposition. Interface Focus. 2012;2:325–36.
49. Singh AV, Vyas V, Patil R, Sharma V, Scopelliti PE, Bongiorno G, et al. Quantitative characterization of the influence of the nanoscale morphology of nanostructured surfaces on bacterial adhesion and biofilm formation. PLoS One. 2011;6:e25029.
50. Campoccia D, Montanaro L, Arciola CR. A review of the biomaterials technologies for infection-resistant surfaces. Biomaterials. 2013;34:8533–54.
51. Yeo IS, Kim HY, Lim KS, Han JS. Implant surface factors and bacterial adhesion: a review of the literature. Int J Artif Organs. 2012;35:762–72.
52. An YH, Bradley J, Powers DL, Friedman RJ. The prevention of prosthetic infection using a cross-linked albumin coating in a rabbit model. J Bone Joint Surg Br. 1997;79:816–9.
53. Rivardo F, Turner RJ, Allegrone G, Ceri H, Martinotti MG. Anti-adhesion activity of two biosurfactants produced by Bacillus spp. Prevents biofilm formation of human bacterial pathogens. Appl Microbiol Biotechnol. 2009;83:541–53.
54. Rodrigues L, Banat IM, Teixeira J, Oliveira R. Biosurfactants: potential applications in medicine. J Antimicrob Chemother. 2006;57:609–18.
55. Hetrick EM, Schoenfisch MH. Reducing implant-related infections: active release strategies. Chem Soc Rev. 2006;35:780–9.
56. Stoodley P, Hall-Stoodley L, Costerton B, DeMeo P, Shirtliff M, Gawalt E, et al. Biofilms, biomaterials, and device-related infections. In: Ratner BD, Hoffman AS, Schoen FJ, Lemons JE, editors. Biomaterials science: an introduction to materials in medicine. Waltham: Academic Press (Elsevier); 2013. p. 565–83.
57. Lemire JA, Harrison JJ, Turner RJ. Antimicrobial activity of metals: mechanisms, molecular targets and applications. Nat Rev Microbiol. 2013;11:371–84.
58. Chernousova S, Epple M. Silver as antibacterial agent: ion, nanoparticle, and metal. Angew Chem Int Ed Engl. 2013;52:1636–53.
59. Mijnendonckx K, Leys N, Mahillon J, Silver S, van Houdt R. Antimicrobial silver: uses, toxicity and potential for resistance. Biometals. 2013;26: 609–21.
60. Noda I, Miyaji F, Ando Y, Miyamoto H, Shimazaki T, Yonekura Y, et al. Development of novel thermal sprayed antibacterial coating and evaluation of release properties of silver ions. J Biomed Mater Res B Appl Biomater. 2009;89:456–65.
61. Panacek A, Kolar M, Vecerova R, Prucek R, Soukupova J, Krystof V, et al. Antifungal activity of silver nanoparticles against Candida spp. Biomaterials. 2009;30:6333–40.
62. Wafa H, Grimer RJ, Reddy K, Jeys L, Abudu A, Carter SR, et al. Retrospective evaluation of the incidence of early periprosthetic infection with silver-treated endoprostheses in high-risk patients: case-control study. Bone Joint J. 2015;97-B(2):252–7.
63. Hardes J, von Eiff C, Streitbuerger A, Balke M, Budny T, Henrichs MP, et al. Reduction of periprosthetic infection with silver-coated megaprostheses in patients with bone sarcoma. J Surg Oncol. 2010;101(5):389–95.
64. Grass G, Rensing C, Solioz M. Metallic copper as an antimicrobial surface. Appl Environ Microbiol. 2011;77:1541–7.
65. Petrini P, Arciola CR, Pezzali I, Bozzini S, Montanaro L, Tanzi MC, et al. Antibacterial activity of zinc modified titanium oxide surface. Int J Artif Organs. 2006;29:434–42.
66. Hodgkinson V, Petris MJ. Copper homeostasis at the host-pathogen interface. J Biol Chem. 2012;287:13549–55.
67. Pelgrift RY, Friedman AJ. Nanotechnology as a therapeutic tool to combat microbial resistance. Adv Drug Deliv Rev. 2013;65:1803–15.
68. Moseke C, Gbureck U, Elter P, Drechsler P, Zoll A, Thull R, et al. Hard implant coatings with antimicrobial properties. J Mater Sci Mater Med. 2011;22:2711–20.
69. Shtansky DV, Gloushankova NA, Bashkova IA, Kharitonova MA, Moizhess TG, Sheveiko AN, Kiryukhantsev-Korneev FV, et al. Multifunctional Ti-(Ca, Zr)-(C, N, O, P) films for load-bearing implants. Biomaterials. 2006;27:3519–31.
70. Arenas MA, Perez-Jorge C, Conde A, Matykina E, Hernandez-Lopez JM, Perez-Tanoira R, et al. Doped TiO2 anodic layers of enhanced antibacterial properties. Colloids Surf B Biointerfaces. 2013;105:106–12.
71. Hu H, Zhang W, Qiao Y, Jiang X, Liu X, Ding C. Antibacterial activity and increased bone marrow stem cell functions of Zn-incorporated TiO2 coatings on titanium. Acta Biomater. 2012;8:904–15.
72. Holinka J, Pilz M, Kubista B, Presterl E, Windhager R. Effects of selenium coating of orthopaedic implant surfaces on bacterial adherence and osteoblastic cell growth. Bone Joint J. 2013;95:678–82.
73. Tran PA, Webster TJ. Selenium nanoparticles inhibit Staphylococcus aureus growth. Int J Nanomedicine. 2011;6:1553–8.

74. Martynkova GS, Valaskova M. Antimicrobial nanocomposites based on natural modified materials: a review of carbons and clays. J Nanosci Nanotechnol. 2014;14:673–93.
75. Tsuchiya H, Shirai T, Nishida H, Murakami H, Kabata T, Yamamoto N, et al. Innovative antimicrobial coating of titanium implants with iodine. J Orthop Sci. 2012;17(5):595–604.
76. Antoci Jr V, King SB, Jose B, Parvizi J, Zeiger AR, Wickstrom E, et al. Vancomycin covalently bonded to titanium alloy prevents bacterial colonization. J Orthop Res. 2007;25:858–66.
77. Alt V, Bitschnau A, Osterling J, Sewing A, Meyer C, Kraus R, et al. The effects of combined gentamicin-hydroxyapatite coating for cementless joint prostheses on the reduction of infection rates in a rabbit infection prophylaxis model. Biomaterials. 2006;27:4627–34.
78. Schmidmaier G, Lucke M, Wildemann B, Haas NP, Raschke M. Prophylaxis and treatment of implant-related infections by antibiotic-coated implants: a review. Injury. 2006;37:S105–12.
79. Fei J, Liu GD, Pan CJ, Chen JY, Zhou YG, Xiao SH, et al. Preparation, release profiles and antibacterial properties of vancomycin-loaded Ca-P coating titanium alloy plate. J Mater Sci Mater Med. 2011;22:989–95.
80. Neut D, Dijkstra RJ, Thompson JI, van der Mei HC, Busscher HJ. A gentamicin-releasing coating for cementless hip prostheses-longitudinal evaluation of efficacy using in vitro bio-optical imaging and its wide-spectrum antibacterial efficacy. J Biomed Mater Res A. 2012;100:3220–6.
81. Shchukin D, Mohwald H. Materials science. A coat of many functions. Science. 2013;341:1458–9.
82. Shi X, Wu H, Li Y, Wei X, Du Y. Electrical signals guided entrapment and controlled release of antibiotics on titanium surface. J Biomed Mater Res A. 2013;101:1373–8.
83. Guillaume O, Garric X, Lavigne JP, Van Den Berghe H, Coudane J. Multilayer, degradable coating as a carrier for the sustained release of antibiotics: preparation and antimicrobial efficacy in vitro. J Control Release. 2012;162:492–501.
84. Tang Y, Zhao Y, Wang H, Gao Y, Liu X, Wang X, et al. Layer-by-layer assembly of antibacterial coating on interbonded 3D fibrous scaffolds and its cytocompatibility assessment. J Biomed Mater Res A. 2012;100:2071–8.
85. Fuchs T, Stange R, Shmidmaier S, Raschke MJ. The use of gentamicin-coated nails in the tibia: preliminary results of a prospective study. Arch Orthop Trauma Surg. 2011;131(10):1419–25.
86. Campbell AA, Song L, Li XS, Nelson BJ, Bottoni C, Brooks DE, et al. Development, characterization, and anti-microbial efficacy of hydroxyapatite-chlorhexidine coatings produced by surface-induced mineralization. J Biomed Mater Res. 2000;53:400e7.
87. Kozlovsky A, Artzi Z, Moses O, Kamin-Belsky N, Greenstein RB. Interaction of chlorhexidine with smooth and rough types of titanium surfaces. J Periodontol. 2006;77:1194e200.
88. Yount NY, Yeaman MR. Emerging themes and therapeutic prospects for anti-infective peptides. Annu Rev Pharmacol Toxicol. 2012;52:337–60.
89. Haney EF, Hancock RE. Peptide design for antimicrobial and immunomodulatory applications. Biopolymers. 2013;100:572–83.
90. Dobson AJ, Purves J, Kamysz W, Rolff J. Comparing selection on S. aureus between antimicrobial peptides and common antibiotics. PLoS One. 2013;8:e76521.
91. Holmberg KV, Abdolhosseini M, Li Y, Chen X, Gorr SU, Aparicio C. Bio-inspired stable antimicrobial peptide coatings for dental applications. Acta Biomater. 2013;9:8224–31.
92. Costa F, Maia S, Gomes P, Martins MC. Characterization of hLF1-11 immobilization onto chitosan ultrathin films, and its effects on antimicrobial activity. Acta Biomater. 2014;10:3513–21. doi:10.1016/j.actbio.2014.02.028.
93. Yang CC, Lin CC, Liao JW, Yen SK. Vancomycin-chitosan composite deposited on post porous hydroxyapatite coated Ti6Al4V implant for drug controlled release. Mater Sci Eng C. 2013;33:2203–12.
94. Jennison T, McNally M, Pandit H. Prevention of infection in external fixator pin sites. Acta Biomater. 2014;10:595–603.
95. Muszanska AK, Rochford ET, Gruszka A, Bastian AA, Busscher HJ, Norde W, et al. Antiadhesive polymer brush coating functionalized with antimicrobial and rgd peptides to reduce biofilm formation and enhance tissue integration. Biomacromolecules. 2014;15:2019–26.
96. Yu Q, Cho J, Shivapooja P, Ista LK, Lopez GP. Nanopatterned smart polymer surfaces for controlled attachment, killing, and release of bacteria. ACS Appl Mater Interfaces. 2013;5:9295–304.
97. Buchholz HW, Engelbrecht H. Depot effects of various antibiotics mixed with Palacos resins. Chirurg. 1970;41:511e5.
98. Engesaeter LB, Lie SA, Espehaug B, Furnes O, Vollset SE, Havelin LI. Antibiotic prophylaxis in total hip arthroplasty: effects of antibiotic prophylaxis systemically and in bone cement on the revision rate of 22,170 primary hip replacements followed 0–14 years in the Norwegian Arthroplasty Register. Acta Orthop Scand. 2003;74:644e51.
99. Gutowski CJ, Zmistowski BM, Clyde CT, Parvizi J. The economics of using prophylactic antibiotic-loaded bone cement in total knee replacement. Bone Joint J. 2014;96-B(1):65–9.
100. Dunbar MJ. Antibiotic bone cements: their use in routine primary total joint arthroplasty is justified. Orthopedics. 2009;32(9):660–3.

101. van de Belt H, Neut D, Schenk W, van Horn JR, van Der Mei HC, Busscher HJ. Staphylococcus aureus biofilm formation on different gentamicin-loaded polymethylmethacrylate bone cements. Biomaterials. 2001;22(12):1607–11.
102. Neut D, Hendriks JG, van Horn JR, van der Mei HC, Busscher HJ. Pseudomonas aeruginosa biofilm formation and slime excretion on antibiotic-loaded bone cement. Acta Orthop. 2005;76(1):109–14.
103. De Grood MP. Pathology, diagnosis and treatment of subdural empyema. Arch Chir Neerl. 1951;3:128e38.
104. Buttaro MA, Pusso R, Piccaluga F. Vancomycin-supplemented impacted bone allografts in infected hip arthroplasty. Two-stage revision results. J Bone Joint Surg Br. 2005;87:314e9.
105. Gautier H, Merle C, Auget JL, Daculsi G. Isostatic compression, a new process for incorporating vancomycin into biphasic calcium phosphate: comparison with a classical method. Biomaterials. 2000;21:243e9.
106. Yamamura K, Iwata H, Yotsuyanagi T. Synthesis of antibiotic-loaded hydroxyapatite beads and in vitro drug release testing. J Biomed Mater Res. 1992;26:1053e64.
107. Overstreet D, McLaren A, Calara F, Vernon B, McLemore R. Local gentamicin delivery from resorbable viscous hydrogels is therapeutically effective. Clin Orthop Relat Res. 2015;473(1):337–47.
108. Pitarresi G, Palumbo FS, Calascibetta F, Fiorica C, Di Stefano M, Giammona G. Medicated hydrogels of hyaluronic acid derivatives for use in orthopedic field. Int J Pharm. 2013;449(1–2):84–94.
109. Heydemann JS, Nelson CL. Short-term preventive antibiotics. Clin Orthop Relat Res. 1986;205:184–7.
110. Antoci Jr V, Adams CS, Hickok NJ, Shapiro IM, Parvizi J. Antibiotics for local delivery systems cause skeletal cell toxicity in vitro. Clin Orthop Relat Res. 2007;462:200–6.
111. Drago L, Boot W, Dimas K, Malizos K, Hänsch GM, Stuyck J, et al. Does implant coating with antibacterial-loaded hydrogel reduce bacterial colonization and biofilm formation in vitro? Clin Orthop Relat Res. 2014;472(11):3311–23.
112. Giavaresi G, Meani E, Sartori M, Ferrari A, Bellini D, Sacchetta AC, et al. Efficacy of antibacterial-loaded coating in an in vivo model of acutely highly contaminated implant. Int Orthop. 2014;38(7):1505–12.
113. Logoluso N, Malizos K, Blauth M, Danita A, Simon K, Romanò C. Anti-bacterial hydrogel coating of osteosynthesis implants: early clinical results from a multi-center prospective trial. Proceeding of eCM XVI Congress on Bone and Implant Infection. 2015.
114. Boot W, Vogely HCh, Nikkels PGJ, Pouran B, van Rijen M, Dhert WJA, et al. Local prophylaxis of implant-related infections using a hydrogel as carrier. Proceeding of eCM XVI Congress on Bone and Implant Infection. 2015
115. Daghighi S, Sjollema J, van der Mei HC, Busscher HJ, Rochford ET. Infection resistance of degradable versus non-degradable biomaterials: an assessment of the potential mechanisms. Biomaterials. 2013;34:8013–7.

Part IX

Future Approaches

The Future of Periprosthetic Joint Infections

29

David A. George and Fares S. Haddad

Abstract

We have highlighted the complexity of periprosthetic joint infections in the previous chapters, specifically the difficulty in preventing, diagnosing, and managing these troublesome complications. The future of periprosthetic joint infections may at first appear bleak. The number of arthroplasty procedures is growing, parallel with an aging population, and if the incidence of infections remains constant, the number of patients suffering will also increase.

However, multiple initiatives and strategies have been, or are being, developed to help improve the fight against these infections. We may be on the brink of reducing the impact these devastating infections have upon our patients, as well as reducing their socioeconomic impact. This chapter reviews many of these encouraging strategies, which gives us hope that all is not as bad as we had first thought.

Keywords

Periprosthetic joint infection • Future • Nano-technology • Next-generation sequencing • Ultra-violet light • Silver • Antibiotic coatings • Antibiofilm coatings • Photodynamic therapy • Magnetic fields • Bioactive glass

Introduction

The previous chapters have highlighted the complexity of periprosthetic joint infections (PJIs) in terms of prevention and risk stratifying of patients, diagnosing the presence of infections via a number of modalities, and the management of patients with acute or established infections by a combination of medical and surgical approaches. Unfortunately, as a profession we have failed to

D.A. George, MBChB, BMedSc, MRCS (Eng)
Department of Trauma and Orthopaedics,
University College Hospital, London, London, UK

F.S. Haddad, BSc, MD(res), MCh, FRCS (Orth) (✉)
Department of Trauma and Orthopaedics, University College London Hospitals NHS Trust, London, UK
e-mail: fsh@fareshaddad.co.uk

D. Kendoff et al. (eds.), *Periprosthetic Joint Infections: Changing Paradigms*,
DOI 10.1007/978-3-319-30091-7_29

eradicate the threat of infection, perhaps we never will.

It is important to continue to develop new strategies to reduce the consequences of infection and control the impact they have upon our patients, as well as the economy. The future for PJI is promising. In this chapter we review a number of emerging, and potentially ground breaking, novel and unique strategies that may revolutionize our approach to fighting these infections. The ultimate goal is to give us the advantage, and improve the overall care we can provide our patients.

Prevention

Preventing the onset of PJI, through a combination of different approaches is key in reducing the burden that we face. Several therapies are being developed that could have a role in preventing contamination and biofilm production during the primary arthroplasty, by acting directly at the implant surface, systemically, or externally.

One of the most focused areas for ongoing research is at the surface of the implant, the site most in contact with the patient, and at risk of biofilm formation. Modifications to the composition of the prosthesis, as well as potential coverings have been explored.

Antibacterial and antibiofilm coatings have been developed to inhibit bacterial adhesion and biofilm formation. When applied directly to the surface of the implant, these agents are able to act locally and higher concentrations can be reached that otherwise would not have been able systemically, with the aim to prevent initial bacterial adhesion and subsequent biofilm formation. The non-adherent bacteria would then be more exposed to systemic and local antibiotics, and host immune defenses, improving eradication [1].

These coatings are either based upon established antibiotics, such as vancomycin [2], gentamicin [3], and levofloxacin [4], or are biologically active compounds.

The antibiotics can be added to the surface of the implant as a biodegradable and non-biodegradable polymer coating (or sleeve), or covalently tethered to the surface [1,5–7]. Biodegradable polymers are advantageous at the time of surgery and in the early postoperative period as they release a high concentration of antibiotics initially, as demonstrated by over two thirds of gentamicin released during the first 3 days following implantation [3]. However, they may be at risk of bacterial resistance and adhesion when the antibiotics levels are low [8].

Non-biodegradable polymers persist for longer periods, releasing antibiotics at a slower rate generally over months [8], whereas covalently tethered antibiotics, such as vancomycin, can be released over years as demonstrated in animal models [1,9].

Success in the application and development of a biodgradable polymer has been shown by Metsemakers et al. [10]. They investigated the efficacy of a biodegradable polymer-lipid encapsulation matrix (PLEX) that was loaded with the doxycycline, and used in cases of implant-associated osteomyelitis. They demonstrated through in-vitro studies that 25 % of the doxycycline was released within the first day, followed by a 3 % release per day up to day 28. It was highly effective against meticillin-sensitive *Staphylococcus aureus* (MSSA) for at least 14 days. In-vivo rabbit model studies with infected titanium PLEX-doxycycline-coated intramedullary nail, demonstrated no growth of doxycycline-sensitive MSSA, and a statistically significant reduction in the number of culture-positive samples for doxycycline-resistant MSSA [10].

Biologically active agents such as deoxyribonuclease (DNase) I and Dispersin B, have shown promising outcomes as antibiofilm agents [11]. As biofilm-dispersing enzymes they interrupt the physical integrity and increases the permeability of the protective biofilm matrix via a number of mechanisms. In-vitro studies have demonstrated increased susceptibility to antibiotics, as they now penetrate this layer, and gain direct access to the bacteria [11,12]. This has been confirmed following in-vivo studies combining Dispersin B and triclosan, with resultant antibiofilm and antibacterial activity against *Staphylococcus aureus* (S. aureus) and *Staphylococcus epidermidis* (S. epidermidis), the main causative organisms of PJI [13].

Table 29.1 Naturally occurring compounds demonstrating antibacterial and antibiofilm properties originating from marine microorganisms [17]

Marine source origin	Compound extracted from the source	Bacteria susceptible to the extracted compounds
Algae Delisea pulchra	Furanone	Escherichia coli
Actinomycetes	Metabolites	Vibrio species
Coral Acropora digitifera	Bacillus horikoshii, Vibrio natriegens, Bacillus pumilus Streptomyces akiyoshinensis (A3)	Streptococcus pyogenes
Pseudoalteromonas species	Exoproducts	Pseudomonas aeruginosa Salmonella enterica Escherichia coli, Staphylococcus epidermidis
Bacillus licheniformis	Polysaccharide	Escherichia coli

Compounds extracted from marine microorganisms [14,15] and peptides from reptiles [16], demonstrate natural antibiofilm and bacteriostatic activity (Table 29.1) [18,19]. Genomic sequencing has taken place to identify the underlying structure of these compounds to enable resynthesis and antimicrobial testing [16]. Further studies may enable greater understanding of these compounds that may 1 day be adapted as biological coatings.

Resistance to antibiotics is becoming increasingly common, and many fear that tethered or antibiotic carriers may exaggerate this further. In response, other anti-infective coatings such as incorporate nanoparticulate metal ions have generated much interest.

The only commercially available metal ion incorporated within the surface of the prosthesis and currently indicated for revision surgery is silver [20]. Silver is known to have broad-spectrum antibacterial properties against otherwise multi-drug resistant organisms [21]. Its mode of action remains relatively unclear with an antibacterial effect seen under aerobic and anaerobic conditions [12,22]. *S. aureus* and *S. epidermidis* are sensitive to silver, with significant bactericidal activity demonstrated in in-vitro studies [23,24]. The rate of eradication is similar to high-dose tetracycline and vancomycin [25]. Similarly, other metals ions, including carbon, zinc, iron, and titanium, have shown potential antimicrobial and antibiofilm in in-vitro testing [26–28].

Within laboratory testing, silver has been successfully applied to the surface of the prosthesis within a polymer coating [23,29], ceramics [30], or combined with other metal ions such as copper [31]. The mid-term results of the commercially available silver implants show significantly lower rates of a recurrence of infection following a two-stage exchange arthroplasty ($p=0.03$) [32].

An alternative to silver being applied to the surface of the implant during the manufacturing process, gels may be used to apply antibacterial coatings at the time of surgery onto the implant immediately prior to insertion. Examples of this include Bactisure Ag.™, a silver-based gel which is in the early stages of development [33] and an implant disposable antibacterial coating (iDAC) [34].

Early results from iDAC in Europe have shown a benefit in both primary and revision procedures [34] and in-vitro tests verify its chemical and physical stability, and safety [35,36]. iDAC is a short-acting biodegradable hydrogel, which combined with broad-spectrum antibiotics at the time of implant insertion, releases antibiotics at the implant surface for up to 96 h [36].

Alternative methods for infection prevention include modifications to the operating theatre layout. Recent data has failed to show a clear benefit for laminar airflow at preventing PJI, which is in widespread use in the United Kingdom [37–39]. In combination with ongoing improvements to ultra-clean ventilation, a potential alternative may be to utilize ultraviolet light. Despite a potential risk to unprotected skin, used appropriately it can disrupt bacterial DNA, and subsequent replication and contamination [40]. Significant improvement of PJI rates have been shown when comparing ultraviolet light to laminar airflow during primary arthroplasty [41], as it can be utilized to eradicate airborne and surface-based sources of pathogens [42,43].

Diagnostics

Diagnosing the presence of infection in an artificial joint can be extremely difficult. A variety of investigations have been discussed in the previous chapters, and often combines a variety of different modalities such as serological markers C-reactive protein (CRP) and erythrocyte sedimentation rate (ESR), radiological investigations such as plain radiographs, computed tomography (CT), or radionuclear imaging, and microbiological cultures of various specimens [44]. No single test is 100 % sensitive for PJI. In the presence of infection, samples often received from either investigative joint aspirations, or as a result of the surgical debridement, may be contaminated and the true pathogen may not be adequately identified.

There is therefore a need to improve our methods of diagnosis. Several new methods to aid in diagnosis, such as sonification of samples within the microbiology laboratory, and Synovasure® used within the operating room, have been discussed in previous chapters and may continue to play an important role in the near future.

A disadvantage of the sonficiation process is the need for dedicated laboratory tools found only in specialist centers, and the risk of contamination due to inappropriate sample handling, damage to containers, and bacterial proliferation in the sonication water [45]. An emerging technology to help improve the bacterial yield from an intraoperative sample or explanted implant, and prevent such contamination, is the use of DL-dithiothreitol (DTT; C4H10O2S2).

DTT is a sulfhydryl compound able to disrupt polysaccharides and proteins and alter the extracellular matrix of biofilm, releasing bacteria from within it. DTT is in common use in liquefying specimens from the respiratory tract, and Drago et al. [46] applied this to explanted implants to determine if the bacteria released from the biofilm would be able to be retrieved and cultivated with traditional methods. Approximately 450 periprosthetic tissue samples and 160 implants were analysed, and compared DTT to sonification and standard tissue culture methods. DTT gave similar results to sonication in terms of bacterial yield, and specificity (94.1 %), but a better sensitivity (85.7 %) [46]. Additional advantages of DTT includes the low toxicity, ease of use, and low relative costs.

The combination of DTT to a closed loop collection system has been developed. This enables the explanted implant or tissue to be placed within a sterile bag, DTT to be added, and the resultant liquid be retrieved in a sterile manner for analysis [47]. This may have a greater importance in the future to optimize sample transport and improve bacterial yield.

Current methods of identifying the presence of infection include identifying the presence of the pathogen via their enzymes, products, or their genes. Pathogen molecular diagnosis is mainly undertaken via polymerase chain reaction (PCR) techniques, the most sensitive of the existing rapid methods to detect microbial pathogens in clinical specimens [48]. PCR use in paediatric patients with culture-negative septic arthritis had improved the detection of bacteria in the joint fluid compared to standard culture. In this retrospective analysis, 68 samples were analysed with PCR, and was positive in 32 cases (47.1 %). Combined with the results from standard blood and joint fluid culture, PCR improved the rate of detection by 15.4 % [49]. However, in the setting of total joint arthroplasties with established biofilm, PCR was less effective at identifying isolated pathogens compared to conventional culture [50], and results were delayed by up to 15 days [49].

Alternatives to standard PCR have helped reduce the delay in diagnosis, and includes pathogen-specific real-time PCR [51] coupled to high-resolution melting curve analysis [52], fluorescence in-situ hybridization using peptide nucleic acid probes [53], direct matrix-assisted laser desorption ionization–time of flight mass spectrometry [54,55], and BioFire Diagnostic's FilmArray system [56]. The main disadvantage of each of these techniques is that they compare the samples to a narrow panel of known targets which includes a variety of the most common bacteria and yeasts [56].

An alternative to these methods is the use of next generation sequencing (NGS) technology to determine the presence of pathogen DNA. NGS refers to non-Sanger-based high-throughput DNA sequencing technologies [57]. This new approach enables billions of DNA strands to be sequenced in parallel, minimising the need for fragment-cloning often used in Sanger-sequencing [57]. Unlike methods based upon PCR, NGS can be used in an 'open' mode which does not rely on set parameters or a panel of targets. No preconceived ideas of the possible responsible pathogens are needed, and NGS searches all known databases for a match. Such technology adapted to infection is in early stages of development, and is led by C. Chiu [58]. He has developed a process of sequencing and identify pathogens using ultra-rapid processes based upon clinical NGS metagenomics data. The process is able to produce results in 10 h to 2 days, a fraction of the time taken in other conventional methods. An alternative to this open approach is the use of NGS with a focused question, where specific genetic sequences relating to known, or likely pathogens, can be sought.

Although not in a clinical phase of testing for orthopaedic-related infections, such technology has been used in other scenarios such as analysing blood in febrile and afebrile children. Wylie et al. [59] identified multiple viruses in plasma that corresponded with febrile children, that would not have been highlighted had PCR been utilized. Other clinical studies applying NGS have included stool samples from patients with diarrhoea [60], and urine samples from patients with suspected urinary tract infections [61].

We believe NGS may revolutionise the diagnostics of PJI, and play an increasing role in identifying pathogens in infection revision cases resistant to antibiotic therapy, help determine the presence of pathogens in presumed aseptic loosening cases, and in identifying multiple pathogens in proven infected cases.

Furthermore the technology can be adapted to analyse patient genetic susceptibility to PJI, which may dictate their inflammatory responses to infection, the implant and indeed their response to antibiotics therapy. Previous attempts have identified specific genotypes that may make a patient susceptible, but due to amounts of data included in the study, these results are just preliminary at present. These studies suggest that C allele and genotype C/C for MBL-550 SNP, genotype A/A for MBL-54 SNP and G allele for MBL-221 SNP increase the risk of PJI, while G allele and genotype G/G for MBL-550 SNP decrease the risk of PJI in Caucasian populations [62]. Further research is required to determine the feasibility of epigenetic manipulation, as a potential route to preventing the development of PJI in genetic susceptible patients.

Treatment

The treatment of acute and chronic infected joints has been discussed in depth in the previous chapters. What is evident is the uncertainty of the various medical and surgical treatments. The multidisciplinary team should be the center of discussions regarding each patient, and each decision individualised based on patient and pathogen factors and reflect the most up to date high-level research. Surgically a variety of options exist to explore and debride the infected joint, with or without an exchange of mobile parts or revision arthroplasty [63], which is combined with medical antibiotic therapy.

Adjuvant therapies, applied alongside core surgical and medical treatments, may be the key to improving rate of eradication in the future. This may include phage or photodynamic therapy, and use of magnetic or electric currents, shockwave treatment, bioactive glass, or simply honey and vinegar applications to the implant.

Phage therapy involves the use of programmed bacteriophages that target specific pathogenic bacteria, and eradicate them [64]. Bacteriophages are able to self-replicate and multiply to maintain a therapeutic level needed to deliver a prolonged antibacterial action specific to their targets [65]. Animal models have utilised linezolid and a broad spectrum lytic bacteriophage to target MRSA [66]. Applied to Kirschner wires, bacterial adhesion was reduced, without any obvious adverse effects [67]. If incorporated into a polymer which is applied to an implant, bacterial adherence, colonization, and subsequent reinfection may be prevented [68,69].

Photodynamic therapy involves the combination of a photosensitive molecule and an activating low-intensity visible light, to form oxygen and hydroxyl radicals [70]. This results in targeted cell death, and can potentially be used to target specific sites adjacent to the implant, specific bacterial pathways, or specific pathogenic DNA [71–73]. Its benefits against infections has been seen in periodontal infections [74], and animal studies have proved its bactericidal effect against the biofilm of *S. aureus* and *S. epidermidis* [75,76] and MRSA [77–79]. Following the uptake of the photosensitizer within the biofilm matrix, neutrophil function is heightened, with a resultant protective role [80,81].

The potential role of photodynamic therapy may be pre- and postoperatively. Preoperatively the focused light on either a virgin or infected joint may help up-regulate neutrophils and improve the host defenses. Postoperatively, if a photosensitizer-coated prosthesis is inserted, the activating light can enable a release of oxygen and hydroxyl radicals directly at the implant-bone or implant-cement surface [17].

Alternatively the surface of the implant may be magnetically or electrically charged prior to insertion. Metal ions, such as iron oxide ions, have magnetic properties and are able to directly disrupt bacterial cell walls [82,83]. The use of an externally placed magnetic field may enable these ions to be focused to a specific area adjacent to the implant to disrupt the biofilm, as demonstrated in animal models [84].

Electronically charged implants may have a role in reducing bacterial adherence to the prosthesis surface as bacteria have an inherent negative charge, important for bacterial adhesion to the implant surface [85]. In vitro studies have demonstrated a significant reduction of bacterial adherence and survival, by alternating microcurrents across platinum electrodes when used in urological catheters [86]. Electronically polarized titanium [87] and bioceramic hydroxyapatite [88] have demonstrated significantly reduced biofilm formation and growth of *S. aureus* and *E. coli* at relatively low voltages (15–30 V). The practical implications of charging implants prior to insertion, or during insertion, has not been explored, and the impact upon ossteointegration is unknown.

Externally focused ultrasonic or laser-generated shockwaves has been shown to physically disrupt biofilm and bacterial adhesion [29]. Laboratory studies have demonstrated the successful use of ultrasound in dislodging *E. coli* off polyethylene disks implanted subcutaneously on the backs of rabbits, and when combined with gentamicin, the bacterial count was significantly reduced [89]. Within a few seconds of focused laser-generated shockwaves, biofilm associated with *P. aeruginosa*, was completely destroyed from the threads of stainless steel screws [90]; however, this has not been assessed against deep seated infection as would be seen in hip PJI.

Bioactive glass (BAG), on the other hand, has been used in clinical trials due to its proven antimicrobial and osteoconductive properties. It can be augmented to be an alternative carrier to antibiotics as it is biodegradable, unlike standard poly (methyl methacrylate) cement. In-vitro and in-vivo studies have combined BAG with teicoplanin and gentamicin in a rabbit tibia osteomyelitis model [91]. The BAG was shown to convert to hydroxyapatite and supported the ingrowth of new bone into the tibia defects within 12 weeks of implantation, whilst the teicoplanin had a sustained release of over the first 9 days [91]. Gentamicin-loaded BAG pellets against *E coli* demonstrated an eradication rate of 81.8 % of infections in rabbits with tibial osteomyelitis, without the simultaneous use of a systemic antibiotic [92]. Not only can the release of antibiotics be sustained, but they also help restore deficient bone.

Drago et al. undertook in-vitro and clinical studies to determine the antimicrobial activity of bioglass BAG-S53P4 against multi-resistant microorganisms without the addition of antibiotics [93]. BAG-S53P4, composed of SiO2-Na2O-CaO-P2O5, was shown to promote antibacterial activity by altering local pH and osmotic pressures with resultant hostility and prevention to bacterial adhesion and proliferation [94,95]. After 72 h of incubation there was a total absence of growth of all pathogens (MRSA, *P. aeruginosa*, methicillin-resistant *S. epidermidis* and *A. baumanni*). The clinical element included a prospectively cohort of 27 patients with clinically and radiologically diagnosed osteomyelitis of the long bones. During the surgical debridement, the bone defect was filled with BAG-S53P4 granules without the addition of local antibiotics were added. As per their protocol the patients received microbe-specific systemic antibiotic therapy for 4–6 weeks postoperatively. At a mean follow-up of 17.8 months (standard deviation 6.1 months) 24 patients (88.9 %) did not demonstrate any recurrence of infection. Plain radiographs showed incorporation of the bioglass within the host bone, with an absence of osteolysis or periosteal reactions even though visible after 2 years from surgery [93]. They have shown that BAG is a viable option in the treatment of chronic osteomyelitis of the long bones, which could potentially be adapted in PJI.

Bioglass is a relatively modern approach in infection treatment. Vinegar (acetic acid) on the other hand has been used for centuries as a means of antisepsis in ulcerations and sores, dating back to the Hippocrates (460–377 BC) [96], and has recently been explored in PJI. It is currently used in ENT for the treatment of ear infections, superficially following wound debridement as part of a closed loop vacuum system [97], and in the treatment of pseudomonal wound infections [98]. Compared to regular antibiotics, 0.5 % acetic acid outshone ampicillin, penicillin, cephalothin and tetracycline against wound infections contaminated with *S. aureus, E coli*, Proteus species and coagulase-negative staphylococci, which was bactericidal to them all [99].

Morgan-Jones et al. are currently exploring its function in revision total knee arthroplasty in a prospective cohort study of complex revision [100]. Following a meticulous debridement of the joint, the area is soaked for 20 min in 3 % acetic acid, prior to reimplantation of the definitive implant or replacement of mobile components. They have noticed no adverse effects in postoperative wound healing. After a mean follow-up of 6.6 months, they have had a recurrence of two infections (11.78 %) in patients undergoing debridement and implant retention. They conclude that acetic acid works best within the first 6 h of surgery to prevent bacterial growth and they have noticed a small but definitive effect [100].

The same team are also exploring the role of honey during complex revision procedures. Honey has also been used for wound care since ancient times. A Cochrane review determining the role honey in topical treatments found honey may reduce time to healing in acute wounds compared with some conventional dressings in partial thickness burns [101]. Surgihoney®, a mechanically processed honey, is freely available and demonstrates antimicrobial properties via the production and release of oxygen free radicals, and is active against gram-positive and gram-negative bacteria, including multi-drug-resistant strains [102]. Morgan-Jones et al. have applied this honey to the implant prior to closure and have early encouraging results [103].

The aforementioned strategies have focused upon novel therapies utilising exogenous methods. There has also been heightened interest to develop vaccines and therapeutic antibodies that focus on antigens key to *S. aureus* pathogenesis, to improve patient active and passive immunity. Anti-staphylococcal immunotherapy has been developed for several decades, with a variety of different antigens being targeted; however, many attempts have failed [104].

Merck V710 is one such vaccine. It inhibits the surface protein IsdB which is believed to play a role in iron uptake [105] and an anti-IsdB vaccine has been protective in animal infection studies against most *S. aureus* strains [106]. Clinical trials are currently ongoing utilizing this vaccine in patients undergoing cardiothoracic surgery and hemodialysis [104]. Alfa-toxin, a polyclonal antibody against specific *S. aureus* capsular polysaccharides, has been successfully used in a mouse lung infection models, infected with both MRSA and methicillin-susceptible strains [107], but clinical trials have not been attempted. A variety of other vaccines and antibodies are in development. Whilst none of these have evaluated their potential role when applied to PJI, we believe the use of these agents to target the infection microenvironment and bridge the innate and adaptive immune response has a promising role in the treatment and prevention of PJI.

Discussion

The number of arthoplasty procedures is increasing worldwide, with similarly increasing numbers of complex revision procedures. Multiple strategies have been successful in preventing and treating PJIs over the years, as shown by a relative low rate of infection. Infection comes at a cost, not only to the patient but the Institute and widespread health service. The successful management of PJI can be challenging, and requires an appreciation of the surgical and microbiological complexities, in light of increasing resistant infecting pathogens.

We have discussed several novel and emerging strategies that have shown promising results, but the majority of these therapies are still in preclinical development at a theoretical, in-vitro or animal testing stage. Others are based on historic ideas but have been adapted to PJI, or have not been explored in this field, such as NGS, but may have a very important role in future management.

However, several barriers exist that may prevent many of these strategies becoming available to be used in the clinical practice for the treatment of PJI. The treatment aims and goals pursued by academics and scientists may not be the same as those administering or receiving them. Strategies must be clinically safe, meet regulatory requirements, and be felt to be profitable by the industry to become established.

Regarding the treatment of infections, the variable, rare and unpredictable nature of PJI means it would be very difficult to demonstrate a significant improvement as a result of a specific strategy. Multiple factors play a role for the infection to become established and present itself, that success in eradicating the infection can rarely be associated to a single intervention, but a combination.

One fundamental future consideration must be the emphasis on education. The education of patients is especially important, as they must be made aware of their individual risk of infection. Patients with known modifiable risk factors should be advised to change their lifestyle to help reduce this risk, such as reducing their weight and improving their nutrition, or stop smoking. The surgical team must understand their role to help prevent infection, by being continual vigilant upon the wards and in theatre to prevent contamination. If the magnitude of PJI gains political and media interest, and is brought into the limelight, greater funding may become available to help these strategies and others become a reality.

References

1. Hickok NJ, Shapiro IM. Immobilized antibiotics to prevent orthopedic implant infections. Adv Drug Deliv Rev. 2012;64(12):1165–76.
2. Lawson MC, Hoth KC, Deforest CA, Bowman CN, Anseth KS. Inhibition of Staphylococcus epidermidis biofilms using polymerizable vancomycin derivatives. Clin Orthop Relat Res. 2010;468:2081–91.
3. Moskowitza JS, Blaissea MR, Samuela RE. The effectiveness of the controlled release of gentamicin from polyelectrolyte multilayers in the treatment of Staphylococcus aureus infection in a rabbit bone model. Biomaterials. 2010;31(23):6019–30.
4. Hart E, Azzopardi K, Taing H, Graichen F, Jeffery J. Efficacy of antimicrobial polymer coatings in an animal model of bacterial infection associated with foreign body implants. J Antimicrob Chemother. 2010;65:974–80.
5. Sinclair KD, Pham TX, Farnsworth RW, Williams DL, Loc-Carrillo C, Horne LA, et al. Development

of a broad spectrum polymer-released antimicrobial coating for the prevention of resistant strain bacterial infections. J Biomed Mater Res A. 2012;100(10):2732–8.
6. Lee CT, Lee CW, Hu CW, Lai KA, Yeh ML. PLGA encapsulating antibiotic loaded titanium prosthesis in osteomyelitis prevention in rats. Presented at the 2012 annual meeting of the Orthopaedic Research Society, San Francisco, 2012.
7. Stewart S, Barr S, Engiles J, Hickok NJ, Shapiro IM, Richardson DW, et al. Vancomycin-modified implant surface inhibits biofilm formation and supports bone-healing in an infected osteotomy model in sheep. A proof-of-concept study. J Bone Joint Surg Am. 2012;94(15):1406–15.
8. Panyam J, Labhasetwar V. Biodegradable nanoparticles for drug and gene delivery to cells and tissue. Adv Drug Deliv Rev. 2012;64:61–71.
9. Antoci Jr V, King SB, Jose B, Parvizi J, Zeiger AR, Wickstrom E, et al. Vancomycin covalently bonded to titanium alloy prevents bacterial colonization. J Orthop Res. 2007;25(7):858–66.
10. Metsemakers WJ, Emanuel N, Cohen O, Reichart M, Potapova I, Schmid T, et al. A doxycycline-loaded polymer-lipid encapsulation matrix coating for the prevention of implant-related osteomyelitis due to doxycycline-resistant methicillin-resistant Staphylococcus aureus. J Control Release. 2015;209:47–56.
11. Kaplan JB. Therapeutic potential of biofilm-dispersing enzymes. Int J Artif Organs. 2009;32:545–54.
12. Arciola CR, Montanaro L, Costerton JW. Editorial. New trends in diagnosis and control strategies for implant infections. Int J Artif Organs. 2011;34(9): 727–36.
13. Darouiche RO, Mansouri MD, Gawande PV, Madhyastha S. Antimicrobial and antibiofilm efficacy of triclosan and DispersinB combination. J Antimicrob Chemother. 2009;64:88–93.
14. Selvin J, Ninawe AS, Kiran GS, Lipton AP. Sponge-microbial interactions: ecological implications and bioprospecting avenues. Crit Rev Microbiol. 2010;36:82–90.
15. Sayem SM, Manzo E, Ciavatta L, Tramice A, Cordone A, Zanfardino A, et al. Anti-biofilm activity of an exopolysaccharide from a sponge-associated strain of Bacillus licheniformis. Microb Cell Fact. 2011;10:74.
16. van Hoek ML. Antimicrobial peptides in reptiles. Pharmaceuticals (Basel). 2014;7(6):723–53.
17. George DA, Gant V, Haddad FS. The management of periprosthetic infections in the future. Bone Joint J. 2015;97-B(9):1162–9.
18. Reed M. Marine nuclease and biofilm: a new approach to periprosthetic infection? Presented at the London knee meeting, London, 2013.
19. Shakir A, Elbadawey MR, Shields RC, Jakubovics NS, Burgess JG. Removal of biofilms from tracheoesophageal speech valves using a novel marine microbial deoxyribonuclease. Otolaryngol Head Neck Surg. 2012;147(3):509–14.
20. Agluna. Accentus Medical Ltd. Oxford, UK. 2014. Available from: www.accentus-medical.com. Accessed 20 May 2014.
21. Ellis JR. The many roles of silver in infection prevention. Am J Infect Control. 2007;35(5): E26.
22. Park HJ, Kim JY, Kim J, Lee JH, Hahn JS, Gu MB, et al. Silver-ion-mediated reactive oxygen species generation affecting bactericidal activity. Water Res. 2009;43:1027–32.
23. Gordon O, Vig Slenters T, Brunetto PS, Villaruz AE, Sturdevant DE, Otto M, et al. Silver coordination polymers for prevention of implant infection: thiol interaction, impact on respiratory chain enzymes, and hydroxyl radical induction. Antimicrob Agents Chemother. 2010;54(10):4208–18.
24. Randall CP, Oyama LB, Bostock JM, Chopra I, O'Neill AJ. The silver cation (Ag+): antistaphylococcal activity, mode of action and resistance studies. J Antimicrob Chemother. 2013;68(1):131–8.
25. Taylor E, Webster TJ. Reducing infections through nanotechnology and nanoparticles. Int J Nanomedicine. 2011;6:1463–73.
26. Colon G, Ward BC, Webster TJ. Increased osteoblast and decreased Staphylococcus epidermidis functions on nanophase ZnO and TiO2. J Biomed Mater Res A. 2006;78A(3):595–604.
27. Puckett SD, Taylor E, Raimondo T, Webster TJ. The relationship between the nanostructure of titanium surfaces and bacterial attachment. Biomaterials. 2010;31(4):706–13.
28. Tobin EJ, Karimy H, Barry JE, et al. Infection-resistant external fixation pins. Trans Soc Biomater. 1997;20:390.
29. Hansen EN, Zmistowski B, Parvizi J. Periprosthetic joint infection: what is on the horizon? Int J Artif Organs. 2012;35(10):935–50.
30. Lee JS, Murphy WL. Functionalizing orthopedic implants with silver nanoparticles to treat infection. Presented at the 2012 annual meeting of the Orthopaedic Research Society, San Francisco, 4–7 Feb 2012.
31. Fiedler J, Kolitsch A, Kleffner B, Henke D, Stenger S, Brenner RE. Copper and silver ion implantation of aluminium oxide- blasted titanium surfaces: proliferative response of osteoblasts and antibacterial effects. Int J Artif Organs. 2011;34(9):882–8.
32. Wafa H, Grimer F, Carter S, Tillman R, Abudu S, Jeys L. Retrospective evaluation of the incidence of early periprosthetic infection with silver-treated custom endoprostheses in high risk patients: case control study. Presented ISOLS Conference, Bologna. 2013.
33. Ferrando M. Zimmer infection management: what's next? Presented at the Milano Biofilm meeting 2015. Implantables and Infection Control: a Promising Future? 19 June 2015, Milan.

34. Romanò CL, Giammona G, Giardino R, Meani E. Antibiotic-loaded resorbable hydrogel coating for infection prophylaxis of orthopaedics implants: preliminary studies. J Bone Joint Surg Br. 2011;93-B:337–8.
35. Romano C. Resorbable hydrogel provides effective antibacterial coating in vitro and in vivo. Presented at the Musculoskeletal Infection Society annual meeting, Philadelphia. 2013.
36. Drago L, Boot W, Dimas K, et al. Does implant coating with antibacterial- loaded hydrogel reduce bacterial colonization and biofilm formation in vitro? Clin Orthop Relat Res. 2014;472:3311–23.
37. Miner AL, Losina E, Katz JN, Fossel AH, Platt R. Deep infection after total knee replacement: impact of laminar airflow systems and body exhaust suits in the modern operating room. Infect Control Hosp Epidemiol. 2007;28(2):222–6.
38. Hooper GJ, Rothwell AG, Frampton C, Wyatt MC. Does the use of laminar flow and space suits reduce early deep infection after total hip and knee replacement?: the ten-year results of the New Zealand Joint Registry. J Bone Joint Surg Br. 2011;93(1):85–90.
39. Breier AC, Brandt C, Sohr D, Geffers C, Gastmeier P. Laminar airflow ceiling size: no impact on infection rates following hip and knee prosthesis. Infect Control Hosp Epidemiol. 2011;32(11):1097–102.
40. Thai TP, Keast DH, Campbell KE, Woodbury MG, Houghton PE. Effect of ultraviolet light C on bacterial colonization in chronic wounds. Ostomy Wound Manage. 2005;51(10):32–45.
41. Ritter MA, Olberding EM, Malinzak RA. Ultraviolet lighting during orthopaedic surgery and the rate of infection. J Bone Joint Surg Am. 2007;89(9):1935–40.
42. Mangram AJ, Horan TC, Pearson ML, Silver LC, Jarvis WR. Guideline for prevention of surgical site infection. Centers for disease control and prevention (CDC) hospital infection control practices advisory committee. Am J Infect Control. 1999;27(2):97–132.
43. Pittet D, Simon A, Hugonnet S, Pessoa-Silva CL, Sauvan V, Perneger TV. Hand hygiene among physicians: performance, beliefs, and perceptions. Ann Intern Med. 2004;141(1):1–8.
44. George DA, Khan M, Haddad FS. Periprosthetic joint infection in total hip arthroplasty: prevention and management. Br J Hosp Med (Lond). 2015;76(1):12–7.
45. Trampuz A, Piper KE, Hanssen AD, Osmon DR, Cockerill FR, Steckelberg JM, et al. Sonication of explanted prosthetic components in bags for diagnosis of prosthetic joint infection is associated with risk of contamination. J Clin Microbiol. 2006;44:628–31.
46. Drago L, Signori V, De Vecchi E, Vassena C, Palazzi E, Cappelletti L, et al. Use of dithiothreitol to improve the diagnosis of prosthetic joint infections. J Orthop Res. 2013;31:1694–9.
47. Drago L, Signori V, De Vecchi E, et al. Use of dithiothreitol to improve the diagnosis of prosthetic joint infections. J Orthop Res. 2013;31(11):1694–9.
48. Yamamoto Y. PCR in diagnosis of infection: detection of bacteria in cerebrospinal fluids. Clin Diagn Lab Immunol. 2002;9(3):508–14.
49. Carter K, Doern C, Jo CH, Copley LA. The clinical usefulness of polymerase chain reaction as a supplemental diagnostic tool in the evaluation and the treatment of children with septic arthritis. J Pediatr Orthop. 2015;36:167–72.
50. Zegaer BH, Ioannidis A, Babis GC, Ioannidou V, Kossyvakis A, Bersimis S, et al. Detection of bacteria bearing resistant biofilm forms, by using the universal and specific PCR is still unhelpful in the diagnosis of periprosthetic joint infections. Front Med (Lausanne). 2014;1:30.
51. Selva L, Esteva C, Gene A, de Sevilla MF, Hernandez-Bou S, Munoz-Almagro C. Direct detection of Streptococcus pneumoniae in positive blood cultures by real-time polymerase chain reaction. Diagn Microbiol Infect Dis. 2010;66:204–6.
52. Jeng K, Gaydos CA, Blyn LB, Yang S, Won H, Matthews H, et al. Comparative analysis of two broad-range PCR assays for pathogen detection in positive-blood-culture bottles: PCR-high-resolution melting analysis versus PCR-mass spectrometry. J Clin Microbiol. 2012;50:3287–92.
53. Hartmann H, Stender H, Schafer A, Autenrieth IB, Kempf VA. Rapid identification of Staphylococcus aureus in blood cultures by a combination of fluorescence in situ hybridization using peptide nucleic acid probes and flow cytometry. J Clin Microbiol. 2005;43:4855–7.
54. Prod'hom G, Bizzini A, Durussel C, Bille J, Greub G. Matrix-assisted laser desorption ionization-time of flight mass spectrometry for direct bacterial identification from positive blood culture pellets. J Clin Microbiol. 2010;48:1481–3.
55. Patel R. Matrix-assisted laser desorption ionization-time of flight mass spectrometry in clinical microbiology. Clin Infect Dis. 2013;57:564–72.
56. Altun O, Almuhayawi M, Ullberg M, Ozenci V. Clinical evaluation of the FilmArray blood culture identification panel in identification of bacteria and yeasts from positive blood culture bottles. J Clin Microbiol. 2013;51(12):4130–6.
57. Definition. Next-generation sequencing. Subject Areas. Nature publishing group, 2015. Available from: www.nature.com/subjects/next-generation-sequencing. Accessed online 2 July 2015.
58. Chiu CY. Viral pathogen discovery. Curr Opin Microbiol. 2013;16:1–11.
59. Wylie KM, Mihindukulasuriya KA, Sodergren E, Weinstock GM, Storch GA. Sequence analysis of the human virome in febrile and afebrile children. PLoS One. 2012:7, e27735.
60. Loman NJ, Constantinidou C, Christner M, Rohde H, Chan JZ, Quick J, et al. A culture-independent

sequence-based metagenomics approach to the investigation of an outbreak of shiga-toxigenic escherichia coli O104:H4. JAMA. 2013;309:1502–10.
61. Hasman H, Saputra D, Sicheritz-Ponten T, Lund O, Svendsen CA, Frimodt-Møller N, et al. Rapid whole-genome sequencing for detection and characterization of microorganisms directly from clinical samples. J Clin Microbiol. 2014;52: 139–46.
62. Zhou X, Yishake M, Li J, Jiang L, Wu L, Liu R, et al. Genetic susceptibility to prosthetic joint infection following total joint arthroplasty: a systematic review. Gene. 2015;563(1):76–82.
63. George DA, Konan S, Haddad FS. Single-stage hip and knee exchange for periprosthetic joint infection. J Arthroplasty. 2015;30:2264–70.
64. Smith HW, Huggins MB, Shaw KM. The control of experimental Escherichia coli diarrhoea in calves by means of bacteriophages. J Gen Microbiol. 1987;133:1111–26.
65. Abedon ST, Kuhl SJ, Blasdel BG, Kutter EM. Phage treatment of human infections. Bacteriophage. 2011;1(2):66–85.
66. Kaur S, Harjai K. Chhibber S. Bacteriophage mediated killing of Staphylococcus aureus In Vitro on Orthopaedic K wires in presence of Linezolid prevents implant colonization. Becker K, ed. PLoS One. 2014;9(3):e90411.
67. Sulakvelidze A, Alavidze Z, Morris J. Bacteriophage therapy. Antimicrob Agents Chemother. 2001;45: 649–59.
68. Chhibber S, Kaur T, Kaur S. Co-therapy using lytic bacteriophage and linezolid: effective treatment in eliminating methicillin resistant Staphylococcus aureus (MRSA) from diabetic foot infections. PLoS One. 2013;8(2), e56022.
69. Yilmaz C, Colak M, Yilmaz BC, Ersoz G, Kutateladze M, Gozlugol M. Bacteriophage therapy in implant-related infections: an experimental study. J Bone Joint Surg Am. 2013;95(2):117–25.
70. Jori G. Photodynamic therapy of microbial infections: state of the art and perspectives. J Environ Pathol Toxicol Oncol. 2006;25:505–19.
71. Hopper C. Photodynamic therapy: a clinical reality in the treatment of cancer. Lancet Oncol. 2000;1:212–9.
72. Salmon-Divon M, Nitzan Y, Malik Z. Mechanistic aspects of photodynamic inactivation by cationic tetra-meso (N-methylpyridyl) porphine. Photochem Photobiol Sci. 2004;3(5):423–9.
73. Schäfer M, Schmitz C, Facius R, Horneck G, Milow B, Funken KH. Systematic study of parameters influencing the action of Rose Bengal with visible light on bacterial cells: comparison between the biological effect and singlet-oxygen production. Photochem Photobiol. 2000;71(5):514–23.
74. Usacheva MN, Teichert MC, Biel MA. Comparison of the methylene blue and toluidine blue photo bactericidal efficacy against Gram-positive and Gram- negative microorganisms. Lasers Surg Med. 2001;29(2):165–73.
75. Sharma M, Visai L, Bragheri F, Cristiani I, Gupta PK, Speziale P. Toluidine blue- mediated photodynamic effects on staphylococcal biofilms. Antimicrob Agents Chemother. 2008;52:299–305.
76. Maisch T. A new strategy to destroy antibiotic resistant microorganisms: antimicrobial photodynamic treatment. Mini Rev Med Chem. 2009;9:947–83.
77. Wilson M, Yianni C. Killing of methicillin-resistant by low-power laser light. J Med Microbiol. 1995;42(1):62–6.
78. Embleton ML, Nair SP, Cookson BD, Wilson M. Antibody-directed photodynamic therapy of methicillin resistant. Microb Drug Resist. 2004;10(2):92–7.
79. Ashkenazi H, Malik Z, Harth Y, Nitzan Y. Eradication of by its endogenic porphyrins after illumination with high intensity blue light. FEMS Immunol Med Microbiol. 2003;35(1):17–24.
80. Hamblin MR, Hasan T. Photodynamic therapy: a new antimicrobial approach to infectious disease? Photochem Photobiol Sci. 2004;3:436–50.
81. Saino E, Sbarra MS, Arciola CR, Scavone M, Bloise N, Nikolov P, et al. Photodynamic action of Trimeso (N- methyl-pyridyl), meso (N-tetradecyl-pyridyl) porphine on Staphylococcus epidermidis biofilms grown on Ti6Al4V alloy. Int J Artif Organs. 2010;33(9):636–45.
82. Zhang L, Jiang Y, Ding Y, Povey M, York D. Investigation into the antibacterial behaviour of suspensions of ZnO nanoparticles (ZnO nanofluids). J Nanopartcle Res. 2007;9(3):479–89.
83. Trana N, Webster TJ. Magnetic nanoparticles: biomedical applications and challenges. J Mater Chem. 2010;20:8760–7.
84. Chertok B, Moffat BA, David AE, Yu F, Bergemann C, Ross BD, et al. Iron oxide nanoparticles as a drug delivery vehicle for MRI monitored magnetic targeting of brain tumors. Biomaterials. 2008;29(4):487–96.
85. Garrett TR, Bhakoo M, Zhang Z. Bacterial adhesion and biofilms on surfaces. Proc Natl Acad Sci U S A. 2008;18(9):1049–56.
86. Gabi M, Hefermehl L, Lukic D, Zahn R, Vörös J, Eberli D. Electrical microcurrent to prevent conditioning film and bacterial adhesion to urological stents. Urol Res. 2011;39(2):81–8.
87. Ercan B, Kummer KM, Tarquinio KM, Webster TJ. Decreased Staphylococcus aureus biofilm growth on anodized nanotubular titanium and the effect of electrical stimulation. Acta Biomater. 2011;7(7):3003–12.
88. Ueshima M, Tanaka S, Nakamura S, Yamashita K. Manipulation of bacterial adhesion and proliferation by surface charges of electrically polarized hydroxyapatite. J Biomed Mater Res. 2002;60(4): 578–84.
89. Rediske AM, Roeder BL, Brown MK, Nelson JL, Robison RL, Draper DO, et al. Ultrasonic enhancement

of antibiotic action on Escherichia coli biofilms: an in vivo model. Antimicrob Agents Chemother. 1999;43(5):1211–4.
90. Krespi YP, Stoodley P, Hall-Stoodley L. Laser disruption of biofilm. Laryngoscope. 2008;118(7):1168–73.
91. Zhang X, Jia W, Gu Y, Xiao W, Liu X, Wang D, et al. Teicoplanin-loaded borate bioactive glass implants for treating chronic bone infection in a rabbit tibia osteomyelitis model. Biomaterials. 2010;31(22):5865–74.
92. Xie Z, Cui X, Zhao C, Huang W, Wang J, Zhang C. Gentamicin-loaded borate bioactive glass eradicates osteomyelitis due to escherichia coli in a rabbit model. Antimicrob Agents Chemother. 2013;57(7):3293–8.
93. Drago L, Romanò D, De Vecchi E, Vassena C, Logoluso N, Mattina R, et al. Bioactive glass BAG-S53P4 for the adjunctive treatment of chronic osteomyelitis of the long bones: an in vitro and prospective clinical study. BMC Infect Dis. 2013;13:584.
94. Munukka E, Leppäranta O, Korkeamäki M, Vaahtio M, Peltola T, Zhang D, et al. Bactericidal effects of bioactive glasses on clinically important aerobic bacteria. J Mater Sci Mater Med. 2008;19:27–32.
95. Stoor P, Söderling E, Salonen JI. Antibacterial effects of a bioactive glass paste on oral microorganisms. Acta Odontol Scand. 1998;56:161–5.
96. Garrison, Fielding H. History of medicine. Philadelphia: WB Saunders; 1966.
97. Kirkterp-Moeller. A new approach to chronic wounds and biofilm. EBJIS Prague, Denmark, Sept 2013.
98. Nagoba BS, Selkar SP, Wadher BJ, Gandhi RC. Acetic acid treatment of pseudomonal wound infections – a review. J Infect Public Health. 2013; 6(6):410–5.
99. Mama M, Abdissa A, Sewunet T. Antimicrobial susceptibility pattern of bacterial isolates from wound infection and their sensitivity to alternative topical agents at Jimma University Specialized Hospital, South-West Ethiopia. Ann Clin Microbiol Antimicrob. 2014;13:14.
100. Morgan-Jones R. Acetic acid lavage in revision total knee replacement. Presented at the EBJIS 2014, Utretch, Sept 2014.
101. Jull AB, Rodgers A, Walker N. Honey as a topical treatment for wounds. Cochrane Database System Rev. 2008;(4):CD005083.
102. Cooke J, Dryden M, Patton T, Brennan J, Barrett J. The antimicrobial activity of prototype modified honeys that generate reactive oxygen species (ROS) hydrogen peroxide. BMC Res Notes. 2015;8:20.
103. Morgan-Jones R. SurgiHoney and alternative novel therapies Condiment surgery, another use for vinegar. Presented at the 6th National Orthopaedic Infection Forum, London, June 2015.
104. Otto M. Novel targeted immunotherapy approaches for staphylococcal infection. Expert Opin Biol Ther. 2010;10(7):1049–59.
105. Torres VJ, Pishchany G, Humayun M, Schneewind O, Skaar EP. Staphylococcus aureus IsdB is a hemoglobin receptor required for heme iron utilization. J Bacteriol. 2006;188(24):8421–9.
106. Kuklin NA, Clark DJ, Secore S, Cook J, Cope LD, McNeely T, et al. A novel Staphylococcus aureus vaccine: iron surface determinant B induces rapid antibody responses in rhesus macaques and specific increased survival in a murine S. aureus sepsis model. Infect Immun. 2006;74(4):2215–23.
107. Bubeck Wardenburg J, Schneewind O. Vaccine protection against Staphylococcus aureus pneumonia. J Exp Med. 2008;205(2):287–94.

Index

D. Kendoff et al. (eds.), *Periprosthetic Joint Infections: Changing Paradigms*,
DOI 10.1007/978-3-319-30091-7

Printed by Printforce, the Netherlands